PROBLEMS OF BIRTH DEFECTS

PROBLEMS OF BIRTH DEFECTS

From Hippocrates to Thalidomide and After

Original papers with commentaries by
T. V. N. Persaud, MD, PhD, DSc, MRCPath, FACOG

Professor of Anatomy and Director,
Teratology Research Laboratory, University of Manitoba;
Consultant in Teratology and Pathology,
Health Sciences Centre, Winnipeg, Canada

UNIVERSITY PARK PRESS

BALTIMORE

Published in USA and Canada by
University Park Press,
Chamber of Commerce Building,
Baltimore, Maryland 21202

Published in UK by
MTP Press Limited
St Leonard's House
Lancaster, Lancs.

Library of Congress Cataloging in Publication Data
Main entry under title:

Problems of birth defects, from Hippocrates to Thalidomide
    and After.

    Bibliography: p.
    1. Abnormalities, Human—Addresses, essays, lectures. 2.
Abnormalities, Human—Etiology—Addresses, essays,
lectures. I. Persaud, T. V. N. [DNLM: 1. Abnormalities.
QS675 P962]

RG626.P75 1977   616'.043   77–6833
ISBN 0–8391–1139–8

Printed in Great Britain

CONTENTS

INTRODUCTION

Surprisingly, the beginning of a modern approach to the problems of birth defects is relatively recent and dates from Gregg's classical report in 1941 that mothers who contracted rubella during the first trimester of pregnancy gave birth to infants with severe multiple anomalies. For the first time, an environmental agent was found to be teratogenic in man and was documented in a thoroughly convincing manner. Since then, many important discoveries and significant developments have been made, particularly in the areas of environmental teratogenesis, hereditary mechanisms, and prenatal diagnosis.

In recent years, there has been an impressive surge of interest in the causes and prevention of birth defects. Undoubtedly this resulted not only from the thalidomide tragedy, but also from the steady decline in infant mortality from other causes, such as infectious and nutritional diseases. The magnitude of the problem is emphasized by a recent report which estimated that at least 6% of all infants are born with some genetic or developmental anomaly. Furthermore, congenital defects contribute to approximately 20% of all neonatal mortality.

This collection of articles and commentaries is an integration of information from many disciplines, and presents a comprehensive survey of both recent and previously reported work related to the major aspects of birth defects. In particular, an attempt has been made to provide a critical assessment of current concepts and to identify areas in need of further investigation.

The scope of this volume and space limitations precluded discussion of and reference to all papers of relevance or importance: a work of the present nature must necessarily be selective. Some good papers have been left out or given relatively little consideration. It is my hope that the list of Further References will be consulted and should compensate for this lack of completeness. The important milestones in the investigation of birth defects are highlighted by the inclusion of the original reports or extracts from them. In some cases, however, more recent articles have been given preference to original scientific papers. These have been selected primarily for their appropriateness and depth of interpretation.

ACKNOWLEDGEMENTS

I am greatly indebted to the authors, editors, and publishers who have granted permission to reprint previously published articles. It is a special pleasure for me to acknowledge their cooperation in making this work possible.

Several colleagues have made valuable suggestions with respect to the commentaries; I am, however, especially grateful to Dr K. L. Moore, Professor and Chairman of the Department of Anatomy, University of Toronto; Dr M. Ray, Associate Professor of Anatomy and Pediatrics (Genetics), University of Manitoba; Dr J. B. Hyde, Associate Professor of Anatomy, University of Manitoba; and my graduate student Ms Lois A. Kennedy.

I wish to thank Mr P. M. Lister, Managing Editor, MTP Press Limited, not only for his advice on editorial matters, but also for providing the original impetus in this undertaking.

Thanks are also due to Mrs Roberta Van Aertselaer for her splendid secretarial help and to Ms Brenda Bell for preparing excellent photographic copies of several articles.

Finally, I am indebted to my wife, Gisela, for her patience and understanding which have been a constant source of encouragement.

PART I

BELIEFS, MYTHOLOGY, MAGIC AND SUPERSTITION

PAPERS 1 AND 2

1. Warkany, J. (1959). Congenital malformations in the past. *J. Chron. Dis.*, **10**, 84–96
2. Barrow, M. V. (1971). A brief history of teratology to the early 20th century. *Teratology*, **4**, 119–130

COMMENTARY

The first two papers deal with the historical aspects of birth defects and serve as an admirable introduction to this collection of articles.

Monstrous deformities present in children at birth have been known since earliest times. Primitive man's interest and fascination with these bizarre phenomena have found expression in drawings, carvings, and sculptures. At various periods in history, children born with severe congenital defects were attributed to astrological factors, divine will, witches, and demons. Magic, superstition, and speculation remained long in control of the field.

The ancient Babylonians predicted future events from the birth of deformed children. As far back as 3000 BC, achondroplasia was depicted by the Egyptians in paintings. Hippocrates (460–377 BC), the father of medicine, has given us the first description of hydrocephalus. Empedocles of Acragas (483–424 BC) and Democritus (460–371 BC) speculated that maternal impressions were responsible for abnormal development. Aristotle (384–322 BC) dismissed as impossible the monsters described in ancient mythology and observed that 'the monstrosity is contrary to nature, not contrary to nature taken absolutely, but contrary to the most usual course of nature'. In his book *De Conceptu et Generatione Hominis*, published in 1554, Jacob Rueff attributed the occurrence of monsters to the direct will of God. The distinguished French surgeon, Ambroise Paré, considered 'the glory of God, a narrow womb, an abundance of seed and overflowing matter, a wayward maternal imagination and the craft and wickedness of the devil as the causes of monsters and prodigies'.

Publication of Harvey's *Exercitatio de Generatione Animalium* in 1651 represented an important milestone in the study of embryonic development. Harvey discussed the significance of environmental influences during development and suggested that narrowness of the uterus and faulty maternal posture may be responsible for certain malformations.

The influence of maternal impressions on prenatal development has long been considered to be an important factor in the aetiology of birth defects. And this concept was widely accepted until recent times. The hybridity theory which assumed interspecies fertility claimed numerous victims during the middle Ages. Both these theories are discussed in considerable detail in Dr Warkany's paper. During the 18th century experimental techniques were introduced in the study of developmental processes. Etienne Geoffroy de Saint-Hilaire (1772–1844) experimentally produced anencephaly and spina bifida in chick embryos which proved a death blow to the preformation hypothesis. He introduced the word 'teratology' and, together with Meckel (1781–1833), Saint-Hilaire advanced the concept of developmental arrest, which explained the fact that in many congenital abnormalities, such as cleft plate, development appeared to have stopped at some stage and the primitive features of that period were retained.

Mendel's work and his laws of inheritance, published in 1865, exerted considerable influence on the speculation regarding the causation of malformations. For the first time, a scientific explanation, that of hereditary mechanisms, provided an apparently satisfactory explanation of the occurrence of developmental defects. For many years, 'congenital' and 'hereditary' were to be regarded as being synonymous.

From the end of the 18th century, morphological studies, particularly those of an embryological nature, eventually provided a scientific basis for the investigation of abnormal development. Animal experiments, designed to elucidate the functional aspects of development, were introduced during the latter part of the 19th century. Although the basis for the scientific study of abnormal development had been established by this time, the first significant observation relating to the causes of human malformations was not made until four decades later.

From J. Warkany (1959). J. Chron. Dis., **10**, 84–96. *Copyright* (1959), *by kind permission of the author and Pergamon Press Ltd*

CONGENITAL MALFORMATIONS IN THE PAST

JOSEF WARKANY, M.D.,*

CINCINNATI, OHIO

From the Children's Hospital Research Foundation, and Department of Pediatrics, University of Cincinnati College of Medicine

(Received for publication June 4, 1959)

TO DISCUSS the past at a conference designed to consider the future of teratology may seem a superfluous task. Yet the uses of the past are clearly demonstrable in the field of teratology, a science that can be traced to the earliest times of human history. From time immemorial, men and women of all continents and countries have been fascinated by monstrous human beings and animals. In fact, they recorded such curiosities before they learned the arts of reading and writing. This is demonstrated in artistic expressions of very primitive peoples. For instance, a rock drawing found in New South Wales, Australia, shows a double-headed human male figure, 9 feet, 6 inches long, with six fingers on the right hand and four on the left, the remarkable work of an Australian aborigine who felt impelled to put on record an unusual human birth. A beautiful carving of chalk from New Ireland in the South Pacific represents a double-headed human figure with two, or probably, three arms, a case of dicephalus dibrachius well known to modern science. A wooden carving from the Solomon Islands suggests conjoined twins of the pygopagus type with union of the bodies and heads and the extremities shortened by achondroplasia (chondrodystrophy), a systemic skeletal malformation. This anomaly, though known to man for millenia, did not become a scientific entity until 1878 when Parrot[17] recognized it as a disorder of cartilage formation and called it "achondroplasia."

The remarkable expressions of primitive Australian man were published in 1943 by Brodsky[4] of Sydney, Australia, who collected many examples of art and legends demonstrating a knowledge of monstrosities and malformations in the native population of Australia and her surrounding islands. The teratologic knowledge of man living in a Stone Age civilization is expressed in such works of art which show remarkable power of detailed observation and description.

Written records of congenital malformations have come down to us from the ancient inhabitants of Babylonia. Such records were found in the form of clay tablets covered with cuneiform characters in a mound near the Tigris River

---

*Professor of Research Pediatrics.

in the nineteenth century. The tablets belonged to the Royal Library of Nineveh which was assembled under the Assyrian King, Asshurbanipal, who lived in the seventh century B.C. It is thought, however, that these records date back to 2,000 B.C. and that the observations on which they are based were much older than this.[3]

The Chaldeans are known as the founders of astrology, the science of divination, the science of foretelling the future from the constellations of the stars, the sun, and the moon. The future was predictable not only from the course of the heavenly bodies, but also from terrestrial events. The flights of birds, the organs of sacrificial animals, and the births of deformed children were included in the calculations which predicted events to come. The abnormalities of newborn children were considered a reflection of stellar constellations and could be used, therefore, to foretell the future with as much accuracy as the stars themselves.

Among the many astrologic and astronomic tablets found in the library of Nineveh there were two which contain a list of sixty-two human malformations with the prophetic meanings attached to them by the Chaldean diviners. Only a few of the forecasts listed by Ballantyne can be given as examples:

When a woman gives birth to an infant
    that has the ears of a lion, there will be a powerful king
        in the country;
    that wants the right ear, the days of the master (king) will
        be prolonged (reach old age);
    that wants both ears, there will be mourning in the country,
        and the country will be lessened (diminished) . . . .

Eleven malformations of the ear are enumerated and their prognostic value is specified. Other malformations are listed that may be of interest to the plastic surgeon:

When a woman gives birth to an infant
    whose nostrils are absent, the country will be in affliction,
        and the house of the man will be ruined;
    that has no lips, affliction will seize upon the land, and the
        house of the man will be destroyed;
    that has no fingers, the town will have no births . . . .
    that has six toes on each foot, the people of the world will
        be injured . . . .

The orthodontist may be interested in an infant
    whose upper lip overrides the lower, the people of the world
        will rejoice . . . .

There are also statements of interest to the urologist and the endocrinologist:

When a woman gives birth to an infant
    that has no well-marked sex, calamity and affliction will seize
        upon the land; the master of the house shall have no happiness;
    that has no penis, the master of the house will be enriched by
        the harvest of his fields . . . .

Many types of twinning were known to these ancient writers such as the con-joined twins carved in wood by the aboriginal Australian:

If a woman gives birth to

twins joined back to back, the gods will abandon the country, the king and his son will abandon the city . . . .[12]

And so it goes through a long list of malformations and their meaning to the master of the house, the king, and the country. The remarkable thing about this catalogue is that, as Ballantyne[3] has pointed out, none of the recorded ano-malies, with one exception, can be regarded as impossible or mythical. Most of the malformations enumerated are known to us today and are listed in modern publications on congenital malformations. Whatever we may think of the con-clusions drawn by the Babylonian priests, we must admit that these founders of the science of teratology were excellent observers and recorders.

The people and the cities of Babylonia disappeared but Babylonian belief in divination has never died. Predictions from the birth of monsters and from other impressive events spread from Babylonia through neighboring lands, through Greece and Rome, and to other countries of Europe. Augury played an enormous role in Roman history, and Cicero[6] devoted two books to a discus-sion of divination in which he argued vigorously against this superstition while he let his brother, Quintus, present the arguments in its favor. From him we learn that the very word "monstra" had been chosen because of the monster's property of demonstrating the future. The stoic philosophers were the chief defenders of the belief that the future could be foretold through careful obser-vation and interpretation of monsters and other portents. They considered those diviners as competent who "having learned the known by observation, sought the unknown by deduction." They believed in an orderly succession of causes, wherein cause was linked to cause. The birth of a hermaphrodite, for instance, was considered an ill omen by the early Romans.[19] Unfortunately they executed such bisexual children. They apparently thought that disaster could be prevented by removal of the monstrum, which, according to the Chal-deans, was merely an indicator, a symptom of the future misfortune. But the Romans mistook the symptom for the cause, an error not unknown to the tera-tologists of today.

During the Middle Ages the interpretation of monsters as portents continued and played an important role during the religious controversies of the Refor-mation. In 1523 Luther and Melanchthon jointly published a work under the title *Der Papstesel* interpreting the significance of a strange asslike monster which had been found floating in the Tiber. The monster was assigned from God, indicating the doom of the Papacy.[22] This prediction was balanced by the birth in 1569 of twins who were conjoined at the chest, with only one of the twins being baptized in time. The physician, Jacques Roy, who performed the autopsy, interpreted this event as intimating that the Catholic faith would survive that of the Huguenots.[13] Belief in the birth of deformed children as omens and por-tents can be followed through many popular pamphlets and broadsheets pub-lished for the entertainment of the public from the fifteenth to the eighteenth century.[9]

To us it is of interest that the Chaldean beliefs crossed the Atlantic and traveled into the New World with its European settlers. Although they seldom come to the surface, they are still transmitted in whispers and have not lost their grip on the human mind. In 1945 a candid autobiography of an American physician, Tryon,[21] appeared in which an account is given of the emotions and thoughts aroused in the author on the occasion of delivery of a monstrous child. The physician, who practiced in a Dutch community of Pennsylvania, was undecided at the time whether to get married or not, and he relates how his decision was influenced: "During this time I delivered a monstrosity and I suppose with all the other things I inherited from my distant German ancestry, was a strong streak of mysticism. The monster became a portent. . . . It was a sign, a portent that I could expect nothing good from the way things were drifting along." This physician's thoughts were probably not very different from those of other people of our time, but his candor and frankness are unusual and permit a glimpse into popular belief. It seems worthwhile to keep in mind that even in our day parents of a monstrous child may be plagued by antiquated views which must be discussed and corrected by an understanding physician.

While the Chaldeans made use of the birth of deformed children to predict the future, other theories are concerned with causation and explanation. These concepts, which represent the answer of the past to the questions of etiology, are less grandiose than those of the Chaldeans and limit their search to terrestrial events.

The belief that psychogenic factors play a role in the causation of congenital malformations is very widespread. This idea appears in many forms, but essentially two subgroups can be distinguished. One belief is that parental mental impressions at the time of conception or mental impressions of the mother during pregnancy influence the formation of the child by producing a kind of photographic effect upon the offspring. A different theory suggests that maternal frights, worries, shock, or stress can produce malformations in the child in a rather unspecific way so that the exciting factor has no direct relationship to the morphology of the defect.

Theories of mental impressions as a cause of malformations and monstrosities were thoroughly discussed by Ballantyne[2] who traces these beliefs from ancient times to the end of the nineteenth century.

The idea that mental impressions have a formative and molding effect upon the fetus apparently originated independently among people who were widely separated geographically as well as culturally. It existed not only among all the peoples of Europe, but also in the Near East, in India, China, Japan, and South America. It developed among the Eskimos and the African Negroes. It seems that this idea is inbuilt in the human brain and finds expression wherever children are observed who do not resemble their parents. This "photographic" theory was not used originally as an explanation of congenital anomalies, but was employed for eugenic purposes with the intention of changing and improving the fruit of man or animal. One of the best known examples is found in the Bible in the story of Jacob (Genesis, Chapter 30) who tried to obtain a large number of speckled offspring in Laban's flocks from which all the ring-streaked and spotted animals had been removed. To this purpose Jacob peeled branches of various trees, thus producing white streaks on the rods which he placed in the watering troughs of the flocks. As the flocks conceived before the troughs, they brought forth ring-streaked, speckled, and spotted offspring. This method was applied chiefly to the stronger animals which went to Jacob, while the feeble, not exposed to the experiment, belonged to Laban. Needless to say, Jacob became exceedingly prosperous by this procedure.

Methods of mental "modification" were used in Greece where expectant mothers were encouraged to look at beautiful statues and pictures so that their children would be strong and beautiful. The method was considered effective by Empedocles[5] and by the Spartans whose law ordered pregnant women to look at statues of Castor and Pollux to make their children well formed and strong. The Romans continued the belief, and Pliny wrote that maternal and paternal thoughts at conception can shape the child.[2]

The idea of maternal impressions was also used in reverse to explain ill-formed children. For instance, the resemblance to monkeys of microcephalic or anencephalic children gave rise to the opinion that it is dangerous for women to look at monkeys during pregnancy. The birth of a black child to white parents was attributed to the picture of a Moor. It is most interesting to trace this concept through the centuries. The French surgeon, Ambroise Paré, considered a wayward maternal imagination as one of his thirteen causes of monsters. In his writings we see that this belief can be combined with scientific knowledge of embryology. Paré mentions that some people believed that after 42 days in the womb, the fetus is not endangered by the mother's imagination because once it has acquired a perfect figure, it cannot be altered by external impressions. Thus, already in the sixteenth century, it was believed by some that the organo-genetic period of the embryo was passed after 6 weeks of gestation and that maternal impressions after that time cannot be accused of deforming the child, which shows that knowledge of embryologic time tables is compatible with superstitious beliefs. The best minds of the sixteenth century adopted the theory of maternal impressions, including the skeptic Montaigne[15] who, in an essay entitled "On the Power of Imagination," explained why this belief was so prevalent. Since man had observed that the mind had definite influence upon such organic functions as yawning, vomiting, potency, and impotence, many unexplained somatic disturbances were attributed to the mind. In the past as well as today psychosomatic influences are blamed for disorders without tangible causes. It was thought that the imagination works not only upon one's own body, but also upon that of others. In the days of Montaigne, transmission of contagious diseases was attributed to visual impressions. "And as an infected body communicates its maladies to those that approach or live near it, as we see in the plague, the smallpox and sore eyes, that run through whole families and cities . . . . so the imagination, being vehemently agitated, darts out infection capable of offending the foreign object." Thus, at a time when neither bacteria nor viruses were known as causative agents of contagious diseases, it was believed that communicable diseases could be transferred by visual exposure. Since imagination and fear could influence involuntary functions of the body, since diseases could be transmitted by visual perception, it seemed very likely that maternal impressions could modify the growth of the developing fetus who is a part of the mother's body. Therefore, Montaigne states, "We know by experience that women impart the marks of their fancy to the bodies of the children they carry in their womb." These thoughts of an enlightened man of the sixteenth century explain why mental factors were and are used in the explanation of disorders for which no visible causes could or can be found. Similarly, we can and must expect that maternal impressions will be employed as explanations for malformations as long as we have no convincing explanations for the birth of defective children.

In the seventeenth and eighteenth centuries the theory of maternal impressions continued to flourish, and one finds the names of many outstanding scientists among its adherents. At the same time, the first voices were heard objecting to its validity and scientific foundation. It was pointed out that in consideration of the multiplicity of maternal impressions during the long 9 months of pregnancy, all children born should have marks and some should be spotted like leopards. It was observed that adverse maternal impressions were not always followed by the birth of defective children and that often abnormal children were born to mothers who did not have frightening experiences. Anatomy had progressed sufficiently to demonstrate that there were no nervous connections between mother and fetus. How could the mother's thoughts or fears be transmitted to her unborn child? It was known that the maternal and fetal circulations were separated. How could images be transmitted through the placenta?[2] During the nineteenth century the theory lost ground continually and German teratologists were particularly opposed to it. It was known then that most malformations are determined in the first weeks of gestation, while the tales of maternal impressions or frights usually referred to events late in pregnancy.

It should be mentioned as a curiosity that in the United States the theory survived throughout the nineteenth century and supporters could be found here among the leading medical authorities. In 1889 Keating's *Cyclopedia of the Diseases of Children*[10] still contained a special chapter on "Maternal Impressions" which is worth reading since it presents in clear and scientific language and by modern tabulation the most naïve credulity in maternal impressions. Ninety instances of defects in children were recorded together with "the cause or nature of the impression" and the "period of pregnancy" in which the impression occurred. Some of these cases are remarkable indeed. In one case the milkman whom the mother saw daily from the time of her marriage had one finger amputated, and the child born subsequently had only four fingers on one hand. In another case the mother lived next door to a man with a harelip and was apprehensive lest her child should be similarly deformed, and the child had a harelip. Another unfortunate mother was in her fourth month of pregnancy when she scuffled with a man who attempted undue liberties with her. The mother noticed that he had but one ear. When the child was born he had but one ear. These examples will suffice to show that the idea of maternal impressions held its own in its most primitive form in the medical literature of the nineteenth century. In our own times it has appeared in modern garb. Since fright can cause a release of adrenal hormones and since cortisone can induce cleft palate in certain strains of mice, a new mechanism has been found for those who want to believe in the ancient theory. However, the evidence for this mechanism as a cause of human malformations is extremely meager to say the least, and it should be emphasized that those who did the experiments mentioned did not propose their application to the theory of mental stress.

In the past there may have been humanitarian reasons for the enlightened and progressive minds to support the theories of maternal impressions. Such theories were rather humane and harmless if compared with some other ancient explanations of birth defects.

There was a widespread belief that members of different species might be fertile with one another and thus produce monstrous offspring. This theory, which was termed the "hybridity theory" by Ballantyne,[2] probably originated in India and Egypt where the transmigration of souls from man to animal was taught, and animals were considered as equal or superior to human beings. A cross between different species was not considered repulsive and if a woman produced a monstrous child who resembled a particular animal, the child was paid the same respect due that animal in the official religion. For instance, at Hermopolis in Egypt the mummy of a human anencephalus was found in a grave reserved for sacred animals. Since the monster seemed to resemble a monkey, it was probably thought to be of animal origin and was embalmed and buried with other sacred creatures. The birth of such sacred monsters, considered the result of unnatural though not sinful cohabitation, did not lead to persecution of the mother.[2] Crosses of human and terrestrial beings also are found in Greek mythology as centaurs, minotaurs, satyrs, and many other more or less respectable personalities, suggesting that fertility between different species was considered possible in those days.

In contrast to these pagan ideas, the Mosaic and Christian laws condemned relations of man with animals as criminal. With the acceptance of these religious laws the hybridity theory became very dangerous to the mother or the suspected father of a monstrous creature. Many examples could be cited, but I shall limit discussion of this unpleasant period to two events which prove the survival of this theory and its cruel consequences to more recent times.

For the first example I am indebted to Professor Walter Landauer of Storrs, Connecticut, who expects to report on it in detail. The story is told in the *Records of the Colony and Plantation of New Haven, From 1638 to 1648*.[8] Three years after the founding of the colony, a monstrous pig was born (in 1641) that had "butt one eye in the middle of the face" and over the eye "a thing of flesh grew forth and hung downe, itt was hollow, and like a mans instrum' of gen'ation." This was obviously a cyclopic pig with a proboscis, a malformation not rare in that species. However, to the good people of New Haven, cyclopia was not known as a spontaneous defect in pigs, and they attributed the birth of this monster to the "unnatureall spell and abominable filthynes" of a servant, George Spencer, who had "butt one eye for vse, the other hath (as itt is called) a pearle in itt" and closely resembled the eye of the miraculous pig. The court procedures, the confessions, and retractions, as well as the testimonies are recorded in great detail. This trial continued from 1641 to 1642, but finally the prisoner was executed on April 8, 1642, after the cyclopic sow had been "slaine in his sight, being run through wth a sworde." On reading this trial one realizes that the hybridity theory of India and Egypt was, with modifications, imported to this country—but also, the proceedings demonstrate that "brain washing" was not invented in recent times.

It is impossible to estimate how many persons became victims of the hybridity belief during the Dark Ages. That punishment was probably not rare may be gathered from the second example to be cited. The Danish anatomist, Bartholin, mentions in his writings that a girl who gave birth to a monster with a "cat's head" was burned alive in the public square of Copenhagen "ob lasciviorem cum fele jocum." This happened in 1683 in a civilized country, only 276 years ago. The fact is reported by Bartholin without criticism or expression of disapproval.[13] The event occurred 12 years after Niels Stensen, another Danish anatomist, had demonstrated his teratologic knowledge by an admirable description of a fetus with tetralogy of Fallot.[23] This is an illustration of the fact that science and coarsest superstition can thrive side by side in the same country at the same time.

Comparisons of malformations with structures seen in animals have been continued to our own times in many languages by the use of such expressions as harelip, bec-de-lièvres, gueule-de-loup, Hasenscharte, Wolfsrachen, phocomelia, and others.

Related to the hybridity theory is the belief that malformations are the result of the association of human beings with demons, witches, and other evil consorts. Especially in Europe during the fifteenth and sixteenth centuries it was believed that the world was populated by demonic creatures, sorcerers, witches, incubi, and succubi who plagued human beings waking or asleep. When a deformed child showed any sign which resembled the imaginary features of the devil, a demonic origin was suggested. Hairy nevi, ichthiosis, club feet, shortening of the upper extremities, long and deformed ears, syndactylism, and similar anomalies could be interpreted as signs of satanic origin. Many pamphlets and broadsheets are existent which show such creatures of unmistakable demonic origin.[9] In these pamphlets the devilish creature shows wings in place of arms, illustrating probably such malformations as phocomelia, syndactylism, or polydactylism. Repeatedly one hears of a monster born in Crakow, Poland, in 1543, whose head was comparable to that of a cat. It had fiery eyes and on each shoulder two small monkey heads. On the arms and knees small dog heads were attached. The fingers and toes were webbed and a tail and a trunk were well developed. The description of this child and his picture were published many times in pamphlets and in books; the monstrosity was ascribed to an evil spirit by some of the learned authors. Whatever the anomalies of this child may have been, they cannot have resembled the description and the pictures reproduced. However, printing and reprinting and a wide distribution made this fabulous child an accepted fact, an example of the power of written or printed records, which with a minimum of factual content can create psychological realities lasting for centuries. In those days demonology with all its ramifications had developed into a pseudoscience incomprehensible to the modern mind and was exacting many sacrifices of human lives.

Of course, sometimes it was observed that honest and pious women gave birth to monstrous children, and such mothers were not punished like the sinners who were burned at the stake. In many broadsheets still existent such unusual births were interpreted as manifestations of the divine anger aroused by the depravity of the world. Man's haughtiness and arrogance, and particularly his innovations were obviously going too far as intimated by the birth of deformed children. Hollaender[9] gives many examples of pamphlets which compare certain malformations with new and foreign fashions, a clear indication of divine disapproval of the prevailing trends.

In justice to the medieval world, it should be said that execution of the deformed child or of the mother did not originate in those rather recent times. Although there are indications that primitive peoples sometimes kept deformed children, twins, or conjoined twins alive and treated them well,[4] there can be little doubt that among many savage tribes deformed children were quickly disposed of. Infanticide was practiced not only on children with malformations,[7] but also on normals when economic or religious causes demanded it. In certain tribes female infants were endangered; in others, males. Twins were sometimes killed together with their mothers.

Infanticide was widespread among the early Greeks and Romans. It was practiced, according to Aristotle[7] when there were too many children, and Plato advocated it for the inferior or deformed in his *Republic*. However, it was in national-socialist Sparta that infanticide was incorporated in the constitution and practiced for the good of the commonwealth[20]—"Lycurgus was of a persuasion that children were not so much the property of their parents as of the whole commonwealth" and if "puny and ill shaped ordered it (the child) to be taken to what was called the Apothetae a sort of chasm under Taygetus." There the child was disposed of "if it did not, from the very outset, appear made to be healthy and vigorous." With such eugenic measures, the Spartans became a courageous, hardy, and ruthless people, but to art and culture they contributed nothing. This is not surprising since they probably threw into the chasm at Mount Taygetus the Spartan equivalents of such weak children as Newton, Darwin, Voltaire, and Rousseau, who, though puny at birth, made important contributions to a later civilization.[11] Lycurgus would have been surprised to learn that another tiny premature developed into Napoleon Bonaparte, a military commander who would have won the admiration of the most virile of Spartans.

In Rome deformed children were sometimes exposed in the Tiber, and it was particularly hermaphrodites that were chosen as victims and were executed. Other monstrous children also were sacrificed, especially in times of danger or when a catastrophe occurred. When the Roman republic was threatened, Arnus, chief of the Etruscan augurs, ordered that all monstrous children be killed and burned.[2] Thus the treatment of deformed children was often unfavorable among savage and pagan peoples, but the hybridity theory and the demonology of the Middle Ages extended the danger to the mother, neighbors, or other persons not conforming to the customs and beliefs of the land.

It would be erroneous to assume that only superstitious and primitive atti-tudes prevailed in the past and that the ideas which we now have about congenital malformations originated entirely in recent times. Biologic theories and expla-nations of deformities that appear rational to us date back to early periods of history. Some ancient concepts are rather similar to our own, although some of the basic facts of human reproduction were then unknown and the terminology has changed. The Greek philosopher, Empedocles, who lived in the fifth century B.C., was apparently so impressed by the existence of human monstrosities that he considered them as the forerunners of man as we know him. He developed a theory of evolution which was somewhat related to the modern one. It as-sumed an accidental appearance of disjointed organs which formed a variety of combinations and permutations with survival of the fittest. On the earth "many heads sprung up without necks and arms wandered bare and bereft of shoulders. . . . Eyes strayed up and down in want of foreheads. . . . Solitary limbs wandered, seeking for union. . . . Many creatures with faces and breasts looking in different directions were born. . . . Some, offspring of oxen with faces of men, while others, again, arose as offspring of men with the heads of oxen, and creatures in whom the nature of women and men was mingled, furnished with sterile parts. . . . But as divinity was mingled still further with divinity, these things joined together as each might chance, and many other things besides them continually arose. . . ." The monstrous forms which came into being by the fortuitous union of these parts soon became extinct, but finally the fit formations survived as animals and men.[2, 5, 16]

Aristotle had a surprising knowledge of teratologic facts. He knew of re-dundance and reduction of the fingers, toes, hands, and feet. He knew of im-perforate anus, absence of the gall bladder, spleen, or one kidney; he mentioned situs inversus, and cases of two spleens. He knew that milder malformations can occur in viable animals and that those which depart more severely from the normal do not live beyond the newborn period. Aristotle's description of a hermaphrodite or pseudohermaphrodite agrees perfectly with present-day obser-vations. His knowledge of, and approach to, malformations represent the height of ancient teratology. The fact that his statements were uncritically repeated and passed on for centuries without verification cannot be held against him. His writings on embryology and teratology were not surpassed for many centuries.

Pliny the Elder, who lived in the first century A.D., mentions many terato-logic curiosities in his *Natural History*. Unfortunately, he was an uncritical writer, so that some fantastic statements are intermingled with pertinent obser-vations and excellent descriptions. He knew that some moles and birthmarks can be transmitted through several generations. He relates that in the Lepidus family three children were born with a membrane over the eye. He knows of sex reversal and hermaphroditism. And he gives a brief description of a boy with precocious sex development and premature growth who was carried off by a sudden attack of paralysis when he turned three. Such cases still occur and one is tempted to venture a diagnosis 1,900 years later. But in contrast to Aristotle, Pliny had no general concepts or explanations for the anomalies he described.

New ideas were also lacking during the following centuries and the decline of teratology as a biologic science during the Middle Ages has been illustrated by the superstitions mentioned before.

It was not until 1,600 years after Pliny, when Harvey's *Exercises on the Generation of Animals* appeared in 1651, that a new biologic explanation was introduced into teratology, the explanation of congenital malformations by arrest of embryonic development. William Harvey had an opportunity to study reproductive processes by direct observation and he acquired a good knowledge of embryology derived from hen's eggs and particularly by dissections of deer, which were available to him during the hunting expeditions of his patron, Charles I. In the treatise concerned with reproduction the following sentences are found: "In the foetuses of all animals, indeed that of man inclusive, the oral aperture without lips or cheeks is seen stretching from ear to ear; and this is the reason, unless I much mistake, why so many are born with the upper lip divided as it is in the hare and camel, whence the common name of harelip for the deformity. In the development of the human foetus, the upper lip only coalesces in the middle line at a very late period."[2] Here for the first time, apparently, the idea of arrest of development during embryonic life is mentioned as a cause of congenital anomalies, and with this thought a new period of teratology began. Although the principle of embryologic arrest was expressed by Harvey, it was not applied by many during the next 150 years, after which this explanation for congenital malformations became most popular.

This brings us to the nineteenth century which represents a peak in the area of teratology. Then malformations were intensively studied in man, and brilliant experiments in lower animals began to supplement morphologic investigations. The teratologists of the past century were generally concerned with the study of environmental modifications of embryos, as germinal concepts had not yet gone beyond the stage of speculation. But in 1866 there appeared a small publication by a monk called Gregor Mendel[14] on plant hybrids which had no direct connection with malformations yet proved of fundamental importance for our science. Again, the seed did not germinate for 40 years until it was found that some malformations in man and in animals are transmitted like normal traits of the garden pea. Thus, genetic explanations made their appearance, indicating that in many instances the origin of malformations dates back to events which occurred generations before conception of the deformed child.

The ancient history of teratology does not teach us much about the origin, prevention, or treatment of congenital malformations; but it tells us a great deal about the human mind and its reactions to unexplained phenomena. If an abnormal child is born in a family or tribe, man insists upon an explanation. He does not put off his question and does not wait until science gives him a satisfactory answer. Considering the millenia of observations, explanations have been relatively few, and most of the theories of the past are now considered superstitions. Knowledge of the old and deep-rooted superstitions is of some practical importance since ancient beliefs often plague the parents even today, as they interpret them as portents or punishments. Such beliefs should be brought out into the open, discussed, and treated as a possible source of emotional disturbances. But let there be no mistake—as long as we cannot explain to a mother why *her* child is deformed, she will retain her own explanation and remain unconvinced by our general statements. It is not easy to define the border line between a superstition and a theory. Superstitions generally are based on a disproportion between knowledge and belief. Since even in our time knowledge concerning the etiology of congenital malformations is limited, and beliefs are free, we must be aware of the possibilities that we can create new superstitions in place of the old. For instance, the fascinating animal experiments to be discussed later in this conference may create new superstitions if applied uncritically to human conditions. If certain congenital malformations can be attributed in certain animals to dietary deficiency, anoxia, cortisone, or genetic constellations, one must not conclude without further proof that comparable malformations in man are due to similar adverse conditions. Such premature conclusions, usually not drawn by the experimentor but by a reader whose imagination and beliefs exceed his knowledge, can create superstitions in modern garb. If such a reader is also a writer with access to medical or popular journals, his unfounded beliefs are carried to millions, whereby new superstitions are established. Considerations of the past have shown how inflexible statements become, once they are written down on clay tablets, papyrus, or paper. A single observation of an abnormal child born to a mother who had been in an automobile accident, becomes, if reported in a popular magazine, psychologically, a hundred thousand observations which seem to establish a causal relationship between the two events. The whispered word is powerful, but the written word endures.

History has shown that scientific knowledge can coexist with crude credulity and primitive reactions to the deformed. In our own time we have witnessed how in the Third Reich the discoveries of genetics were distorted, misinterpreted, and transformed into a law which entirely failed to prevent defective offspring. To popularize insufficient knowledge does not pay.

Superstitions disappear quickly when replaced by scientific theories which lead to preventive or curative measures. When the "King's Evil," the "French disease," and childbed fever, which only yesterday also were surrounded by crude superstitions, were eliminated by scientific methods, the superstitions associated with them disappeared rapidly. Since malformations and monstrosities will be with us for some time to come, a knowledge of the beliefs about their origin, ancient or modern, ridiculous or rational, is still a necessity in dealing with the parents and the public.

REFERENCES

1. Aristotle: Generation of Animals, trans. by A. L. Peck, Cambridge, Mass., 1943, Harvard University Press.
2. Ballantyne, J. W.: Manual of Antenatal Pathology and Hygiene. The Embryo, Edinburgh, 1904, W. Green & Sons.
3. Ballantyne, J. W.: The Teratological Records of Chaldea, Teratologia **1**:127, 1894.
4. Brodsky, I.: Congenital Abnormalities, Tetratology and Embryology: Some Evidence of Primitive Man's Knowledge as Expressed in Art and Lore in Oceania, Med. J. Australia **1**:417, 1943.
5. Burnet, J.: Early Greek Philosophy, ed. 4, London, 1930, A. & C. Black, Ltd.
6. Cicero: De senectute, de amicitia, de divinatione, trans. by W. A. Falconer, Cambridge, Mass., 1908, Harvard University Press.

7. Encyclopaedia Britannica, Vol. 14, ed. 11, Cambridge, England, 1910.
8. Hoadley, C. J., Editor: Records of the Colony and Plantation of New Haven, From 1638 to 1649, Hartford, Conn., 1857, Case, Tiffany & Company.
9. Hollaender, E.: Wunder, Wundergeburt und Wundergestalt in Einblattdrucken des fünfzehnten bis achtzehnten Jahrhunderts, Stuttgart, 1922, Ferdinand Enke.
10. Keating, J. M.: Cyclopaedia of Diseases of Children, Philadelphia, 1889, J. B. Lippincott Company.
11. Laughlin, R. A.: Famous Premature Babies, Hygieia 17:203, 1939.
12. Leix, A.: Babylonian Medicine, Ciba Symposium 2:663, 1940.
13. Martin, E.: Histoire des monstres depuis l'antiquité jusqu'a nos jours, Paris, 1880, Reinwald et Cie.
14. Mendel, G.: Versuche an Pfanzen-Hybriden, Verhandl. Naturforsch. Ver. Brünn 4:3, 1886.
15. Montaigne, M. E.: Essays, trans. by C. Cotton; ed. by W. C. Hazlitt, New York, 1892, A. L. Burt Co.
16. Osborn, H. F.: From the Greeks to Darwin, New York, 1899, The Macmillan Company.
17. Parrot, M. J.: Sur la malformation achondroplasique et le dieu Ptah, Bull. Soc. d'anthrop. de Par. (series 3) 1:296, 1878.
18. Plato: Dialogues of Plato, trans. by B. Jowett, Vol. 1, The Republic, book 5, New York, 1937, Random House.
19. Pliny the Elder: Natural History, trans. by H. Rackham, Cambridge, Mass., 1939, Harvard University Press, Vol. 2, lib. 7.
20. Plutarch: Lives of the Noble Grecians and Romans, trans. by J. Dryden, New York, 1934, Modern Library.
21. Tryon, L. R.: Poor Man's Doctor, New York, 1945, Prentice-Hall, Inc.
22. White, A. D.: A History of the Warfare of Science With Theology in Christendom, New York, 1955, George Braziller, Vol. 2, p. 306.
23. Willius, F. A.: An Unusually Early Description of the So-Called Tetralogy of Fallot, Proc. Staff Meet. Mayo Clinic 23:316, 1948.

From M. V. Barrow (1971). Teratology, **4**, 119–130. *Copyright* (1971), *by kind permission of the author and the Wistar Institute Press*

A Brief History of Teratology to the Early 20th Century [1]

MARK V. BARROW

Division of Cardiology, Department of Medicine, University of Florida College of Medicine, Gainesville, Florida 32601

Beginning with the recorded accounts of such entities as clubfoot and achondroplasia in Egyptian wall paintings of as early as 5000 years ago (Martin, 1880; Steindorff, '39) mankind's intense interest in malformed individuals — human beings and animals — has spanned the centuries. Primitive peoples throughout the world, including Australia, the South Pacific islands and North and South America, have left traces of their preoccupation with monstrosities in their carvings and reliefs (Ballantyne, 1895; Born, '47; Brodsky, '49). Giants, dwarfs, one-eyed monsters, and mermaids have existed in the fairy tales of many nations (Schatz, '01; Graves, '57). Schatz ('01) pointed out that many mythological monsters may have arisen from observations of developmental abnormalities. For example, in his view Polyphemus perhaps represented a cyclopic monster, Siren, a sympodial fetus, Janus, a diprosopus one, while an infant with occipital encephalocele represented Atlas and one with exomphalos stood for Prometheus.

The Babylonian belief that the future was foretold by the stars, that abnormal infants were reflections of the stellar constellations, and hence presaged the future since they indicated the stars' positions (Ballantyne, 1894; Gordan, '49), was carried into the Greek and Roman civilizations (Ossequente, 1554). Thus the Latin word *monstrum*, from *monstrare* (to show) or *monere* (to warn) (Ballantyne, 1896), is derived from this concept of a monster's property of foretelling the future. Typical is the following excerpt from a 1554 edition of Julius Obsequens' *Prodigiorum Liber* (Ossequente, 1554); originally written in the 4th century, this book preserves Livy's history, now lost, of prodigies covering the period from about 200 to 12 B.C.: "In Venice a baby boy was born with two heads and in Sinvessa one with only one hand and in Osino a girl infant was born with teeth. At noon, out of a clear sky, a rainbow appeared. In a square in Rome three suns shown together and in the following night masses of fire fell from the sky. The same year [215 B.C.] the Carthagians swore, with the cities of Greece, an alliance against Rome." Such prophetic notions persisted despite Hippocrates' and Aristotle's efforts to seek natural explanations (Ballantyne, 1895; Aristotle, trans. by Peck, '53; Hippocrates, trans. by Jones, '57).

In the 6th century A.D. appeared the first extant pseudoscientific treatise on monsters, by Isidore of Seville (Sharpe, '64). He described numerous abnormalities and tried to give natural explanations of their occurrence, although he did not discount supernatural causes.

From the mid-16th to the mid-17th centuries several books on monstrous births were published (Rueff, 1554; Lycosthenes, 1557; Licetus, 1616; Ambrosinus, 1642; Paré, 1649; Bartholinus, 1654–61; Schott, 1662). These were descriptive texts filled with absurdities but splashed through with sound observations.

During the next 150 years John and William Hunter, Albrecht von Haller and Caspar Friedrich Wolff published their anatomical studies, while Graff, Malpighi, Maitre-Jan, Scharig, and Spallanzani delved into the flowering science of embryology (Meyer, '39; Gabriel and Fogel, '56; Bodenheimer, '58; Needham, '59; Singer, '59; Sirks and Zirkle, '64). A variety of collections of monstrous births appeared during this period (Buffon, 1749; Walter, 1775; Blumenbach, 1791; Sömmerring,

---

[1] Part of the library research for this paper was done while the author was preparing his doctoral dissertation.

1791) and significant discussions on the cause of monsters were given by Wolff (1759), Haller (1768), and Hunter (1775) in their anatomical treatises. In addition, one of the first reliable monographs on fetal diseases (Düttel, 1702) and a paper on the permeability of the placenta to smallpox (Watson, 1749) were presented.

By the early part of the 19th century the subject of malformations became a field in its own right (Zimmer, 1806; Jouard, 1807; Moreau, 1808), while Meckel (1812) first applied embryological principles in studying abnormal development. Experimental approaches to studying malformations was begun by Etienne Geoffroy Saint-Hilaire with his physical insults to chick embryos. He also showed an interest in human beings with malformations (Saint-Hilaire, 1822). These studies and a classification of monsters were well described by his son Isidore, who also is credited with coining the term "teratology" (Saint-Hilaire, 1832–37). Expanded descriptive works also appeared with regularity (Regnault, 1808; J. Breschet, 1829; G. Breschet, 1829; Beale, 1830; Gurlt, 1831-32; Bischoff, 1842; Vrolik, 1849, 1852).

During the latter half of the 19th century malformations were produced by various experimental means and experimental embryology was firmly founded. Numerous publications describing an almost infinite variety of malformations appeared (Panum, 1860; Chance, 1862; Förster, 1865; Ahlfeld, 1880-82) reaching their pinnacle with Taruffi (1881–94), although similar but smaller encyclopedic volumes were also published (Hirst and Piersol, 1891–93; Ballantyne, 1885, '02–'05; Schwalbe, '06–'37).

With the interest engendered by both the experimental teratologists and experimental embryologists during this period teratology now began to be approached not so much in descriptive terms, although books in this area continued being published (Broman, '11; Birnbaum, '12), as in terms of etiology of malformations. An indication of this change is found in Mall ('08), although development of the science of genetics contributed to the concern about etiologies. Thus, with the emphasis on mechanism, the irradiation experiments

of the first few decades (Bagg, '22; Muller, '27), Spemann's ('38) proof of induction in the embryo, Stockard's ('21) classic studies on the minnow, and Streeter's ('30) human embryological studies made their entrance. These studies, together with the experiments of the 1940s, including those of Wolff ('36, '48), Ancel ('50), and Landauer ('54) in the chick, and the nutritional experiments in mammals of Warkany, Giroud, and others (see Kalter and Warkany, '59; Giroud, '60), and the observations on the teratogenicity of the rubella virus by Gregg ('41), opened paths previously untraveled in the study of teratology.

Several excellent histories of teratology (Martin, 1880; Tarrufi, 1881–94; Ballantyne, 1896; Schwalbe, '06–37; Gruber, '64) are available which discuss the various works of teratology in detail. As one reads these works several theories on the causation of malformations tend to emerge. Although there is much overlap in these concepts and the speculations frequently blend into one another an attempt at subdividing them is helpful in understanding the development of many of today's ideas and beliefs.

THEORIES ON THE ETIOLOGY OF CONGENITAL ANOMALIES

The theory of supernatural causes including the diabolical (prehistory to present)

The monsters of early times were often deified. In Egypt the god Ptah resembled an achondroplastic dwarf, while the Greek god Polyphemus was cyclopic (Schatz, '01). The Babylonians, who saw portents in numerous objects, also used abnormal infants as predictors of the future, a practice followed well into the Renaissance as indicated by Lycosthenes (1557) and Aldrovandi (Ambrosinus, 1642). The Hebrews credited cohabitation with the Devil as responsible for monsters (Caffaratto, '65). Antediluvian statues and pottery, worshiped as gods by many primitive tribes, depicted malformations such as harelip and bone abnormalities (Kleiss, '64). St. Augustine, in the 5th century A.D., described a monster with a double head, "created by God," and Martin Luther considered malformed infants as omens (Martin, 1880). Paracelsus (1493), Jacob Rueff (1554), and Ambroise Paré (1649) suggested that the Devil's craft or God's punishment caused many of the gross abnormalities they encountered in their practices.

It is significant, however, that these later writers also included various physical causes as "possibilities." Certain religious sects of this country (e.g., Assembly of God) today regard malformations as "God's Will."

Early theories of natural causes (4th century B.C.)

The classical Greeks, notably Aristotle, looked for purely physical causes of monstrosities and found them in disturbances of the natural phenomena of reproduction. They saw monstrosities as accidents of nature and a lack of fulfilling "a potential" (Aristotle, trans. by Peck, '53). It is difficult to apply their vague terms and concepts to modern ideas of embryology but, importantly, they sought explanations in natural causes.

Theory of maternal impressions (biblical to modern times)

In Genesis 30 Jacob was credited with causing streaks and spots in the progeny of Laban"s sheep and goats by having pregnant animals of the heard look at stripped limbs of hazel or poplar trees. Maternal impressions have been accepted over much of the world as a cause of abnormalities, very likely before, and surely ever since. Hippocrates and Empedocles mentioned such thoughts in their works, Aristotle advised pregnant women to observe beautiful statues to increase the child's beauty, and Pliny the Elder expressed his support of prenatal influences (Martin, 1880).

The belief in maternal impressions was prevalent past the Middle Ages as indicated by Paracelsus, Paré, Montaigne, Descartes, and Robert Boyle in works in which they mention them (Martin, 1880; Ballantyne, 1896). Interestingly, John Hunter, after doing a prospective study in the late 18th century, presented scientific evidence against maternal impressions (Warkany and Kalter, '62), and Vrolik strongly opposed such beliefs in 1849.

Nevertheless, from 1886 to 1900, numerous supporting articles on maternal impressions appeared in *The Journal of the American Medical Association* (Barker, 1886; Jessup, 1888; Fort, 1889; Schneck, 1892; Batman, 1896; Courtright, 1898), and during the same period Keating (1889) in his *Cyclopaedia of Diseases of Children* listed 90 instances of such occurrences. Gould and Pyle (1896) in their *Anomalies and Curiosities of Medicine* strongly supported them.

By the 1920s, in part because of Ballantyne's (1895, '02–'05) and Mall's ('08) scientific studies, much doubt began to be cast on the validity of this belief. However, even today certain socioeconomic groups of this country firmly believe in the existence of prenatal psychological influences, as Ross ('65) delightfully expressed in recounting his experience with midwives, and as I vividly recall from my boyhood in a northwest Florida country town. Although most teratologists would agree today that gross malformations do not result from maternal impressions, some behavioral scientists consider that prenatal events such as maternal stress can affect fetal development (Joffe, '65). Might this not be still another form of belief in maternal impression?

Hybrid theory (prehistory to 18th century)

The view that hybridization between species could result in monstrous animals flourished long ago. The Hebrews, as mentioned previously, believed cohabitation with the Devil produced monsters (Caffaratto, '65). A well-known hybrid, the Egyptian Sphinx, is familiar to to all. Though Aristotle reasoned that hybrid mixtures were impossible because gestation periods were of different lengths, and various animals' natures were incompatible, Greek mythology is rife with hybrids (Graves, '57). Centaurs and Satyrs are readily recalled as well as the Minotaur, a result of the Goddess Pasiphaë's union with Poseidon in the form of a bull (Graves, '57). In a 9th century treatise on poisons a method was presented for producing a hybrid between a man and a cow, which could kill on sight (Levey, '66).

The belief in hybrids as a cause of monsters persisted through the Dark Ages. In 1493 Paracelsus described the Basilisk, a mixture between a cock and a toad, as well as other animals capable of killing a man at a glance. A Prodigy, half animal and half man, was pictured in Boaistuau's book of 1560. In 1616 Licetus still expressed a belief in hybrids, but Aldovandi was doubtful of their existence (Ambrosinus, 1642). Nevertheless, the belief persisted, for in New Haven in America (Hoadley, 1857) and in Denmark (Landauer, '61) a man and a woman, respectively, were executed in the mid-17th century for producing hybrid monsters by supposedly cohabiting with animals.

With the increase in knowledge of embryology in the 18th century and Spallanzani's unsuccessful cross-species breeding experiments (Meyer, '39) the belief in hybrids between species as a frequent cause of congenital malformations gradually declined. But it should be pointed out that several biologists at the turn of the 20th century interbred amphibians of different species to produce hybrids and more recently nonviable rabbit-hare hybrid embryos and viable ferret-polecat hybrids as well as many other hybrids have been produced (Hamburger, '47; Gray, '54). And, of course, the mule, a donkey-horse hybrid, with sterility, as its "malformation," is familiar.

Mechanical theories including adnexal disorders (16th century to present)

The idea that intrauterine trauma or pressure by an abnormally shaped uterus could cause malformations actually originated with Hippocrates and Aristotle but became a prominent theory after Paré's (1649) propounding this possibility. Such things as falling, faulty posture, and narrow uterus were thought to cause malformations, while the umbilical cord, amniotic bands, or adhesions were said to cause amputation. E. G. Saint-Hilaire (1832–37), after noting adhesions around malformed chick embryos, proposed them as a possible cause of most malformations. Later, Dareste's (1877) experiments, in which raised or lowered temperatures of the incubator produced malformed chicks without adhesions, dealt the adhesion concept

a blow. The idea that amniotic pressure acting alone could cause malformations without invoking adnexal diseases was tenaciously upheld, however, and even Dareste accepted this.

Thus, at the close of the 19th century amniotic pressure and to a lesser extent amniotic adhesions were popular theories (Ballantyne, '02–'05). Mall ('08), a few years later, in a classic report, pointed out that many so-called amputations had bits of fingers or nails attached distally. He suggested that faulty germ plasm was responsible for many monsters. He called these "merosomatous terata." Nevertheless, he noted that "other monsters in which more or less of the foetus is destroyed . . . are not germinal but are produced in some mechanical way which usually interferes with the nutrition of the embryo." He went on to say that these latter monsters "are produced by external influences upon normal ova which affect the nutrition of the embryos due to faulty implantation," and attributed this faulty implantation to inflammation (see below). Streeter ('30) discounted most, if not all, abnormalities explained on the basis of adnexal amputations.

The idea persists as accounting for certain malformations, however. Recently Torpin ('68) published cases of several fetuses with complete intrauterine amputation of limbs. Since he noted a ruptured amnion in these cases and recovered the amputated limb he concluded that amniotic bands were the cause, although he admitted this is a very rare occurrence. The view that intrauterine spatial pressure, or membranous perforations of adnexal tissues produce such malformations as clubfoot, scoliosis, and various joint dislocations was recently defended by Browne ('67).

Fetal disease theory (18th century to present)

The theory that fetal disease could occur in utero was probably first mentioned in an account by Watson (1749), describing smallpox infection in human infants in utero. Later Morgagni and others advanced the concept that fetal disease may also cause malformations (Mall, '08). Thus, hydrocephalus was thought to produce anencephaly, fetal peritonitis to cause abdominal abnormalities, and afflictions of the cerebrospinal system to result in a variety of nervous system malformations. Workers of the 19th century, such as Virchow, the pathologist, and His, the embryologist, pointed out that this theory, by and large, was founded on an erroneous conception of embryogenesis (see Mall, '08). Mall ('08), who disregarded adnexal causes after having studied 163 pathological human embryos, concluded, however, that fauty implantation and inflammation might well be involved in causing malformations not due to faulty germ plasm. Later, Corner, Huber, and Robinson suggested that inflammation was an effect of the malformation rather than its cause when they observed defective embryos before implantation (Corner, '61). With the emergence of the genetic theory in the next decade (discussed below) the fetal-disease concept gradually waned until Gregg's ('41) startling report of the teratogenic action of rubella virus in humans. Since then it has been accepted that not only rubella but also *Toxoplasma gondii, Treponema pallidum,* and cytomegalovirus may affect the human fetus in utero to produce congenital abnormalities (Horstmann, '69). Other agents such as influenza virus and mumps have also been incriminated, though no conclusive experimental or statistical proof of the teratogenicity of these agents exists at present (Horstmann, '69).

Embryological or developmental arrest theory (17th century to present)

The embryological or developmental arrest theory of teratogenesis was first forecast by William Harvey, who, in 1651, described early deer embryos. He later pointed out that harelip in human infants was very similar to the normal condition in early embryos. In the 18th century Haller (1768) and Wolff (1759) extended the idea of arrested development to explain ectopia cordis and gastroschisis since the embryo at certain stages of development has these conditions normally. Interestingly, Haller was initially an outspoken advocate of preformation of the embryo, an idea diametrically opposed to the epigenetic concept on which the developmental arrest theory rests.

Later this concept was used to account for nearly every type of malformation, thus gradually supplanting the theories of fetal and adnexal disease, mechanical factors, and abnormal amniotic development. Meckel (1812–18) in the 19th century pointed out that some of these "developmental arrests," which occurred in human beings, seemed to represent conditions found in lower animals, thus giving rise to the idea that the parallel between phylogeny and ontogeny was helpful in explaining malformations that resemble no earlier stage in human embryogenesis, such as a supernumerary tail and transposition defects. He is credited as the chief force in the early evolution of this theory.

It should be noted that this theory was adopted well before the cellular origin of sperm and ovum and the details of early development of the embryo were elucidated, since these discoveries were not to come until the middle and late 19th century. When they were made they merely strengthened the concept.

Dareste's (1877) temperature experiments with chick embryos and Mall's ('08) and Streeter's ('30) painstaking descriptive works added credence, but it was Stockard's ('21) experiments of the first 20 years of this century that thoroughly entrenched the arrest theory. Using a marine minnow, *Fundulus heteroclitus,* and varying the temperature and chemical content (especially oxygen) of the medium in which the eggs were developing, he produced a wide variety of complicated abnormalities. He observed that the type of monster produced depended on the stage during development when the treatment was administered. He further observed that the same abnormality could be produced by a number of experimental manipulations if given at the same stage. From these observations he devised the concept that developmental arrest or lowered rate of development explained all malformations except those of hereditary origin. This idea held until the 1940s when Ancel ('50), Landauer ('54), and others pointed out that different agents administered at the same stage of chick embryo development tended to produce their own unique syndrome of malformations.

Today the concept of arrest or delay of development may sometimes explain some gross defects, but numerous others cannot be understood in this way.

Genetic theory
(16th century to present)

When Mendel's (1865) laws were independently rediscovered in 1900 by Correns, Vries, and Tschermak (Peters, '59) it was realized that animals including man were probably subject to genetic rules and that genetic causes might therefore account for malformations. Although not understood, familial diseases and inherited anomalies had been recognized for many centuries prior to the present one. Paré (1649) mentioned that "crookt-back begets crookt-back," John Hunter (1775) commented on hereditary diseases, and numerous other authors throughout the Middle Ages speak of the same (see Mayer, '61). A more substantial footing for the genetic theory as a cause of malformations was gradually gained with Baer's discovery of the ovum in the 1820s and August Weismann's emphasis on the germ-plasm in the 1880s (Mayer, '61).

Several achievements of the first decade of the 20th century assured the acceptance of the genetic theory as having a role in malformation. This included Garrod's ('63) book on inborn metabolic errors, Farabee's study of five successive generations of brachydactyly in an American family (Haws and McKusick, '63), Cuenot's ('07) discovery of a lethal gene in mice, reports of defective blastocysts in mammals before implantation (Corner, '61), and numerous genetic experiments with *Drosophila melanogaster* (Mayer, '61). Thus, the genetic theory gradually supplanted the others thus far mentioned, especially when it was coupled with the concept that genetic disorders may produce generalized or local arrests of essential stages, as expressed by Streeter ('30). And, although some environmental mammalian teratogens were already known, Murphy ('47) still emphasized, in his book *Congenital Malformations*, that genetic causes probably account for the majority of malformations, at least in human beings. With the irradiation and nutritional-deficiency experiments in chicks and mammals (see below) and the

rubella studies in man prior to World War 2 it has become obvious that purely genetic causes still do not explain most malformations. Nevertheless, genetic causes per se are still a very important area of consideration and investigation today and their modifying influence on environmental, maternal, or local factors cannot be overemphasized. McKusick ('68) has catalogued the known Mendelian conditions in man.

THE DEVELOPMENT OF EXPERIMENTAL TERATOLOGY

Were it not for the generations of foregoing scientists making observations, asking questions, formulating theories, and gradually supplanting outworn ideas with new knowledge the time may not have been ripe for the rapid growth of experimental teratological studies that has occurred in the past 25 years.

Yet the experimental or scientific approach to the problem of congenital malformations is not really new. Democritus in the 4th century B.C. reasoned that two different semens might produce malformations (Aristotle, trans. by Peck, '53). As previously indicated, however, Aristotle can be credited with first adopting the scientific approach, since his advanced thinking led him to believe that congenital malformations resulted from abnormal growth, not from magic or hybridization of species.

During the 17th century the first mention of the artificial production of monsters, albeit accidental production, is found in several agricultural and historical works by Serres, Plot, Birch, Jacobi, Jouard, and Paris (see Needham, '59; Landauer, '67). In describing the initial attempts at reviving the old Greek and Chinese art of artificial incubation of chick eggs Landauer ('67) pointed out that many of the artificially incubated chicks had abnormalities.

Probably the first experiment in altering growth and development was reported in 1744 by Abraham Trembley (Baker, '54; Trembley, 1744), who produced multiheaded monstrous hydras by cutting through the upper part of the organism. Only 5 years later, it will be recalled, Watson (1749) described in utero smallpox, and although this was not an experimental report it revealed interest in pathological embryos.

Etienne Geoffroy Saint-Hilaire was the first experimental teratologist of any note. During the first third of the 19th century he systematically subjected chick eggs to jarring, pricking, inversion, and abnormal atmospheres, thereby producing a variety of abnormal offspring. These studies were reported by his son Isidore (Saint-Hilaire, 1832–37).

Later investigators continued this work (Panum, 1860). Lereboullet and Coste (see Oppenheimer, '68) observed abnormal development in artificially inseminated pike and other fish eggs in 1855. Dareste (1877) began his experimental work about this same time and over a 22-year period performed various manipulations on chick eggs to produce abnormalities. These treatments included varnishing portions of the egg, varying the temperature of incubation, and administering an electric shock to the embryo.

Féré ('09) also performed a wide variety of physical maneuvers and injected numerous chemicals into chick eggs and described the various abnormalities produced.

Other investigators began treating invertebrate, fish, frog, and chick eggs in various ways to produce abnormal embryos and fetuses (see Hirst and Piersol, 1891–92; Mall, 08; Stockard, '09, '21; Corner, '61, Oppenheimer, '68). A few of the more significant experiments were: destroying one cell of two-cell blastomeres to produce half embryos (Morgan, 1895); shaking apart blastomeres to produce abnormal double embryos (Driesch, 1891; Wilson, 1893); constricting blastomeres to produce conjoined twins (Spemann, '03); altering the salt or mineral content of the incubation medium of sea urchin and frog eggs to produce various abnormalities (Loeb, 1893; Wilson, 1897; Morgan, 1899; Hertwig, '05); and irradiating embryos (Baldwin, '19–'20). Cyclopia was also produced by various operative procedures on the head of minnow embryos or by changing the lithium or magnesium content in the culture medium (Stockard, '21). Many of these studies were performed in an effort to study normal development (experimental embryology), but, as Oppenheimer ('68) has pointed out, areas of experimental embryology and teratology are often intimately related one to another.

Experiments using various physical insults to gain insights into mechanisms of normal and abnormal development persisted into the mid-1940s. For technical reasons nearly all these investigations were carried out in fish, amphibians, or chicks and not in mammals. Stockard's ('21) investigations have to be called the zenith of such studies and gave rise to the previously mentioned developmental-arrest theory of malformations, although Spemann ('38) advanced from these efforts to his elegant induction experiments some years later.

How the significant genetic discoveries and breeding experiments using the fruit fly and various mammals came to the forefront in the first part of the present century and how these contributed to the field of experimental teratology have been discussed. Irradiation of the fruit fly for the study of mutations and irradiation of mammalian embryos for studying malformations were also begun during this period (Kalter, '68).

Experimental mammalian teratology evolved rapidly following this epoch. Hale ('33, '35) produced anophthalmia and cleft palate in pigs by long-term depletion of vitamin A; and in the 1940s and 50s many other teratologists began publishing the results of experiments on pregnant mammals and their fetuses. These experiments included the use of physical agents (irradiation, temperature changes, hypoxia, etc.), hormones (estrogens, androgens, cortisone, etc.), and nutritional deficiencies (riboflavin, vitamin A, folic acid, etc.) and excesses, such as vitamin A, etc. These studies were rapidly expanded to include investigations of the effects of drugs and other chemicals during pregnancy, especially growth inhibitors.

During the past 25 years numerous publications describing environmental factors, genetic factors, and combinations of these as a cause of malformations in animals have appeared. Since excellent reviews summarizing these efforts are available (Wolff, '36; Warkany, '45, '47; Gruenwald, '47; Wolff, '48; Ancel, '50; Fraser and Fainstat, '51; Duraiswami, '52; Giroud, '59; Kalter and Warkany, '59, '61; Giroud and Tuchmann-Duplessis, '62; Fave, '64;

Cahen, '64, '66; Kalten, '68) no attempt will be made to cover the recent studies.

In spite of the many experiments in experimental teratology and of many clinical and genetic studies the elucidation of the multiple and intertwined causes of human malformations is still in an early stage. Nevertheless only through such understanding will prevention become a reality.

LITERATURE CITED

Ahlfeld, F. 1880–82 Die Missbildungen des Menschen. 2 vol. Grunow, Leipzig.

Ambrosinus, B. 1642 Ullysis Aldrovandi's Monstrorum historia. Tebaldini, Bologna.

Ancel, P. 1950 La Chimiotératogenèse. Realisation des Monstruosités par des Substances Chimiques chez les Vertébrés. Doin, Paris.

Aristotle Generation of Animals, Translation by A. L. Peck, 1953, Harvard Univ. Press, Cambridge, p. 417.

Bagg, H. J. 1922 Disturbances in mammalian development produced by radium emanation. Am. J. Anat., 30: 133–161.

Baker, J. R. 1954 Abraham Trembley, Scientist and Philosopher, 1710–1784. Arnold, London.

Baldwin, W. M. 1919–20 The artificial production of monsters conforming to a definite type by means of X-rays. Anat. Rec., 17: 135–164.

Ballantyne, J. W. 1885 The Diseases and Deformities of the Foetus. Oliver and Boyd, Edinburgh.

———— 1894 The teratological records of Chaldea. Teratologia, 1: 127–143.

———— 1895 Antenatal pathology in the Hippocratic writings. Teratologia, 2: 275–287.

———— 1896 Teratogenesis. An inquiry into the causes of monstruosities. Edinburgh Med. J., 41: 593–603; 42: 1–12, 240–255, 307–314.

———— 1902–05 Manual of Antenatal Pathology and Hygiene. 2 vol. Wood, New York.

Barker, F. 1886 The influence of mental impressions on the foetus. J. Am. Med. Ass., 7: 441–442.

Bartholinus, T. 1654–61 Historiarum anatomicarum et medicarum rariarum. Centuria V et VI. Hafniae.

Batman, W. F. 1896 Maternal impressions. J. Am. Med. Ass., 27: 1031–1032.

Beale, L. 1830 A Treatise on Deformities Exhibiting a Concise View of the Nature and Treatment of Principal Distortions and Contractions of the Limbs, Joints and Spine. London.

Birnbaum, R. 1912 Clinical Manual of the Malformations and Congenital Diseases of the Foetus. Translated by G. Blacker. Blakiston, Philadelphia.

Bischoff, T. L. W. von 1842 Entwicklungsgeschichte mit besonderen Berüchsichtigung der Missbildungen. In: Handwörterbuch des Physiologie. R. Wagner, ed. Braunschweig, pp. 860–928.

Blumenbach, J. R. 1791 Über den Bildungstrieb (nisus formatiuus) and seinen Einfluss auf die Generation und Reproduction. Göttingen.

Boaistuau, P. 1560 Histoires Prodigieuses les Plus Memorables oui Avent Esté de Surveys Observés, Depuis la Nativité de Jésus Christ. Paris.

Bodenheimer, F. S. 1958 The History of Biology. Dawson, London.

Born, W. 1947 Monsters in art. Ciba Symp., 9: 684–696.

Breschet, G. 1829 Études Anatomiques, Physiologiques et Pathologiques de l'Oeuf dans l'Espèce Humaine et dans Quelq-unes des Principales Familles des Animaux Vertébrés, pour Servir de Matériaux a l'Histoire Générale de l'embryon et du Foetus, ainsi qu'a Cell des Monstruosités ou Déviations Organiques. Paris.

Breschet, J. 1829 Essai sur les Monstres Humains. Paris.

Brodsky, I. 1943 Congenital abnormalities, teratology and embryology: some evidence of primitive man's knowledge as expressed in art and lore in Oceania. Med. J. Aust., 1: 417–435.

Broman, I. 1911 Normale und abnorme Entwicklung des Menschen. Ein Hand und Lehrbuch der Ontogenie und Teratologie. 2 vol. Bergmann, Wiesbaden.

Browne, D. 1967 A mechanistic interpretation of certain malformations. Adv. Terat., 2: 12–37.

Buffon, C. L. L. de 1749 Sur les Monstres. In: Histoire Naturelle de l'Homme. Paris.

Caffaratto, T. M. 1965 I Mostri Umani. Fantasie d'Altri Tempi e Realtà Attuali. Minerva, Turin.

Cahen, R. L. 1964 Evaluation of the teratogenicity of drugs. Clin. Pharmacol. Ther., 5: 480–514.

———— 1966 Experimental and clinical chemoteratogenesis. Adv. Pharmacol., 4: 263–349.

Chance, E. J. 1862 On the Nature, Causes, Variety and Treatment of Bodily Deformities. n.p.

Corner, G. W. 1961 Congenital malformations: the problem and the task. In: First International Conference on Congenital Malformations. Lippincott, Philadelphia, pp. 7–17.

Courtright, G. S. 1898 Monstrosities vs. maternal impressions. J. Am. Med. Ass., 30: 1231.

Cuenot, L. 1907 L'hérédité de la pigmentation chez les souris (5e note). Arch. Zool. Exp. Gén., 4e ser., 6: i–xii.

Dareste, C. 1877 Récherches sur la Production Artificielle des Monstruosités, ou Essais de Tératogénie Expérimentale. Reinwald, Paris.

Driesch, H. 1891 The potency of the first two cleavage cells in echinoderm development. Experimental production of partial and double formations. Z. Wiss. Zool., 53: 160–178, 183–184. Reprinted and translated in: Foundations of Experimental Embryology. B. H. Willier and J. M. Oppenheimer, eds., Prentice Hall, Englewood Cliffs, New Jersey, 1964, pp. 38–51.

Duraiswami, P. K. 1952 Experimental causation of congenital skeletal defects and its significance in orthopaedic surgery. J. Bone Jt. Surg., 34B: 646–698.

Düttel, P. J. 1702 De morbis foetum in utero materno. Thesis, Univ. of Halle.

Fave, A. 1964 Le embryopathies provoquées chez les mammifères. Thérapie, 19: 43–164.

Féré, C. 1909 Index des travaux de Ch. Féré. Normandie Med., 24: 313–314.

Förster, A. 1865 Die Missbildungen des Menschen Systematisch Dargestellt. Mauke, Jena.

Fort, J. M. 1889 Do maternal impressions affect the foetus in utero? J. Am. Med. Ass., 12: 541–547.

Fraser, F. C., and T. D. Fainstat 1951 Causes of congenital defects. Am. J. Dis. Child., 82: 593–603.

Gabriel, M. L., and S. Fogel, eds. 1956 Great Experiments in Biology. Prentice Hall, Englewood Cliffs, New Jersey.

Garrod, A. E. 1963 Inborn Errors of Metabolism. Reprint of 1909 edition with supplement by H. Harris. Oxford Univ. Press, London.

Giroud, A. 1960 The nutritional requirements of embryos and the repercussions of deficiencies. World Rev. Nutr. Diet., 1: 231–263.

Giroud, A., and H. Tuchmann-Duplessis 1962 Malformations congénitales. Role des facteurs exogènes. Path. Biol. 10: 119–151.

Gordan, B. L. 1949 Medicine Throughout Antiquity. Davis, Philadelphia, p. 158.

Gould, G. M., and W. L. Pyle 1896 Anomalies and Curiosities of Medicine. London.

Graves, R. 1957 The Greek Myths. Brazilin, New York.

Gray, A. P. 1954 Mammalian Hybrids; a Checklist with Bibliography. Commonwealth Agriculture Bureaux, Bucks., England.

Gregg, N. M. 1941 Congenital cataract following German measles in the mother. Tr. Ophth. Soc. Aust., 3: 35–40.

Gruber, G. B. 1964 Studien zur Historik der Teratologie. Zbl. Allg. Path., 105: 219–237; 106: 512–562.

Gruenwald, P. 1947 Mechanisms of abnormal development. Arch. Path., 44: 398–436, 495–530, 648–725.

Gurlt, R. 1831–32 Handbuch de pathologische Anatomie der Hassäugethiere. Berlin.

Hale, F. 1933 Pigs born without eyeballs. J. Hered., 27: 105–106.

——— 1935 The relation of vitamin A to anophthalmos in pigs. Am. J. Ophth., 18: 1087–1093.

Haller, A. von 1768 Operum anatomici argumenti minorum, tomus tertius. Grasset, Lausanne.

Hamburger, V. 1947 Monsters in nature. Ciba Symp., 9: 666–683.

Harvey, W. 1651 Exercitationes de generatione animalium. Jansson, Amsterdam.

Haws, D. V., and V. A. McKusick 1963 Farabee's brachydactylous kindred revisited. Bull. Johns Hopkins Hosp., 113: 20–29.

Hertwig, O. 1894–95 Beitrage zur experimentellen morphologie und Entwicklungsgeschichte. Arch. Mikr. Anat., 44: 285–344.

Hippocrates Translation by W. H. S. Jones, 1957, Harvard Univ. Press, Cambridge, pp. 131, 347.

Hirst, B. L., and G. A. Piersol 1891–93 Human Monstrosities. 4 vol. Lea, Philadelphia.

Hoadley, C. J., ed. 1857 Records of the Colony and Plantation of New Haven from 1638 to 1649. Case Tiffany, Hartford.

Horstmann, D. M. 1969 Viral infections in pregnancy. Yale J. Biol. Med., 42: 99–112.

Hunter, J. 1775 On monsters. In: Essays and Observations on Natural History, Anatomy, Physiology, Psychology and Geology. Revised in 1861 by R. Owen, ed. 2 vol. Van Voorst, London, pp. 239–251.

Jessup, R. B. 1888 Monstruosities and maternal impressions. J. Am. Med. Ass., 11: 519–520.

Joffe, J. M. 1965 Genotype and prenatal and premating stress interact to affect adult behavior in rats. Science, 150: 1844–1846.

Jouard, G. 1807 Des monstruosités et bizarreries de la nature. Paris.

Kalter, H. 1968 Teratology of the Central Nervous System. Univ. of Chicago Press, Chicago, p. 91.

Kalter, H., and J. Warkany 1959 Experimental production of congenital malformations in mammals by metabolic procedures. Physiol. Rev., 39: 69–115.

Keating, J. M. 1889 Cyclopaedia of Diseases of Children. Lippincott, Philadelphia.

Kleiss, E. 1964 Historia de la Embriologia y Teratologia en la Antiquedad y Epocas Precolombinas. Talleres Graficos Universitarios, Merida, Venezuela.

Landauer, W. 1954 On the chemical production of developmental abnormalities and of phenocopies in chicken embryos. J. Cell. and Comp. Physiol., 43, Suppl. 1: 261–280.

——— 1961 Hybridization between animals and man as a case of congenital malformations. Arch. Anat. 44, Suppl.: 155–164.

——— 1967 The Hatchability of Chicken Eggs as Influenced by Environment and Heredity. Univ. Conn. Agr. Exp. Sta. Monograph 1 (Revised), Storrs, Connecticut.

Levey, M. 1966 Medical Arabic toxicology. Tr. Am. Phil. Soc., 56: 1–130.

Licetus, F. 1616 De monstrorum, causis, natura et differentiis. Frambottum, Padua.

Loeb, J. 1893 Ueber die Entwicklung von Fischembryonen ohne Kreislauf. Arch. Ges. Phys. Mensch. Tier., 54: 525–531.

Lycosthenes (Konrad Wolffhart) 1557 Prodigiorum ac ostentorum chronicon. Froschorerum, Basel.

Mall, F. P. 1908 A Study of the Causes Underlying the Origin of Human Monsters. Wistar Inst. Press, Philadelphia. Also J. Morph., 19: 1–368.

Martin, E. 1880 Histoire des Monstres: Depuis l'Antiquité Justqu'a Nos Jours. Reinwald, Paris.

Mayer, C. F. 1961 History of genetics. In: De Genetica Medica. L. Gedda, ed. Mendel Inst., Rome.

McKusick, V. A. 1968 Mendelian Inheritance in Man. Catalogs of Autosomal Dominant, Autosomal Recessive, and X-linked Phenotypes. 2nd Ed. Johns Hopkins Press, Baltimore.

Meckel, J. F. 1812–18 Handbuch der pathologischen Anatomie. 2 vol. Reclam, Leipzig.

Mendel, G. 1865 Experiments in Plant Hybridization. In: Classic Papers in Genetics. J. A. Peters, ed. Prentice Hall, Englewood Cliffs, New Jersey, 1959.

Meyer, A. W. 1939 The Rise of Embryology. Stanford Univ. Press, Stanford.

Moreau, J. L. 1808 Description des principales monstruosités. n.p.

Morgan, T. H. 1895 Half embryos and whole embryos from one of the first two blastomeres of the frog's egg. Anat. Anz., 10: 623–628.

——— 1899 The action of salt solution on the unfertilized eggs of Arbacia and other animals. Arch. Entwickl., 8: 448–540.

Muller, H. J. 1927 Artificial transmutation of the gene. Science, 66: 84–87.

Murphy, D. P. 1947 Congenital Malformations. 2nd Ed. Lippincott, Philadelphia.

Needham, J. 1959 A History of Embryology. Abelard-Schumann, New York.

Oppenheimer, J. M. 1968 Some historical relationships between teratology and experimental embryology. Bull. Hist. Med., 62: 145–159.

Ossequente, G. 1554 De Prodigii. Giovan di Tournes, Lione.

Panum, P. L. 1860 Untersuchungen über die Entstehung der Missbildungen zunächst in der Eiern der Vögel. Reimer, Berlin.

Paracelsus 1493 De animalibus natis ex sodomia. n.p.

Paré, A. 1649 The Works of that Famous Chirugion, Ambrose Parey. Translation of 1573, T. Johnson, ed. Clark, London.

Peters, J. A., ed. 1959 Classic Papers in Genetics. Prentice Hall, Englewood Cliffs, New Jersey.

Regnault, N. F. 1808 Descriptions des Principles Monstruosités. Paris.

Ross, R. A. 1965 Old midwife tales. Bull. Sch. Med. Univ. N. C., 13: 24–30.

Roux, W. 1888 Contributions to the developmental mechanics of the embryo. On the artificial production of half embryos by destruction of the first two blastomeres and the later development (post generation) of the missing half of the body. Virchow Arch. Path. Anat., 114: 113–153, 289–291. Reprinted and translated in Foundations of Experimental Embryology. B. H. Willier, and J. M. Oppenheimer, eds. Prentice Hall, Englewood Cliffs, New Jersey, pp. 2–37.

Rueff, J. 1554 De conceptu et generatione hominis. Tigurin.

Saint-Hilaire, E. G. 1822 Philosophie anatomique des monstruosités humaines. Riqnoux, Paris.

Saint-Hilaire, I. G. 1832–1837 Histoire générale et particulière des anomalies de l'organisation chez l'homme et les animaux, ouvrage comprenant des recherches sur les caractères, la classification, l'influence physiologique et pathologique, les rapports généraux, les lois et les causes des monstruosités, des variétés et vices de conformation, ou traité de tératologie. 3 vol. and atlas. Baillière, Paris.

Schatz (n.f.) 1901 Die griechischen Götter und die menschlichen Missgeburten. Bergman, Wiesbaden.

Schenck, J. 1892 A child without arms or legs: maternal impressions. J. Am. Med. Ass., 18: 314–315.

Schott, G. S. J. 1662 Physica curiosa, sive mirabilia naturae et artis. Book V: de mirabilibus monstrorum. Endter and Wolff, Herbipoli.

Schwalbe, E., ed. 1906–37 Die Morphologie de Missbildungen des Menschen und der Tiere. 3 vol. Fischer, Jena.

Sharpe, W. D. 1964 Isidore of Seville: the Medical Writings. American Philosophical Soc., Philadelphia.

Singer, C. 1959 A History of Biology. Abelard-Schumann, New York.

Sirks, M. J., and C. Zirkle 1964 The Evolution of Biology. Ronald Press, New York.

Sömmerring, S. T. 1791 Abbildungen und Beschreibungen einiger Missgeburten. Mainz.

Spemann, H. 1903 Entwickelungsphysiologische Studien Am Triton-E. Arch. Entwickl., 16: 551–631.

——— 1938 Embryonic Development and Induction. Yale Univ. Press, New Haven.

Steindorff, G. 1939 Physicians and medicine in ancient Egypt. Ciba Symp., 1: 299–330.

Stockard, C. R. 1909 The development of the artificially produced cyclopean fish — the magnesium embryo. J. Exp. Zool., 6: 285–340.

——— 1921 Developmental rate and structural expression. An experimental study of twins, "double monsters" and single deformities, and the interaction among embryonic organs during their origin and development. Am. J. Anat., 28: 115–277.

Streeter, G. L. 1930 Focal deficiencies in fetal tissues and their relations to intrauterine amputation. Contr. Embryol. Carnegie Inst., 126: 1–125.

Taruffi, C. 1881–94 Storia della Teratologia. 8 vol. Regia Tipografia, Bologna.

Torpin, R. 1968 Fetal Malformations Caused by Amnion Rupture during Gestation. Thomas, Springfield.

Trembley, A. 1744 Memories Pour Servira l'Histoire d'une Genre de Polypes d'Ear Douce a Bras en Terme de Corner. Leiden.

Vrolik, W. 1849 Tabulae ad illustrandam embryogenes in hominis et mammalium tam naturalem quam abnormem. Amsterdam.

——— 1852 Teratology. In: Cyclopedia of Anatomy and Physiology. 4 vol. R. B. Todd, ed. London, pp. 942–976.

Walter, J. G. 1775 Observationes Anatomicae, Historia Monstrii Bicorporis duobis Capitibus . . . de Anastomosi Tubulorum Lactiferorum Mammae Muliebris. Berlin.

Warkany, J. 1945 Manifestations of prenatal nutritional deficiency. Vit. Horm., 3: 73–103.

——— 1947 Etiology of congenital malformations. Adv. Pediat., 2: 1–63.

Warkany, J., and H. Kalter 1961 Congenital malformations. New Eng. J. Med., 265: 993–1001, 1046–1052.

——— 1962 Maternal impressions and congenital malformations. Plast. Reconstr. Surg., 30: 628–637.

Watson, W. 1749 Some accounts of the fetus in utero being differently affected by the smallpox. Phil. Tr. Roy. Soc. 46: 235–240.

Wilson, C. B. 1897 Experiments on the early development of the amphibian embryo under the influence of Ringer's and salt solution. Arch. Entwickl., 5: 615–649.

Wilson, E. B. 1893 Amphioxus and the mosaic theory of development. J. Morph., 8: 579–638.

Wolff, C. F. 1759 Theoria generationis. Halle.

Wolff, E. 1936 Les bases de la tératogénese expérimentale des vertébrés amniotes, d'après les résultats de méthodes directes. Arch. Anat., 22: 1–382.

——— 1948 Le Science des Monstres. Gallimard, Paris.

Zimmer, J. C. 1806 Physiologische Untersuchungen über Missgeburten. Rudolstadt.

PART II

EPIDEMIOLOGY OF BIRTH DEFECTS

PAPER 3

3. Christiansen, R. L. *et al.* (1975). Classification and nomenclature of morphological defects. *Lancet*, **i,** 513

COMMENTARY

There is general agreement that the terms used to describe human malformations, as well as the system for classifying them, are far from ideal. *Congenital anomalies* is an all encompassing term used to describe structural, functional, metabolic, behavioural, and hereditary defects present at birth. If the defect is structural, then it is called a *malformation*. Congenital malformations may be either gross or microscopic; single or multiple; external or internal; major or minor.

The most widely used reference guide for classifying human malformations is the *International Classification of Diseases* of the World Health Organization. It is recognized, however, that no single classification schedule could have a universal appeal. Each is limited, having been designed for a specific purpose.

Because of this situation and the rapid increase of information in the field of birth defects, an international meeting of experts drawn from many disciplines was recently convened at the National Institutes of Health in Bethesda, Maryland. The objectives were to 'suggest a flexible, practical, but specific nomenclature which could be used by clinicians as the basis of a universal classification'. It was hoped that such a nomenclature would provide a basis for improving the identification of malformations and for the storage and search of information.

A summary of the proposals, which have evolved from this meeting, forms the basis of this report. The suggestions are straightforward and sound. Undoubtedly, these provisional guidelines will be modified to suit particular requirements, but their adoption by workers in the field of birth defects appears almost certain.

Special Article

CLASSIFICATION AND NOMENCLATURE OF MORPHOLOGICAL DEFECTS

A MEETING, initiated by Dr Richard L. Christiansen, was held on Feb. 10 and 11 at the National Institutes of Health, Bethesda, Maryland, to discuss further the tentative suggestions for classification and nomenclature of malformations published last year.[1]

Suggested definitions:

1. (*a*) *Malformation*, a primary structural defect that results from a localised error of morphogenesis (e.g., cleft-lip). This is distinguished from (*b*) *deformation*, an alteration in shape and/or structure of a previously normally formed part (e.g., torticollis).

2. *Anomalad*, a malformation together with its subsequently derived structural changes (e.g., Robin anomalad).

3. Malformation *syndromes*, recognised patterns of malformation presumably having the same ætiology and currently not interpreted as the consequence of a single localised error in morphogenesis (e.g., Down syndrome).

4. An *association*, a recognised pattern of malformations which currently is not considered to constitute a syndrome or an anomalad. As knowledge advances, an association may be re-classified as a syndrome or as an anomalad (e.g., hemihypertrophy with Wilms tumour).

Proposed classification of multiple malformations:

I. Syndromes:
  A. Known ætiology:
    (1) Chromosome abnormality.
    (2) Gene abnormality:
      known biochemical defect;
      no known biochemical defect.
  B. Ætiology not established. C. Environmental
II. Anomalads.
III. Associations. factor
IV. Combination of malformations not assigned to any of the above categories.

Proposal for naming single malformations: utilise adjective or descriptive term and the name of the structure or the classical equivalent in common use (e.g., small mandible or micrognathia).

Proposal for naming patterns of malformations:

(1) When the ætiology is known and easily remembered, utilise the appropriate term to designate the disorder.

(2) Continue time-honoured designations unless there is good reason for change.

(3) In the absence of a reasonably descriptive designation, eponyms, some of them multiple, may be used until the basic defect for the disorder is recognised. However, usage of an eponym should, in the future, be limited to one proper name.

(4) The possessive use of an eponym should be discontinued, since the author neither had nor owned the disorder.

1. *Lancet*, 1974, i, 798.

(5) Designation of a disorder by one or more of its manifestations does not necessarily imply that they are either specific or consistent components of that disorder.

(6) Avoid names which may have an unpleasant connotation for the family and/or affected individual.

(7) The syndrome should not be designated by the initials of the originally described patients.

(8) Names which are too general for a specific syndrome should be avoided.

(9) Avoid acronyms unless extremely pertinent or appropriate.

Considerable discussion centred on names for many of the more common patterns of malformations. While there was often unanimity in the choice of a name, it was not always possible to obtain agreement by strict observance of the above guidelines because of preference for time-honoured designations. The group generally expressed the hope that the guidelines would be observed in future naming of patterns of malformation and that consideration be given to incorporating these proposals in the next revision of the International Classification of Disease.

Examples of recommended names:

Syndromes:
  Chromosome abnormality (subclassified by karyotype):
    Trisomy 21, or Down syndrome
    Trisomy 18 syndrome
    Trisomy 13 syndrome
    Turner syndrome
    Klinefelter syndrome
  Gene abnormality:
    Neurofibromatosis
    Tuberous sclerosis
  Environmental:
    Congenital rubella syndrome
    Congenital alcohol syndrome
  Ætiology not established:
    deLange or Cornelia deLange syndrome
    Russell-Silver syndrome
    Noonan syndrome
    Beckwith-Wiedemann syndrome
    Williams syndrome
    Prader-Willi syndrome
  Anomalads:
    Abdominal muscle deficiency anomalad
    Holoprosencephaly anomalad
    Robin anomalad

It was hoped that in the future attention will be given to nomenclature for less common patterns of malformation, and for single anomalies. Interest was shown in the possibilities of the application of new methods in taxonomy for the analysis of birth defects.

Comments concerning these guidelines should be directed to Dr Richard L. Christiansen, Chief, Craniofacial Anomalies Program, National Institute of Dental Research, Westwood Building, Room 520, Bethesda, Maryland 20014, U.S.A.

PAPERS 4, 5 AND 6

4. Kennedy, W. P. (1967). Epidemiologic aspects of the problem of congenital malformations. *Birth Defects, Orig. Artic. Ser.*, **III**, No. 2, 1–18
5. Stevenson, A. C., Johnston, H. A., Stewart, M. I. P. and Golding, D. R. (1966). Congenital malformations. A report of a study of series of consecutive births in 24 centres. *Bull WHO*, **34** (Suppl.), pp. 9 and 100–102. (Extracts)
6. Polani, P. E. (1973). The incidence of developmental and other genetic abnormalities. *Guy's Hosp. Rep.*, **122**, 53–63

COMMENTARY

These three papers deal with the magnitude of the problem of developmental anomalies in different populations. Many studies of this nature have been reported, based on either retrospective (newborn records, death certificates, or questionnaires) or prospective work (see Part IX). It is seldom possible to compare the results of epidemiological surveys of birth defects. Some data are derived from follow-up studies extending beyond a year; others may terminate after only a few days. What should be considered a malformation is not always clear. Because of differences in definition and terminology, the actual reporting of birth defects may vary considerably. The criteria used for assessment are unlikely to be the same, and minor abnormalities are not included in all studies. In most retrospective studies, the population sample is uncontrolled as are the diagnostic criteria. The problems are greater when information is obtained from hospital records. These are invariably inadequate or incomplete, and because much must be rejected the sample is biased. In contrast, a prospective study carefully defines the population sample ahead of time and establishes exact protocols for the examination of the infants and the reporting of the abnormalities.

Kennedy's paper represents one of the most comprehensive surveys of the world's literature on the frequency and geographic distribution of congenital malformations. It is based on 238 studies, published during the period 1901 to 1966, reporting more than 20 million births. The *overall* percentage of congenital malformations was found to be 1·08, ranging from 0·83 (data obtained from hospital records, birth certificates, and retrospective questionnaires) to 4·50 (intensive examination of children). Not surprisingly, congenital malformations contributed significantly to neonatal deaths and a high incidence of defects was detected in abortions and stillbirths.

Dr Kennedy emphasized some of the difficulties involved in interpreting the data which were caused by varying terminology and differences in diagnostic criteria (see Paper 3). For these reasons, the overall frequency of reported birth defects may be of little value and comparison of different studies is definitely difficult. Of even greater merit than the extensive data summarized in this work is the recognition of the serious 'variability of the reporting methods and the inconsistency of diagnostic criteria'.

The report by Stevenson and his colleagues (Paper 5) is a detailed survey of 421 781 pregnancies from 24 centres in 16 countries. The work was done under the auspices of the World Health Organization, using standardized techniques for obtaining and recording the data. The enormous amount of information obtained has been analysed with respect to the incidence, pattern, and geographic variations of specific types of malformations. Of considerable interest is the further discussion of these extensive data in relation to consanguinity of parents.

From all pregnancies reported, there were 416 695 single and 5086 multiple births resulting in 426 932 live- or stillborn offspring. The overall frequency of major and minor malformations in the singletons was 12·7 and 4·6 per 1000 births, respectively. A high percentage of malformed infants, particularly with neural tube defects, were born to related parents. This WHO report is widely used for purposes of comparison with other data and as a reference source.

It seems appropriate here to draw attention to two recent prospective studies (Collaborative Perinatal Project) which surveyed the epidemiological characteristics of congenital malformations occurring in 53 394 consecutive single births (Myrianthopoulos and Chung, 1974) and in 1197 twin births (Myrianthopoulos, 1975). All information was obtained and recorded in a uniform manner according to pre-established guidelines. Up to the end of the first year of life, malformations were detected in 15·56% of all singletons, including the malformations observed in 1004 fetal deaths. Multiple malformations were present in 2·59% of the offspring, the highest frequency (78·41%) being associated with the cardiovascular system. Male infants had a higher incidence of major and multiple malformations. The incidence of minor malformations was higher in negroes than whites (see also Wynter and Persaud, 1972). Because no more than a third of all malformations were detected at the time of birth, the need for follow-up studies is most evident.

A higher incidence (18·33%) of congenital malformations was found among the twins, compared to the singletons. This difference was attributed entirely to monozygosity. Multiple malformations were present in 3·25% of the offspring. Male and negro infants showed relatively more malformations than female and white infants, respectively.

Thus, in both singletons and twin births there is a definite racial difference in the frequency of congenital malformations.

The frequency of malformations which is detected at birth depends on the incidence of genetic anomalies at conception and on early embryonic loss. Taking into consideration that at least 20% of all pregnancies terminate in spontaneous abortion, due largely to faulty embryonic development, the actual levels of developmental anomalies should be considerably higher. The paper by Polani is therefore of particular interest. A conservative estimate based on the available data indicates that at least 6% of all newborns show genetic and developmental abnormalities. These include congenital defects (about 4%), single gene abnormalities (1·3—1·7%), major chromosomal anomalies with imbalance (0·5%), and cerebral palsy (0·1%).

Major malformations are present in *at least* 2% of all live-born infants, and such malformations account for approximately 20% of all neonatal deaths. Of all known causes of perinatal mortality, it would be most difficult to influence the occurrence of congenital malformations in terms of prevention and management. The magnitude of the problems involved and their importance can hardly be over-emphasized.

REFERENCES

Myrianthopoulos, N. C. (1975). Congenital malformations in twins: Epidemiologic survey. In D. Bergsma (ed.). *Birth Defects, Orig. Artic. Ser.*, Vol. XI, No. 8. (Miami: Symposia Specialists for the National Foundation—March of Dimes)

Myrianthopoulos, N. C. and Chung, C. S. (1974). Congenital malformations in singletons: Epidemiologic survey. In D. Bergsma (ed.). *Birth Defects, Orig. Artic. Ser.*, Vol. X, No. II. (Miami: Symposia Specialists for the National Foundation—March of Dimes)

Wynter, H. H. and Persaud, T. V. N. (1972). Results of a three-year study of birth defects in Jamaica. *J. Trop. Pediatr. Environ. Child Health*, **18**, 293–295

From W. P. Kennedy (1967). Birth Defects. Orig. Artic. Ser., **III**, *No. 2, 1–18.*
Copyright (1967), by kind permission of the author and the National Foundation

Epidemiologic Aspects of the Problem of Congenital Malformations

W. P. KENNEDY. Ph.D.. F.R.C.P. (Glas.). F.R.S.E.*

Increasing interest in congenital defects raises the question of their incidence. No extensive examination of the world literature was found so an attempt was made to provide a broad conspectus of the available data. This shows great variety of procurement and recording, and underreporting appears to be probable. The need for agreement on standardized diagnostic criteria and recording methods is emphasized.

As other causes of pregnancy wastage are being brought under control, congenital malformations are rapidly emerging as one of the major worldwide problems in this field. Yet, though aware that this is so, we are at present unaware of the actual size of the problem. There is no standardization of recording or reporting, and for this and other reasons many epidemiologic problems remain unsolved. While reviewing the world literature on the incidence of congenital malformations, the paper does not attempt to answer these questions for the evidence is still insufficient. The aim is rather to summarize the published data, and so to highlight the importance of this group of disorders, and to indicate that more comparable and extensive statistics are needed for the elucidation of the many problems.

Until recently the main area of epidemiologic research has been the infectious diseases, but successes in the control of epidemic and endemic fevers have widened the field so that in 1960 MacMahon and his colleagues in their standard textbook[123] were able to define epidemiology as "the study of the distribution and determinants of disease prevalence." This concept places the responsibility on the epidemiologist of illuminating by his technics those aspects of human disorders which are generally less accessible to clinician or pathologist. To these the patient is an individual subject for investigation, while to the epidemiologist he is a statistical unit, part of a population sample providing data for wide generalizations. Of course, the two attitudes to research are not antithetical; they are (or at least ought to be) cooperative and indeed, interdependent, each assisting and at the same time gaining from the other's advances.

From the earliest times the problems of congenital defects have puzzled and troubled man, first because of magic and theologic ideas, then from the practical difficulties of affected survivors and the distress and often guilt feelings of the parents. Lately the medical aspects of causation have been studied more intensively, and the topic of possible prevention is being explored. These developments point the need for an epidemiologic approach for several reasons:

1. Congenital anomalies are relatively common, occuring in 1 to 5% (or even more) of live births according to the criteria used.

2. The incidence of these defects is proportionately higher in stillbirths and abortions, and there is clearly a causal interrelation. In essence this is part of the general problem of pregnancy wastage.

3. Congenital malformations rank high among the causes of neonatal death, and the numbers in this category have not shared in the decrease in neonatal and infantile death rates seen in all medically advanced countries.

4. Since any organ or organs may be affected, and to a degree ranging from inconsequential anomalies to complete failure of development, the variety of congenital abnormalities is immense, and the incidence of many types is so low that even the assiduous investigator can see only a few cases. As a result, nomenclature and classification are still unsatisfactory. The epidemiologist must bring to the attention of the administrative authorities and even of some of his clinical brethren the need for greater precision in this area so that he — and they — may tackle the many problems more efficiently. In particular the appropriate sections of national and international "Nomenclature of Disease" need revision and addition.

5. Epidemiologic analysis of large populations is an indispensable tool to the understanding of causation because of the low incidence of many anomalies, be-

*Honorary Lecturer, Department of Obstetrics and Gynaecology, Edinburgh University.

cause such a variety of noxae have been accused — though not always convicted — and because the problem of origins must be solved before prevention is even a possibility.

6. Most cases included in reports of incidence require surgical or other treatment, or else are handicapped in some way, often permanently. Hence they make demands on medical and social services; indeed increasingly so, the more therapeutic and palliative technics advance, for example, operations for cardiac septum defects, and powered limb prostheses. It is notable that public dismay over the "thalidomide epidemic" brought to light how little had been done for the even greater number of children with minus malformations of the limbs, or amputations following accidents. This apparent neglect may have been due to some lack of appreciation of the size of the problem that in turn stemmed from the lack of the adequate epidemiologic studies essential for large scale planning.

7. As nearly all congenital defects are unsuspected till the moment of birth, and in many instances for long after it, investigation into individual causation must be mainly retrospective, which reduces the reliability of the evidence. This further emphasizes the need for statistical investigations.

8. Two quotations epitomize the situation. In 1961 Lamy and his colleagues said, "Up to now we have at our disposal only very fragmentary facts on the incidence of congenital malformations. They suffice to show the importance of the problems they set before doctors and public health authorities. But they are too incomplete for any searching etiologic studies."[105] Then the terms of reference of the Canadian National Advisory Committee, 1962 state: "The epidemiologic approach has already led to a better understanding of such chronic diseases as lung cancer, coronary heart disease, dental caries, congenital malformations, and others." But it may be commented that the increase of information on congenital malformations so obtained is by no means as complete as it could have been.

A search of the world literature on the incidence of congenital malformations confirmed the view expressed by many authorities that the state of knowledge is less than satisfactory. Primarily it is difficult, if not indeed impossible, adequately to compare reports because of differences in methods of ascertainment, of sampling, of nomenclature and diagnostic criteria. Secondly many authors have been interested only in particular aspects such as prematurity, anencephaly, lethal anomalies and so on. This is well brought out by Green who reviews the literature under several of these heads, including 22 papers on the incidence of malformations in general.[64] Another important contribution is that of Sievers who reviews the German statistics for the period of 1912-1960, analyzing the figures of 14 authors in detail.[179]

It seemed that there was need for a more extensive survey of the overall picture to discover what information in general there was on the incidence of congenital anomalies. This would be useful in itself and also a possible aid to more detailed studies. The establishment of basic data on prevalence furnishes a standard of reference for investigations on the problems of regional and seasonal variation in frequencies, the relationship to social class, race, parental age, parity, genetic pattern, nutritional states, epidemics, and many other environmental factors. The data from 238 reports have been collated and summarized in the tables.

As had already been shown by other authors the mode of ascertainment of the data is most important. On *a priori* grounds it would be expected that centrally collected government statistics would give a lower figure than that from hospital records, even when those were examined retrospectively, and these in turn would provide lower figures than data obtained from examinations by specialist teams specifically interested in malformations. Similarly one would have anticipated that figures from abortuses, stillbirths, neonatal deaths and prematures would be higher than those from viable live births, and that autopsied material would disclose more instances of anomalies than would external examinations. These expectations were correct.

Again examination at the time of birth would not discover all defects, many of which would not be evident till much later. Some cardiac, renal, aural anomalies etc., are unsuspected till their physiopathologic effects appear in due course. But reassessment even at the age of one month gives higher incidence rates than those obtained in the first 24 hours.

The data were divided territorially (Tables I to V) taking Britain alone (because of national interest), and separating Germany from the rest of Europe as this group of papers was large, and German medical teach-

ABOUT THE AUTHOR

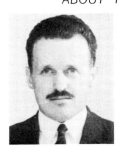

Scots-born W. P. Kennedy, B.Sc., Ph.D. of Edinburgh, qualified in medicine in 1929, and was Lecturer in Physiology and Clinical Assistant in Gynecology there. In 1932 he went to Baghdad, Iraq, as Professor of Physiology. In 1938 he joined the British Ministry of Health as a Pharmacologist, and after sixteen years turned to occupational medicine. "Fascinated by too many subjects," he says, his publications range from reproductive physiology and pathology to health education, and he is now working on thalidomide. Dr. Kennedy is an Honorary Lecturer in Obstetrics at Edinburgh University, a Fellow of the Royal College of Physicians of Glasgow and a Fellow of the Royal Society of Edinburgh.

ing and methods are so homogeneous that separation of this block was justified; the United States and Canada were taken together. Table VI summarizes the data on the basis of modes of procurement: —

1. Birth certificates and other official records;

2. hospital and clinic records; and

3. those in which there had been some more searching examination, say by consultant pediatricians, or follow up after weeks or months.

Just as the final draft of this paper was completed, a most important report of a study on a series of consecutive births in 24 centers was published by A. C. Stevenson and his colleagues under the auspices of the World Health Organization.[191] This report is required reading for all interested in the field. Because of the unified direction of the work in the individual centers, and the same recording methods being used throughout, an unusually high degree of comparability was attained. The gross incidence of the malformations in single births has been incorporated in Table VI, and accorded a separate grouping because of the uniformity of technics just mentioned. The figures for the individual centers are quoted in Tables I, II, and V, and also included in the summary groupings by regions in Table VI.

The grouping we adopted according to method of ascertainment was perforce arbitrary as the source of the data was not always clearly stated, but at least it tended to confirm the correctness of the expectations that the three groups would differ in completeness of reporting. Many papers had restricted data, such as "significant anomalies," "major malformations only," "live births only," "single births," or "birth weight over 500 g." This made the three categories still more arbitrary, but more subdivision would have only further complicated the confused picture. Such class restrictions mean considerable underreporting of the total incidence, but apart from this, many authors say that their figures are understated because of failure to diagnose at the time of birth, or to record the diagnosis accurately, or at all. In some states in the U.S.A. birth certificates have a tear-off attachment for such data as congenital malformations which are confidential to the Medical Officer of Health, and not given to the parents, and it is stated that these forms are not always completed as fully as they could be (Lilienfeld *et al*[217]; Barret, Bock and Zimmerman[216]). But there is no need to detail the causes of underreporting. They are familiar to everyone who has worked on records. It is considered safe to conclude that almost all the papers understate the real incidence. It is true that occasionally an author goes outside the customary usages and includes such conditions as phimosis, undescended testis and atelectasis among congenital malformations, but this is rare and additions of this kind are far outweighed by the omissions.

Few of the papers reviewed provided any data of follow-up examinations, and hence many cardiopathies, renal, aural, and cerebral defects could not have been recorded. No congenital biochemical anomalies such as phenylketonuria were included in this survey which was concerned with anatomical malformations, and in any case little information is yet available of large scale investigations of the former. There is, however, increasing evidence that congenital physiologic anomalies add appreciably to the total of infants born with some inherent handicap.

The tables summarizing the data must be allowed to speak for themselves. Detailed comparisons of the individual data within the groups are in fact impossible because of the diversities of procurement and criteria mentioned above. Of this, one has become too well aware as the collection of the material has progressed, but until it had been gathered together it was not possible to say just how varied it was. Again, any attempt to comment on the individual researches would extend this paper to an impractical length. The aim here was to draw a large scale map of the area, and to go deeply into detail, however interesting, would have detracted from the panoramic nature of the survey.

This review of the world literature covers 20 million births, and gives some indication of the size of this group of problems. Taking into consideration the evidence of underreporting in the greater part of the data, we must conclude that not less than two percent of all births have some degree of congenital defect. This of course includes minor anomalies, but it must be remembered that many defects classified as minor can have serious effects on their possessors. It is enough to mention one example — how facial disfigurement can lead the sufferer therefrom into antisocial attitudes and delinquency as has been shown by Sheldon amongst others.[178] By inference this underlines the amount of human suffering involved, as well as the implications for social and medical services. The phrase "group of problems" is used above with intent since in view of the undoubtedly multifactorial etiology, it would seem to be unreasonable from the epidemiologic point of view to speak of the problem of congenital malformations any more than the problem of cancer.

Nevertheless, estimates of total incidence of congenital anomalies, while therefore of limited value in determining etiology or suggesting methods of remedy for the various conditions, may be of use in several ways.

Perhaps their greatest value is in highlighting the variability of reporting methods and the inconsistency of diagnostic criteria. Here a further analogy may be drawn with cancer as a group of diseases. Fifty years ago one referred to the problem of cancer because knowledge of its various forms was so limited especially in the fields of etiology and epidemiology — and possibly even in morbid anatomy. This is the position today in regard to congenital abnormalities, and progress in this field will depend primarily in gathering more consistent taxonomic data in such a way that legitimate statistical comparisons can be made, *inter alia*, for different disorders in different races, areas, and environmental conditions, and at varying periods of time.

For valid statistical comparability the first essential is standardization of diagnostic criteria and the second, standardization of the point of time at which the diagnosis is made. An indication of the importance of this point is the fact that it will be seen from Table VI (p. 14) that the total incidence of the congenital malformations recorded ranges from 0.15% when the resources of the recording are birth certificates and "official records"; through a mean of 1.26% when the data are derived from hospital records; and to 4.50% when the information was obtained by special examinations. The last figure was considerably raised by the inclusion of several American reports which covered a wide range of minor anomalies. The overall mean percentage was 1.08% but it is considered that for many reasons there was underreporting in each group, and that therefore the real incidence must be at least 2%, even when "trivial" defects such as minor rudimentary digits are excluded. It may indeed, be significantly higher.

Wacker in his review has defined a congenital malformation as "any gross developmental defect which is apparent on inspection at the time of birth or within the first few weeks of life."[202] Metabolic abnormalities and anomalies which, though present at birth, do not manifest themselves for months or years, are excluded, and even within the relatively precise terms of his definition there is room for subjective differences in interpretation. His "gross" defects include for example, pilonidal cysts but not sinuses, and there is no mention of accessory auricles. Yet study of these "minor" developmental anomalies may be equally important in the investigation of etiologic factors. It is not only for the purposes of epidemiologic and etiologic research that so-called "minor" abnormalities may be of importance. As Le Vann has pointed out, a "minor" defect such as a facial hemangioma may have major repercussions for the growing child's psyche, and one might add, serious implications in the sphere of medical care.[113]

Many reports give no indication of the diagnostic criteria used, while as noted in the tables, still others have been concerned only with a few specific abnormalities.

The importance of the point of time at which diagnosis is made has been mentioned. In most of the papers in this survey diagnosis has been made at birth or within a few days thereafter, or in the case of lethal deformities, at the time of death, but there is no uniformity in this matter, and such uniformity is essential for statistical comparison. Moreover, in many instances no information is given as to when the diagnosis was made, or by whom, and such lacunae in the reports are regrettable. It is manifestly impossible that the same standardized time of recording could be made applicable to all deformities, but there would seem to be no insuperable obstacle to coming to an internationally agreed decision in respect of each anomaly, and incorporating this in the "International Classification of Diseases." The determination of the most appropriate time for reporting of each anomaly may be most difficult in some conditions such as congenital heart disease where a diagnosis may be made with some confidence at birth, only to be discarded some months or even years later.

Standardization of method of reporting is of equal relevance. For some inevitably lethal anomalies such as anencephaly, death and stillbirth, registration can give an accurate picture of incidence, but while it is self-evident that other methods of reporting are necessary for nonlethal deformities, it may not always be appreciated that in cases of lethal anomalies which are not immediately fatal, death certification alone may give an incomplete picture.

One final difficulty may be impossible to resolve. In respect of some orthopedic deformities, including talipes equinovarus and dislocation of the hip (especially the latter), remediable treatment undertaken within the first ten days of life is so easy and so satisfactory that one would foresee an increasing tendency to report and treat "probable" cases in which, because of the treatment, it will never be possible to establish an unequivocal diagnosis. Overreporting on an increasing scale may take place and accurate statistical evaluation of either incidence or trends may therefore be impossible.

In summary therefore, this review has:

1. Emphasized the universality and the size of the problems of congenital abnormalities today.

2. Underlined the wide diversity in criteria of diagnosis and in methods of reporting.

3. Emphasized the desirability of, indeed the necessity for, international agreement for standardization of diagnosis so that statistically accurate incidence rates may be recorded, trends estimated and a sound basis laid for epidemiologic and etiologic research into the many possible causes of these widespread and damaging conditions.

Acknowledgement

Grateful thanks are due to Dr. N. M. B. Dean of the Department of Social Medicine, for his counsel and aid in preparing this paper, and to Professor R. J. Kellar of the Department of Obstetrics and Gynecology, Edinburgh University, for his encouragement.

W. P. Kennedy, Ph.D.

TABLE I BRITAIN

Authors	Locality	Period	Source of Statistics	No. of Births	Number Affected	Percentage Affected	Remarks
Slater et al[183]	England	1963	College of G.P. Survey	1,038	23	2.21	January results only: LB and SB
Emerson[49]	Aldershot	1961	Hospital records	1,374	25	1.81	
Stevenson et al.[190]	Belfast	1957	Examination and re-examination after one year	8,519	120	1.40	LB and SB. Gross anomalies
Cheeseman and Froggat[191]	Belfast	1960-61	W.H.O. forms	28,091	544	1.93	Quoted by Stevenson et al[191]
McKeown and Record[122]	Birmingham	1950-52	Special cards	56,760	1,231	1.73	1,221 SB
Charles[30]	Birmingham	1949	Special cards	19,711	357	1.81	"Probable underreporting"
Leck[109]	Birmingham	1957-63	Hospital records and Home Visitors' reports	147,500	1,238	0.84	
Leck and Millar[110]	Birmingham	1957-61	Hosp. and Pub. Hlth. Dept. records, H.V. reports	102,042	939	0.92	LB and SB
Corner[26]	Bristol	1960-61	Hospital records	8,059	236	2.92	
Coffey and Jessop[32]	Dublin	1953-54	Questionnaire and exams.	12,552	204	1.63	
Coffey and Quinn[33]	Dublin	1965	Hospital deliveries / Home deliveries	18,971 / 2,276	260* / 30*	1.37 / 1.27	
(Simpson Maternity Hosp.[182])	Edinburgh	1938-48 / 1955-63	Annual Reports	66,532	2,088	3.14	LB 63,666 CM 1706 or 2.68% SB 2866, CM 382 or 13.32%
(Elsie Inglis Hospital[47])	Edinburgh	1948-49	Annual Reports	676	55	8.13	
Dean[41]	Edinburgh		Individual examination	11,548	348	3.05	
Nelson[144]	Edinburgh		Individual examination	8,648	496*	5.74 / 1.50	Total / Major
Ward and Irvine[206,207]	Exeter	1954-62	Welfare clinics and special enquiries	10,599	343	3.21	"Substantial abnormalities"
Landsman et al[107]	Glasgow	1960-61	Hospital records and follow-up	2,542 / 48	45 / 11	1.77 / 22.91	LB / SB
Craig[37]	Leeds	1947-64	Hospital records	35,750	1,074	3.00	
Moss[138]	Leicester	1953-62	Midwives, HVs and Clinic	46,312	921	1.99	77 had more than one severe CM
Malpas[125]	Liverpool	1923-32	Hospital records	13,964	294	2.11	
Smithells[184]	Liverpool	1960-61	Hospital observation	2,688	88*	3.27	
Carter[29]	London	1943-49	Hospital observation	14,283	219	1.47	LB and SB
Landtman[108]	London	1945-48	Hospital observation	3,593	73	2.03	
Böök and Fraccaro[21]	London	1947-51	Maternity registers	20,151	609	3.02	Two hospitals
Pleydell[158]	Northamptonshire	1944-57	Special register	60,890	603	0.99	Only 6 major groups CM included
Griffin and Sorrie[67]	Reading	1958-63	Varied	12,951	393	3.04	
Stark[188]	South Shields	1944-50	Hospital records	4,444	62*	1.39	
McDonald[120]	Watford, St. Albans	1952-55	Personal Interviews	3,216	50 / 72	1.58 / 2.37	Major / Minor

Note: CM = Congenital malformation.   LB = live births   SB = stillbirths   NND = neonatal death   * signifies the figure has been calculated from the authors' data

TABLE II

EUROPE, excepting GERMANY

Authors	Locality	Period	Source of Statistics	No. of Births	Number Affected	Percentage Affected	Remarks
Reiffenstuhl[167]	Austria, Graz	1946-51	Hospital records	38,687	105	0.27	Gross cases, "visible without special examination."
Fink[55]	Austria, Vienna	1934-53	University Obstetric Clinic	35,999	413	0.74	679 twins, 10 triplets
Elsner-Mackay[48]	Austria, Wels	1945-62	Hospital records	30,000	81*	0.27	Major cases
Derom[45]	Belgium	1945-62	Hospital records	29,696	366	1.61	
Heyne[75]	Belgium	1958-62	Inspector of Hygiene and Doctors' reports	554,703 / 186,253	3,363 / 1,632	0.61 / 0.88	
Radanov et al[164]	Bulgaria			8,022	118	1.47	
Bovev et al[72]	Bulgaria, Sofia	1954-61	Hospital records	16,276	200	1.22	
Houštĕk et al[80]	Czechoslovakia	1958-60	Registration	39,000	559	1.43	LB only
Kucera[102]	Czechoslovakia		Clinic records	678,132	7,526	1.10	
Kucera et al[191]	Czechoslovakia	1960-61	W.H.O. study	20,074	348	1.73	Quoted from Stevenson, A.C., et al[191]
Schnellerova et al[172]	Czechoslovakia, Brno	1957-60	University Neonatal Clinic	19,305	329	1.70	
Biering-Sorensen[15]	Denmark, Copenhagen	1962	Health visits or supervision	6,485	75	1.16	
Büchi[23]	Denmark, Copenhagen	1911-49		167,940	2,619	1.56	Quoted by Bóók and Fraccaro[21]
Pedersen et al[152]	Denmark, Copenhagen	1959-60		1,212	26	2.14	
Villumsen and Zachau-Christiansen[201]	Denmark, Copenhagen	1959-61	Pediatrician's examination	1,707	61	3.57	
Stähler[187]	Europe	1959	40 Clinic records in different countries	65,758	942	1.43	
Hirvensalo and Hjelt[76]	Finland			14,091	606*	4.30	
Saxen and Härö[169]	Finland	1957-62	Official questionnaire to maternity hospitals	504,742	9,398	1.86	Includes 7,777 SB with 1,038 CM, 13.34%
Klemetti[94]	Finland, Keski Soumi	1963-64	Maternity Health Centers	3,674	103	2.80	Diagnosis by M.D. and/or pediatrician
Alison[3]	France	1953-59	18 Maternity Hospitals	4,479	221	4.93	13 Parisian hospitals 5 provincial
Ravina et al[165]	France	1945-52	Hospital records	18,303	167	0.91	
Baron et al[12]	France, Dijon	1950-58	Maternity register	13,403	162	1.21	
Azer[10]	France, Lyon	1927-40	Maternity register	23,841	296	1.13	
Turpin[198]	France, Paris	1941-50	Maternity register	78,844	622*	0.84	
Tholen[195]	Holland, The Hague	1944-46	Obstetric Clinic	1,833	66	3.60	
Kovacs and Mackay[101]	Hungary, Baja	20 years	Hospital records	12,232	158	1.29	
Horn et al[78]	Hungary, Budapest	1953-62	Clinic records	22,592	111	1.16	Major CM, single births
Nagy et al[140]	Hungary, Debrecen	1947-58	Hospital records	42,988	774	1.84	
Cocozza and Tiso[31]	Italy		Clinic records	3,200	52	1.62	
Nobili[147]	Italy	1950-63		8,227	148	1.79	
Vignali[200]	Italy, Brescia	1943-60	Hospital records	28,170	231	0.82	
Leone[111]	Italy, Cagliari	1935-60	Hospital records	33,682	245	0.73	
Campli and Pedone[27]	Italy, Foggia	1937-59	Hospital records	14,672	172	1.17	

Reference	Location	Years	Method	Total	Cases	Rate	Notes
Greco et al[63]	Italy, Gargano	1957-61	Special examination	1,435	48	3.35	
Beolchini[14]	Italy, Milan	1942-62	Hospital records	85,976	1,185	1.35	
Toricelli et al[197]	Italy, Milan	1950-61		24,004	617	2.57	Quoted by Avezzu and Vinci[9]
Avezzu and Vinci[9]	Italy, Milan	1960-64	University Clinic	35,390	162	0.45	Major cases only
Ferrario and Fortuna[53]	Italy, Novara	1930-49	Hospital records	9,474	72	0.76	Quoted by Böök and Fraccaro[21]
Carollo et al[28]	Italy, Palermo	1957-64	Clinic records	6,669	99	1.48	
Spoto[186]	Italy, Parma	1938-47		8,228	70	0.85	Quoted by Böök and Fraccaro[21]
Piccioni[156]	Italy, Rome	1936-50	Obstetric Clinic	53,567	418	0.78	
Livadiotti et al[117]	Italy, Rome	1949-62	Hospital records	37,853	742	1.96	
Calvani[26]	Italy, Rome	1956-60	Hospital observation	15,233	359	2.35	
Maggiore[124]	Italy, Rome	1956-58	Official records	2,660,990	4,120	0.15	1311 SB or NND
Bologna[19]	Italy, Rome		Hospital records	38,812	299	0.77	Major cases only
Aicardi et al[2]	Italy, Sassari	1936-65	Clinic records	18,676	262	1.40	
Dellepiane and Colla[43]	Italy, Torino	1949-55		7,991	61	0.76	Quoted by Böök and Fraccaro[21]
Avanzini and Girando[8]	Italy, Torino	1953-58	Hospital records	6,465	88	1.36	
Morra and Cremona[136]	Italy, Torino	1956-62	Hospital records	20,908	240	1.14	
Morandi and Marchesoni[135]	Italy, Trento	1960-62	Hospital records	4,085	38	0.93	
Colucci and Tosolini[34]	Italy, Udine	1950-63	Hospital records	16,217	94	0.57	
Kolbas[100]	Jugoslavia, Croatia		Special examination	1,706	119	6.97	All babies at birth; nurslings 9.5%
Cupic et al[191]	Jugoslavia, Ljubljana	1960-61	W.H.O. study	8,888	171	1.92	Quoted from Stevenson, A.C., et al[191]
Kesic and Sestak[191]	Jugoslavia, Zagreb	1960-61	W.H.O. study	8,416	107	1.27	Quoted from Stevenson, A.C., et al[191]
Bjøro and Iversen[17]	Norway	1944-58		39,848	394	0.98	
Mosing[137]	Poland	1955-61	Hospital records	5,535	70	1.26	
Kobielowa et al[97]	Poland, Krakow	12 years	Clinic records	18,000	47	0.26	
Zytkiewicz et al[215]	Poland, Lublin	10 years	Clinic records	18,537	617	3.32	
Jaworska[86]	Poland, Warsaw	1947-58	Clinic records	17,767	474	2.66	LB and SB
Roszkowski and Kietlinka[168]	Poland, Warsaw		Clinic records	10,971	221	1.94	
Popa and Iliescu[161]	Rumanian	1960-63	Clinic records	6,890	177	2.5	
Gonzalez-Coviella[61]	Spain, Madrid	1963-64	Clinic records	20,221	271	1.34	
Monero et al[191]	Spain, Madrid	1960-61	W.H.O. study	19,714	264	1.32	Quoted from Stevenson, A.C., et al[191]
Fiuza Perez[56]	Spain, Santander		Two Pediatric Institutions	31,500	690	2.19	31,500 children in the Institutions, obviously no lethal defects involved.
Hedberg et al[71]	Sweden, Göteborg	1954-58	Prenatal Care Center	2,952	61	2.06	
Böök[20]	Sweden, Lund	1927-46	Maternity Register	44,109	589	1.33	
Pfiffer[155]	Switzerland, Basel	1920-33	Hospital records	25,241	370	1.46	Quoted by Sievers[179]
Da Rugna[39]	Switzerland, Basel	1953-62	Inspection with consultation	37,484	313	0.83	Severe cases only
Pomerants and Chukanina[159]	U.S.S.R., Andizhan	9 years		30,034	382	1.27	Mostly limbs affected
Deduhk and Lankovits[42]	U.S.S.R., Moscow		Hospital records	47,936	448	0.93	

Note: CM = Congenital malformation.   LB = live births   SB = stillbirths   NND = neonatal death   * signifies the figure has been calculated from the authors' data

TABLE III
GERMANY

Authors	Locality	Period	Source of Statistics	No. of Births	Number Affected	Percentage Affected	Remarks
Mischel[132]	Altona	1930-61	Hospital records	40,270	636	1.58	
Pereyma[153]	Bamberg	1940-48		18,995	220	1.16	
Eichmann and Gesenius[46]	Berlin and environs	1911-50	Hospital records	474,950	3,016	0.63	55 Hospitals
Präger[162]	Berlin	1928-37	Hospital records	23,132	311	1.34	Quoted by Sievers[179]
Kühnelt and Rotter-Pool[104]	Berlin	1934-54	Hospital records	44,291	514	1.11	
Ockel and Klemm[149]	Berlin	{1956-63 {1960-64	Potsdam Hospital Friedrichsheim	12,320 15,922	145 57	1.18 0.36	
Schenk[170]	Berlin	1938-41	Hospital records	11,077	366	3.30	
Winter and Pätz[208]	Berlin and environs	1950-56	Hospital and Clinic records	201,692	1,775	0.88	
Schubert[173]	Berlin Moabit	1950-57	Inspection, pediatric consultation, obligatory P.M.s	5,314	112	2.10	
Buurman et al[25]	Bonn, Celle, Gottingen, Leipzig	1901-56	Maternity register	240,691	2,667	1.11	
Nowak[148]	Chemnitz	1945-59	Hospital records	21,384	237	2.40	
Klosterkötter[95]	Cologne	1931-44	Hospital records	22,905	300	1.31	
Naujoks[142]	Cologne	before 1938	Obstetric clinics	17,800	236	1.33	
Soergel[185]	Dortmund	1947-58	Hospital records	17,830	181	1.02	No postmortems were done
Hohlbein[77]	Dresden	1921-58	Hospital records	129,382	748	0.58	
Hohlbein[77]	Dresden-Friedrichstadt	1915-50	Hospital records	41,067	324*	0.79	
Prediger[163]	Essen	1934-58	Hospital records	27,033	304	1.14	
Anon.[77]	Frankfurt-a.M.	1925-35	Univ. Obstetric Clinic	13,927	38	0.27	Quoted by Hohlbein[77]
Anon.[77]	Freiburg i.Br.	1906-20	Univ. Obstetric Clinic	14,650	25	0.17	Quoted by Hohlbein[77]
May[130]	Freiburg i.Br.	1945-53	Univ. Obstetric Clinic	12,304	80	0.65	
Worm[210]	Griefswald	1930-50	Hospital records	14,611	148	1.01	

Lindemann[116]	Halle	1929-50	Univ. Obstetric Clinic	20,126	102	0.51	
Zuschlag[214]	Hamburg	1914-49	Hospital records	111,217	1,137	1.02	
Mestwerdt[129]	Hamburg-Barmbek	1960-61	Inspection by obstetricians and pediatricians	3,202	76	2.37	
Pfau and Täger[154]	Heidelberg	1928-57	Univ. Obstetric Clinic	39,712	321	0.80	LB and SB, externally visible defects at birth.
Stein[189]	Kiel	1937-47	Hospital records	17,698	145	0.85	Quoted by Böök and Fraccaro[21]
Manzke and Falck[126]	Kiel	1948-61	Hospital records	27,080	522	1.92	Quoted by Sievers[179]
Rechenberger[166]	Leipzig	1926-31	Hospital records	21,420	143	0.67	Quoted by Sievers[179]
John[87]	Leipzig	1932-41	Hospital records	38,442	328	0.85	Quoted by Sievers[179]
Aresin and Somer[7]	Leipzig	1936-48	Maternity register	43,647	399	0.91	
Schlosser[171]	Ludwigshafen	1956-61		2,582	26	1.01	
Baucks[13]	Marburg	1936-60	Hospital records	24,489	450	1.83	Babies all over 600g.
Hegnauer[72]	München	1907-50	Hospital records	141,706	951	0.67	
Strohofer[193]	München	1912-31	Hospital records	67,063	333	0.44	Quoted by Sievers[179]
Klabanov and Hegenauer[93]	München	1919-47	Univ. Obstetric Clinic	1,430	58	4.05	
Oster[150]	Nuremberg	1939-53 / 1954-58		16,955 / 2,885	492 / 81	2.90 / 2.80	
Lewin and Fischer[115]	Offenbach/Main	1950-56	City Obstetric Clinic	4,182	51	1.22	
Niemetz[146]	Rostock	1926-35	Hospital records	7,187	97	1.35	Quoted by Sievers[179]
Lork[118]	Rostock	1935-49		17,397	209	1.20	
Kühne[103]	Rostock	1960-62	Univ. Obstetric Clinic	8,373	161	1.92	29.8% of cases lethal
Herrmann[74]	Stuttgart	1915-37		18,830	272	1.45	Quoted by Sievers[179]
Maurer[128]	Tübingen	1917-33		16,429	208	1.26	Quoted by Sievers[179]
Knörr[96]	Tübingen	1940-62	Hospital records	35,802	829	2.32	
Götz[62]	Würzburg	1941-58	Hospital records	25,185	645	2.56	
Cretius and Fuchs[38]	Würzburg	1941-61	Univ. Obstetric Clinic	28,894	757	2.62	All births after 28 weeks

Note: CM = Congenital malformation.   LB = live births   SB = stillbirths   NND = neonatal death   * signifies the figure has been calculated from the authors' data

TABLE IV
NORTH AMERICA

Authors	Locality	Period	Source of Statistics	No. of Births	Number Affected	Percentage Affected	Remarks
Le Vann[113] Le Vann[113] Le Vann[114]	Alberta Alberta Alberta	1959 1961 1962	Questionnaire survey	33,874 38,353 38,400	257 344 416	0.776 0.89 1.08	
Leonski[112]	Manitoba, Winnipeg	?	Nursery records	4,433	95	2.26	Major cases only
Greenhill[66]	Canada and U.S.A.	to 1937	Hospital records	369,597	3,474	0.94	Figures from 26 clinics
Yerushalmy et al[213]	Calif., San Francisco	1960-64	Intensive study	7,447	701	9.41	Single births only: white
Newton and McLean[145]	Connecticut	before 1947		15,421	130*	0.84	Quoted by Neel[143] Major cases only
Anon.[11]	Connecticut			16,080 1,953	798 63	4.94 3.19	White Quoted by Baird[11] Nonwhite
Kohl[98]	Connecticut	1957-59	Intensive study	23,840	596	2.50	Lethal 124 0.5% Consequential 260 1.1% Inconsequential 212 0.9%
Altemus and Ferguson[5]	District of Columbia	1952-62		79,842	4,655	5.83	Negro
Burge[24]	Illinois, Evanston	1940-49	Hospital records	12,000	289	2.42	110 major, 179 less severe.
Davis and Potter[40]	Illinois, Chicago	1941-55	Hospital records Special examination	53,847 5,000	242* 336	0.45 6.73	Lethal cases only, SB and LB, all CM included
Wacker[202]	Illinois, Chicago	1950-59	Hospital records	19,615	296	1.50	
Lucy[119]	Indiana	1942-47	Hospital records	11,881	195*	1.64	
Miller[131]	Kansas		Univ. Med. Center histories	4,095	66	1.61	
Frazier[57]	Maryland, Baltimore	1954-58	Birth certs. with addenda	71,032 49,095	477 389	0.68 0.79	White Nonwhite
Stevenson S.S. et al[192]	Massachusetts, Boston	1930-41	Hospital records	29,024	677	2.33	
Evans and Brown[51]	Michigan, Ann Arbor	1943-62	Hospital records	23,898	823	3.49	"Prolonged observation not possible, doubtless a number of cases not recorded"
Hautau[70]	Michigan	1958	Birth certs., official records	205,791	3,297	1.6	3101 SB
Kleinman et al[92]	Minnesota	1958	Public Health Nurse interviews	10,109	419	4.14	39.6% diagnosed at birth 60.4% in first year
Hartman and Kennedy[69]	Minnesota, Rochester			1,237	65	5.25	

Silberg et al[180]	Missouri	1953-64	Birth certificates	1,135,156	8,407	0.74	LB only
Segall et al[174]	New England	1952-61	Hospital records	87,184	2,070	2.37	LB and SB: P.M. results included
Javert and Stander[85]	New York City	1932-40	Hospital records	27,000	793	2.93	LB, SB, and NND
McIntosh et al[121]	New York City	1946-53	Hospital records	5,964	433	7.26	
Greenberg et al[65]	New York City	1947	Hospital questionnaire Child Health Stature exams	6,358	98	1.54	
Sesgin and Stark[175]	New York City	1949-58	Hospital records	27,087	511	1.85	Includes only most frequent CM in all viable neonates
Wallace et al[204]	New York City	1951	Birth certificates	162,755	1,501	0.92	
Shapiro et al[176]	New York City			5,984	280	4.67	
Shapiro et al[177]	New York City	1958-60	Health Insurance Plan Study	5,123	280	5.46	"Significant congenital anomalies"
Shapiro et al[176]	New York City	1952-55	Hospital charts, birth to seven days	30,398	640	1.99	
Conway and Wagner[35]	New York City	1952-62	Birth certificates	1,823,244	21,804	1.19	
Wallace et al[205]	New York City	1953	Birth certificates	161,499	1,438	0.89	"Significant anomalies making a difference to life and needing attention"
Erhardt and Nelson[50]	New York City	1958-59	Birth certificates	344 542	5,152	1.49	
De Porte and Parkhurst[44]	New York State	1940-42		273,604	5,283	1.93	
Gentry et al[58]	New York State	1948-55	Birth certificates	1,242,744	13,248	1.07	
Hendricks[73]	Ohio, Cleveland	1953	Birth certificates with addenda	210,727	1,560	0.74	LB
Osterud et al[151]	Oregon		Birth certificates	186,579	1,493	0.80	
Murphy[139]	Penna., Philadelphia	1929-33	Maternity register plus examinations	130,132	807	0.62	
Ivy[82]	Penna., Philadelphia	1951-55	Birth certificates	1,195,976	9,827	0.82	
Ivy[83]	Penna., Philadelphia	1956-60	Birth certificates	1,240,540	14,143	1.14	
Ivy[84]	Penna., Philadelphia	1961	Birth certificates	240,145	2,761	1.14	
Ingals and Kleinberg[81]	Penna., Philadelphia			131,000	1,179	0.90	Authors state there was underreporting
Wulf et al[211]	Vermont, Chittenden			1,775	238	13.40	12-year followup
Marden et al[127]	Wisconsin, Madison	1960-62	Direct examination	4,412	609 / 91	13.8 / 2.06	Minor / Major

Note: CM = Congenital malformation.   LB = live births   SB = stillbirths   NND = neonatal death   * signifies the figure has been calculated from the authors' data

TABLE V

OTHER COUNTRIES

Authors	Locality	Period	Source of Statistics	No. of Births	Number Affected	Percentage Affected	Remarks
Alpen[4]	Australia, South	1954-62	Hospital records	17,502	366	2.09	Not all SB and NND included
Farrer and Mackie[52]	Australia, Carringbah	1961	Special examination	1,835	225	12.33	
Pitt[157]	Australia, Melbourne	1955-57	Hospital records	22,364	400*	1.79	
Townsend[191]	Australia, Melbourne	1960-61	W.H.O. study	7,844 / 3,921	148 / 68	1.88 / 1.73	Royal Womens Hospital / Queen Victoria Hospital — Quoted from Stevenson, A.C., et al[191]
De Araujo[6]	Brazil, Ipiranga			19,293	1,486	7.70	SB and NND excluded 981 cases were minor
Delascio et al[191]	Brazil, São Paulo	1960-61	W.H.O. study	14,421	231	1.60	Quoted from Stevenson, A.C., et al[191]
Figueroa and Manterola[54]	Chile	1949-58	Hospital records	63,340	892	1.40	LB only
Avendano[191]	Chile, Santiago	1960-61	W.H.O. study	23,720	224	0.94	Quoted from Stevenson, A.C., et al[191]
Saenez et al[191]	Colombia, Bogotá	1960-61	W.H.O. study	18,812	315	1.67	Quoted from Stevenson, A.C., et al[191]
Chica[191]	Colombia, Medellin	1960-61	W.H.O. study	20,459	229	1.11	Quoted from Stevenson, A.C., et al[191]
Toppozada and Abul-Einen[191]	Egypt, Alexandria	1960-61	W.H.O. study	9,598	111	1.15	Quoted from Stevenson, A.C., et al[191]
Karim et al[90]	Egypt, Cairo	1963-64	CM Investigation Center	2,093	46	2.19	
Boldt[18]	Ethiopia, Addis Ababa	Not stated	Not stated	7,500	84	1.12	
Bierman et al[16]	Hawaii, Kauai	1954-56	Special examination	1,963	149*	7.59	
Emerson[49]	Hong Kong	1960-61	Hospital records	1,030	28	2.71	European women only
Chun and Kan[191]	Hong Kong	1960-61	W.H.O. study	9,872	114	1.15	Quoted from Stevenson, A.C., et al[191]
Ghosh and Bali[59]	India	1959-62	Hospital records	4,353	147	3.37	276 SB included
Kolah, et al[99]	India, Bombay	1960-62-63	Hospital records	29,553	413	1.04	CM incidence LB 1.02 SB 9.44 and NND 9.24
Purandare[191]	India, Bombay	1960-61	W.H.O. study	39,498	340	0.86	Quoted from Stevenson, A.C., et al[191]
Mitra[191]	India, Calcutta	1960-61	W.H.O. study	19,191	59	0.30	
Nair and Mathai[141]	India, Calicut	2 years	Hospital records	3,721	50*	1.34	
Yassin et al[212]	Iraq, Mosul	1964	CM Investigation Center	296	22	7.43	4 months records only
Halevi[68]	Israel	1959-60	Notifications by hospitals and a few doctors	89,580 / 1,213	1,111 / 84	1.24 / 6.92	LB / SB

			Physical examination soon after birth				
Neel[143]	Japan, Hiroshima Kure, Nagasaki	1948-54	Physical examination soon after birth	64,569	659*	1.02	Major defects
Tabuchi et al[194]	Japan, Hiroshima	1961-62	Immediate inspection in hospital	1,344	{ 10 } 13	0.74 0.97	Major Further 37 NND Minor
Miyamoto[134]	Japan, Iwate Univ. Hosp.	1960-63	Hospital examination	1,923	28	1.45	
Kaminura[89]	Japan, Niigata	1953-63	Hospital and obstetric questionnaire	48,015	413	0.86	
Mitani[133]	Japan, Tokyo	1922-52	Hospital records	80,435	729	0.91	Quoted by Böök and Fraccaro[21]
Khan, A. A.[91]	Kenya, Nairobi	1963-64	Immediate inspection in hospital	3,016	54	1.79	Major cases only: 6 months recording
Abou-Daoud[1]	Lebanon, Beirut	1953-64	University Clinic	12,146	139*	1.15	
Llewellyn Jones[191]	Malaysia, Kuala Lumpur	1960-61	W.H.O. study	15,937	167	1.05	Quoted from Stevenson, A.C., et al[191]
Lean[191]	Malaysia, Singapore	1960-61	W.H.O. study	39,683	343	0.76	Quoted from Stevenson, A.C., et al[191]
Wong Hock Boon[209]	Malaysia, Singapore	1961-63	Hospital records	128,223	187*	0.14	
Equiluz and Urrusti[191]	Mexico City	1960-61	W.H.O. study	24,700	364	1.47	Quoted from Stevenson, A.C., et al[191]
Viezca and Ayala[191]	Mexico City	1960-61	W.H.O. study	14,083	155	1.10	Quoted from Stevenson, A.C., et al[191]
Bissot et al[191]	Panama City	1960-61	W.H.O. study	15,852	329	2.07	Quoted from Stevenson, A.C., et al[191]
Landazuri Fuentes[106]	Peru, Lima		Hospital records	40,158	432*	0.99	
Jongco et al[191]	Philippines	1960-61	W.H.O. study	29,669	252	0.85	Quoted from Stevenson, A.C., et al[191]
Jongco et al[88]	Philippines		Hospital records	46,025	258*	0.56	
Vasquez et al[191]	Philippines	1961-63	Hospital records	26,663	369	1.28	
Craig[191]	S. Africa, Cape Town	1960-61	W.H.O. study	3,051	26	0.85	Quoted from Stevenson, A.C., et al[191]
Horner and Lanzkowsky[79]	S. Africa, Cape Town	no date	Exam. by pediatric registrar	{ 2,807 } 3,695	100* 83*	3.57 2.25	White 54 SB 1.92% Colored 145 SB 3.92%
Wallace[203]	S. Africa, Durban	1963-65	Hospital records	5,000	82	1.64	Consecutive deliveries, Europeans
Samson[191]	S. Africa, Johannesburg	1960-61	W.H.O. study	11,176	252	2.25	Quoted from Stevenson, A.C., et al[191]
Glietenberg[40]	S. Africa, Johannesburg	1961-65	Hospital observation	22,672	585	2.57	Consecutive deliveries
Geldenhuys[191]	S. Africa, Pretoria	1960-61	W.H.O. study	10,025	129	1.28	Quoted from Stevenson, A.C., et al[191]
Thom[196]	S. Africa, Pretoria	1964	Hospital records	4,524	45*	0.99	Karl Bremer Hospital
Ping Wen Wei et al[191]	Taiwan		Hospital records	14,834	129	0.87	Quoted from Stevenson, A.C., et al[191]
Simpkiss and Lowe[181]	Zambia, Kampala	1956-57	Hospital observation	2,068	122	0.85	Major defects; 114 SB, Africans

Note: CM = Congenital malformation.   LB = live births   SB = stillbirths   NND = neonatal death   * signifies the figure has been calculated from the authors' data

EPIDEMIOLOGIC ASPECTS OF THE PROBLEM OF CONGENITAL MALFORMATIONS

TABLE VI

SUMMARY

Region	No. of Reports	Births	Cases of Malformations	Percentage of Malformations
I Data based on official records, birth certificates, retrospective questionnaires				
Belgium	1	740,956	4,995	0.67
Italy	1	2,660,990	4,120	0.15
U.S.A. and Canada	17	8,784,188	92,604	1.05
Totals	19	12,186,134	101,719	0.83
II Hospital and Clinic Records				
Britain and Eire	17	640,413	7,593	1.18
Europe (excluding Germany)	54	2,560,937	35,103	1.37
Germany	43	2,154,964	21,046	0.97
U.S.A. and Canada	18	876,835	17,210	1.95
Other Countries	22	652,462	6,463	0.99
Totals	154	6,885,611	87,415	1.26
III W.H.O. Investigations				
	24	416,695	5,290	1.27
IV More Intensive Examinations				
Britain	10	170,224	4,914	2.88
Europe (excluding Germany)	10	78,610	2,334	2.96
Germany	2	8,516	188	2.20
U.S.A.	10	144,769	12,690	8.76
Other Countries	9	121,264	3,467	2.85
Totals	41	523,383	23,593	4.50
V Regional Totals				
Britain and Eire	28	838,728	13,051	1.55
Europe (excluding Germany)	70	6,098,585	47,442	0.77
Germany	45	2,154,964	21,234	0.98
U.S.A. and Canada	45	9,805,792	122,504	1.24
Other Countries	50	1,105,238	13,786	1.24
Totals	238	20,011,823	218,017	1.08

REFERENCES*

1. Abou-Daoud, K. T.: Congenital malformations observed in 12,146 births at the American Hospital of Beirut. *J. méd. liban.* **19**:113-121, 1966.

2. Aicardi, G.; Rugati, S. and Acinelli, G.: [Congenital malformations seen in the Obstetric and Gynecological Clinic of Sassari, 1936 to 1965. Note 1. Statistical considerations.] *Minerva pediat.* **18**:73-79, 1966.

3. Alison, F.: [Enquiry on embryopathies and diseases of pregnancy.] *Rev. Hyg. Méd. soc.* **7**:97-105, 1959

4. Alpen, H. U. H. von: Congenital abnormalities. A survey of abnormalities encountered at the Q.E.M.H. from opening in 1954 to December, 1962. *S. Austral. Clin.* **1**:167-170, 1965.

5. Altemus, L. A. and Ferguson, A. D.: Comparative incidence of birth defects in negro and white children. *Pediatrics* **36**: 56-61, 1965.

6. Araujo, J. de: [Congenital malformations.] *Pediat. prát. (S. Paulo)* **34**:131-138, 1963.

7. Aresin, N. and Somer, K. H.: [Malformations and environmental factors.] *Zbl. Gynäk.* **72**:1329-1336, 1950.

8. Avanzini, P. and Girando, G.: [Incidence of congenital malformations consequent on pandemic influenza.] *Minerva pediat.* **12**:120, 1960.

9. Avezzu, G. and Vinci, G. W.: [Fetal malformations and conditions possibly due to various teratogenic causes.] *Ann. Ostet. Ginec.* **88**:49-72, 1960.

10. Azer, V.: [Contribution to the study of fetal and congenital malformations.] Thesis, Lyons 1944, quoted by Lamy *et al.*

_____

* Titles in brackets have been translated

W. P. Kennedy, Ph.D.

11. Baird, Sir Dugald: Variations in fertility associated with changes in health status. *J. chron. Dis.* **18**:1109-1124, 1965.

12. Baron, F.; Michiels, Y. and Rochas, J. E.: [Influenza and fetal malformations, statistical considerations.] *Gynéc. et Obstét.* **59**:271-276, 1960.

13. Baucks, K. D.: [Child malformations.] *Geburtsh. u. Frauenheilk.* **22**:144-155, 1962.

14. Beolchini, P. E.: [Statistical and genetic research on congenital malformations. II. The frequency of malformations seen at the Milan Maternity Hospital in 85,976 babies between 1942 and 1946.] *Acta Genet. med. (Roma)* **13**:203-215, 1964.

15. Biering-Sørensen, K.: Congenital malformations and antihistamine drugs. *Bull. Soc. roy. belge Gynéc. Obstét.* **33**:87-93, 1963.

16. Bierman, S. M.; Siegel, E.; French. F. E. and Simonian, K.: Analysis of the outcome of all pregnancies in a community. *Amer. J. Obstet. Gynec.* **91**:37-45, 1965.

17. Bjøro, K. and Iversen, S.: [Survey of congenital malformations from an obstetric point of view.] *T. norske Laegeforen.* **79**:1308-1312, 1959.

18. Boldt, H. D.: Congenital malformations in Ethiopia. *Ethiopian Med. J.* **4**:43-45, 1965.

19. Bologna, V.: [Congenital malformations of the fetus. Report of 299 cases.] *Clin. ostet. ginec.* **56**:268-291, 1955.

20. Böök, J.A.: The incidence of congenital diseases and defects in a South Swedish population. *Acta genet. (Basel)* **2**:289-311, 1951.

21. Böök, J.A. and Fraccaro, M.: Research on congenital malformations. *Neo-Natal Studies.* **5**:39-54, 1956.

22. Bovev Velichkova; Markova and Iordanav: [Incidence, types and etiology of congenital malformations in children.] *Sũvr. Med.* **14**:8-17, 1963.

23. Büchi, E. C.: *Bull. Schweiz. Ges. Anthrop. Ethnol.* **26**:11, 1950, quoted by Böök and Fraccaro.

24. Burge, E. S.: Relationship of threatened abortion to fetal abnormalities. *Amer. J. Obstet. Gynec.* **61**:615-621, 1951.

25. Buurman, G.; Langendörfer, G.; Noack, J. and Witt, H. J.: [Occurrence of congenital abnormalities in the last 55 years.] *Zbl. Gynäk.* **80**:1432-1442, 1958.

26. Calvani, M.: [Statistical data on 359 cases of congenital malformations in newborn babes.] *Infanzia* **11**:520-524, 1961.

27. Campli, C. and Pedone, G.: [Review of the malformations in Foggia Maternity Hospital.] *Minerva ginec.* **11**:99-103, 1962.

28. Carollo, F.; Fiorino, S. and Candela, G.: [Congenital malformations seen in the Obstetric and Gynecological Clinic of Palermo University. Clinical and statistical study.] *Sicilia sanit.* **11-12**:1-48, 1964.

29. Carter, C. O.: Maternal states in relation to congenital malformations. *J. Obstet. Gynaec. Brit. Emp.* **57**:897-911, 1950.

30. Charles, E.: Statistical utilization of maternity and child welfare records. *Brit. J. prev. soc. Med.* **5**:41-61, 1951.

31. Cocozza, G. and Tiso, E.: [Clinico-statistical contribution on embryopathic malformations.] *Pediatria (Napoli)* **63**:822-844, 1955.

32. Coffey, V. P. and Jessop, W. J. E.: Congenital abnormalities. *Irish J. med. Sci.* 30-48, 1955.

33. Coffey, V. P. and Quinn, P.: Domiciliary deliveries in Dublin. *J. Irish med. Ass.* **59**:44-54, 1966.

34. Colucci, G. and Tosolini, G. C.: [Fetal malformations in the Obstetrical and Gynecological Department of the Civil Hospital of Udine.] *Attual. Ostet. Ginec.* **9**:1-22, 1963.

35. Conway, H. and Wagner, K. J.: Congenital abnormalities reported on birth certificates in New York City 1952-1962. *N. Y. St. J. Med.* **65**:1087-1090, 1965.

36. Corner, B. D.: Congenital anomalies, clinical considerations. *Med. J. S.-W.* **77**:46-52, 1962.

37. Craig, W. S.: Care of the newly born infant. 3rd edn., Livingston, Edinburgh, 1965.

38. Cretius, K. and Fuchs. R.: [Report on the unusual increase in micromelia and amelia in 1961 in the Obstetric Clinic, Würzburg University.] *Med. Klin.* **57**:923-927, 1962.

39. Da Rugna, D.: [Frequency of severe congenital malformations in the Women's Hospital, Basel.] Medikamentöse Pathogenese fetale Missbildungen. Symposium in Liestal, 29/30 March, 1963. 116-123. Karger, Basel, 1964.

40. Davis, M. E. and Potter, E. L.: Congenital malformations and obstetrics. *Pediatrics* **19**:719-724, 1957.

41. Dean. N. M. B.: in press.

42. Dedukh. L. G. and Lankovits, A. V.: [Some data on developmental defects in the newborn.] *Vop. Okhrany Materin. Dets.* **10**:65-68, 1965.

43. Dellepiane, G. and Colla, G.: [On the etiopathogenesis of congenital dysmelias.] *Minerva ginec.* **14**:1029-1040, 1962.

44. De Porte, J. V. and Parkhurst, E.: Congenital malformations and birth injuries among children born in N.Y. State 1940-1942. *N. Y. St. J. Med.* **45**:1097-1100, 1945.

45. Derom, R.: [New statistics on the frequency of certain malformations in Belgium.] *Bull. Soc. roy. belge Gynéc. Obstét.* **33**:143-148, 1963.

46. Eichmann, E. and Gesenius, H.: [The increase in congenital malformations in Berlin and environs after the war.] *Arch. Gynäk.* **181**:168-184, 1952.

47. Elsie Inglis Hospital, Edinburgh, Annual Report 1948-1949.

48. Elsner-Mackay, P.: [Exogenous malformations.] *Wien. klin. Wschr.* **76**:181-189, 1964.

49. Emerson, R. G.: Obstetric practice in the tropics. *Trans. roy. Soc. trop. Med. Hyg.* **58**:589-592, 1965.

50. Erhardt, C. L. and Nelson, F. G.: Reported congenital malformations in New York City 1958-1959. *Amer. J. publ. Hlth* **54**:1489-1506, 1964.

51. Evans. T. N. and Brown, G. C.: Congenital anomalies and virus infections. *Amer. J. Obstet. Gynec.* **87**:749-761, 1963.

52. Farrer, J. F. and Mackie, I. J.: Survey of possible causes of congenital malformations. *Med. J. Aust.* **ii**:702-704, 1964.

53. Ferrario, E. and Fortuna, A.: [Clinical and statistical data on fetal malformations seen in the Novaro Commune Maternity Hospital in the last twenty years.] *Minerva ginec.* **2**:248-257, 1950.

54. Figueroa, M. J. and Manterola, A. A.: [Some considerations on malformations seen in 63,340 viable children in 10 years in the Barros Luco Hospital.] *Pediatria (Santiago)* **3**:331-334, 1960.

55. Fink, A.: [Malformations and their correlation with the mother's age.] *Z. Geburtsh. Gynäk.* **147**:214-226, 1956.

56. Fiuza Perez, L.: [Genetic and hereditary factors in the development of congenital malformations. Study of 690 cases.] *Acta pediát. esp.* **16**:367-382, 1958.

57. Frazier, T. M.: A note on race specific congenital malformation rates. *Amer. J. Obstet. Gynec.* **80**:184-185, 1960.

58. Gentry, J. T.; Parkhurst, E. and Bulin, E. V., Jr.: Epidemiological study of congenital malformations in New York State. *Amer. J. publ. Hlth* **49**:497-513, 1959.

59. Ghosh, S. and Bali, L.: Congenital malformations in the newborn. *Indian J. Child Hlth* 448-452, July, 1963.

60. Glietenberg, H.: Congenital malformations from the obstetricians point of view. *S. Afr. med. J.* 161-164, February 18, 1967.

61. Gonzales-Coviella, L.: [Incidence of congenital malformations in 20,221 newborn babes.] *Rev. esp. Pediat.* **21**:767-776, 1965.

62. Götz, G.: [The problem of malformations. Report on 645 cases.] *Med. Klin.* **55**:577-583, 1960.

63. Greco, E.; Landi, E. and Rubino, S.: [The high incidence of congenital malformations in Gorgano.] *Clin. pediat. (Bologna)* **44**:96-126, 1962.

64. Green, C. R.: The incidence of human maldevelopment. *Amer. J. Dis. Child.* **105**:301-312, 1963.

65. Greenberg, M.; Yankauer, A.; Krugman, S.; Osborn, J. J.; Ward, R. S. and Dancis, J.: The effect of smallpox vaccination during pregnancy on the incidence of congenital malformation. *Pediatrics* **3**:456-467, 1949.

66. Greenhill, J. P.: Increased incidence of fetal abnormalities in cases of placenta previa. *Amer. J. Obstet. Gynec.* **37**:624-633, 1939.

67. Griffin, G. V. and Sorrie, G. S.: Congenital abnormalities in Reading 1958-1963. *Med. Offr* **112**:197-198, 1964.

68. Halevi, H. S.: Congenital malformations in Israel. *Brit. J. prev. soc. Med.* **21**:66-77, 1967.

69. Hartman, E. E. and Kennedy, R. L. J.: Illness in the first trimester, its lack of significance in relation to congenital anomaly of prematurity and still birth. *J. Pediat.* **38**:306-309, 1951.

70. Hautau, E. R.: Congenital malformations in infants born to Michigan residents in 1958. *J. Mich. med. Soc.* **59**:1833-1836, 1960.

71. Hedberg, E.; Holmdahl, L. K.; Pehrson, S. and Zackrisson, U.: On the relationship between maternal conditions during pregnancy and congenital malformations. Preliminary report. *Acta paediat.* **52**:353-360, 1963.

72. Hegnauer, H.: [Frequency of malformations and age of mother.] *Geburtsh. u. Frauenheilk.* **11**:77-92, 1951.

73. Hendricks, C. H.: Congenital malformations. Analysis of 1953 Ohio records. *Obstet. and Gynec.* **6**:592-598, 1955.

74. Hermann, F.: Inaugural Dissertation. Tübingen, 1939, quoted by Sievers.

75. Heyne, D.: [Initial statistical elements relative to congenital malformations in Belgium.] *Arch. belges Méd. soc.* **21**:186-198, 1963.

76. Hirvensalo, M. and Hjelt, L.: [Incidence of congenital malformations in a Finnish Maternity Hospital.] *Duodecim (Helsinki)* **79**:798-803, 1963.

77. Hohlbein, R.: [Malformation frequency in Dresden.] *Zbl. Gynäk.* **81**:719-731, 1959.

78. Horn, B., Csordas, T.; Dömötöri, J. and Kiszel, J.: [Developmental anomalies.] *Zbl. Gynäk.* **87**:1180-1189, 1965.

79. Horner, R. and Lanzkowsky, P.: Incidence of congenital abnormalities in Cape Town. *S. Afr. med. J.* **40**:171, 1966.

80. Houštek, J.; Kucera, J. and Kotzmanova, J.: [Incidence of congenital malformations in the Stredocesky Kraj.] *Čs. Pediat.* **17**:458-468, 1962.

81. Ingals, T. H. and Kleinberg, M. A.: Congenital malformations. Clinical and community considerations. *Amer. J. med. Sci.* **249**:316-344, 1965.

82. Ivy, R. H.: Congenital anomalies as recorded on birth certificates in the Division of Vital Statistics of the Pennsylvania Department of Health for the period 1951-1955 inclusive. *Plast. reconstr. Surg.* **20**:400-411, 1957.

83. Ivy, R. H.: The influence of race on the incidence of certain congenital anomalies. *Plast. reconstr. Surg.* **30**:581-585, 1962.

84. Ivy, R. H.: Congenital anomalies as recorded on birth certificates in the Division of Vital Statistics of the Pennsylvania Department of Health for 1956-1960. *Plast. reconstr. Surg.* **20**:361-367, 1963.

85. Javert, C. T. and Stander, H. J.: Plasma vitamin C and prothrombin concentrations in pregnancy and in threatened and spontaneous abortions. *Surg. Gynec. Obstet.* **76**:115-122, 1943.

86. Jaworska, M.: [Statistical analysis of congenital defects.] *Pol. Tyg. lek.* **17**:209-212, 1962.

87. John, J.: Inaugural Dissertation. Leipzig, 1942, quoted by Sievers.

88. Jongco, A. P.; Carlos, F. C. and Fernandez, E. V.: Congenital anomalies in Filipinos. *J. Philipp. med. Ass.* **41**:57-60, 1965.

89. Kaminura, K.: [Incidence of gross malformations at birth surveyed by the mail questionnaire method.] *Jap. J. Pub. Hlth.* **12**:135-140, 1965.

90. Karim, M. *et al*: Congenital deformities in the U. A. R. and Iraq. *J. Iraqui med. Prof.* **13**:57-61, 1965.

91. Khan, A. A.: Congenital malformations in African neonates in Nairobi. *J. trop. Med. Hyg.* **68**:272-274, 1965.

92. Kleinman, H.; Prince, J. T.; Mathey, W. E.; Rosenfeld, A. B.; Bearman, J. E. and Syverton, J. T.: Echo 9 virus infection and congenital abnormalities. A negative report. *Pediatrics* **29**:261-269, 1962.

93. Klebanov, D. and Hegenauer, H.: [The question of secondary germinative ovarian insufficiency.] *Zbl. Gynäk.* **73**:50-53, 1951.

94. Klemetti, A.: Relationship of selected environmental factors to pregnancy outcome and congenital malformations. Academic Dissertation, pp. 70, Helsinki, 1966. (and as Supplement 26 to *Ann. Paediat. Fenn* 26, 1966).

95. Klosterkötter, W.: Inaugural Dissertation. Cologne, 1943, quoted by Sievers.

96. Knörr, K.: [The incidence of congenital anomalies considered in relation to their observation and recording.] *Geburtsh. u. Frauenheilk.* **22**:1291-1293, 1962.

97. Kobielowa, Z.; Kucharska, A. and Ostrowski, A.: [Statistical analysis of congenital defects.] *Pol. Tyg. lek.* **17**:213-216, 1962.

98. Kohl, S. K.: Community obstetrical study. Hartford County, Connecticut 1960, quoted by Baird.

99. Kolah, P. J.; Master, P. A. and Sanghvi, L. D.: Congenital malformations and perinatal mortality in Bombay. *Amer. J. Obstet. Gynec.* **97**:400-406, 1967.

100. Kolbas, V.: [Congenital defects among infants in a region of Croatia.] *Liječn. Vjesn.* **86**:675-682, 1964.

101. Kovacs, I. and Makay, L.: [Problems of the etiology of abnormalities.] *Zbl. Gynäk.* **82**:1335-1341, 1960.

102. Kucera, J.: Personal communication, 1967.

103. Kühne, D.: [Anamnestic investigation of mothers of malformed babes at Rostock University Clinic for Women, 1960-1962.] *Zbl. Gynäk.* **85**:1475-1480, 1963.

104. Kühnelt, H. J. and Rotter-Pool, P.: [Malformations in the Women's Clinic of Berlin University in the light of embryopathy.] *Zbl. Gynäk.* **77**:893-400, 1955.

105. Lamy, M. and Frezal, J.: The frequency of congenital malformations. First International Conference on Congenital Malformations. 1960. 34-44. Lippincott, Philadelphia.

106. Landazuri Fuentes, H.: [Congenital anomalies, study of 40.000 births in Obrero Hospital, Lima.] *Acad. peru. Cirug.* **17**:119-125, 1964.

107. Landsman, J. B.; Grist, N. R. and Ross, C. A. C.: Echo 9 virus and congenital malformations. *Brit. J. prev. soc. Med.* **18**:152-156, 1964.

108. Landtman, B.: On the relationship between maternal conditions during pregnancy and congenital malformations. *Arch. Dis. Childh.* **23**:237-240, 1948.

109. Leck, I.: Examination of the incidence of malformations for evidence of drug teratogenesis. *Brit. J. prev. soc. Med.* **18**:196-201, 1964.

110. Leck, I. and Millar, E. L. M.: Short term changes in the incidence of malformations. *Brit. J. prev. soc. Med.* **17**:1-12, 1963.

111. Leone, A.: [Malnutrition of the mother as a cause of malformation of the child.] *Ann. ital. Pediat.* **15**:143-160, 1962.

112. Leonski, E. F.: A consideration of the incidence of common major congenital malformations in a Winnipeg Nursery. *Manitoba med. Rev.* **42**:602-604, 1962.

113. Le Vann, L. J.: Congenital abnormalities in children born in Alberta during 1961: a survey and a hypothesis. *Canad. med. Ass. J.* **89**:120-126, 1963.

114. Le Vann, L. J.: Congenital abnormalities in children born in Alberta during 1962. A further communication. *Alberta med. Bull.* 1-10, August, 1965.

115. Lewin, H. and Fischer, G.: [Report on congenital malformations.] *Zbl. Gynäk.* **80**:413-429, 1958.

116. Lindemann, G.: [Incidence of malformation in Halle.] *Zbl. Gynäk.* **74**:876, 1962.

117. Livadiotti, M.; Formato, R. and La Femina, R.: [Clinico-statistical reports on congenital malformations in St. Camillo de Lellis Maternity Hospital, Rome, 1949-1962.] *Infanzia* **14**:5-25, 1964.

118. Lork, E. C.: [Incidence of malformations in Rostock.] *Zbl. Gynäk.* **74**:877, 1952.

119. Lucy, R. E.: Study of congenital malformations. *J.-Lancet* **69**:80-81, 1949.

120. McDonald, A. D.: Maternal health and congenital defect. *New Engl. J. Med.* **258**:767-775, 1958.

121. McIntosh, R.; Merritt, K. I.; Richards, M. R.; Samuels, M. H. and Bellows, M. T.: Incidence of congenital malformations, a study of 5,964 pregnancies. *Pediatrics* **14**:505-522, 1954.

122. McKeown, T. and Record, R. G.: Malformations in a population observed for five years after birth. Ciba Symposium on Congenital Malformations, London. 2-16, 1960.

123. MacMahon, B.; Pugh, T. F. and Ipsen, J.: Epidemiological methods. London, 1960.

124. Maggiore, L.: [Statistics of human congenital malformations in Italy 1956-1958.] *Acta Genet. med. (Roma)* **12**:276-290, 1960.

125. Malpas, P.: The incidence of human malformations and the significance of change in the maternal environment in their causation. *J. Obstet. Gynaec. Brit. Emp.* **44**:434-454, 1937.

126. Manzke, H. and Falck, H. R.: [Malformations in the birth record of Kiel University Obstetric Clinic 1948-1961.] *Geburtsh. u. Frauenheilk.* **23**:1088-1098, 1963.

127. Marden, P. M.; Smith, D. W. and McDonald, M. J.: Congenital anomalies in the newborn, including minor variations. *J. Pediat.* **64**:357-371, 1964.

128. Maurer, E.: Inaugural Dissertation, Tübingen, 1935, quoted by Sievers.

129. Mestwerdt, G.: [Frequency of malformations in Hamburg Barmbeck.] *Geburtsh. u. Frauenheilk.* **23**:196-197, 1963.

130. Mey, R.: [Hyperemesis gravidarum as a possible exogenous cause for congenital malformations.] *Zbl. Gynäk.* **80**:1785-1791, 1955.

131. Miller, H. C.: Scope and incidence of congenital malformations. *Pediatrics* **5**:320-324, 1950.

132. Mischel: [Frequency of malformations in Altona Obstetric Clinic.] *Geburtsh. u. Frauenheilk.* **23**:196, 1963.

133. Mitani, S.: Malformations of the newborn and fetus. International Congress Gynecology and Obstetrics. S. A. Sandoz, Basel, 1954.

134. Miyamoto, K.: [Congenital malformations: 4 year study.] *J. Jap. obstet. gynaec. Soc.* **16**:531-535, 1964.

135. Morandi, E. and Marchesoni, M.: Incidence of congenital malformations following meclizine therapy in the first three months of pregnancy. *Bull. Soc. roy. belge Gynéc. Obstét.* **33**:139-142, 1963.

136. Morra, C. and Cremona, G. F.: [Problems connected with fetal malformations. Incidence and clinical aspects of fetal malformations observed at the S. Anna Maternity Hospital in Turin.] *Minerva ginec.* **15**:779-783, 1963.

137. Mosing, K.: [An unusual case of ectromelia and developmental defects of newborn infants.] *Pol. Tyg. lek.* **19**:227-230, 1962.

138. Moss, B. J. L.: Congenital abnormalities in Leicester, 1953-1962. *Med. Offr* 79-82, 31 July, 1964.

139. Murphy, D. P.: Congenital defects. Incidence among siblings of first congenitally malformed children in 275 families. *J. Amer. med. Ass.* **106**:457-458, 1936.

140. Nagy, T.; Bazso, J. and Lampe, L.: [Frequency of malformations in the clinical records of our hospital.] *Zbl. Gynäk.* **83**:866-880, 1961.

141. Nair, N. S. and Mathai, N. M.: Congenital malformations in the newborn at Calicut. A preliminary report. *Antiseptic* **61**:823-829, 1964.

142. Naujoks, H.: [Occurrence and treatment of malformations and birth injuries in the newborn.] *Arch. Gynäk.* **166**:445-455, 1938.

143. Neel, J. W.: A study of major congenital defects in Japanese infants. *Amer. J. hum. Genet.* **10**:398-445, 1958.

144. Nelson, A. M.: in press.

145. Newton, L. and McLean, T.: Microcephaly in three successive pregnancies. *Conn. med. J.* **11**:617-619, 1947.

146. Niemetz, K.: Inaugural Dissertation. Rostock, 1938, quoted by Sievers.

147. Nobili, F.: [External causes of congenital malformations.] *Minerva ginec.* **15**:1137-1151, 1963.

148. Nowak, J.: [Frequency of congenital malformations after the war years, 1945-1949.] *Zbl. Gynäk.* **72**:1313-1328, 1950.

149. Ockel, E. and Klemm, P.G.: [Epidemiological study of the malformation problem.] *Santé publ. (Buc.)* **7**:413-431, 1965.

150. Oster, H.: [Incidence of malformations and anlage disorders in newborn infants.] *Kinderärztl. Prax.* **27**:28-32, 1959.

151. Osterud, H. T. and Menashe, V. D.: The congenitally malformed. I. The problem. *Northw. Med. (Seattle)* **64**:337-341, 1965.

152. Pedersen, L. M.; Tygstrup, I. and Pedersen, J.: Congenital malformations and maternal diabetes. *Lancet* i:1124-1126, 1964.

153. Pereyma, K.: Inaugural Dissertation. Erlangen, 1950, quoted by Sievers.

154. Pfau, P. and Täger, F.: [Statistical observations on the increase of congenital malformations in the Obstetric Clinic, Heidelberg University, 1927-1957.] *Z. Geburtsh. Gynäk.* **158**:229-236, 1962.

155. Pfiffer, L.: Inaugural Dissertation. Basel, 1935, quoted by Sievers.

156. Piccioni, V.: [Deficiencies of maternal nutrition and congenital fetal malformations.] *Clin. ostet. ginec.* **57**:24-37, 1955.

157. Pitt, D. B.: Study of congenital malformations. *Aust. N. Z. J. Obstet. Gynaec.* **2**:23-27, 1962.

158. Pleydell, M. J.: Ancephaly and other congenital abnormalities. An epidemiological study in Northamptonshire. *Brit. med. J.* **1**:309-314, 1960.

159. Pomerants, S. A. and Chukanina, L. K.: [Congenital defects in development.] *Med. Zh. Uzbek.* **9**:53-56, 1966.

160. Poole, T. R.: Congenital malformations in West Virginia. *W. Va. med. J.* **56**:16-21, 1960.

161. Popa, S. and Iliescu, A.: [Some factors producing congenital malformations.] *Rev. med.-chir. (Jassy)* **70**:607-614, 1966.

162. Präger, E.: Inaugural Dissertation. Berlin, 1940, quoted by Sievers.

163. Prediger, F.: [Contribution to the question of the increase of congenital malformations.] *Zbl. Gynäk.* **83ii**:1053-1060, 1961.

164. Radanov, D.; Stojanov, S. and Sachariev, B.: [Incidence and cause of malformations in the newborn.] *Dtsch. Gesundh.-Wes.* **19**:392-395, 1964.

165. Ravina, J.; Daunay, J. J. and Benamour, P.: [One hundred and fifty-two malformations: their relative frequency at certain times of the year.] *Bull. Féd. Soc. Gynéc. Obstét. franç.* **6**:91-121, 1954.

166. Rechenberger, H. G.: Inaugural Dissertation. Leipzig, 1945, quoted by Sievers.

167. Reiffenstuhl, G.: [Malformations of the newborn in Graz University Maternity Clinic 1946-1961.] *Zbl. Gynäk.* **86**:889-895, 1964.

168. Roszkowski, I. and Kietlinska, Z.: Etiology of congenital malformations in the newborn. A clinical study. *Obstet. and Gynec.* **23**:893-897, 1964.

169. Saxen, L. and Härö, S.: [Congenital malformations of newborn infants in Finland, 1957-1962.] *Duodecim (Helsinki)* **80**:257-263, 1964.

170. Schenk, H.: [Malformations in the years 1938-1941 in the Womens Clinic of Berlin University.] *Zbl. Gynäk.* **46**:2078, 1942.

171. Schlosser, G. A.: [On the problem of the frequency of malformations.] *Med. Klin.* **57**:1616-1621, 1962.

172. Schnellerova, M.; Nováková, M. and Dufková, V.: [Incidence of congenital defects in the Neonatal Department of the University Hospital in Brno in 1957-1961.] *Čs. Pediat.* **19**:193-197, 1964.

173. Schubert, E. V.: [The inadequacy of malformation statistics from maternity hospitals.] *Geburtsh. u. Frauenheilk.* **19**:475-490, 1959.

174. Segall, A.; MacMahon, B. and Hannigani, I.: Congenital malformations and background radiation in Northern New England. *J. chron. Dis.* **17**:915-932, 1964.

175. Sesgin, M. Z. and Stark, R. B.: The incidence of congenital defects. *Plast. reconstr. Surg.* **27**:261-267, 1961.

176. Shapiro, R. N.; Eddy, W.; Fitzgibbon, J. and O'Brien, G.: Incidence of congenital anomalies discovered in the neonatal period. *Amer. J. Surg.* **96**:396-400, 1958.

177. Shapiro, S.; Ross, L. J. and Levine, H. S.: Relationship of selected prenatal factors to pregnancy outcome and congenital anomalies. *Amer. J. publ. Hlth* **55**:268-282, 1965.

178. Sheldon, W. H.: Varieties of delinquent youth. Harper, N.Y. 1949.

179. Sievers, G.: [Problem of the frequency of congenital malformations.] *Med. Klin.* **60**:1761-1768, 1965.

180. Silberg, S. L.; Marienfield, C. J.; Wright, H. and Arnold, R. C.: Surveillance of congenital anomalies in Missouri 1953-1964. *Arch. environm. Hlth* **13**:641-644, 1966.

181. Simpkiss, M. and Lowe, A.: Congenital abnormalities in the African newborn. *Arch. Dis. Childh.* **36**:404-406, 1961.

182. Simpson Maternity Hospital, Edinburgh, Annual Reports, 1938-1948; 1955-1963.

183. Slater, B. C.; Watson, G. I. and McDonald, J. C.: Seasonal variations in congenital abnormalities. *Brit. J. prev. soc. Med.* **18**:1-7, 1964.

184. Smithells, R. W.: The Liverpool congenital abnormalities registry. *Devel. Med. Child Neurol.* **4**:320-324, 1962.

185. Soergel, W.: [The increase of deformities of limb and ear since 1960 with reference to exogenous factors.] *Geburtsh. u. Frauenheilk.* **22**:1473-1481, 1962.

186. Spoto, P.: [Clinical and statistical data on fetal malformations.] *Lattante* **18**:338, 1947.

187. Stähler, F.: [Geographical differences in frequency of malformations in children.] *Geburtsh. u. Frauenheilk.* **22**:1288-1291, 1962.

188. Stark, A. M.: A report of two cases of iniencephalus. *J. Obstet. Gynaec. Brit. Emp.* **58**:462-464, 1951.

189. Stein, W.: Inaugural Dissertation. Kiel, 1950, quoted by Sievers.

190. Stevenson, A. C. and Warcock, H. A.: Observations on the result of pregnancies in women resident in Belfast. I. Data relating to all pregnancies ending in 1957. *Ann. hum. Genet.* **23**:382-394, 1959.

191. Stevenson, A. C.; Johnston, H. A.; Stewart, M. I. P. and Golding, D. R.: Congenital malformations. A report of a series of consecutive births in 24 centres. *Bull. Wld Hlth Org.* **34**:Suppl. 1-127, 1966.

192. Stevenson, S. S.; Worcester, J. and Rice, R. G.: Congenital malformed infants associated gestational characteristics. I. General considerations; II. Parental factors. *Pediatrics* **6**: 37-50; 208-222, 1950.

193. Strohofer, M.: Inaugural Dissertation. München, 1933, quoted by Sievers.

194. Tabuchi, A. *et al*: Study on epidemiological factors affecting the frequency of occurrences of congenital anomalies. *Hiroshima J. med. Sci.* **11**:143-158, 1962.

195. Tholen, A.: [Congenital malformations with special reference to rubella during pregnancy.] *Geneesk. Gids* **24**:338-340, 1946.

196. Thom, J. C.: [4524 babies: statistical review of all live born babies in the Karl Bremer Hospital, 1961-62. *S. Afr. med. J.* **38**:548, 1964.

197. Torricelli, C., *et al*: *Minerva nipiol.* **12**:2, 1962, quoted by Avezzu and Vinci.

198. Turpin, R.: [Etiology of malformations.] *Presse méd.* **3**: 857-860, 1955.

199. Vasquez, L.-A.; Pascual-Problete, E. and Jongco, A: Congenital malformations in the newborn. *J. Philipp. med. Ass.* **41**:294-304, 1965.

200. Vignali, M.: [Statistical studies of the pathogenetic factors of fetal abnormalities. Clinical and statistical research on malformations 1943-1960.] *Folia hered. path. (Milano)* **11**:257-275, 1962.

201. Villumsen, A. L. and Zachau-Christiansen, B.: Incidence of malformations in the newborn in a prospective child health study. *Bull. Soc. roy. belge Gynec. Obstét.* **33**:95-105, 1963.

202. Wacker, M. N.: Congenital abnormalities. *Amer. J. Obstet. Gynec.* **86**:310-320, 1963.

203. Wallace, H.: Personal communication, 1967.

204. Wallace, H. M.; Baumgartner, L. and Rich, H.: Congenital malformations and birth injuries in New York City. *Pediatrics* **12**:525-534, 1953.

205. Wallace, H. M.; Hoenig, L. and Rich, H.: Newborn infants with congenital malformations or birth injuries. *Amer. J. Dis. Child.* **91**:529-541, 1956.

206. Ward, I. V. and Irvine, E. D.: Incidence of congenital abnormality in infants born in Exeter 1954-1960 inclusive. *Med. Offr* **106**:381-383, 1961.

207. Ward, I. V. and Irvine, E. D.: Incidence of congenital defects in infants born to Exeter mothers. *Med. Offr* **108**: 195-196, 1963.

208. Winter, G. F. and Pätz, A: [Malformation frequency in Berlin and environs in 1950-1956.] *Arch. Gynäk.* **190**:404-418, 1958.

209. Wong Hock Boon: Congenital malformations in Singapore. *Bull. Kandang Kerbau Hospital Singapore* **3**:1-12, 1964.

210. Worm, M.: [Frequency of malformations at Womens Clinic, University of Greifswald from 1930-1950.] *Geburtsh. u. Frauenheilk.* **12**:443-447, 1952.

211. Wulf, R.; Gibson, T. C. and Meyer, R. J.: Congenital abnormalities in a Vermont County: detection and medical care. *New Engl. J. Med.* **274**:861-868, 1966.

212. Yassin, S. M. and Al-Taei, M. S.: Congenital malformations in Mosul, Iraq. *Ein. Shams Med. J. (Cairo)* **1**:1964.

213. Yerushalmy, J.; Van Den Berg, B. J. and Erhard, T.: Birth weight and gestation as indices of "immaturity." Neonatal maturity and congenital anomalies of the "immature." *Amer. J. Dis. Child.* **109**:43-57, 1965.

214. Zuschlag, H. G.: Inaugural Dissertation. Hamburg 1950, quoted by Sievers.

215. Zytkiewicz, A.; Bokiniec, M. and Czarkowska, D.: [Statistical analysis of fetal malformations with consideration of certain causes.] *Pol. Tyg. lek.* **20**:1420-1422, 1965.

ADDENDUM

216. Barret, Bock H. and Zimmerman, J. H.: Study of selected congenital anomalies in Pennsylvania. *Publ. Hlth Rep. (Wash.)* **82**:446-450, 1967.

217. Lilienfeld, A. M.; Parkhurst, E.; Patton, R. and Schlesinger, E. R.: Accuracy of supplemental medical information on birth certificates. *Publ. Hlth Rep. (Wash.)* **66**:191-198, 1957.

*From A. C. Stevenson et al. (1966). Bull. WHO., **34** (Suppl.), pp. 9, 100–102.*
Copyright (1966), by kind permission of the authors and the World Health Organization

Congenital Malformations
A Report of a Study of Series of Consecutive Births in 24 Centres

A report is presented of a study of births in 24 centres in 16 countries with respect to the occurrence and type of congenital malformations found in stillborn and liveborn infants. In all, the outcomes of 421 781 pregnancies are investigated (416 695 single births, 5022 sets of twins, 63 sets of triplets, and one set of quadruplets). The frequencies of malformations of specific types or of groups of malformations are considered with particular reference to geographical variations and associations with consanguinity of parents. The evidence relating to clinical and etiological heterogeneity is considered, as well as that on the genetical contribution to congenital malformations and perinatal mortality. The data are presented in considerable detail in tables and in addition there is available on request to the authors a 400-page companion booklet of basic tables for each centre.

Among the findings of particular interest are : the large contribution of neural tube defects to foetal wastage in most countries and the significant correlations of frequencies of these defects over the 24 recording centres ; the unexplained correlation in frequency between neural tube defects and dizygous twinning ; the marked association of consanguinity of parents with increased stillbirth rates and frequency of early death of the infant, these frequencies being highest where parents are most closely related ; and the demonstration that, if malformations known to be due to the expression of single recessive gene mutations are ignored, consanguinity of parents is demonstrably associated in these data with neural tube defect frequencies only.

A number of interesting observations, either novel or confirmatory of views derived from different approaches, emerge in respect of specific groups of malformations. This is so particularly in respect of harelip and cleft palate, malformations of the gut, malformations of the urogenital tract and multiple malformations occurring in the same child. The findings in respect of twin births are of interest for the light which they throw on the relative contributions of monozygous and dizygous pairs to the total variance of twinning frequencies in the different centres. Estimates are made of the effects of monozygosity on survival of infants and of the occurrence of malformations.

1. INTRODUCTION

ORIGINS OF THE STUDY

In 1958, in the course of discussions in which the World Health Organization took part on needs in medical research, a prospective study of congenital malformations in different countries was suggested as an example of an undertaking which it would be difficult to carry out except under the auspices of the Organization. It was further suggested that a simple and unambitious study would be useful in a field where there were big gaps in knowledge and that much useful experience in the methodology of international studies would accrue.

Subsequently, at an informal meeting at Ann Arbor, Michigan, USA, in April 1959, Professor J. V. Neel, Professor W. J. Schull, Dr J. A. Fraser Roberts and Dr A. C. Stevenson considered, at the request of WHO, all the suggestions for genetic research which had been put forward at the 1958 discussions. It was again recommended that a simple prospective study of the malformations occurring in a consecutive series of births in hospitals in several countries should be undertaken. The limitations of such data, inevitably determined by the biasses introduced by recording hospital births only, were fully recognized. It was realized also, however, that in many of the areas where it would be of great interest to have data there was no possibility of getting adequate information about home births.

This recommendation was accepted and one of us (A.C.S.) was asked to organize and carry out the study from the Population Genetics Research Unit of the Medical Research Council of Great Britain, as facilities were available there for collection and analyses of the not inconsiderable amount of data which would be assembled. Thereafter the authors of this report were responsible for the conduct of the study.

ORGANIZATION AND CONDUCT OF THE STUDY

It was decided that a minimum of about 10 000 consecutive births from each centre was desirable to yield a sufficient number even of the commonest malformations to be of value for analysis. It was also realized that it would be unreasonable to ask the medical staff of busy maternity hospitals to continue the recording over a long period, perhaps more than two years, as changes of staff and diminishing interest in routine recording would be bound to interfere with efficiency. These limitations determined a search for hospitals or groups of hospitals which had a minimum of 10 000 births in two years. By European standards therefore these maternity hospitals would have to be rather large. There are relatively few University hospitals throughout the world of sufficient size and in countries in eastern Europe the " Mother and Child Institutes " usually have only about 100 beds and perhaps 2000 births per year. As will be seen from the data, these limitations resulted in some smaller series of recordings being arranged—on the principle that some data are better than none.

Large hospitals with so many births each year are inevitably very busy places and invariably are understaffed, so that it would have been unrealistic to expect recording of elaborate information about births. Further, uniform recording seemed essential. It was necessary, therefore, to decide what was the maximum amount of information which could reasonably be expected to be recorded in these hospitals which had the minimum facilities.

After consultations at the World Health Organization in Geneva with medical officers who had personal knowledge of many countries, letters were sent by the Organization to the Ministries of Health of a number of countries explaining what was proposed and asking for co-operation. Following this, a visit was paid to each country, except Australia, by a member of the staff of the Population Genetics Research Unit. It was not necessary to visit Australia as there were already close contacts with obstetricians in Melbourne and it was known that the system of recording there was very similar to that in the United Kingdom.

It proved possible in most, although not all, of the countries visited to find hospitals or groups of co-operating hospitals where there were sufficient numbers of births per year and where obstetricians and paediatricians were interested and willing to participate in a joint study. The centres at which recording was started and completed are listed at the front of this publication. In each case the name of the person directly responsible for the local arrangements is indicated, but it will be realized that there are many others—persons in Ministries of Health, obstetricians and paediatricians—whose co-operation was essential. It was made clear to the physicians at each centre visited that the data assembled belonged to them and could be published as desired. It was agreed that no publication of their findings would be made until they had seen the tabulated data from their own hospital and had given permission for their inclusion in a general report. The writers wish to make it clear that in presenting this report they are acting only as co-ordinating agents for many colleagues in all these centres.

Recording of births began at different times and its duration varied between centres. Completion of record forms began in the first centre in October 1961 and ended in the last centre in December 1964.

RECORDING, TRANSMISSION AND HANDLING OF DATA

The simple information which was recorded is shown in Annex 1. A 5-inch by 8-inch white card (12.5 cm × 20.5-cm) was used for each single birth, and there were similar cards—yellow in colour— with a place for the second member of a twin pair, or the second and third members of triplets on the front and back. These cards were printed in Oxford in English, Spanish, Serbo-Croat and Czech. They were serially numbered and then posted in batches to the various centres. Starting on a fixed date in each hospital every livebirth and stillbirth of over 28 weeks' duration of pregnancy was recorded. When completed, cards were returned in batches of one or two thousand to Oxford. The intention was that the cause of death and up to six malformations in each child would be coded and the whole information from each birth transferred to a punch card.

In practice the complexities of types of malformations and the difficulties of interpreting descriptions determined that the ultimate listing and sorting of malformations recorded were done by hand. Further, as might have been anticipated, no use could be made of the causes of death as recorded. As is well known, it is impossible to specify the underlying or the proximate causes of death in many perinatal deaths and the "causes" of death recorded reflected this difficulty.

The exceptions to the above system of recording were in Czechoslovakia and Northern Ireland. Dr V. Matousek, from the Biological Institute of the Czechoslovak Academy of Sciences, spent three weeks in this Unit prior to the study, familiarizing himself with the methodology of analysis which we were pursuing and, at the end of the period of recording, the paediatrician in charge, Dr J. Kucera, came to Oxford, bringing with him the information about all recorded malformations; these were listed in this Unit with his help. In this way a maximum degree of comparability could be achieved. The recording of the Northern Ireland data was started by one of us (A.C.S.) in 1957 when at Queen's University, Belfast. Although the recording system at Belfast was much more elaborate than that used in the present study, it was easy to take from the punched cards most of the information which was being collected in the other centres and it was felt that the inclusion of these data, which had been carefully collected over a number of years, was worth while.

In Oxford, the cards returned were hand-checked for discrepancies and omissions and, as far as possible, these were repaired by writing to the countries concerned. Once it had been confirmed that each card where the child was recorded as having a malformation (including "minor" malformations—considered below) had been correctly coded, the cards were sent for punching to the Statistical Section of this Unit. Thereafter the original cards of all children with malformations were returned to the main Unit for further consideration.

When a basic analysis of the data from each centre had been completed, 15 basic tables and lists of malformations in a form previously agreed were sent out to each centre. The approval of the organizing physician was sought and he was asked to give permission for circulation of these tabulations to all the other centres.

Liaison was maintained with and between the centres by a series of bulletins which were sent out at intervals over the period of the study. These reported progress and called attention to difficulties being encountered in interpreting the returned cards, and were used to send out data and seek approval for the proposed form of their presentation.

ADMINISTRATIVE PROBLEMS

Inevitably, in dealing with so many centres in different parts of the world, many difficulties were encountered. Inexplicable postal delays in both directions were not uncommon whenever the package was of such a size that parcel post had to be employed and a customs declaration completed. Several outgoing batches of cards were returned for no apparent reason by customs authorities; others just never arrived. This was troublesome but could be remedied by dispatching further batches. More serious was the loss of many thousands of completed cards being returned to Oxford or the delay in whole or part of batches of boxes for many months. Several thousand cards sent by Dr Chow of the Kowloon Hospital never arrived, so that no data can be included from there. In addition some boxes from Santo Tomás Hospital, Panama, and from the Maternity Hospital, Kuala Lumpur, arrived too late to be included in the report. The date for final compilation of tables was repeatedly deferred in the hope that they might arrive but in the end the decision to proceed with assembly of the data could not further be delayed without serious disruption of the time-table of the work in this Unit.

20. DISCUSSION AND SUMMING-UP

THE FINDINGS OF THE STUDY IN PERSPECTIVE

The very large amount of information made available by this study and set out in preceding sections has precisely the values and deficiencies which were anticipated when the project was first discussed. The findings give support to many views based on previous evidence. They are not compatible with some others. Some of the data presented are unique, perhaps in particular those relating to consanguinity of parents.

The study was intended to be exploratory, and to stimulate further work by defining some problems better and in so doing indicating where and how *ad hoc* studies might profitably be pursued. It is difficult for those responsible to judge how far these limited objectives have been achieved. However inadequate may be the comments and limited interpretations of the data which have been presented, this report, in conjunction with the Basic Tabulations by Centres booklet, provides, for interpretation by anyone interested, more detailed information in a form suitable for analysis than has ever previously been made available in respect of malformations occurring in a large series of births.

THE WAYS IN WHICH THE DATA HAVE BEEN PRESENTED

Throughout this report the data accumulated in the study have been set out in simple tabular form. There are large numbers of tables, and the information given in them is comprehensive. Further detail has been discussed in the text only where it seemed essential to explain or to stress what seemed of particular interest or importance. It was impracticable, before publication, to circulate the whole report and to seek comments from the organizers at all the centres. Under these circumstances, it was decided that the text should avoid, in so far as possible, controversial interpretations of their data.

The literature on congenital malformations is very large, and descriptions of many birth series with some specification of those malformed have been published. However, these accounts vary very greatly in size and few present the information in sufficient detail to permit even the simplest of comparisons with the present data. To have attempted a review of this literature would have required enorm-ous effort, and would have increased greatly the size of the report.

The only large study in which the nature of the malformations was reported in any detail, and in which information on consanguinity was available, was the investigation sponsored by the United States Atomic Bomb Casualty Commission in Japan. The most complete information on this excellent work, in respect of the malformation data derived from all births in the populations, is in papers by Neel (1958) and Schull (1958). These authors set out the findings in 720 malformed infants occurring in 26 012 births in Hiroshima, 30 240 births in Nagasaki, and 7544 births in Kure, between 1948 and 1954. The over-all consanguinity rate was about 7%. References to these findings are made in several places in this report.

THE TYPES OF CONGENITAL DEFECTS RECOGNIZED AT BIRTH AND THEIR ETIOLOGY

Malformations recognized at birth are predominantly of types which are suspected to have complex genotypic as well as environmental contributions to their etiology, and the nature neither of the environmental nor of the genotypic contributions is understood. It has to be remembered in order to see these malformations in biological perspective (*a*) that those affected are the survivors of a much larger number of zygotes which were malformed and eliminated before or shortly after implantation or as recognized pre-28th week abortions; (*b*) that, as noted in section 2, there is ample evidence that the over-all frequency of malformations present at birth would, if all the children were followed up for a few years, be increased by about 50%, although the numbers " missed " at birth depend on the type of malformation and vary from zero upwards; (*c*) that the very small number of single-gene traits detected in this and other birth series reflects the small proportion of these traits which present as developmental defects recognizable by inspection of the child at birth; (*d*) that only a small proportion of infants who have gross chromosomal defects are detectable at birth by clinical methods only.

Quantitative aspects of these phenomena are reviewed in the report to the International Commission on Radiation Protection (1966). It is important to realize that the remaining types of defects, which constitute a very high proportion of those reported in this study, are not associated with any specifiable genotypic or karyotypic situation, and, however we may speculate about the genotypic contribution and its interaction with environment, at best we are forced to postulate sufficiently simple genotypic and population genetic models and then to see how far the observed facts fit these models.

We know that insult to the embryo by radiation, rubella and possibly other virus infections and by certain chemical agents (including hormones) will determine malformations of these types and there is considerable time- as well as agent-specificity. However, we certainly have no means of identifying more than 1% or 2% of all these defects as being so caused.

There is, however, much to suggest that the environment is extremely important in determining many malformations. The variation by socio-economic class and the somewhat conflicting evidence for seasonal variation of neural tube defects have been most studied, mainly because the numbers of these are sufficiently large. It is doubtful whether, except possibly for harelip and cleft palate and for ulnar polydactyly, any variation by ethnic group can be substantiated. This is mainly because of the difficulty of separating out the effects of geographical location, social class and ethnic origins.

Most of these defects of complex etiology occur in sibs of index cases, with a frequency 5-10 times as great as that in the general population. As most, but not all, of them preclude the affected subjects having children or effectively limit their fertility it cannot be shown in these instances whether the frequency in other first-degree relatives of index cases is equally high.

There has been much controversy about the genetical theory involved and, in particular, about the interpretation of the excess mortality and the possibility of occurrence of malformations not readily recognized being due to homozygosity for single-gene mutations in the offspring of consanguineous parents. A " black-and-white " description of the basis of this controversy is that at one extreme the protagonists believe that almost all the excess mortality and malformation frequency is determined by homozygosity at specific loci, while at the other extreme there are those who consider that homozygosity at specific loci, although not always identifiable, is relatively unimportant. It is thought that the genotypes of importance in determining

most developmental failures are determined at many gene loci and that the precipitating cause is often an unfavourable intra-uterine environment.

The controversies have been " spelt out " with some enthusiasm, particularly from one point of view by Schull & Neel (1965), and among other key references to the theory under discussion which should be consulted are the works of Lerner (1954), Dobzhansky (1955), Morton, Crow & Muller (1956), and Crow (1958). The very large number of consanguineous marriages reported in the present study makes a substantial contribution to the total information available on the relationship between consanguinity, perinatal mortality, and type and frequency of malformation.

SOME FINDINGS OF PARTICULAR INTEREST

Variations and associations of frequencies of neural tube defects and their relationships to consanguinity

The data on neural tube defects are discussed in section 4. There seems to be no doubt that there are real variations in the frequencies of anencephalus and of the other common neural tube defects in different parts of the world. This has long been known, and in particular, the remarkably high frequency of all these defects in Belfast has previously been reported. In this study Alexandria and Bombay also had very high frequencies.

The ten possible frequency comparisons between anencephalus alone, anencephalus with spina bifida, hydrocephalus alone, hydrocephalus and spina bifida, and spina bifida alone all show positive correlations over the 24 centres and these are all significant at least at a 5% level. This finding is of considerable interest and contradicts suggestions that some of the neural tube defect frequencies are negatively correlated. It also suggests that, whatever differing etiological factors there are for the different defects, there are some which are common to all. Apart from the findings of Polman (1951), no association of anencephalus or other neural tube defects with consanguinity had been reported. In this study there are significant associations between consanguinity and these defects in Alexandria and Bombay. Even when these two are excluded from the data, there is a non-significant association with consanguinity in the remainder. The numbers in Alexandria and Bombay are large and the associations highly significant. An explanation (other than that the relationship is causal) which occurs to the writers is that high consanguinity and neural tube defects may both be more common to the lower socio-economic groups of mothers admitted to the hospitals in Alexandria and Bombay. However, it seems unlikely that this could explain all the association.

It would appear that, over the 22 centres for which the consanguinity data are available, there is a significant positive correlation between the frequency of neural tube defects and the estimated frequencies of dizygous twinning. No explanation can be offered for this phenomenon.

Harelip (G1), harelip and cleft palate (G2) and cleft palate (G3)

The high proportion of males in G1 and G2 and the correlation of frequencies of these two in various centres, significant at a 5% level, suggest a common etiology and support other evidence for such a supposition. In contrast, there is no excess of males in cases of cleft palate alone, and the correlations of G1 and G3, G2 and G3, and G1 + G2 and G3 are all negative and of borderline significance. This finding does not support the suggestion which has sometimes been made that, in spite of other evidence for heterogeneity in etiology, the frequency of cleft palate alone tends to be high in communities where the frequency of harelip and cleft palate is also high. It is noted that the disturbance of the sex proportion in the harelip and cleft palate group which is found when these are the only reported abnormalities is also found even when these are associated with other malformations, and so the cases were placed in the N group.

The frequencies of harelip and harelip and cleft palate are as high in several centres as those found in the Japanese study, when the comparisons are made either where these were the only defects or when they were associated with other malformations. It has to be remembered, however, that the Japanese data did not represent hospital cases only and the condition may be more common in hospital births. The frequencies in Chinese and Malays are high, and the relatively few data suggest a high frequency in European births in Johannesburg. There are also some centres in South America with relatively high frequencies. There is no evidence that the frequency is high in the offspring of mothers who were American Indians; however, the numbers are rather small.

The twinning data

When appropriate calculations are made it seems clear that (a) there is no significantly higher frequency of malformations in twins than in single-born infants; (b) the mortality and over-all malformation rates in monozygous twins are both higher than in dizygous twins and the more frequent death or malformation of both of monozygous twins does not fully account for this phenomenon.

There is confirmatory evidence of the homogeneity of the frequency of monozygous twinning over the range of centres, but highly significant heterogeneity of frequency of dizygous twinning so that the latter frequency is the predominant modifier of the over-all twinning rate. The dizygous twinning rate appears to be low in South-East Asia and very high in Alexandria and Belfast.

The consanguinity data

14 000 of the single-born infants in this study had consanguineous parents, and the over-all frequencies of consanguinity in these children varied from over 30% in Alexandria to less than 0.1% in Zagreb. These variations are so large that the summed data have to be interpreted with considerable care.

In families where the children were not malformed, there was strong evidence for a higher mortality (SB + LBD) in the offspring of consanguineous marriages, and it is demonstrated that the mortality is higher in closely related than in less closely related parents. No more detailed analysis of this mortality has been made, but the full data available to the authors are there for anyone who wishes to make the appropriate calculations and express the over-all detriment in terms of " lethal equivalents " or in other ways thought to be more appropriate or meaningful.

It is of interest to note that there was no contribution to the over-all increased mortality in the offspring of related parents in Alexandria, where both consanguinity and perinatal mortality were high. Presumably the amount of concealed inbreeding in Alexandria is high and the effects of inbreeding as identified in parents are masked by the high proportion of deaths primarily caused by poor socio-economic conditions.

From P. E. Polani (1973). Guy's Hosp. Rep., 122, 53–63. *Copyright* (1973),
by kind permission of the author and Guy's Hospital

THE INCIDENCE OF DEVELOPMENTAL AND OTHER GENETIC ABNORMALITIES*

PAUL E. POLANI

Paediatric Research Unit, Guy's Hospital Medical School, London SE1 9RT

SUMMARY

Possibly **6 per cent** of all new born infants have a developmental anomaly—sometimes severe, sometimes relatively mild, at times treatable but often not. The commonest anomalies are those of the central nervous and of the cardiovascular systems and of mentation. Biochemically defined errors, though singly rare, are relatively frequent in the aggregate and chromosome disorders with variable degrees of developmental anomaly are even more frequent. In addition many conceptuses that are chromosomally abnormal are spontaneously aborted and quite a few die in the perinatal period.

Single gene abnormalities account for about one-third of developmental errors discovered or present at birth and chromosome errors for about one-twelfth. In a further substantial proportion of developmental errors the cause is not a single gene anomaly: multiple genes and their alleles interact between themselves and with the environment to produce abnormal development and the relative contributions of nature and nurture can vary a great deal.

IT is a truism that in advanced communities the impact of developmental disorders and malformations, whether environmental or inherited or resulting from a proportionally variable interaction of the two, is greater now that many disorders, particularly of nutrition and from infection, have been largely controlled. However, this must be qualified because in many large and modern cities malnutrition, in children especially, is by no means eradicated, nor is a subtle form of what can be called intrauterine malnutrition; and we have some way to go in the control of virus infections, a far from negligible cause of morbidity. Nevertheless, the general trend towards the increasing importance of developmental and genetically determined disorders is clearly recognizable; statistics are the only way of assessing this in relation to the planning of services and judging the efficacy of therapeutic and preventive efforts.

When the infant mortality rate in the last 4 years of the nineteenth century was 156 per thousand live births, the proportion of infants dying from congenital malformation was about 1 in 35; with the drop of infant mortality by 1970 to about 18.5 per thousand, the number of those dying from congenital malformations has fallen but little, so that now they represent 1 in 5 of the causes of infant death.

However, the problem of malformation is obviously much more serious than that fraction of malformations that are responsible for infant mortality, and the obstetricians were the first to become concerned with

* Expanded from a paper given to the Royal Society of Medicine, Section of Obstetrics and Gynaecology with Section of Paediatrics, on 23 March 1973.

prevalence and causation studies. Since Malpas' original obstetric survey (Malpas, 1937) which estimated the rate of congenital malformations in newborns in Liverpool at over 2 per cent, many surveys have in essence confirmed these figures, while the retrospective work of Murphy (1947) in Philadelphia, based on death certificates, attempted to analyse the origins of congenital abnormalities. McIntosh and his colleagues (1954) in New York gave prevalence figures of over 3 per cent and Nelson and Forfar (1969) in Scotland dealing with survivors gave overall figures of nearly 5 per cent; however, about only 1.3 per cent were of a 'major' nature. Difficulties and differences arise from the method of study and the discipline of the student, but some are related to the population scrutinized. For example, only some 60 per cent of all malformations are reported on birth or death certificates or are similarly recorded. Further-more, even experienced observers are unable to diagnose a proportion of malformations at birth, proportions ranging from 30 to 50 per cent depending on the type of malformation. Be this as it may, that the problem is a serious one has been stressed by many and it has been estimated (Bierman *et al.*, 1965) that perhaps 10 per cent of survivors, by the time they are past infancy, require specific medical or educational provisions for mental, physical or combined handicaps. Further evidence of the impact of genetic diseases and malformations, many of which can be treated by surgery, diet, drugs or by the avoidance of drugs, is the estimate that they account for one-third, or more, of admissions to children's hospitals, for example, in North America, and for an important proportion of bed occupancy and hospital expenditure. Figures from the Toronto Children's Hospital, for example, show that some 10 per cent of all admissions were for single gene or chromosomal disorders, or for conditions with a multi-factorial basis due to polygenic determination with a variable environ-mental component, and a further 20 per cent for congenital anomalies of the type which sometimes are thought to be of multi-factorial origin (W.H.O., 1972).

Perhaps a useful way of considering developmental and other genetic abnormalities is to look at them individually and in some detail before considering the aggregate load of these disorders.

The commoner malformations are listed in Table I wherein are included some lethal ones, as anencephaly almost always is, some mild ones like inguinal hernia, some disabling ones, some eminently treatable ones and some that are almost untreatable. Looking at some of these in detail, anencephaly and spina bifida can be alternative forms of the same type of major CNS anomaly in different members of the same family and spina bifida may have a relative frequency some 20 per cent higher than that of anencephaly. It is well known that the incidence of anencephaly varies in different countries and in these isles it ranges from about 1.5 per thousand in south-east England to about 2.5 per thousand in northern England, 3.0 per thousand in Scotland and Wales, 4.0 per thousand in

INCIDENCE OF MALDEVELOPMENT

TABLE I
POPULATION FREQUENCIES OF THE COMMONER ANOMALIES OF DEVELOPMENT

Condition	Population frequency (per cent)
Anencephaly	0.20–0.30
Spina bifida cystica	0.30
Serious mental defect	0.35+
Congenital heart disease	0.80 (+0.4%*)
Hypertrophic pyloric stenosis	0.30
Idiopathic scoliosis	0.22
Club foot	0.12
Congenital dislocation of the hip	0.10
Cleft lip + cleft palate	0.10
Cleft palate only	0.04
Hirschsprung's disease	0.02
Inguinal hernia	1.0 approx.

* Bicuspid aortic valve (Campbell, 1973).

Northern Ireland and up to 6.0 per thousand in Eire (Carter, 1969). It is also of interest that this is one of the conditions, like a number of others in Table I, for which a multi-genic multi-factorial origin is postulated. The recently propounded hypothesis (Renwick, 1972) that the condition may be due to an effect of some teratogens produced (or released) in spoilt potatoes would, however, throw a greater, or perhaps a preponderant. responsibility on environmental factors but more recent work has failed to provide support for the hypothesis (Clarke et al., 1973; Lorber et al., 1973). Major central nervous system anomalies are an example of the difficulties which one faces when trying to sort out the relative contributions of genetic and environmental factors in the aetiology, for example, of congenital anomalies; at the extremes of the scale things are relatively black or white but in the intervening territory there is much blurring and marked interaction of genes and environment. An aspect which is quite interesting in both theory and practice, about multi-factorial disorders, is that they often show unusual sex ratios of those affected, as in anencephaly, hypertrophic pyloric stenosis, etc.

Serious mental defect (with an approximate I.Q. of less than 50) is best revealed by studies of older children, in common with, say, inguinal hernia and certain types of congenital heart disease, and, like mild intellectual subnormality, it is detected especially during school age when its prevalence could be 3.5 per thousand or higher (Kushlick and Cox, 1973). The assessed general population prevalence for all ages may be somewhat less than 2 per thousand. Excluding mongolism which is comprised within this estimate, and other known causes of severe intellectual defect resulting from central nervous system infections, trauma, etc., some 88 per cent of cases appear to be sporadic and, on the whole, not due to single gene defects. In the remaining 12 per cent of cases there is good evidence of recessive inheritance (Dewey *et al.*, 1965) and, making a number of assumptions, it has been estimated that the total number of gene loci that may be involved in contributing to severe mental deficiency is large: just more than 100 gene loci would certainly be considered a very conservative under-estimate and 300 may be nearer the mark. But I stress that this genetic contribution still accounts for only a proportion of the causes of severe subnormality, and though the figure of genes that could be implicated may seem large it must be viewed against the background of 1800 or so proven or putative genetic disorders known in Man, of which some 900 are more or less proven autosomal dominants, some 800 are proven or likely autosomal recessives and about 150 are proven or presumptive sex-linked (McKusick, 1971a). There is a different way of looking at the above points about the causes of mental defect and some think that the genetic contribution can be emphasized in a different way than I have just stated. It is estimated that about 35 per cent of the causes of mental defect are genetic. Chromosome anomalies on the one hand and the combined action of multiple genes on the other account each for 40 per cent of the genetic causes and the remaining 20 per cent is attributable to mutant major genes of large effect, mostly recessive. Clear cut environmental causes are responsible for one-fifth while in more than two-fifths of cases the origin of mental defect is unassigned. Most of the inheritable conditions due to so-called single genes of large effect are rare, singly, but obviously relatively common when taken all together and Table II lists a number of different biochemical defects, some treatable and some not; some are identifiable at birth and those marked with an asterisk are potentially identifiable prenatally by the study of amniotic fluid and/or cells and indeed some have been so identified.

Two points should be made. The first is that many of these disorders are genetically heterogeneous (Childs and Der Kaloustian, 1968) and often this can be shown clinically and biochemically. To take three

TABLE II

POPULATION FREQUENCIES OF SOME OF THE COMMONER GENETIC ERRORS OF METABOLISM

Condition	Per 100 000
Maple syrup urine disease*	0.3
Classical phenylketonuria	7.0
Benign hyperphenylalaninaemia	3.0
Homocystinuria*	3.0–8.0
Cystinuria*	7.0
Histidinaemia*	6.0
Arginosuccinicaciduria*	0.5
Mucopolysaccharidoses*	4.0
Galactosaemia*	1.5–2.5

* Conditions which are potentially identifiable pre-natally (modified from W.H.O. 1972).

examples: galactosaemia seems to be caused by either of two different enzyme variants, but there is a third, seemingly non-morbid variant of the enzyme galactose-l-phosphate-uridyl-transferase, specified by another mutant allele; in classical phenylketonuria three different phenotypes can be recognized by their response to phenylalanine; the Ehlers-Danlos syndrome seems to resolve, at present, into six different disorders (sex-linked, autosomal dominant and recessive) of which only one is bio-chemically characterized (Beighton, 1970; McKusick, 1972). Other examples of heterogeneity could be given and their detection may require very sophisticated studies. For example, in xeroderma pigmentosum the DNA repair defect produced by different alleles may show quantitative differences which cell hybridization techniques can demonstrate, albeit laboriously. Genetic heterogeneity suggests either the activity of different alleles at the same locus or different genes at different loci and the distinc-tion can be of practical importance. Firstly, the heterogeneity makes prenatal diagnosis of biochemical errors an even more delicate proposition and secondly, it has to be taken into account in the, admittedly rare, examples of marriage counselling between possible carriers of genes for the same disorders. Nor is the problem of heterogeneity confined to rare genetic conditions as the experience with the Tay Sachs 'syndrome' in Jews testifies. Indeed, it has been suggested that even fibrocystic disease of the pancreas, a commonly 'lethal' genetic disorder in, for example, Anglo-Saxon people is genetically heterogeneous. Some of the hetero-geneity in genetic disease is revealed by enzyme protein differences which can be detected biochemically and is due to homozygosis for different alleles at one or more loci. Each pairwise combination of these different alleles can produce a specific effect and an identifiable biochemical phenotype. In other cases, however, the heterogeneity may result from the interaction of different mutant alleles at the same locus combining in pairs in a person who thus is heterozygous. However, the resulting abnormal phenotype almost simulates homozygosity for the one or the other allele. In this situation the heterogeneity is even greater than in the first case and may result in a graded as opposed to a step-wise variation in phenotype. The existence of different alleles in the population as the cause of a given genetic disease may, in fact, account for the difficulties in detecting a proportion of heterozygotes even in cases when these are strongly suspected on genetic grounds, i.e. even when dealing with obligatory heterozygotes.

The second point can also be introduced from considering phenyl-ketonuria. This disorder may be some four times more common in Scotland than shown in Table II for example (Lindsay, 1970) and conversely appears to have a much lower frequency in Jews.

Table III lists a number of genetic biochemical disorders whose fre-quencies are known to vary widely in different regions and populations. The explanation usually given for most of this variation is a non-random

TABLE III

Some of the Genetic Biochemical Defects Which Show Marked Regional Variation

Condition	Per 100 000	Region or population group
Galactokinase deficiency* ..	1.0 2.0 0.4 6.2	North America Massachusetts, U.S.A. Manitoba, Canada
Hereditary tyrosinaemia*.. ..	30.0 0.4	Quebec isolate, Canada N.E. U.S.A. and Eastern Canada
Tay Sachs disease*	30.0 0.3	Ashkenazi Jews Sephardic Jews, Gentiles
Cystic fibrosis	50.0	Europeans
Adrenogenital syndrome* ..	1.5 20.0	North America Switzerland
Thalassaemia	1000.0	Mediterranean, etc.
Sickle cell anaemia	1000–2000	Africans

* Conditions which are potentially identifiable prenatally (modified from W.H.O., 1972).

distribution of genes among originally small populations often concurrent with migration, due to those forms of sampling variation that do under the names of 'drift' and of the 'founder principle'. However, in some cases, as for example in the recessive disorders cystic fibrosis of the pancreas or in sickle-cell anaemia the frequency of the given genetic disease, that is to say, the frequency of the homozygous affected person, is very high in some populations and yet the disorder itself is lethal or nearly so. In view of this high frequency, recurrent mutation cannot be the means whereby the disease is maintained at this high level in a population. The gene, as opposed to the disease, must be maintained in the population by the healthy heterozygous carriers of the gene from whom the affected homozygotes derive. In these circumstances one looks for some advantage that these so-called 'recessive genes' may confer upon the heterozygous carriers and make them genetically fitter than the persons homozygous for the 'normal' (wild type) gene in question. One is trying to detect an advantage, often quite small, which allows the population frequency of the gene to increase to a certain level in spite of its rapid loss from the population through the many diseased, lethal or near lethal homozygotes. As a result of the selective advantage conferred upon its carriers, the gene in question is maintained at an equilibrium which is set at a high level, a balance between mutation and selective advantage on the one hand, and loss on the other. In the case of sickle-cell anaemia the advantage appears to be protection from malaria in zones of high endemicity. Another example is Tay Sachs cerebro-macular degeneration, a disease prevalent in, especially, North American Jews of North European, but not South

European stock. The disease, with a high frequency of about 1 : 3000 infants, is lethal but the carriers—about 1 in 30 of the given population— are alleged to have a possible selective advantage in being relatively resistant to tuberculosis, a factor that clearly would have a considerable survival value in a ghetto (Myrianthopoulos and Aronson, 1972). It is interesting to consider the effect which human selection, as opposed to selection by bacteria, would have on the gene frequency if the authorities who screened the immigrant population selected the immigrants for freedom from active tuberculosis or even from past tuberculous infection. In the case of fibrocystic disease of the pancreas a selective advantage which may even not have reached equilibrium as yet, has been attributed to increased fertility of the carriers (Knudson *et al.*, 1967) but this sugges- tion awaits confirmation.

To these and other genetic disorders whose biochemical basis has been worked out—perhaps 15 per cent of all genetic conditions—we may add a number whose biochemical basis is obscure or completely unknown. The latter conditions are often morphologically striking, often detrimental and equally often inherited in an autosomal dominant manner.

Perhaps a comment is required on the differences between autosomal recessive and dominant disorders. There is a tendency to attribute the latter to different types of genes and mutations, compared with the former. A general view of recessivity is that it is due to the presence of a single dose of a mutant allele which, in essence, produces an abnormal enzyme component or fails to produce it altogether. However, it is assumed that the working margin of enzymes in standard conditions is wide and thus a partial enzyme deficiency is not necessarily revealed. Hence the heterozygote generally behaves as the homozygote normal except when the biochemical step which is involved can be selectively stressed. In dominants instead, it is held (McKusick, 1971b) that the gene at fault is responsible for an irreplaceable component of a tissue aggregate and that the presence of faulty elements in the tissue fabric weakens its whole texture. Hence the presence of a single dose of such a mutant gene, in the heterozygote, is revealed and the effect is dominant. Of this type could be the connective tissue disorder of Marfan's syndrome or the red cell membranes in elliptocitosis (Fraser, 1972). Another possibility for dominance is a mutant allele whose produce may be qualitatively inadequate to remove a metabolic waste or may produce a molecule which itself, through insolubility or other property, cannot be satis- factorily turned over and causes cell and tissue damage by its presence. Finally, it is possible that some dominant mutations are small chromosome deficiencies, i.e. errors in chromosome structure rather than point muta- tions, as for example happens in some cases of retinoblastoma.

Taken all together, disease caused by mutant genes of large effect may affect almost 0.8 per cent of births and, in addition, malformation due to single mutant genes might affect 0.5 per cent of newborns. Furthermore, erythroblastosis, based on genetic inequalities, may involve 0.4 per cent of infants. A total figure for single gene disorders could thus be between 1.3 and 1.7 per cent.

In this estimate are included genetically determined forms of blindness and of deafness (Fraser, 1966). Approximately half the cases of these sensory disorders are of genetic origin, the rest being caused by pre-, peri-, or post-natal events. It has been estimated that, taking autosomal dominant, recessive and X-linked conditions together, some 35 different gene loci can be involved in causing different types of genetic deafness and some 60 gene loci in producing genetically determined forms of blindness. But these are minimal estimates. For example, recent lists of hereditary deafness suggests that some 70 different types exist (Konigsmark, 1969; McKusick, 1971c) and these may be caused by mutation at different loci or by alternative alleles at a smaller number of loci.

Leaving aside point mutational genetic abnormalities let us now consider those abnormalities which result from chromosome mutations. These may be numerical, or structural, or sometimes a combination of the two. In the aggregate they affect about one in 180 or more infants surviving at birth though imbalance does not always result from structural chromosome changes. At least one in 200 infants have a chromosome anomaly with imbalance and perhaps a little more than half the anomalies are of the autosomes and the rest of the sex chromosomes (Court-Brown, 1967; Gerald and Waltzer, 1970; Hamerton *et al.*, 1972; Lubs and Ruddle, 1970; Ratcliffe *et al.*, 1970; Sergovich *et al.*, 1969; and Turner and Wald, 1970).

The most common autosomal anomaly and the best known is Down's Syndrome or mongolism caused by trisomy 21. Trisomies 13 and 18 are much rarer with frequencies of the order of 1 in 6000 to 1 in 10 000 of newborn infants. It is well known that the incidence of Down's Syndrome shows an overall rise with maternal age, though the aetiological relationship with maternal age is obscure and probably not caused by a single biological phenomenon. However, there are forms of this condition which are aetiologically independent of maternal age, for example, translocation Down's Syndrome: 3.5 per cent of the 1 in 600 incidence of mongolism.

Of the more common sex chromosome anomalies XYY males and XXY males are probably 1 in 700 male infants and XX males (who may be considered as examples of sex inversion) may be four times rarer in males than in XO females among females (one in 2500, say), XY females being rarer. Mosaicism for sex chromosomes or autosomes could be relatively not uncommon. One in 1400 female infants is XXX.

Another point of interest concerns the fact that chromosomally abnormal survivors are the tip of the iceberg of all chromosome anomalies. As is well known about a quarter to half of all spontaneous abortions are chromosomally abnormal and the distribution of anomalies is different from that in survivors. Sex chromosome trisomic abortuses, XXX, XXY and XYY must be exceptionally rare but the XO is the single commonest chromosome anomaly (0.8 per cent to 1.0 per cent of all conceptions). Autosomal trisomies in the aggregate are commoner than XOs and triploids are also quite common (perhaps 0.5 per cent of all conceptions).

From these data it can be estimated that at least 4 per cent of all human conceptions with a recognizable pregnancy are chromosomally abnormal but that some 85 to 90 per cent of them are selectively eliminated as spontaneous abortions. Some more that are chromosomally abnormal never embed or never lead to a recognizable pregnancy of some duration. Additional weeding out of chromosomally abnormal conceptions occurs perinatally. Studies at Guy's (Machin, 1973) show that about 5 per cent of perinatal deaths—one in 20 compared to one in 200 survivors—are chromosomally abnormal with a frequency which is almost five times higher in macerated than in fresh stillbirths. Interestingly, and unlike what happens in abortions, sex chromosomal as well as autosomal trisomies are among the anomalies found.

In conclusion, to the various developmental anomalies, which amount to about 4 per cent (including inguinal hernia) some mild, some severe, could be added 1.3 to 1.7 per cent for major single gene defects and genetic inequalities with resulting abnormality, 0.5 per cent for major chromosomal anomalies with imbalance in surviving infants and about 0.1 per cent for cerebral palsy. The total figure would be of a 6 per cent or greater load of genetic and developmental anomalies of all types.

Omitted from consideration have been a number of other conditions of variable causation (Table IV) which arise in later life, but in which genetic factors appear to play an important role.

TABLE IV

A LIST OF RELATIVELY COMMON CONDITIONS IN WHICH GENETIC FACTORS MAY PLAY A VARIABLE ROLE

Condition	Approximate population frequency (per cent)
Schizophrenia	1.0
Cyclothymia	0.4
Diabetes mellitus	1.0
Epilepsy	0.5

REFERENCES

Beighton, P. (1970) *The Ehlers-Danlos Syndrome.* Heinemann Medical Books, London, p. 194.
Bierman, J. M., Siegal, E., French, F. E. and Simonian, K. (1965) Analysis of the outcome of all pregnancies in a community: Kauai pregnancy study. *American Journal of Obstetrics and Gynaecology,* **91,** 37.
Campbell, M. (1973) Incidence of cardiac malformations at birth and later, and neonatal mortality. *British Heart Journal,* **35,** 189.
Carter, C. O. (1969) Spina bifida and Anencephaly: a problem in genetic-environmental interaction. *Journal of Biosocial Science,* **1,** 71.

Childs, B. and Der Kaloustian, V. M. (1968) Genetic heterogeneity. *New England Journal of Medicine*, **279**, 1205 and 1267.

Clarke, C. A., McKendrick, O. M. and Sheppard, P. M. (1973) Spina bifida and potatoes. *British Medical Journal*, **3**, 251.

Court-Brown, W. M. (1967) *Human Population Cytogenetics*. (North-Holland Research Monographs, 'Frontiers of Biology', Vol. 5.) North-Holland Publishing Co., Amsterdam.

Dewey, W. J., Barrai, I., Morton, N. E. and Mi, M. P. (1965) Recessive genes in severe mental defect. *American Journal of Human Genetics*, **17**, 237.

Fraser, G. R. (1966) The role of Mendelian inheritance in the causation of childhood deafness and blindness. In: *Mutation in Population*. Proceedings of a Symposium held in Prague, 9–11 August 1965. Edited by R. Honcariv, p. 129. Academia, Prague.

Fraser, G. R. (1972) Unsolved Mendelian disease. In: *The Biochemical Genetics of Man*. Edited by D. J. H. Brock and O. Mayo, p. 639. Academic Press, London and New York.

Gerald, P. S. and Waltzer, S. (1970) Chromosome studies of normal new-born infants. In: *Human Population Cytogenetics*. Edited by P. A. Jacobs, W. H. Price and P. Law, p. 143. Edinburgh University Press, Edinburgh.

Hamerton, J. L., Ray, M., Abbott, J., Williamson, C. and Ducasse, G. C. (1972) Chromosome studies in a neonatal population. *Canadian Medical Association Journal*, **106**, 776.

Knudson, A. G., Wayne, L. and Hallett, W. Y. (1967) On the selective advantage of cystic fibrosis heterozygotes. *American Journal of Human Genetics*, **19**, 388.

Konigsmark, B. W. (1969) Hereditary deafness in man. *New England Journal of Medicine*, **281**, 713, 774 and 827.

Kushlick, A. and Cox, G. (1973) Epidemiology of mental handicap. *Developmental Medicine and Child Neurology* (in press).

Lindsay, G. (1970) In: Society for the Study of Inborn Errors of Metabolism. Proceedings of the seventh annual symposium, Glasgow, 1969. *Errors of Phenylalanine, Thyroxine and Testosterone metabolism*. Edited by W. Hamilton and F. P. Hudson, p. 8. Livingstone, Edinburgh.

Lorber, J., Stewart, C. R. and Milford-Ward, A. (1973) Alpha-fetoprotein in antenatal diagnosis of anencephaly and spina bifida. *Lancet*, i, 1187.

Lubs, H. A. and Ruddle, F. H. (1970) Applications of quantitative karyotype to chromosome variation. In: *Human Population Cytogenetics*. Edited by P. A. Jacobs, W. H. Price and P. Law, p. 119. Edinburgh University Press, Edinburgh.

Machin, G. (1973) Personal communication.

Malpas, P. (1937) The incidence of human malformations and significance of changes in the maternal environment in their causation. *Journal of Obstetrics and Gynaecology (British Empire)*, **44**, 434.

McIntosh, R., Merritt, K. K., Richards, M. R., Samuels, M. H. and Bellows, M. T. (1954) The incidence of congenital malformations: a study of 5,964 pregnancies. *Paediatrics*, **14**, 505.

McKusick, V. A. (1971a) *Mendelian Inheritance in Man*. 3rd edition, p. ix. The Johns Hopkins Press, Baltimore and London.

McKusick, V. A. (1971b) *Mendelian Inheritance in Man*. 3rd edition, p. xi. The Johns Hopkins Press, Baltimore and London.

McKusick, V. A. (1971c) *Mendelian Inheritance in Man*. 3rd edition, p. xxiii. The Johns Hopkins Press, Baltimore and London.

McKusick, V. A. (1972) The Ehlers-Danlos syndrome. In: *Heritable Disorders of Connective Tissue*. 4th edition, p. 292. C. V. Mosby Company, Saint Louis.

Murphy, D. P. (1947) *Congenital Malformations*. 2nd edition. J. B. Lippincott Company, Philadelphia.

Myrianthopoulos, N. C. and Aronson, S. M. (1972) Population dynamics of Tay-Sachs disease. II. What confers the selective advantage upon the Jewish heterozygote? In: *International Symposium on Sphingolipids, Sphingolipidoses and Allied Disorders*. 4th, New York, 1971. Edited by B. W. Volk and S. M. Aronson, p. 561. Plenum Press, New York and London.

Nelson, M. M. and Forfar, J. O. (1969) Congenital abnormalities at birth: their association in the same patient. *Developmental Medicine and Child Neurology*, **11**, 3.

Ratcliffe, S. G., Stewart, A. L., Melville, M. M., Jacobs P. A. and Keay, A. J. (1970) Chromosome studies on 3,500 newborn male infants. *Lancet*, i, 121.

Renwick, J. H. (1972) Hypothesis: anencephaly and spina bifida are usually preventable by avoidance of a specific but unidentified substance present in certain potato tubers. *British Journal of Preventive and Social Medicine*, **26**, 67.

Sergovich, F., Valentine, G. H., Chen, A. T. L., Kinch, R. A. H. and Smout, M. S. (1969) Chromosome aberrations in 2159 consecutive newborn babies. *New England Journal of Medicine*, **280**, 851.

INCIDENCE OF MALDEVELOPMENT

Turner, J. H. and Wald, N. (1970) Chromosome patterns in a general neonatal population. In: *Human Population Cytogenetics*. Edited by P. A. Jacobs, W. H. Price and P. Law, p. 153. Edinburgh University Press, Edinburgh.

World Health Organization (1972) *Genetic Disorders: Prevention, Treatment and Rehabilitation*. World Health Organization Technical Report Series No. 497, Geneva.

PART III

TERATOLOGICAL MECHANISMS

7. Roberts, C. J. and Powell, R. G. (1975). Interrelation of the common congenital malformations. Some aetiological implications. *Lancet*, **ii**, 848–850

COMMENTARY

The precise mechanisms of abnormal development are unknown. Several theories have been proposed, but so far these have provided little insight into the actual problem. That certain hereditary and environmental factors may adversely affect the development of the embryo, in both man and experimental animals, is well documented. However, the initial reaction of the conceptus to a teratogen, its further responses in terms of metabolic and morphological alterations, and the subsequent events which occur prior to the manifestation of the congenital defect have hardly been investigated. Indeed, the great emphasis has been only to study the definitive results at the end of gestation without attempting to grasp their significance.

Recently, two interesting theories of teratogenesis, both concerned with fundamental mechanisms, have been advanced. McCredie (1973, 1974) found that the radiological changes in the bones and joints of children with thalidomide deformities were similar to the trophic changes present in adult sensory peripheral neuropathy. A mechanism of neural-crest cell damage has been proposed as a 'unifying concept' to account for many apparently unrelated birth defects, including the thalidomide abnormalities. The results of teratological studies with vitamin A and cadmium in laboratory animals do not, however, lend support to this hypothesis. More recently, Hughes (1975) emphasized the importance of the 'inorganic metabolism' of the embryo. The observation was made that sodium ions accumulated in chick embryos in cases of neural tube defects. A basic teratological mechanism, not depending on a single teratogen, but on the inhibition of sodium extrusion from the embryo at gastrulation stages, was proposed to account for developmental defects, in particular those involving closure of the neural tube.

The paper by Roberts and Powell (1975) also advances a novel concept directly related to the primary causes of teratogenesis. From a study of 90 921 single births, they found a strong interrelation between specific congenital malformations, i.e. the occurrence of two or more defects in the same individual was encountered more frequently than one would have expected by chance. On this basis, it was argued that multiple external factors are unlikely to be responsible for human malformations, and a 'single cause' theory was proposed. In particular, this hypothesis advanced 'intrinsic mutagenesis' as the underlying mechanism and considers developmental anomalies as survivors of a continuous stream of mutants, produced at random.

Interesting as it may be, this hypothesis is unacceptable for several reasons. It cannot account for *all* malformations (see Holmes *et al.*, 1976). Indeed, the group of malformations suggested by Roberts and Powell as resulting from a single cause should be considered aetiologically heterogeneous (monogenic disorders with pleiotropic effects; polygenic inheritance; cytogenetically undetectable deletions or duplications; environmentally induced; and chance association) as pointed out by Cohen (1976). Furthermore, the role of environmental influences may very well be underestimated.

An acceptable alternative is the concept of 'environmental preconditioning' proposed by Janerich (1975). Environmental factors become teratogenic depending on maternal susceptibility. It is also on this basis of differences in teratogenic susceptibility and specificity that the lack of time-clustering of congenital malformations may be explained.

REFERENCES

Cohen, M. M. (1976). Interrelationships between common congenital malformations. *Lancet*, **i**, 147

Holmes, L. B., Driscoll, S. G. and Atkins, L. (1976). Etiologic heterogeneity of neural-tube defects. *N. Engl. J. Med.*, **294**, 365–369

Hughes, A. (1975). Teratogenesis and the movement of ions. *Dev. Med. Child. Neurol.*, **17**, 111–114

Janerich, D. T. (1975). Female excess in anencephaly and spina bifida: possible gestational influences. *Am. J. Epidemiol.*, **101**, 70–76

McCredie, J. (1973). Thalidomide and congenital Charcot's joints. *Lancet*, **i**, 1058–1061

McCredie, J. (1974). Embryonic neuropathy: a hypothesis of neural crest injury as the pathogenesis of congenital malformations. *Med. J. Aust.*, **1**, 159–163

From C. J. Roberts and R. G. Powell (1975). Lancet, **ii**, 848–850. *Copyright* (1975), *by kind permission of the authors and The Lancet Ltd*

INTERRELATION OF THE COMMON CONGENITAL MALFORMATIONS
SOME ÆTIOLOGICAL IMPLICATIONS

C. J. ROBERTS   R. G. POWELL*

Department of Community Medicine, Welsh National School of Medicine, Cardiff

Summary   Analysis of congenital defects in a population of 90 921 singleton births revealed a strong interrelation between malformations: for example, 84% of lung defects, 70% of kidney defects, 34% of eye defects, 19% of cleft palate, and 15% of spina bifida coexisted with other defects which could not be designated as subsequently derived structural changes. The strength and intimacy of these interrelations casts doubt on the notion that multiple external factors are involved in the causation of human malformations.

Introduction

SCIENTIFIC inferences may concern events which are retrospective (ætiological) or prospective (predictive) to the process of classification. When malformations are classified so as to allow inferences to be drawn upon ætiology, judgment must be exercised in the selection of an "appropriate" dimension for classification. The failure of epidemiological investigation to identify any significant causal agent in spina bifida is usually explained by saying that the correct causal factor has not yet been selected for investigation—in other words, that the *ætiological* classifications used have been inappropriate. But has enough attention been paid to the propriety of the effect (disease) classification? Should spina bifida and anencephaly be considered separately or together? Those who favour separate investigation argue that combined study of neural-tube defects may mask an association with a factor which is causal for one but not for the other. As a compromise, epidemiologists have tended to study spina bifida and anencephaly both together and

separately, but this approach lacks any intrinsic logic. What real justification is there for considering neural-tube defects separately from (say) cleft palate? The only logical explanation (in relation to ætiological inferences) is that each has a different ætiology; but what evidence is there for this? One argument is that the epidemiology of cleft palate differs substantially from that of neural-tube defect. Given that this is true, should an observation, made after and deriving out of the classification, be accepted as prior justification for that classification, in the absence of independent and convincing evidence that cleft palate and neural-tube defects do in fact have separate ætiologies? A second and more pragmatic view is that their distinct anatomical and pathological features justify their consideration as separate entities. Whilst such an approach may be valuable for making prognostic inferences, past experience suggests that this does not necessarily apply to considerations of ætiology (congenital heart-disease and deafness have the same ætiology in rubella embryopathy). It may be necessary then to consider seriously the notion that, in the sphere of human malformations, classes of proven value for making prognostic clinical judgments may bear little relation to those necessary for appropriate ætiological investigation.

Materials and Methods

This investigation is based on the South Wales Congenital Malformation Study which has been described in detail elsewhere.[1] It covered the years 1964–66 inclusive and involved all births occurring in Monmouthshire, Glamorganshire, and the county boroughs therein (Cardiff, Swansea, and Newport), during this period. Out of a total 90 921 singleton births, 3242 were recorded as having congenital defects by the second anniversary of their birth. An examination of all recorded congenital malformations was carried out which revealed a total of 325 infants with two or more recorded defects (10% of the series). Of these, 232 (7%) were found to have two or more of the defects specified in the accompanying table. Certain categories of defect were excluded from the analysis: limb defects (other than those specified), owing to inadequate description at the time of recording; skin and miscellaneous defects, because of their minor nature; anomalads (a malformation together with its subsequently derived structural changes—e.g., Robin anomalad); and deformations (alteration in shape and/or structure of a previously normally formed part—e.g., torticollis—because they were not strictly malformations but rather primary structural defects arising from a localised error or morphogenesis). Case-finding was restricted to information collected by the second birthday, and not all the subjects came to routine necropsy, with the result that internal malformations such as kidney defect, diaphragmatic hernia, congenital heart-disease, and congenital dislocation of the hip are likely to be under-reported. The results that follow reflect a conservative estimate of the interrelation between the common congenital malformations recorded by the second birthday of a large population, most of whom came to necropsy if they died of a congenital malformation during this period.

Results

The cases included in this investigation all had two or more of the defects specified in the table. Fig. 1 shows the interrelations of the 232 cases included in this study. Each line represents a case possessing the two defects joined by that line. Where more than two defects coexisted, the defect with the highest percentage of associated defects (see table) was used as a base from which several lines were drawn. Since only one possible combination of lines is shown, fig. 1 is a conservative illustration of the extent of interrelation observed in this study.

FREQUENCY OF AND INTERRELATION BETWEEN CONGENITAL DEFECTS IN SOUTH WALES (1964–66)*

Abnormality	No. of cases	Rate/1000 singleton births	No. with assoc. defects	% with assoc. defects
Lung defect	19	0·21	16	84
Kidney defect	59	0·65	41	70
Other brain defects	106	1·16	55	52
Imperforate anus	44	0·48	22	50
Exomphalos	50	0·55	20	40
Œsophageal atresia/ tracheo-œsophogeal fistula	46	0·51	16	35
Eye defect	58	0·64	20	34
Single umbilical artery	32	0·35	9	28
Congenital dislocation of hip	77	0·85	19	25
Diaphragmatic hernia	49	0·54	11	22
Cleft lip/cleft palate	187	2·06	35	19
Congenital heart-disease	398	4·38	65	16
Spina bifida	356	3·92	54	15
Ear defect	135	1·48	19	14
Finger defect	140	1·53	17	12
Hypospadias	110	1·21	13	12
Anencephaly	281	3·09	25	9

*Excluding limb defects (unless specified), skin and miscellaneous defects, and all those with a frequency of less than 0·01%.

Fig. 2 gives a clearer view of the defects involved in fig. 1. Defects are depicted on orbits which indicate their rates of occurrence and each line joining two defects denotes an association which could have occurred by chance *more* frequently than once per 250 000 births. The likelihood that any combination of defects given on the figure could have occurred by chance can be calculated by multiplying the rates of occurrence on the related orbits. For example, the coexistence of a kidney defect and an imperforate anus in a single child is almost certain to be a syndrome since its chance occurrence is only once in 3×10^6 births.

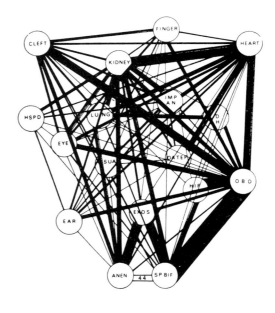

Fig. 1–Interrelations of defects in 232 cases.
For explanation, see text. HSPD = hypospadias; ANEN = anencephaly; EXOS = exomphalos; SP. BIF. = spina bifida; SUA = single umbilical artery; IMP. AN. = imperforate anus; OATEF = œsophageal atresia/tracheal fistula; D.H. = diaphragmatic hernia; O.B.D. = other brain defects.

Discussion

Many more malformed individuals have multiple defects than would be the case if all combinations were fortuitous (16% of a Birmingham series of 2527 malformed children had more than one defect,[2] as did 7% of the present series). It is now believed that between 30% and 80% of all malformations are aborted[3][4] and, since it would also be reasonable to assume that the more serious (or complex) the misfortune the greater is the likelihood of its abortion, the rates of interrelation shown in the table (and those reported by previous workers) are probably minimum estimates.

What are the likely explanations? First, that a malformation of one part of the body may lead to maldevelopment of another (e.g., the Robin anomalad); as far as

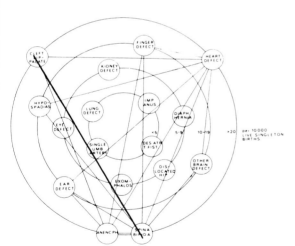

Fig. 2–Interrelation predictor, assuming that associations occur by chance.
For explanation, see text.

possible we excluded all combinations of this kind from our analysis, and this cannot explain a major, or even a substantial part of the relations shown in fig. 1. Second, that chromosomal malformations usually lead

to syndromes rather than single defects; and third, that environmental teratogens have multiple targets. The second implies that conception is abnormal from the outset and the third that the conception is normal but suffers some subsequent misfortune. The last explanation assumes that the misfortune is extrinsically determined, and carries with it the implication that prevention may be possible. The second, whilst it could arise from extrinsic teratogenic action on gametes, allows an alternative and conceptually quite different explanation—namely, that the defect may have arisen from some intrinsic accident. We believe that the strong interrelation of common malformations throws some light on the question of whether the misfortune is extrinsically or intrinsically determined.

Given any number of anatomically defined defects, the only justification for their separate investigation (for ætiological purposes) would be the prior assumption that each had a separate ætiology. Any subsequent indication that they were strongly interrelated would undermine this assumption, and imply instead that they shared some common ætiological factor. The intensity and the intimacy of the interrelations observed in this study suggest that there may well be only one extrinsic factor responsible for most malformations, and the susceptibility of one organ as opposed to another could be explained just as well by chance and/or, say, critical time of impact, as by the existence of several extrinsic teratogens.

However, the evidence that environment is in some way responsible for the ætiology of the common serious malformations is itself tenuous and circumstantial, and derives largely from work in laboratory animals. Although hope is rekindled each time a new extrinsic teratogen is identified, it should be borne in mind that all the teratogens thus far identified account for less than 5% of all human malformations. The cause for the remainder, which includes all the common and important defects, continues to elude discovery despite intensive international investigation spanning forty years.

Thus far we have suggested not only that, if serious human malformations are extrinsically determined, the cause could equally well be unifactorial as multifactorial, but also that if there were just one extrinsic cause it is surprising that it has never been identified. An alternative and possibly more plausible option is that this "single" factor is not extrinsic but intrinsic. Once the notion that the pattern presented in fig. 1 could have arisen from a single extrinsic cause is accepted then (in the light of evidence that exists at the moment), the notion that the pattern could also have arisen from a single intrinsic cause assumes at least an equal probability.

In our view, the current absence of any strong evidence that conventional physical and chemical teratogens are substantially involved in the causation of human malformations, together with the observation that common malformations are highly interrelated, favours the hypothesis that there is "one single cause" for most human malformations and that this is likely to be "intrinsic" rather than "extrinsic". In the absence of evidence to the contrary, the notion of intrinsic mutagenesis is an obvious candidate for this role. To quote from Sir Macfarlane Burnet's book on the subject[5]— "the concept of intrinsic mutagenesis is no more than the formal expression of the opinion that the commonly accepted environmental causes of mutation are, in normal circumstances, quantitatively unimportant and for the most part effective only through their influence on errors of DNA replication of intrinsic origin". Most congenital malformations, then, may be the survivors of a continuous supply of mutations which are (and have been throughout time) randomly produced to allow the species to "adjust to changes in the ecosystem, or to occupy new niches which may become available".

We acknowledge with gratitude the generous grant from the Association for the Aid of Crippled Children, New York, which made this investigation possible. R. G. P.'s part in the work was done during a student elective attachment to the department.

REFERENCES

1. Richards, I. D. G., Lowe, C. R. *Br. J. prev. soc. Med.* 1971, **25**, 59.
2. Leck, I., Record, R. G., McKeown, T., Edwards, J. H. *Teratology*, 1968, **1**, 263.
3. Hertig, A. T., Rock, J., Adams, E. C. *Am. J. Anat.* 1956, **98**, 435.
4. Roberts, C. J., Lowe, C. R. *Lancet*, 1975, i, 498.
5. Burnet, F. M. Intrinsic Mutagenesis: A Genetic Approach to Ageing. Lancaster, 1974.

PAPER 8

8. Saxén, L. (1970). Defective regulatory mechanisms in teratogenesis. *Int. J. Gynaecol. Obstet.*, **8,** 798–804

COMMENTARY

Embryogenesis is an explicitly and highly coordinated process of remarkable regularity. It involves complex interactions between genetic and exogenous factors as well as a series of interrelated cellular and biochemical events. These include the proliferation and determination of cells; induction; cell aggregation; morphogenetic movement of cells; cellular growth; and the phenomenon of programmed cell death. The mechanisms directing these processes are largely unknown. There is, however, sufficient experimental evidence to indicate that their derangement may lead to abnormal morphogenesis.

The present article rightly deals with birth defects as an embryological problem. It provides a logical starting point for the interpretation and understanding of the mechanisms of dysmorphogenesis. In this excellent paper, current concepts of major intercellular and intracellular processes during embryonic development are reviewed. In addition, the regulatory mechanisms of embryogenesis and how their derangement may affect the subsequent development of the concepts are briefly discussed.

From L. Saxén (1970). Int. J. Gynaecol. Obstet., **8**, 798–804. *Copyright* (1970), *by kind permission of the author and the Williams & Wilkins Co*

Defective Regulatory Mechanisms in Teratogenesis

Lauri Saxén, M.D., Phil. Lic.

Our 16th century colleagues, the animalculists, believed that the germ(cell), the egg or the sperm, carried a small, complete embryo and that its further development merely involved growth of the preformed organism. We may today agree with their basic assumption: the fertilized egg does, in fact, contain all of the informative material for building an individual and no additional instructions are required from outside. Instead of pure growth, however, the development of the zygote involves the gradual expression of the genetic information stored in its DNA, which leads to the specialization of a variety of cell types and tissue complexes with specialized metabolism, form, and structure. As we shall soon see, this synchronous, well timed sequential differentiation is controlled by a great number of different built-in regulatory mechanisms responsible for the creation of a harmonious organism.

Deviations from the normal may occur at any step of this progressive segregation of the organism; the genetic code of the zygote may be defective or misleading at some point and may result in abnormal development at the stage of embryogenesis where this particular locus is normally expressed. Or, some exogenous factor may affect this expression at any step in the chain of events beginning with the transcription of the genomic information and ending in the formation of complex organs. Consequently, our ideas on the formation of defects should be based on knowledge of normal developmental events, and especially of the regulatory mechanisms of embryogenesis.

In what follows, an endeavor is made to provide a very brief summary of our present, still fragmentary knowledge of certain major developmental events and their control mechanisms, and to outline how these could be affected so as to result in abnormal embryogenesis and congenital defects. For further details,

From the Third Department of Pathology, University of Helsinki, Helsinki, Finland.

the reader is recommended to consult the following reviews: Zwilling,[33] Lash,[15] DeHaan,[6] and Saxén and Rapola.[26]

CONTROL OF NORMAL GROWTH AND DEVELOPMENT

To illustrate some steps in normal development and the control systems regulating them, the ontogenesis of a completely hypothetic organ is illustrated in Figure 1.

Before they can express their developmental capacities, the cells in a certain population have to create a certain *minimal mass or minimal density*, below which no differentiation takes place.[12, 27] Two fundamentally different ways of achieving this goal can be suggested: *multiplication* and/or *aggregation* of cells in a certain colony. Both mechanisms seem to operate during normal development and both seem to be controlled by environmental mechanisms. Several growth-controlling factors have been detected or suggested, including, in addition to hormones, such target-specific devices as erythropoietin, nerve growth-promoting factor, and epidermal chalone(s),[2, 16, 32] and morphogenetic tissue interactions which seem to involve mitotic stimulation.[25, 30] Aggregation at an early stage of development apparently results from changes in the cell surface leading to altered adhesive properties, creating dense populations; here, too, it has been suggested that there is an exogenous triggering of such changes.[11, 28]

In our hypothetic developmental model (Fig. 1), aggregation was preceded by *determination* transmitted through *inductive stimuli*. In a great variety of developmental processes and steps, such determinative interactions between tissues have been detected, suggesting that differentiation of a particular cell population is triggered or controlled by the neighboring tissues, the inductors.[10, 25] Inside these induced, determined cell colonies, different types of kinetic processes can now take place: the ran-

DEFECTIVE REGULATORY MECHANISMS

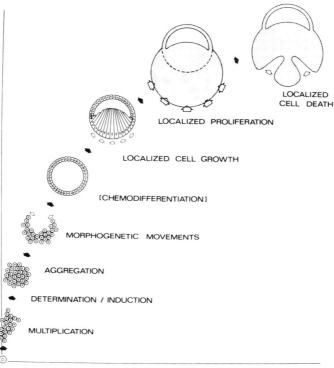

LOCALIZED
CELL DEATH

LOCALIZED PROLIFERATION

LOCALIZED CELL GROWTH

[CHEMODIFFERENTIATION]

MORPHOGENETIC MOVEMENTS

AGGREGATION

DETERMINATION / INDUCTION

MULTIPLICATION

FIG. 1

domly moving cells may be trapped in particular aggregation centers, they may selectively move toward certain points, or the whole cell cluster may show oriented migrations. Again, environmental conducting systems are known to exist.[5, 29] In our model organ, such oriented migrations of cells lead to the formation of a vesicle or closure of a tube and this stage is followed by processes creating asymmetry of this luminated mass.

Again, different ways of reaching this goal can be suggested. One would be *local enlargement or elongation of the cells*, as seen during the development of the vertebrate lens, and another would be *local growth by mitotic stimulation*, as shown in the early development of the central nervous system. In both of these cases, as might be expected, the stimulatory action of the neighboring mesenchymal tissue has been established.[14, 20]

Finally, a most interesting developmental event is included in our scheme. *Localized cell death*, leading to the shaping and carving out of embryonic organs, is known to play a cen-

tral role in the development of various structures, for example in limb morphogenesis. As this necrosis must take place at a strictly defined time and place, it is not surprising to find that the event is, again, controlled by exogenous factors, such as certain hormones and neighboring tissues.[22, 24]

In conclusion, we may state that normal embryogenesis consists of a series of sequential events at subcellular, cellular, and tissue levels, where the species-specific information of the genomic DNA is expressed, but only after having been triggered by epigenetic factors and only under the strict control of its micromilieu. We may now ask whether there are any examples, proven or suspected, in which defects in these major events and their regulatory mechanisms ultimately lead to abnormal development. When trying to answer this question, I shall use the hypothetic organ model already illustrated in Figure 1 but shall, in addition, make an effort to find illustrative examples from experimental teratology and fetal pathology.

DEFECTIVE REGULATIVE MECHANISMS

Proliferation, Determination, and Aggregation

Experimental work employing mitotic inhibitors (irradiation, radiomimetic drugs) has shown that blocking proliferation at certain sensitive periods may totally prevent further differentiation and, hence, lead to *agenesis* of the organ in question. If applied during later stages, when the cells have undergone their terminal mitosis and have reached the number and density required for the "critical mass," although differentiation need not be affected, the actual growth of the anlage is prevented. Here the resulting *hypoplasia* is not attributable to small abnormal cells, as in malnourished infants, but to an actually decreased number of cells. Analogously, Naeye and Blanc[18] have concluded that the hypoplastic organs of infants with congenital rubella contain a subnormal number of cells. This, again, seems not to be attributable to loss of cells during infection but rather to an inhibitory action of the virus on cell multiplication. Agenesis of an organ may also be traced back to lack of an inductive stimulus, as can easily be demonstrated experimentally in Amphibian embryos. In a certain anophthalmic strain of mice thoroughly analyzed by Chase and Chase[3] in 1941, 90% of the embryos are born eyeless. During the early development of these embryos, the optic cup is seemingly normal but soon becomes definitely retarded in its growth and does not reach the overlying epidermis, the presumptive lens. Since the formation of the latter is triggered by an inductive stimulus supplied by the optic cup, no lens develops in these embryos and this again seems to affect the differentiation of the optic vesicle, which remains small and rudimentary. The example thus demonstrates a defect apparently attributable to a complex mechanism, where retarded growth is the primary (?) defect resulting in distorted inductive interactions and, consequently, agenesis.

A variety of other mutants have been detected in the chick and the mouse, where defective interactive processes, resulting from lost activity of the inductor, lack of contact, or lost responsiveness of the target tissue, lead to congenital defects.[15, 26, 33]

As already stated, the critical mass or density required for the expression of the developmental capacities of a given cell population may be obtained not only through increased proliferation but also through aggregation or condensation of the cells (as in some colonies of unicellular organisms) (Fig. 2). Distortion at this stage may lead to abnormally small, dispersed aggregates instead of to a single, solid organ anlage. Consequently, two alternative courses of development may be expected: ei-

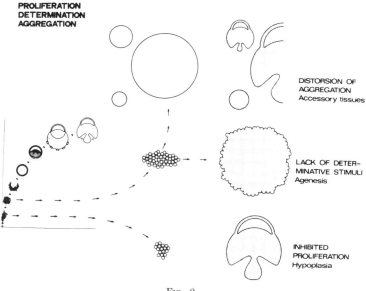

PROLIFERATION
DETERMINATION
AGGREGATION

DISTORSION OF AGGREGATION
Accessory tissues

LACK OF DETERMINATIVE STIMULI
Agenesis

INHIBITED PROLIFERATION
Hypoplasia

Fig. 2

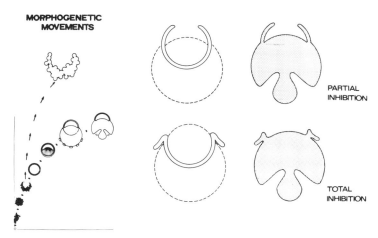

FIG. 3

ther the accessory masses are below the critical one and do not differentiate, or they develop into small, hypoplastic accessory organs. Whether this is the actual mechanism behind the many accessory tissues and organs known to every pathologist cannot yet be decided, however.

Abnormal adhesiveness of cells might, in addition, affect development in another way. Ede and Agerbak[8] have recently analyzed this in the talpid[3] mutant chick, which has abnormally shaped wing buds. Observations on the aggregation pattern of disaggregated wing bud cells from mutant chicks, as compared to that of cells from wild-type embryos, suggested an increased mutual adhesiveness of the mutant cells. This may, in fact, affect the normal migrations of cells in the mesodermal blastema and thus lead to abnormally shaped wings. Such inhibited movements and migrations of cells and cell clusters have been shown to be the causal mechanism in some other defects as well, as will be discussed in the next section.

Morphogenetic Movements

The migratory process of the cells in our model organ may bear a resemblance to the closure of the neural tube, and the defects illustrated in Figure 3 would correspondingly represent different degrees of the defect myeloschisis. Another common defect probably attributable to incomplete morphogenetic movements is cleft palate.[9]

An elegant experimental demonstration of the causative role of prevented migratory processes in teratogenesis has been presented by

DeHaan.[4] The vertebrate heart is formed from a paired mass of precardiac mesodermal cells, which migrate from their lateral position to the ventral midline, where they fuse. The oriented migration of these clusters can be followed by time-lapse cinematography and experimental evidence suggests that the movement is guided by the underlying entoderm. Treatment of the explant with chelating agents, which remove the divalent cations from the cell periphery, apparently prevents migration through interference with cell contacts and results in a paired heart, cardia bifida. Addition of calcium ions in concentrations equimolar to that of the chelating agent abolishes the teratogenic action of the latter.

Localized Cell Growth and Multiplication

Asymmetry in our model organ was created through uneven distribution of growth (elongation) and proliferation of the cells. The scheme in Figure 4 illustrates some hypothetic consequences of inhibited, misplaced, or excessive elongation of the cells, but there are no examples where this mechanism has been convincingly shown to be of causal significance. It may be of interest, however, to quote some recent observations from my laboratory.[13] When lens primordia of 25- to 35-somite mouse embryos are separated from their normal control system (see above) and cultivated in vitro, all of the types illustrated in the scheme are frequently detected.

Inhibition of cell multiplication has already been mentioned in connection with the early proliferation preceding organogenesis. More

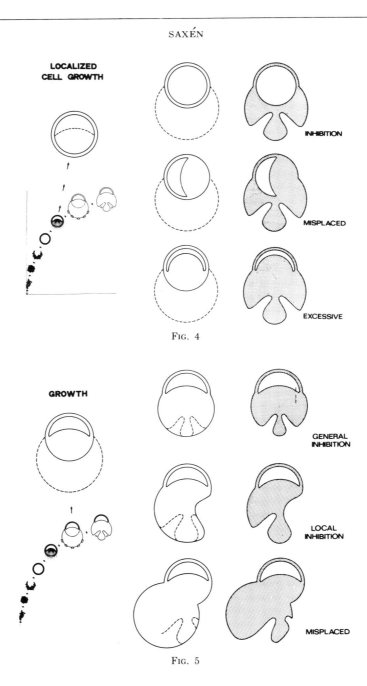

LOCALIZED
CELL GROWTH

INHIBITION

MISPLACED

EXCESSIVE

FIG. 4

GROWTH

GENERAL
INHIBITION

LOCAL
INHIBITION

MISPLACED

FIG. 5

selective effects, affecting only a certain organ anlage or part of it, are obtained during organogenesis as a result of the different sensitive periods of the various tissues involved. If a whole embryo is irradiated during different periods of development, the results vary greatly and apparently tissues of high mitotic activity are preferentially affected.[1, 21] If our model organ is irradiated during its period of rapid growth, a general inhibition and hypoplasia would result (Fig. 5). The microcephalic babies born to the survivors of the atomic bombings in Japan may be included in this group of defective development.[35]

85

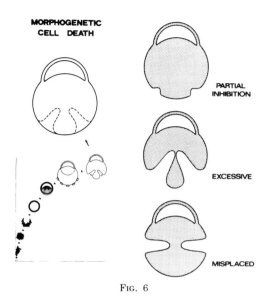

MORPHOGENETIC CELL DEATH

PARTIAL INHIBITION

EXCESSIVE

MISPLACED

FIG. 6

More localized inhibition, as illustrated in Figure 5, may, at least theoretically, be obtained by strictly localized inhibitors (e.g. viruses affecting cell multiplication). Experimentally, these are extremely difficult to produce, despite some technics by which the embryo is irradiated and partially shielded. As one of the defects probably resulting from such local growth inhibition, septal defects of the heart may be mentioned, although the same end result may be brought about by other mechanisms (such as extensive resorption, to be discussed below).[6]

Quantitatively normal but misplaced growth should be considered as a third possibility of abnormal proliferation. An example, in all probability related to this mechanism, will be given, where growth at an abnormal site has caused a complicated "syndrome" of malformations. The partitioning of the truncus arteriosus is achieved through the development of two opposing folds, dividing the truncus into the pulmonary artery and the aorta. If this division takes place unequally through misplaced growth of one of the folds, the result is a defect known as the tetrad of Fallot: a small pulmonary trunk and a large aorta overriding the interventricular septum.[19]

Finally, a generalized, systemic overgrowth may be mentioned (not included in the scheme). Generalized hypertrophy of the skeleton occurs in the condition known as multiple exostoses and a corresponding general hypertrophy of a particular organ has been de-

scribed in the mutant mouse strain t^{w18}. Here, the primitive streak shows excessive growth, causing malformations in the derivatives of the overlying ectoderm.[7]

Morphogenetic Cell Death

Total or partial inhibition of the interdigital necroses, leading to separation of the digits and carving of the normal hand or foot, should result in soft-part syndactyly. Treatment of chick embryos with Janus green prior to the onset of this localized cell death does, in fact, cause such syndactyly, and analysis of the development of these embryos indicates that the normal necrotic process was inhibited.[17, 23] In human pathology, a great many developmental vestiges are known which apparently result from inhibited normal resorption, but their causal mechanisms are wholly obscure.[31]

One example will be given of excessive "normal" cell death leading to maldevelopment. The knee joint, during normal organogenesis, is delineated by a zone of necrotic cells. When chick embryos are treated with insulin during the early stages of limb development, this normal zone of dying cells is widened and leads to micromelia, as shown by Zwilling.[34] Whether some defects in human embryos, such as atrial septal defects or certain skeletal malformations, can be attributed to excessive spread of normal necrotic foci remains to be studied. The same is true of the misplaced morphogenetic necrosis, included in Figure 6 as a theoretic possibility.

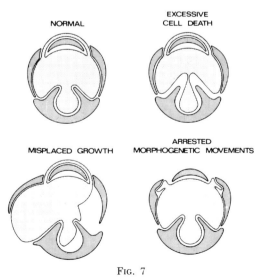

NORMAL   EXCESSIVE CELL DEATH

MISPLACED GROWTH   ARRESTED MORPHOGENETIC MOVEMENTS

FIG. 7

COMMENTS ON THE COMPLEXITY OF THE PROBLEM

As stated in the introductory comments on normal developmental mechanisms, organogenesis involves a great variety of sequential events, each controlled by the microenvironment provided by the neighboring tissues in the complex organism. Hence, it is always difficult and unjustifiable to extract a single step or a single tissue from this progressive development and to pinpoint this as the causative event underlying maldevelopment. Inhibition of growth or morphogenetic migration leads to profound disorganization of the particular sites in the embryo, as illustrated in Figure 7, and this will definitely affect further tissue interactions controlling differentiation, growth, and resorption of the interactants. This extreme complexity of the situation and the dynamic nature of the developing organism under exploration may explain our poor and fragmentary knowledge of the genesis of congenital malformations and the defects in the normal control mechanism.

REFERENCES

1. Brent, R. L. The effect of irradiation on the mammalian fetus. Clin. Obstet. Gynec., 3: 928, 1960.
2. Bullough, W. S. Mitotic and functional homeostasis. A speculative review. Cancer Res., 25: 1683, 1965.
3. Chase, H. B., and Chase, E. B. Studies on an anophthalmic strain of mice. I. Embryology of the eye region. J. Morph., 68: 279, 1941.
4. DeHaan, R. L. Cell migration and morphogenetic movements. In McElroy, W. D., and Glass, B.: The Chemical Basis of Development. Johns Hopkins Press, Baltimore, 1958, p. 339.
5. DeHaan, R. L. Cell interactions and oriented movements during development. J. Exp. Zool., 157: 127, 1964.
6. DeHaan, R. L. Development of form in the embryonic heart. An experimental approach. Circulation, 35: 821, 1967.
7. Dunn, L. C., and Bennett, D. Abnormalities associated with a chromosome region in the mouse. I. Transmission and population genetics of the t-region. II. Embryological effects of lethal alleles in the t-region. Science, 144: 260, 1964.
8. Ede, D. A., and Agerbak, G. S. Cell adhesion and movement in relation to the developing limb pattern in normal and talpid mutant chick embryos. J. Embryol. Exp. Morph., 20: 81, 1968.
9. Fraser, F. C. Some genetic aspects of teratology. In Wilson, J. G., and Warkany, J.: Teratology, Principles and Techniques. University of Chicago Press, Chicago, 1965, p. 21.
10. Grobstein, C. Inductive tissue interaction in development. Advances Cancer Res., 4: 187, 1956.
11. Grobstein, C. Interactive processes in cytodifferentiation. J. Cell. Comp. Physiol., 60: Suppl. 1, 35, 1962.
12. Grobstein, C., and Zwilling, E. Modification of growth and differentiation of chorio-allantoic grafts of chick blastoderm pieces after cultivation at a glass-clot interface. J. Exp. Zool., 122: 259, 1953.
13. Jääskeläinen, M., unpublished data.
14. Källen, B. Contribution to the knowledge of the regulation of the proliferation processes in the vertebrate brain during ontogenesis. Acta Anat. (Basel), 27: 351, 1956.
15. Lash, J. W. Normal embryology and teratogenesis. Implications for pathological development from experimental embryology. Amer. J. Obstet. Gynec., 90: 1193, 1964.
16. Levi-Montalcini, R. The nerve growth factor. Its mode of action on sensory and sympathetic nerve cells. Harvey Lect., 60: 217, 1966.
17. Menkes, B., and Deleanu, M. Leg differentiation and experimental syndactyly in chick embryo. II. Experimental syndactyly in chick embryo. Rev. Roumaine Embriol. Cytol., 1: 69, 1964.
18. Naeye, R. L., and Blanc, W. Pathogenesis of congenital rubella. J. A. M. A., 194: 1277, 1965.
19. Patten, B. M. Varying developmental mechanisms in teratology. In Warkany, J.: Congenital Malformations. Pediatrics, Suppl. 19, 734, 1957.
20. Philpott, G. W., and Coulombre, A. J. Cytodifferentiation of pre-cultured embryonic chick lens epithelial cells in vitro and in vivo. Exp. Cell Res., 52: 140, 1968.
21. Russell, L. B., and Russell, W. L. An analysis of the changing radiation response of the developing mouse embryo. J. Cell. Comp. Physiol., 43: Suppl. 1, 103, 1954.
22. Saunders, J. W., Jr. Death in embryonic systems. Science, 154: 604, 1966.
23. Saunders, J. W., Jr., and Fallon, J. F. Cell death in morphogenesis. In Locke, M.: Major Problems in Developmental Biology. Academic Press, New York, 1966, p. 289.
24. Saunders, J. W., Jr., and Gasseling, M. T. Ectodermal-mesenchymal interactions in the origin of limb symmetry. In Fleischmajer, R., and Billingham, R. E.: Epithelial-Mesenchymal Interactions. The William & Wilkins Co., Baltimore, 1968, p. 78.
25. Saxén, L., and Kohonen, J. Inductive tissue interactions in vertebrate morphogenesis. Int. Rev. Exp. Path., 69: 57, 1969.
26. Saxén, L., and Rapola, J. Congenital Defects. Holt, Rinehart and Winston, Inc., New York, 1969.
27. Saxén, L., and Toivonen, S. Primary Embryonic Induction. Academic Press, London, 1962.
28. Saxén, L., and Wartiovaara, J. Cell contacts and cell adhesion during tissue organization. Int. J. Cancer, 1: 271, 1966.
29. Trinkaus, J. P. Morphogenetic cell movements. In Locke, M.: Major Problems in Developmental Biology. Academic Press, New York, 1966, p. 125.
30. Wessells, N. K. Tissue interaction and cytodifferentiation. J. Exp. Zool., 157: 139, 1964.
31. Willis, R. A. The Borderland of Embryology and Pathology. Butterworth & Co., Ltd., London, 1958.
32. Wilt, F. H. The control of embryonic hemoglobin synthesis. Advances Morph., 6: 89, 1967.
33. Zwilling, E. Teratogenesis. In Willier, B. H., Weiss, P. A., and Hamburger, V.: Analysis of Development. W. B. Saunders Co., Philadelphia, 1955, p. 699.
34. Zwilling, E. Micromelia as a direct effect of insulin. Evidence from in vitro and in vivo experiment. J. Morph., 104: 159, 1959.
35. Yamazaki, J. N., Wright, S. W., and Wright, P. M. A study of the outcome of pregnancy in women exposed to the atomic bomb blast in Nagasaki. J. Cell. Comp. Physiol., 43: Suppl. 1, 319, 1954.

PAPER 9

9. Wilson, J. G. (1972). Mechanisms of teratogenesis. *Am. J. Anat.*, **136**, 129–132

COMMENTARY

The primary objectives of all teratological investigations are the identification of causal teratogenic agents, the elucidation of the mechanisms whereby these agents produce their effects, and the prevention, where possible, of birth defects. Although congenital malformations have been induced in experimental animals by a wide range of teratogens (Shepard, 1976), attempts to locate the cellular and biochemical sites of action have not been intensively pursued.

Several theories of teratogenesis have been proposed. In most cases, these are either speculative or based on insufficient experimental data. The exact mechanisms by which drugs and other environmental factors interfere with embryonic development and so produce abnormalities remain obscure.

The paper by Wilson (1972) is a brief review of *possible* mechanisms of abnormal development. It is derived from the voluminous literature of experimental teratology, and whether similar mechanisms are involved in man is difficult to ascertain at the present time. The teratological responses and mechanisms discussed represent significant alterations in fundamental biological processes. These are likely to be primary lesions, but their relative importance may very well change with the accumulation of more information.

As pointed out by Wilson, this listing of teratological mechanisms is incomplete and should be considered as being provisional. Nonetheless, these guidelines provide a basis for the interpretation and elucidation of most developmental defects in terms of cellular and subcellular mechanisms.

REFERENCE

Shepard, T. H. (1976). *Catalog of Teratogenic Agents.* (Baltimore: The Johns Hopkins University Press)

From J. G. Wilson (1972). Am. J. Anat., **136**, 129–131. *Copyright* (1972),
by kind permission of the author and the Wistar Institute Press

EDITORIAL

Mechanisms of Teratogenesis

Man's early pictorial and written records make it clear that he was aware of and curious about the structural defects that from birth afflicted some of his fellow men. His attitudes about these congenital variants have ranged widely in different cultures: from romanticizing them in mythology, to using them as portent of coming events, to accepting them as divine retribution for wrongdoing, to simply regarding them as manifestations of witchcraft. Historical medical writings contain descriptions of the more bizarre malformations but explanations as to their genesis, if not always as fanciful as those seated in popular superstition, were equally fatalistic in outlook.

The rediscovery of Mendel's laws of genetics at the beginning of the present century, while providing a scientific explanation for some developmental abnormality, may actually have hampered a full appreciation of the causes of maldevelopment. A new form of fatalism resulted from the easy assumption that all abnormal development was determined by the genes, an attitude which dominated medical thought during the first half of the century.

German measles, thalidomide and a spate of experimental studies have made it unequivocally clear that maldevelopment is also initiated by environmental factors, as well as by these interacting with genetic factors. It has also become apparent that the recognition of hundreds of new causative factors has not provided much insight into the underlying mechanisms of abnormal development. How does an adverse influence in the environment initiate a sequence of changes within an embryo or a germ cell that will ultimately lead to a structural or functional deviation in development? Modern teratology accepts the view that the final defect, whether intrauterine death, malformation, growth retardation, or functional deficiency, is preceded by a series of abnormal events in embryogenesis which in total comprise the pathogenesis of deviant development. But which of these events is the key in determining the nature and incidence of the final defect?

It has been suggested that the first reaction within an embryonic or a germinal cell to an adverse influence from the environment is important, not only in initiating, but also in determining the direction of subsequent pathogenesis. Difficulty arises, however, in identifying this initial reaction, which probably most often lies at the molecular level. Until the events in pathogenesis are better known, therefore, it is prudent to apply the term *mechanism of teratogenesis* tentatively to the earliest recognizable event thought to have played a primary role in abnormal development.

EDITORIAL

On sifting through the literature of experimental teratology, it is possible to deduce that there are perhaps eight or ten general types of reactions by which developing cells might respond to environmental stimuli in ways that could lead to deviations in later embryogenesis. Such of these as can at present be supported by scientific evidence or by strong logical presumption are proposed as mechanisms of teratogenesis, in the loose sense stated above.

1. *Mutation* is the mechanism by which the nucleotide sequence in nuclear DNA strands is altered in such a way as to change the developmental potential of progeny cells. If the change occurs in a germinal cell, it is heritable and is called a germinal mutation; if in developing somatic cells, it is not heritable, is called a somatic mutation, and may cause a developmental defect or possibly a neoplasm, but only in that individual.

2. *Chromosomal aberrations*, including nondisjunction and loss or translocation of parts of chromatids, result in visible excess or deficiency of chromatin material in progeny cells. A high percentage of affected individuals do not survive to term but those that do often show both structural and functional abnormality.

3. *Mitotic interference* is a term of convenience to include the several ways in which proliferative rate can be changed by disturbing the cell cycle. Among the known ways are reduced DNA biosynthesis (replication), interference with formation or separation of chromatids (e.g., "stickiness" seen after irradiation) and failure of formation or maintenance of the microtubules necessary for the mitotic spindle (e.g., colchicine effect).

4. *Altered nucleic acid synthesis and function*, exclusive of the above effects on DNA, includes the means by which several antibiotic and antineoplastic drugs interfere with the expression of genetic information during development. For the most part this mechanism concerns the synthesis or translation of one or another variety of RNA.

5. *Lack of precursors, substrates, and coenzymes for biosynthesis* is the mechanism by which nutritional deficiency leads to abnormal development. Failure of absorption or inadequate transport can also result in an insufficient supply of the anabolites needed in development.

6. *Altered energy sources*, aside from the shortage of extrinsic anabolites just noted, includes other interference with the uninterrupted supply of energy necessary for biosynthesis, proliferation and other developmental processes. In addition to the direct means of disrupting anaerobic and aerobic metabolism, analogues of the coenzymes required for cellular energy production, e.g., 6-aminonicotinamide and galactoflavin, are teratogenic as well as embryolethal.

7. *Enzyme inhibition* of specific enzymes, such as dihydrofolate reductase, thymidylate synthetase and carbonic anhydrase, is thought to be primarily involved in initiating abnormal development by interfering in particular metabolic activities. On the other hand, more general enzyme poisons in sufficient dose would likely result in immediate embryonic death.

EDITORIAL

8. *Osmolar imbalance* can be readily induced and has been shown to act as a primary mechanism of teratogenesis by altering fluid pressures, viscosities and composition in different compartments of the embryo. Embryos appear to lack much of the homeostatic regulation available to fetal or postnatal animals.

9. *Changed membrane characteristics* can lead to osmolar imbalance, as above, but probably also can interfere with essential transport functions across cell membranes, or even across the placenta, without appreciable alteration of fluid or osmolite balance.

Additional mechanisms will probably be recognized, just as some of those now proposed will doubtless be found to be secondary to more important primary reactions, but one cannot wait for the final list to be compiled. Research toward better understanding of underlying mechanisms must be intensified if prevention of developmental defects is in any measure to be achieved. The anticipation of teratological risks in today's rapidly changing environment becomes an endless succession of screening tests of individual agents (new drugs, pesticides, food additives, radiations, etc.) unless a knowledge of mechanisms can lead to shortcuts. Furthermore, the application of animal test data to the evaluation of human teratological risk becomes more than empirical only as the degree of comparability of mechanisms between man and animal is better understood.

JAMES G. WILSON

Children's Hospital Research Foundation
and Departments of Pediatrics and Anatomy,
University of Cincinnati College of Medicine

PAPER 10

10. Dunn, P. M. (1972). Congenital postural deformities: perinatal associations. *Proc. R. Soc. Med.*, **65**, No. 8, 735–738.

COMMENTARY

Hippocrates had postulated that intrauterine mechanical influences could disturb fetal growth and development and so produce certain malformations. A similar hypothesis was proposed by Harvey. In more recent times, Sir Dennis Browne (1967), Torpin (1968), and Dunn (1976, and Paper 10) have advocated that mechanical factors are responsible for certain congenital deformities, such as talipes, sternomastoid torticollis, postural scoliosis, and dislocation of the hip. Malposition or the prolonged folding of the fetus in an abnormal position, decreased intrauterine space, and increased mechanical pressure were considered to be the primary causes for this 'intrauterine moulding' of the fetus.

In contrast, others (see Streeter, 1930; Torpin, 1968) have suggested that the formation of amniotic bands, following rupture of the amniotic cavity, and the constrictive effect of these bands on fetal parts, were the causes of some malformations, in particular, reduction abnormalities of the limbs. Streeter (1930), who studied a large number of human limb malformations, concluded that spontaneous amputations were due to 'focal deficiencies or inferior quality of the limb mesenchyme'.

The involvement of mechanical mechanisms in certain congenital deformities is now widely accepted, and from this standpoint Dunn's paper is of considerable interest. Based on his own extensive clinical observations, Dunn argues convincingly that certain non-teratological congenital deformities, i.e. defects arising after embryogenesis is completed from previously normally formed parts, could be caused by mechanical factors acting on the fetus. He suggested that the frequency of these postural congenital defects is influenced by the growth rate of the fetus, fetal plasticity and fetal mobility, in addition to fetal compression. These types of congenital abnormalities are present in approximately 2% of all newborns, but in the majority of cases correct themselves spontaneously after birth.

Dunn (1974, 1976) has also recently reported that a significant association exists between the different groups of congenital postural defects and that these are related to several maternal and fetal characteristics. These include primigravidity, maternal hypertension, breech-presentation, utero-placental insufficiency, fetal growth retardation, polyhydramnios, and oligohydramnios.

Oligohydramnios appeared to be of considerable importance because a large number of cases of congenital deformities were found in association with this condition. Moreover, the malformed infants tended to be small-for-dates and malnourished with signs of fetal distress. For this reason, impairment of uteroplacental function was proposed as an underlying mechanism not only for the oligohydramnios, but also the resulting fetal abnormalities. Polyhydramnios is also frequently associated with major congenital malformations, such as oesophageal atresia, where circulation of amniotic fluid is impaired. Fetal postural anomalies, such as arthrogryposia multiplex congenita, have also been directly attributed to the increased hydraulic pressure resulting from excessive fluid accumulation.

REFERENCES

Browne, D. (1967). A mechanistic interpretation of certain malformations. In D. H. M. Woollam (ed.). *Advances in Teratology*, Vol. 2, pp. 11–36. (New York: Academic Press)

Dunn, P. (1974). Congenital postural deformities: Further perinatal associations. *Proc. R. Soc. Med.*, **67**, 1174–1178

Dunn, P. M. (1976). Congenital postural deformities. *Br. Med. Bull.*, **32**, 71–76

Streeter, G. L. (1930). Focal deficiencies in fetal tissues and their relation to intra-uterine amputations. *Contr. Embryol. Carneg. Instn.*, **22**, 1–44

Torpin, R. (1968). *Fetal Malformations Caused by Amnion Rupture During Gestation*. (Springfield, Ill.: Charles C. Thomas)

From P. M. Dunn (1972). *Proc. R. Soc. Med.,* **65,** *No.* 8, 735–738. *Copyright* (1972), *by kind permission of the author and the Royal Society of Medicine*

Congenital Postural Deformities: Perinatal Associations

by Peter M Dunn MA MD
(*University of Bristol,
Department of Child Health,
Southmead Hospital, Bristol, BS10 5NB*)

The belief that certain congenital anomalies might be caused by mechanical factors *in utero* dates back to Hippocrates and has been readvanced in our own times by Browne (1936, 1955) and Chapple & Davidson (1941). However, the hypothesis was for the most part based on anecdotal clinical evidence and, at any rate by 1960, had failed to gain wide support (Browne 1960, Corner 1960). In that year I commenced a number of clinicopathological studies on this subject which were brought together in a thesis in 1969. In this paper I shall summarize some of the epidemiological data collected between 1960 and 1963. Before doing so, however, it is necessary to draw a distinction between congenital malformations and deformations. I use the term 'malformation' to describe defects that are likely to have arisen during the period of organogenesis, while 'deformation' is reserved for defects arising *after* the embryonic period that appear to be alterations in a previously normally formed part. Thus, while the former are essentially teratological embryopathies (Fig 1A), the latter are nonteratological fœtopathies (Fig 1B). Some of the main characteristics and differences between these two groups are shown in Table 1.

In my thesis (Dunn 1969) I reached the conclusions that quite gentle forces, *if persistently applied*, were capable of producing deformities; that such deformation occurred much more readily in the presence of growth; that the fœtus

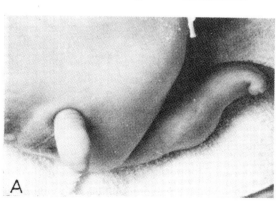
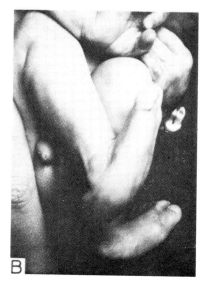

Fig 1 *Typical malformation and deformation* (see text). A, *phocomelia of left lower limb – a teratological embryopathy.* B, *talipes calcaneovalgus – a nonteratological fœtopathy*

Proc. roy. Soc. Med. Volume 65 August 1972

Table 1

Some contrasting characteristics of congenital
malformations and congenital postural deformities

	Malformations	Postural deformations
Incidence before 20th week	5 %+ ●	0.1 % ■
Incidence after 28th week	3.7 % ▲	2.0 % ▲
Perinatal mortality	41 % ▲	6 % ▲
Structural changes	Usual	Rare
Spontaneous correction	Very rare	Usual
Correction by 'posture'	Not possible	Usually possible

● approximate estimation
■ Nishimura (1970)
▲ Dunn (1969)

was particularly vulnerable because of its extremely rapid rate of growth (approximately 50 times faster than in childhood) and because of its relative plasticity; that while prenatal deforming forces might on occasion be of intrinsic origin due to muscle imbalance, most foetuses were exposed to extrinsic forces in the later weeks of pregnancy because of their increasing size and the diminishing volume of amniotic fluid; and that, while some 2 % of newborn infants exhibited one or more musculoskeletal deformities such as talipes, congenital dislocation of the hips (CDH), postural scoliosis or sternomastoid torticollis, the great majority of these deformities either resolved spontaneously after birth or responded to early postural correction.

During 1960 and 1961 personal clinical records were made on all 4754 infants born in the Birmingham Maternity Hospital (BMH) and correlated with data concerning the mothers' medical and pregnancy history and the infants' follow-up records. I examined 97 % of these infants myself. Post-mortem examination was undertaken on 98 % of infants dying during the perinatal period (Dr H G Kohler). In brief, 4486 (94.4 %) of the infants were normally formed, 170 (3.6 %) were malformed (with or without additional deformities) and 98 (2.0 %) had simple postural deformities.

If the various postural deformities have a common mechanical origin, then one would anticipate

finding a proportion of infants with multiple deformities. This was so in the BMH study; 151 distinct deformities were noted among the 98 infants, 33 % of whom had 2 or more deformities ($P<0.001$). The results of a statistical analysis of the BMH data (combined in some instances with additional data from a similar study made in South Warwickshire during 1962–3 involving 2002 infants, 40 of whom exhibited deformities) are shown in Table 2. They demonstrate the highly significant clinical association between the main groups of postural deformities.

Among the 170 malformed infants were 13 (7.6 %) that were also deformed ($P<0.001$). The associations between certain malformations and deformations are worth emphasizing: 11 % of the 54 infants with CNS malformations were deformed ($P \ll 0.001$); 28.6 % of the 28 infants with spinal anomalies (including spina bifida) were deformed ($P \ll 0.001$); likewise, 28.6 % of the 21 infants with just spina bifida were deformed ($P \ll 0.001$); after excluding spina bifida, none of the remaining 33 infants with CNS malformations was deformed. Of the 15 infants with urinary tract malformations 26.7 % were deformed ($P \ll 0.001$). While all 3 infants with bilateral renal anomalies were deformed, none of the 4 with unilateral renal anomalies had deformities ($P=0.028$); in an extended study (Dunn 1969) the significance of this finding was increased to $P \ll 0.001$. While deformities associated with spinal anomalies were almost invariably confined to the lower limbs, those occurring in association with urinary tract malformation involved the upper half of the body as frequently as the lower half ($P \ll 0.001$). Infants with 4 or more deformities were more often found among those with urinary tract anomalies than among those with spinal malformations ($P=0.019$). Only 1 (0.7 %) of the 131 malformed infants without either spinal or urinary tract anomalies was also deformed (an infant with syndactyly) ($P \ll 0.001$).

The association between deformities and certain malformations can be readily explained within the

Table 2

Statistical analysis of studies made during 1960–63 of the
clinical associations between certain congenital postural deformities (*see text*)

	Facial deformities	Plagiocephaly	Mandibular asymmetry	Sternomastoid contracture	Scoliosis (postural)	CDH	Talipes
Facial deformities	—	S	S+	S	S+	S+	S+
Plagiocephaly	S	—	S+	S+	S+	S+	N
Mandibular asymmetry	S+	S+	—	S+	N	S+	S+
Sternomastoid contracture	S	S+	S+	—	S+	N	S+
Scoliosis (postural)	S+	S+	N	S+	—	S+	S
CDH	S+	S+	S+	N	S+	—	S+
Talipes	S+	N	S+	S+	S	S+	—

N, not significant. S, $P<0.05$. S+, $P<0.001$

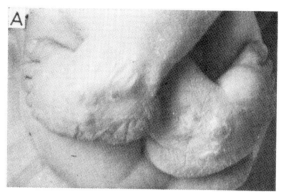

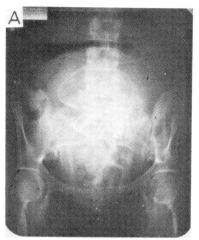

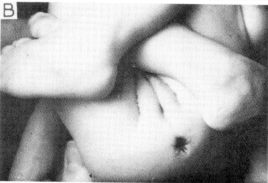

Fig 2 *Bilateral talipes equinovarus associated with fœtal cross-legged position (confirmed by prenatal X-ray).* A, *due to extrinsic pressure: severe maternal oligohydramnios and breech presentation; infant also had deformities of skull, and jaw and a left CDH; note characteristic pressure atrophy and dimpling over external malleoli.* B, *due to intrinsic pressure: maternal polyhydramnios; infant had lumbar spina bifida; legs partially paralysed; note also patulous anus and absence of skin changes over ankles*

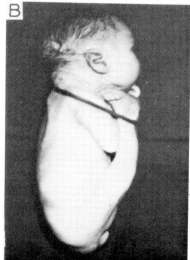

mechanical theory. The legs of infants with spina bifida and other spinal anomalies may be partially paralysed and the resulting muscular imbalance may give rise to an intrinsic deforming force. In addition, paralysis of the lower limbs may deprive the fœtus of its ability to kick and hence change its position *in utero* and alter the direction along which any potentially deforming extrinsic force may be acting. Certainly all prenatal circumstances that might be expected to impair or deprive the fœtus of its ability to move *in utero* have, in my experience, a highly significant association with congenital deformation. Even normal infants are prone to deformation if their legs are folded or trapped in such a way as to make kicking difficult. The best examples of this are the cross-legged position (Fig 2A, B) and the breech presentation with extended legs (Fig 3A, B) (Dunn 1969). Further studies have also demon-

Fig 3A, *prenatal and,* B, *postnatal views of female infant with bilateral renal agenesis. Note oligohydramnios and compressed appearance with breech presentation and extended legs. The baby weighed 1930 g at delivery at 37 weeks and died on the first day of life. Deformities included dolichocephaly, Potter's facies and bilateral CDH*

strated the association of other less common congenital disorders of neuromuscular function with congenital deformation (including, as an extreme form, arthrogryposis multiplex congenita). Another prenatal circumstance which will tend to prevent the fœtus from moving and at the same time expose it to extrinsic pressure is oligohydramnios. There can be no doubt that this is the main cause of the generalized com-

Proc. roy. Soc. Med. Volume 65 August 1972

pression of infants with bilateral renal anomalies; for oligohydramnios is the rule rather than the exception in such cases. Among the multiple deformities found in such infants are congenital dislocation of the hip in approximately 60% of cases (Dunn 1971a) and a characteristic form of compression facies, first described by Potter (1946), in 100%. 'Potter's syndrome' originally described the association of this facies and other limb deformities with bilateral renal agenesis but, in fact, similar signs of prenatal compression are found with bilateral renal hypoplasia and multicystic kidneys as well as with urethral atresia and urethral valves (Dunn 1969).

Maternal oligohydramnios may also arise as a result of premature rupture of the membranes (PRM) with continued drainage of amniotic fluid, often for several weeks before delivery. The infant in Fig 1B is an example; born 18 weeks after PRM, his deformities included plagiocephaly, Potter's facies, a postural scoliosis, flexion deformities of the knees and talipes calcaneovalgus. In the BMH study, 11 infants were born to mothers with PRM; while none was malformed, 10 were deformed ($P \ll 0.001$). Among the 23 deformities shared among them were 5 examples of Potter's facies, 6 of CDH and 4 of talipes. These and further cases have been discussed elsewhere (Dunn 1971b). Similar observations have been reported by Bain *et al.* (1964).

If oligohydramnios favours deformation, polyhydramnios should protect the foetus from extrinsic pressure. In the BMH study, 103 infants were born to mothers considered to have an excess of amniotic fluid; 71 were normally formed and 32 were malformed. No infant was deformed except one with lumbar spina bifida (Fig 2B) (Dunn 1969). Indeed, in twelve years' study I

have not yet seen a deformed (non-malformed) singleton born to a woman with hydramnios.

I have touched on the four main prenatal factors influencing the incidence of congenital deformation – pressure, whether extrinsic or intrinsic in origin, foetal plasticity including hormonal joint laxity, foetal mobility and the rate of foetal growth. All these factors are, of course, themselves directly or indirectly under the influence of heredity and are involved in a dynamic interplay throughout foetal life. Nature plays her hand to the limit. The price we pay for a larger and more mature infant at birth, better able to withstand the stresses of extrauterine life, is a 2% incidence of congenital postural deformities. Perhaps we ought rather to marvel at the fact that 98% of infants are not deformed at birth and that 90% of those that are will correct themselves spontaneously after birth; with early postural assistance this last figure may be brought near to 100%.

Acknowledgments: I am indebted to Dr B S B Wood and Dr M E MacGregor for permission to study infants in their care and also to the Van Neste Foundation for financial support.

REFERENCES
Bain A D, Smith I I & Gauld I K
(1964) *British Medical Journal* ii, 598
Browne D
(1936) *Proceedings of the Royal Society of Medicine* 29, 1409
(1955) *Archives of Disease in Childhood* 30, 37
(1960) *British Medical Journal* ii, 1806
Chapple C C & Davidson D T
(1941) *Journal of Pediatrics* 18, 483
Corner B (1960) Prematurity. Cassell, London; p 300
Dunn P M
(1969) MD Thesis, Cambridge
(1971a) *Archives of Disease in Childhood* 46, 878
(1971b) *Teratology* 4, 487
Nishimura H (1970) In: Congenital Malformation. Ed. F C Fraser & V A McKusick. Excerpta Medica, Amsterdam; p 275
Potter E L
(1946) *American Journal of Obstetrics and Gynecology* 51 885

PART IV

CYTOGENETIC AND CHROMOSOMAL STUDIES

PAPERS 11 AND 12

11. Barr, M. L. and Bertram, E. G. (1949). A morphological distinction between neurones of the male and female, and the behaviour of the nucleolar satellite during accelerated nucleoprotein synthesis. *Nature (London)*, **163**, 676–677
12. Moore, K. L., Graham, M. A. and Barr, M. L. (1953). The detection of chromosomal sex in hermaphrodites from a skin biopsy. *Surg. Gynecol. Obstet.*, **96**, 641–648

COMMENTARY

In 1949, Barr and Bertram (Paper 11) reported a nuclear sex difference in mammalian cells. The female cells showed a darkly staining chromatin mass in contact with the nuclear membrane; this observation, first made in cat neurones, was confirmed by other workers in 21 of 27 mammalian species studied (Moore, 1960). The sex chromatin (often called the Barr body) is considered to arise from random genetic inactivation of one of the two X-chromosomes in the interphase nucleus of female cells.

Moore *et al.* (Paper 12) were the first to describe the clinical application of the sex chromatin utilizing the skin biopsy test, in two cases of hermaphroditism. Moore and Barr (1955) subsequently found that sex chromatin is also demonstrable in the nuclei of cells obtained by scraping the inside of the cheek. Because the buccal smear technique is relatively simple to perform, it is widely used clinically to determine chromosomal sex.

In 1955, the antenatal determination of fetal sex based on the absence or presence of sex chromatin in amniotic fluid cells was reported. The management of certain severe X-linked genetic diseases, such as haemophilia, Duchenne's or Hunter's syndrome, is dependent upon prenatal determination of fetal sex. The deleterious X-linked recessive genes are expressed in the male, but suppressed in females. If the mother is a heterozygote, 50% of all male offspring may be affected with the condition. Because useful treatment is not available to deal with these conditions, the pregnancy may be terminated by parental consent if the fetus is of the high-risk sex.

In 1970, fluorescent staining of the Y-chromatin with quinacrine has been reported (Pearson, 1970), thereby providing a highly reliable technique for the positive recognition of male fetuses from uncultured amniotic fluid cells. This fluorescent technique together with the sex chromatin test permit the exact number of sex chromosomes present in the fetus to be determined.

The overall accuracy of antenatal sex determination by these two methods ranges from 95 to 100% (see Persaud, 1976); some of their limitations should, however, be pointed out. The sex chromatin is not demonstrable in all normal female cells (46,XX) and it is also absent in persons with Turner's syndrome (45,XO). In addition, the long arm of the Y-chromosome is partially deleted in some males and does not produce an intense fluorescence on staining with quinacrine hydrochloride. It is therefore suggested that the results of sex chromatin and fluorescent Y-bodies be confirmed by subsequent chromosomal analysis in cultured amniotic fluid cells, particularly in cases of high-risk fetuses where termination of pregnancy is contemplated.

REFERENCES

Moore, K. L. (1960). Sex, intersex and the chromatin test. *Mod. Med.*, **15**, 71–80

Moore, K. L. and Barr, M. L. (1955). Smears from the

oral mucosa in the detection of chromosomal sex. *Lancet*, **ii**, 57–58

Pearson, P. L. (1970). A fluorescent technique for identifying human chromatin in a variety of tissues. *Bull. Eur. Soc. Hum. Genet.*, **4**, 35–38

Persaud, T. V. N. (1976). Prenatal diagnosis and its pathologic confirmation. In H. S. Rosenberg and R. P. Bolande (eds.). *Perspectives in Pediatric Pathology*, Vol. 3. (Chicago: Year Book Medical Publishers Inc)

From M. L. Barr and E. G. Bertram (1949). Nature (London), **163**, 676–677.
Copyright (1949), *by kind permission of the authors and Macmillan (Journals) Ltd*

A Morphological Distinction between Neurones of the Male and Female, and the Behaviour of the Nucleolar Satellite during Accelerated Nucleoprotein Synthesis

GENETICISTS have long emphasized that 'maleness' and 'femaleness', so far as chromosome content is concerned, are projected from the fertilized ovum into the morphologically and functionally specialized somatic cells. It appears not to be generally known, however, that the sex of a somatic cell as highly differentiated as a neurone may be detected with no more elaborate equipment than a compound microscope following staining of the tissue by the routine Nissl method.

The observations to be recorded here apply to the cat primarily, since the cat is used routinely in this laboratory for investigations in experimental neurocytology. The nuclei of nerve cells contain a prominent nucleolus which stains readily with such basic dyes as cresyl violet and thionin. The difference in nuclear structure between neurones of adult male and female cats rests on the degree of development of a second body, which is much smaller than the nucleolus. The latter body is more or less intimately associated with the nucleolus and, like the latter, stains well with basic dyes. It has been described by many authors under various names. The term 'nucleolar satellite' will be used in this report, in the hope that students of chromosome morphology will not object too strenuously to the use of the word 'satellite' in this connexion.

Typically, nerve cells of mature *female* cats contain a well-developed nucleolar satellite which is located, as a rule, immediately adjacent to the nucleolus (Fig. 1). A single satellite is usually present; but two may be encountered. The satellite, if more deeply stained than the nucleolus, may be seen in all nerve cells which are sufficiently large to have a prominent nucleolus. More often, the intensity of staining of the nucleolus and its satellite is similar. Under these conditions, the satellite is seen in approximately 30–40 per cent of cells, being invisible when eclipsed by the nucleolus.

As a rule, nerve cells of mature *male* cats (Fig. 2) contain a poorly developed nucleolar satellite, seen only infrequently. When visible, it is situated adjacent to the nucleolus and is near the limit of resolution with an oil-immersion objective.

In a small proportion of animals of both sexes, nucleolar satellites of intermediate size are present.

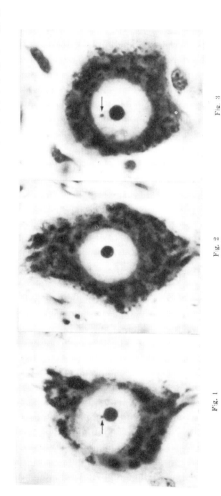

Fig. 1. Normal motor neurone from the hypoglossal nucleus of a mature female cat showing the usual morphology of the nucleolar satellite (indicated by arrow) in the female. Cresyl violet stain, × 1,400

Fig. 2. Motor neurone from the hypoglossal nucleus of a mature male cat. The nucleolar satellite is absent, the typical condition in the mature male. Cresyl violet stain, × 1,400

Fig. 3. Motor neurone from the hypoglossal nucleus of a mature female cat 108 hours following electrical stimulation of the corresponding hypoglossal nerve for a period of 8 hours. Associated with intense synthesis of cytoplasmic ribose nucleoproteins, the nucleolar satellite (indicated by arrow) tends to move away from the nucleolus. Cresyl violet stain, × 1,400

These exceptional cases raise several interesting questions which are now under investigation.

The morphological distinction, therefore, between neurones of the mature male and female cat is so clear that sections from the brain, spinal cord or sympathetic ganglia of animals of both sexes may be readily sorted into two groups without prior knowledge of the sex, with only an occasional section remaining in which the distinctive morphological feature is of an intermediate character.

That there should be a morphological difference in the inter-mitotic nucleus of mature, differentiated cells, according to their sex, is not surprising in view of what is known concerning the relation of the nucleolus to the chromosomes. The nucleolar chromosomes are frequently the sex chromosomes[1]. One may postulate that such is the case in the cat. The nucleolar satellite may be derived from the heterochromatin of the sex chromosomes. Further, the cells of the female cat, because of the duplicated X-chromosomes, may be endowed with a greater quantity of nucleolar associated heterochromatin than are the cells of the male cat. Caspersson and Schultz[2] noted a difference in the absorption curves obtained with ultra-violet light, indicating a difference in nucleoprotein content, in cells of male and female *Drosophila*. These comments suggest the importance of taking the sex into consideration in cytochemical studies of nucleoprotein metabolism.

A preliminary examination of sympathetic ganglia of human males and females indicates that a similar sex difference in nuclear morphology exists in the human. Whether or not such sex differences in nuclear structure will be found in a given species would probably be determined, in part, by the relationship of the nucleolus to the sex chromosomes and by the disparity in size and composition between the X- and Y-chromosomes. It is probable that somatic cells of various tissue, characterized by large nucleoli, will display similar distinctive nuclear differences according to the sex.

We wish to emphasize that these observations apply to mature animals. The influence of the age factor and other aspects of the nucleolar satellite under normal and experimental conditions will be published in later reports.

It is of interest to experimental neurocytologists that the position of the satellite relative to the nucleolus is a useful aid in assessing the physiological state of the cell. In a series of experiments, to be reported in detail elsewhere, depletion of the Nissl material of motor neurones was produced by prolonged electrical stimulation of the hypoglossal nerve. The nucleolus enlarges during the recovery phase, coincident with the re-appearance of abundant Nissl material in the cytoplasm. This observation is in agreement with the views of Caspersson and his co-workers, who regard the nucleolus and the nucleolar associated chromatin as instrumental in the synthesis of ribose nucleoprotein, an important component of the Nissl substance (see Hydén[3] for references). It is of particular interest in the present connexion that the satellite moves away from the nucleolus during the period of intense ribose nucleoprotein synthesis (Fig. 3). The satellite may, in these circumstances, lie in contact with the nuclear membrane. The movement of the nucleolar satellite may be passive, resulting from the outpouring of materials (nucleotides or nucleic acids?) from the region of the nucleolus. On the other hand, complex factors, such as forces of an electrical nature, may be at work. In any case, the position of the satellite is another item for observation, in addition to the appearance of the Nissl substance, in attempting to assess the physiological state of the neurone under experimental conditions. This criterion may be applied to best advantage, of course, only to the cells of female cats. The nucleolar satellite is occasionally found free in the nucleoplasm in control cells. This is regarded as a further indication of the variation in the physiological state of members of a nerve-cell population under normal conditions.

It is hoped that this brief preliminary report may encourage closer attention to the nucleolar satellite in the abundant material available to laboratories of neuropathology in which the Nissl method is constantly in use as a routine staining technique. The possibility that fundamental alterations in the nucleolar associated chromatin may have an important bearing on malignancy gives added interest to these observations.

These observations were made in the course of experiments on the effect of activity on the neurone being done in this laboratory for the Institute of Aviation Medicine, Royal Canadian Air Force. The senior author wishes to thank various members of the staffs of the Department of Neuropathology, University of Toronto, and of the Montreal Neurological Institute, for very helpful discussions.

MURRAY L. BARR
EWART G. BERTRAM

Department of Anatomy,
University of Western Ontario,
London, Canada.
March 3.

[1] Gates, R. R., *Bot. Rev.*, **8**, 337 (1942).
[2] Caspersson, T., and Schultz, J., *Proc. U.S. Nat. Acad. Sci.*, **26**, 507 (1940).
[3] Hydén, H., *Symp. Soc. Exp. Biol.*, **1**, 152 (1947).

From K. L. Moore et al. (1953). Surg. Gynecol. Obstet., **96**, 641–648. *Copyright* (1953),
by kind permission of the author and Surgery, Gynecology and Obstetrics

THE DETECTION OF CHROMOSOMAL SEX IN HERMAPHRODITES FROM A SKIN BIOPSY

KEITH L. MOORE, M.Sc., MARGARET A. GRAHAM, M.Sc., and
MURRAY L. BARR, M.D., London, Ontario, Canada

A CASE of hermaphroditism presents to the physician an exceedingly difficult problem. The tragic status of the patient demands that measures be taken to correct the developmental error, in so far as this is possible. There is little agreement, however, concerning the etiology of hermaphroditism, the criteria on which a decision as to the dominant sex are to be based, or the management of individual cases. In brief, the problem of hermaphroditism appears to have reached an impasse and a new approach is desirable.

Painter, and Evans and Swezy have shown that in humans, females have an XX chromosome combination while males have XY chromosomes as the sex chromosomes. The Y chromosome is small relative to the size of the X chromosome. We have found that the nature of the sex chromosomes (XX or XY) in an individual may be detected by examining the epidermal nuclei in a small biopsy of skin. This technique offers a new approach to the vexatious problem of hermaphroditism.

NORMAL SEX DIFFERENTIATION

Sex is determined at fertilization depending on whether the ovum, with its single X chromosome, is fertilized by a sperm bearing an X or a Y chromosome. Sex differentiation does not begin until the seventh or eighth week of intrauterine life when the previously indifferent gonads show signs of developing into ovaries or testes. Both sex chromosomes and certain autosomes (chromosomes other than the sex chromosomes) bear genes which are concerned with gonadal differentiation. The balance between genes, with a sex-determining function, on the XX chromosomes and similar genes on the autosomes causes the indifferent gonads to develop into ovaries, while the balance between sex-determining genes on the XY chromosomes and autosomes directs indifferent gonads toward development of testes.

A wolffian or male genital duct system and a müllerian or female genital duct system both appear during early embryonic development. The external genitalia develop from sexually indifferent structures. There is disagreement concerning the factors which direct the development of wolffian or müllerian derivatives and the appropriate maturation of the anlage of the external genitalia in later stages. Since the classical work of Lillie on the freemartin in cattle, the majority of biologists have adopted the view that sex hormones of the fetal gonads are responsible for the differentiation of the genital system, once definitive ovaries or testes have been formed. This view is summarized well by Greene (7). Moore (12), on the other hand, was unable to reproduce the freemartin condition by experimental treatment of embryos with sex hormones. He expresses the minority opinion that the gonads do not produce sex hormones during fetal life and that sex differentiation during the intrauterine period is a genetically controlled process without the intervention of sex hormones. Resolution of this problem will be helpful in the eventual understanding of the etiology of developmental sex abnormalities.

TYPES OF HERMAPHRODITISM AND ABNORMAL SEX DIFFERENTIATION

In reviewing the literature on hermaphroditism one is impressed by the kaleidoscopic nature of the condition, produced by many variables appearing in diverse combinations. The Klebs classification, whatever its shortcomings may be, is in common use and has served to systematize this complex developmental abnormality.

From the Department of Anatomy, Faculty of Medicine, University of Western Ontario, London, Canada.
This work was made possible by grants-in-aid to one of the authors (M.L.B.) from the National Cancer Institute and the National Research Council of Canada.

According to the Klebs classification there are true hermaphrodites and pseudo hermaphrodites. The criterion of true hermaphroditism is the presence of ovarian and testicular tissue, either as an ovotestis or as a separate ovary and testis. There is great variability in the anatomy of the external and internal genitalia, in body form and in psychosexual outlook. Such cases are rare, about 50 histologically proved cases of true hermaphroditism having been recorded in the literature.

Pseudohermaphrodites are classified as "male" or "female" depending on whether the gonads are testes or ovaries. The male pseudohermaphrodite group is further subdivided into internal and external types, the former having müllerian duct derivatives in addition to whatever abnormality may be present in the external genitalia. As in the true hermaphrodite group, pseudohermaphrodites show great variation in the morphology of the genital organs, in body form, breast development, growth of hair, as well as in their psychosexual manifestations. Pseudohermaphroditism appears to be more common than is usually thought, the incidence being, according to Young, 1 in 1,000 of the population.

The primary importance which is attached to the gonads is a disquieting feature of this classification. The secondary sex characteristics in pseudohermaphrodites often run counter to the type of gonad. Absurdities result if the Klebs nomenclature is carried over literally into the management of certain cases. It is possible that a new and more reliable classification, based on the sex chromosomes, will arise out of the present work.

The etiology of hermaphroditism in general is not sufficiently well known to merit comment at this time. Two points, however, do stand out clearly. First, regardless of whether or not homones participate in normal fetal sex differentiation, it is certain that some types of hermaphroditism are caused by hormonal dysfunction during fetal life. This applies especially to the large proportion of female pseudohermaphrodites showing the adrenogenital syndrome. In these cases, hyperplasia of the fetal adrenal cortex with excessive production of androgens (often at the expense of other cortical hormones) directs the maturation of the genitalia in a female fetus in the male direction. An androgen-producing tumor in the mother may also cause female pseudohermaphroditism in the child, although such cases are necessarily rare. An especially interesting example was described by Bretnall, the tumor in this instance being an arrhenoblastoma of the ovary. The second well established fact in etiology is the genetic basis of many cases of hermaphroditism of all types, as shown by their familial incidence. A thorough study of the genetics of hermaphroditism would be well worth while. With the exception of the role of the adrenal cortex in one group of cases and the genetic background of many cases of hermaphroditism the etiology of the abnormality is obscure in most important aspects.

PRELIMINARY INVESTIGATIONS WHICH LEAD TO THE DETECTION OF CHROMOSOMAL SEX IN MAN FROM SKIN BIOPSIES

The following brief summary will show that the detection of chromosomal sex in man rests on a firm basis of animal observations.

Tissues of the cat have been studied most extensively. Nerve cell nuclei are most suitable for this work because they are large and vesicular. Nuclear details are obscured in small, pycnotic nuclei. In nerve cell nuclei of the female cat there is, in addition to the large nucleolus, a chromatin mass about 1 micron in diameter. A chromatin body of similar size is seldom seen in nerve cell nuclei of male cats. The chromatin mass is called the sex chromatin in view of its size relation to sex. This sex difference in nuclear morphology is seen to best advantage in larger neurons which are less likely to contain multiple chromatin particles in their nuclei, which make the identification of sex chromatin more difficult. Typical female and male neurons of the cat are illustrated in Figure 1 a and b. The sex chromatin is most frequently adjacent to the nucleolus, as shown in Figure 1 a, but it may be free in the nucleoplasm or adjacent to the nuclear membrane. The sex chromatin gives positive cytochemical tests for desoxyribose nucleic acid. Further details concerning nuclear morphology in nerve cells of the cat have been recorded by Barr, Bertram, and Lindsay.

MOORE ET AL.: SEX IN HERMAPHRODITES BY SKIN BIOPSY

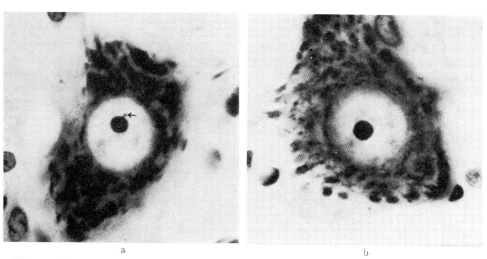

a   b

Fig. 1. a, Motor neuron in the ventral horn of the spinal cord of a *female* cat. The sex chromatin, indicated by the arrow, is adjacent to the nucleolus. Cresyl violet, ×1,000. b, Motor neuron in the ventral horn of the spinal cord of a *male* cat. There is no visible sex chromatin. Occasional male nerve cells show a small mass of chromatin which may be sex chromatin but it is not as large as the typical sex chromatin of female nerve cells. Cresyl violet, ×1,000.

Graham and Barr showed that a similar sex difference in nuclear morphology is present in tissues and organs of the cat generally. In cells other than neurons, however, the sex chromatin takes the form of a planoconvex body with its flattened surface against the nuclear membrane. Moore and Barr (13) made a comparative study of nerve cell nuclei in several mammals. A sex difference in the nuclei, similar to that noted for the cat, was found in the following species—dog, mink, marten, ferret, raccoon, skunk, goat, and deer. The rodents which were studied (guinea pig, rat, mouse, hamster, and ground hog) and the rabbit (a lagomorph) are nonconformists in this regard. Their nerve cell nuclei contain multiple chromatin bodies, adjacent to the nucleolus as a rule, and a sex difference could not be detected. Prince demonstrated a sex difference in nuclear morphology throughout the nervous system of Macacus rhesus. A preliminary general survey of human tissues indicates that the distinctive nuclear morphology, according to sex, is present in man as in many lower animals. With this background, a systematic study of nuclei in human skin was made, because of the availability of this tissue as a biopsy in clinical medicine.

There are good reasons for inferring that the sex chromatin is derived from the sex chromosomes, although direct proof is lacking. The desoxyribose nucleic acid content of the sex chromatin relates it to the chromosomes, which also contain the desoxyribose type of nucleic acid. The sex chromosomes tend to remain compact and deeply staining (i.e. they are heteropycnotic or heterochromatic) when the other chromosomes or autosomes are so diffuse that it is difficult or impossible to identify them individually. This heterochromatic behavior of the sex chromosomes has long been known in developing male germ cells, as shown by Painter for man. Further, Geitler has clearly demonstrated a sex difference in nuclear morphology in somatic cells of insects, on the basis of the heterochromatic property of their sex chromosomes. It is likely, therefore, that in many mammals, including man, the heterochromatic portions of the two X chromosomes of female cells fuse to form a mass of chromatin which is sufficiently large to be readily visible. The small size of the Y chromosome is probably contributory to the minute size of the sex chromatin in male nuclei, rendering it an inconspicuous nuclear constituent with standard microscopic equipment. In general, therefore, it is possible to establish whether nuclei contain XX or XY sex chromosomes on the basis of the size of the sex chromatin and the ease with which it can be identified in a representative sample of nuclei.

THE SEX CHROMATIN OR CHROMOSOMAL SEX IN HUMAN SKIN

Materials and methods. Since others may wish to apply this method of determining chromosomal sex the methods used will be described in some detail.

Specimens of skin from 50 female and 50 male subjects were studied. There were 20 biopsy specimens (10 female and 10 male). The remaining specimens were obtained mainly at autopsy; a few came from the operating room. The genital systems of all subjects were normal to the best of our knowledge. The ages of the subjects ranged from the newborn to 90 years.

The biopsies were taken from staff and students by Dr. W. E. Pace. Although the region from which the biopsy is taken seems unimportant for this work, the extensor surface of the forearm was used as a matter of routine. The area was anesthetized by subcutaneous infiltration of procaine. A small piece of skin, about 0.3 by 0.6 centimeter, was removed and the wound closed with 2 dermal sutures.

Of the various fixatives tried, the following proved most satisfactory. The specimens were fixed for 24 hours in a modified Davidson's solution which has the following formula: formalin 20 parts, 95 per cent alcohol 30 parts, glacial acetic acid 10 parts, and distilled water 30 parts (the 10 parts of glycerine in the original Davidson's solution are omitted). The specimens were then immersed for 24 to 48 hours in 70 per cent alcohol with several changes of solution. A biopsy should be in 70 per cent alcohol for mailing to a distant laboratory, if this is necessary. Routine embedding in paraffin was followed by sectioning at 5 microns.

Sections stained with hematoxylin and eosin are quite satisfactory for the identification of sex chromatin. Best results were obtained by preparation of the hematoxylin according to the method of Harris as described by Gatenby

and Beams (4, section 288). The Feulgen technique, as outlined by Stowell, is also useful since the sex chromatin gives a positive Feulgen reaction because of its desoxyribose nucleic acid content. The nucleolus, containing ribose nucleic acid, is Feulgen-negative.

The sections were studied with an oil immersion objective, attention being directed toward the nuclei of the malpighian layer of the epidermis. A work sheet containing 100 circles representing nuclear outlines is useful. The sex chromatin is drawn in the circle when it can be identified. A minimum of 100 nuclei, selected at random, should be examined in this way and the incidence of visible sex chromatin recorded as a percentage figure.

OBSERVATIONS

Female specimens (Fig. 2 a, b, and c). In most nuclei the sex chromatin is a single, planoconvex body lying against the nuclear membrane. Occasionally the sex chromatin is free in the nucleoplasm or adjacent to the nucleolus. The sex chromatin stains deeply with hematoxylin but there may be a minute pale area within the chromatin mass. In the 50 specimens examined the sex chromatin was visible in from 52 to 85 per cent of nuclei, with an average incidence of 69 per cent. In general it may be said that the sex chromatin can be identified in about two-thirds of the nuclei in 5 micron sections of female epidermis. The real incidence is undoubtedly higher since the sex chromatin will be excluded from the section in some nuclei.

The sex chromatin is recognized most easily when it lies at the periphery of the optical section through the nucleus. With some experience the sex chromatin can also be identified when it lies against a part of the nuclear membrane which is oblique or perpendicular to the optical axis of the microscope. The sex chromatin is Feulgen-positive and stains with methyl green showing that its nucleic acid content is mainly of the desoxyribose type. In addition to one or more nucleoli, which stain less darkly than the sex chromatin, the nucleus contains particulate chromatin with the same staining properties as the sex chromatin. The sex chromatin can be distinguished from unrelated chromatin particles because of its

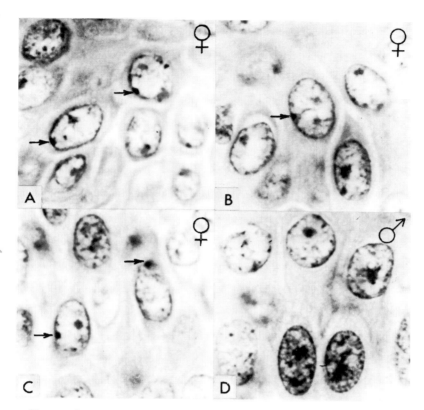

Fig. 2. a, b, and c, Photomicrographs of the malpighian layer of human *female* epidermis. The sex chromatin is indicated by the arrows. By focusing through the thickness of the section, two-thirds of the nuclei are found to contain a mass of sex chromatin located at the periphery of the optical section through the nucleus, as illustrated, or oriented in a different manner. Hematoxylin and eosin, ×1,600. d, Photomicrograph of the malpighian layer of human *male* epidermis. Sex chromatin is not visible in the nuclei and this illustration is characteristic of all focal planes through the section. Hematoxylin and eosin, ×1,600.

larger size, its planoconvex outline when lying against the nuclear membrane as seen in optical section and, at times, the small pale area within the chromatin mass. As noted before, the data available at this time indicate that the sex chromatin of female cells is formed by fusion of heterochromatic regions of the two X chromosomes.

Typical female nuclei are illustrated in Figure 2 a, b, and c, the sex chromatin being indicated by arrows. It is unusual to encounter more than one or two sex chromatin masses in exactly the same focal plane of a field under the high magnification necessary for this work. By focusing through the entire thickness of the section sex chromatin can be seen in about two-thirds of the nuclei, located at the periphery of the optical section of the nucleus as shown, or oriented in a different way.

Male specimens (Fig. 2 d). Nuclei of male epidermis do not contain a chromatin mass which is comparable in size to the sex chromatin of female cells. In the 50 specimens studied from 1 to 14 per cent of nuclei (average 5 per cent) showed a small chromatin mass at the nuclear membrane which may be sex chromatin, although it is difficult to be certain on this point. The evidence available to date indicates that the single X chromosome and the small Y chromosome of male nuclei fail to form a chromatin mass of sufficient size to be distinguished from the general particulate chromatin in most cells. The nucleoli and particulate chromatin are the same in the two sexes. Typical nuclei of male epidermis are illustrated in Figure 2 d. This photomicrograph is characteristic of all focal planes through the section.

With some experience in this work there is no difficulty in sorting sections of skin correctly into male and female groups on the basis of nuclear morphology alone.

THE SEX CHROMATIN IN SKIN BIOPSIES OF HERMAPHRODITES

Severinghaus identified the XY chromosomes in developing germ cells of the testis in a case of male pseudohermaphroditism and Greene and associates (8) identified the XY chromosomes in similar cells in a case of true hermaphroditism. These seem to be the only previous cases in which the particular combination of sex chromosomes has been detected in intersexuality.

It has been our privilege to examine skin biopsies from 2 cases of hermaphroditism. CASE 1. (Courtesy of Drs. W. A. Dafoe and E. A. Morgan.) This is a case of female pseudohermaphroditism with the adrenogenital syndrome. A skin biopsy was studied at the age of about 14 months. The nuclei of the malpighian layer showed a characteristic female morphology, the sex chromatin being visible in 75 per cent of nuclei in a 5 micron section. The sex chromatin was identical with that of the 50 sexually normal females studied earlier, with respect to size, position in the nucleus, and staining properties. This child, therefore, bears the female XX sex chromosome complex, as is to be expected from the clinical diagnosis. The essential points in the case history are as follows.

An enlarged clitoris, absence of labia minora and vaginal introitus, and labia majora rather larger than normal were noted at birth. The infant was registered as a girl. Signs of adrenal cortical insufficiency occurred at the age of 1 month and were brought under control with cortical extract.

The child was admitted to hospital at the age of about 14 months for a more thorough study of the genital system. The clitoris was 3/4 of an inch in length. The urethral meatus was in the usual position for a female but no vaginal introitus could be found. Gonads could not be palpated in the labia or inguinal regions. At laparotomy the uterus, tubes, and ovaries appeared to be normally developed for a child of this age. A biopsy from one gonad showed typical ovarian structure on histologic examination. The adrenals seemed to be of normal size, in so far as this could be determined by palpation.

The adrenogenital syndrome accounts for a considerable proportion of female pseudohermaphrodites. Examination of a skin biopsy is a useful confirmatory diagnostic test and should largely eliminate the necessity of visualizing the internal genitalia by laparotomy in those cases which are still doubtful after urethroscopy and rectal examination. These cases present a serious problem as to management since the virilism is often progressive. The work of Wilkins and associates with cortisone offers some hope that a means of controlling the output of androgen from the hyperplastic adrenal cortex may be found, thus enabling the patient to adopt a life pattern in keeping with her chromosomal sex.

CASE 2. (Courtesy of Drs. W. Kerr and P. Crassweller.) This is probably a case of male pseudohermaphroditism, of the external type predominantly. True hermaphroditism cannot be rigorously excluded without extensive histologic examination of both gonads, although the chances are against such a diagnosis. A skin biopsy was studied when the patient was 24 years old. The morphology of the nuclei in the malpighian layer was indistinguishable from that of the 50 sexually normal males as described previously. A chromatin mass, which may be sex chromatin, was seen in only 4 per cent of nuclei. This individual, therefore, bears the male XY sex chromosomes. Summary of the case history follows.

Abnormal genitalia were noted at birth but the details are not known. The patient was raised as a boy. He was one of a family of 14 children and 1 sibling is said to have external genitalia similar to those of the patient. The patient has been studied in hospitals at distant centers and the complete records are not available. Bilateral mastectomy was performed at the age of 14 and an exploratory laparotomy was done at the age of 15. No ovaries or tubes were found but a testicular element was seen in the left inguinal canal. The following observations pertain to the most recent hospitalization.

The patient was admitted with complaints of tender swellings in the groins and monthly pelvic distress lasting about 8 days, associated with hematuria. The patient was of indeterminate build with no important masculine or feminine characteristics. There was no growth of hair on the face and the distribution of the pubic hair was feminine. The phallus was small. The urethra opened at the base of the phallus and a shallow groove lined with mucous membrane extended from the urethral orifice to the perineal body. The urinary excretion of 17-ketosteroids was 16.6 milligrams in 24 hours.

No evidence of a prostate could be seen on cystoscopic examination. A longitudinal cleft on the enlarged verumontanum lead to a prostatic utricle about 2.5 centimeters long. The floor of this cavity showed fronds which appeared not unlike endometrial tissue. It was believed that this was the source of the periodic bleeding. The enlarged utricle was demonstrated by a urethrogram.

At a later date the gonad (grossly a normal testicle) was removed from the left inguinal region. The gonad on the right side was also exposed. It appeared to be a testicle and was replaced deeply in the inguinal canal after taking a biopsy. Microscopic examination showed the left gonad and the biopsy of the right gonad to consist of testis tissue. The patient is now receiving testosterone.

Although this patient has, we believe, male XY sex chromosomes there appears to have been a genetic factor, in view of the sibling with a similar anomaly, which directed sex differentiation along abnormal lines. If the influence of female sex hormones was involved one cannot say whether they originated in the fetal gonad, adrenal or in the placenta, or whether they may have been of maternal origin. The complex male pseudohermaphrodite group may prove especially profitable in the application of the skin biopsy test of chromosomal sex. The possibility that the nature of the gonads may not always correspond with the chromosomal sex must be entertained. It will be of equal interest to learn the type of sex chromosomes in the rare cases of true hermaphroditism.

DISCUSSION

Although the application of the skin biopsy technique to hermaphrodites is in a preliminary stage, it appears that chromosomal sex is as clear in somatic cell nuclei of hermaphrodites as it is in normal individuals. It is unnecessary to emphasize the possible importance of this observation in the investigative and practical aspects of the complex subject of hermaphroditism.

The term "chromosomal sex" has been used in this report rather than the more common expression "genetic sex." There is no serious objection to the alternative use of these terms when applied to individuals with normal sex development. In the present state of our knowledge it appears inadvisable to use the terms chromosomal sex and genetic sex interchangeably when referring to hermaphrodites. The indications are that it will be possible to establish whether an intersex patient has the female XX or the male XY sex chromosomes. However, this forward step is far removed from detecting the nature of the sex-influencing genes on these chromosomes or on the autosomes. It is evident from the familial incidence of hermaphroditism that the sex-influencing genes are inadequate for normal sex development in many cases. Our hope is that the chromosomal sex will prove to be a reliable indication of the *dominant* sex of the patient as a whole. Such a development would be the more valuable since the dominant sex could be detected *in infancy* by a relatively simple procedure.

Since many female pseudohermaphrodites and possibly a proportion of male pseudohermaphrodites are caused by endocrinologic dysfunction, the question arises as to whether the morphology of the sex chromatin is influenced by sex hormones. Unpublished observations in this laboratory indicate that this is not the case. One of us (M.A.G.) has demonstrated a sex difference in nuclear morphology in cat embryos before the stage of gonadal differentiation into testes or ovaries. Further, Mr. Hugh Lindsay was unable to alter the sex chromatin in neurons of the cat by orchectomy or oophorectomy in early life or by the administration of the opposite sex hormone to such animals. To the best of our knowledge the sex chromatin is a stable component of the nucleus whose morphology is not influenced by sex hormones. The morphology of the sex chromatin is believed, therefore, to be a reliable indication of chromosomal sex in hermaphrodites.

Certain remote possibilities are to be kept in mind in this work. For example, it is theoretically possible that a case of true hermaphroditism with an ovary on one side and a testis on the other might be a gynandromorph, the term being used in the restricted sense of an individual in whom one side of the body is female, the other male. A bilateral biopsy would be indicated should such a possibility arise. It is also possible that some cases of hermaphroditism may be the result of a multiple combination of sex chromosomes, such as XXY. Such remote possibilities as these would seem to have no important bearing on the problem as it is now visualized.

In view of the unsatisfactory state of the subject of hermaphroditism it becomes a duty to establish the chromosomal sex in as large a series as possible. The authors wish, therefore, to make a special plea for the application of the skin biopsy technique in all cases of doubtful sex. It is especially important to do a skin biopsy test of chromosomal sex in the cases which have been described so thoroughly in the recent clinical literature. A sufficiently large series is required to permit a comparison of the chromosomal female hermaphrodites with the chromosomal male hermaphrodites. Such a comparison must include all the variables from the type of gonad to the psychosexual outlook of the patient. Only a thorough study of this nature, requiring the cooperation of many physicians, will permit an evaluation of the importance of chromosomal sex in hermaphroditism. Those who have faced the problem of treating these unfortunate patients will sympathize with the note of urgency in this appeal which reiterates a similar request made recently by Greenhill (9, p. 552).

SUMMARY

1. A study of skin specimens from 50 females and 50 males of normal sex development demonstrates a difference in nuclear structure, according to sex, in cells of the malpighian layer of the epidermis.

2. Nuclei of female specimens contain a mass of sex chromatin which is seldom seen in nuclei of male specimens. The sex chromatin is believed to be derived from heterochromatic parts of the sex chromosomes. The XX chromosomes of the female produce a chromatin mass sufficiently large to be identified, while the XY chromosomes of the male fail to produce a chromatin mass of sufficient size to

be distinguished from the general particulate chromatin.

3. This method of detecting the chromosomal sex of an individual has been applied to 2 cases of hermaphroditism. One case proved to be a chromosomal female, the other a chromosomal male.

4. The extension of this study to other cases of intersexuality is urged in the hope of clarifying the complex problem of hermaphroditism. The potential importance of the skin biopsy technique lies in the possibility that it may prove to be a simple method of detecting the *dominant sex in infancy*, in cases of doubt.

REFERENCES

1. BARR, M. L., BERTRAM, L. F., and LINDSAY, H. A. The morphology of the nerve cell nucleus, according to sex. Anat. Rec., 1950, 107: 283.
2. BRETNALL, C. P. A case of arrhenoblastoma complicating pregnancy. J. Obst. Gyn. Brit. Empire, 1945, 52: 235.
3. EVANS, H. M., and SWEZY, O. The chromosomes in man. California Univ. Mem., 1929, 8: 1.
4. GATENBY, J. B., and BEAMS, H. W. Microtomist's Vade-Mecum. London: J. & A. Churchill Ltd., 1950.
5. GEITLER, L. Kernbaus und der Kernteilung der Wasserläufer Gerris lateralis und Gerris lacustris. Zschr. Zellforsch., 1937, 26: 641.
6. GRAHAM, M. A., and BARR, M. L. A sex difference in the morphology of metabolic nuclei in somatic cells of the cat. Anat. Rec., 1952, 112: 709.
7. GREENE, R. R. Embryology of sexual structure and hermaphroditism. J. Clin. Endocr., 1944, 4: 335.
8. GREENE, R., MATTHEWS, D., HUGHESDON, P. E., and HOWARD, A. A case of true hermaphroditism. Brit. J. Surg., 1952, 40: 263.
9. GREENHILL, J. P. The 1952 Year Book of Obstetrics and Gynecology. Chicago: The Year Book Publishers, Inc., 1952.
10. LILLIE, F. R. The free-martin; sex hormones in the foetal life of cattle. J. Exp. Zool., 1917, 23: 371.
11. LISCHER, C. E., and BYARS, L. T. True hermaphroditism. Ann. Surg., 1952, 136: 864.
12. MOORE, C. R. Embryonic Sex Hormones and Sexual Differentiation. Springfield, Ill.: Charles C Thomas, 1947.
13. MOORE, K. L., and BARR, M. L. Morphology of nerve cell nuclei in mammals. J. Comp. Neur., in press.
14. PAINTER, T. S. The sex chromosomes of man. Am. Natur., 1924, 58: 506.
15. PRINCE, R. H. Sex and the cell nucleus. M. Sc. thesis, Univ. West. Ontario, 1952.
16. SEVERINGHAUS, A. E. Sex chromosomes in a human intersex. Am. J. Anat., 1942, 70: 73.
17. STOWELL, R. E. Feulgen reaction for thymonucleic acid. Stain Techn., 1945, 20: 45.
18. WILKINS, L., LEWIS, R. A., KLEIN, R., GARDNER, L. I., CRIGLER, J. F., JR., ROSENBERG, E., and MIGEON, C. J. Congenital adrenal hyperplasia treated with cortisone. J. Clin. Endocr., 1951, 1: 1.
19. YOUNG, H. H. Genital Abnormalities, Hermaphroditism and Related Adrenal Diseases. Baltimore: Williams & Wilkins Co., 1937.

PAPER 13

13. Tjio, J. H. and Levan, A. (1956). The chromosome number of man. *Hereditas*, **42**, 1–6

COMMENTARY

Human chromosomes were first described in 1891 by von Hansemann; the number present, however, remained unsettled for many years. In 1923, Painter reported that the chromosome number was 48; this became accepted over the next three decades until Tjio and Levan (Paper 13) conclusively demonstrated that the diploid chromosome complement for man is 46, including the two sex chromosomes. This important observation was made in human embryonic lung fibroblasts using hypotonic treatment and more refined tissue culture techniques. Shortly afterwards, Ford and Hamerton (1956) reported that the haploid number of chromosomes in human germ cells was 23, confirming the findings of Tjio and Levan. These observations marked the beginning of modern genetics and led to the recognition of certain major genetic disorders and malformation syndromes.

In 1959, several important chromosomal disorders were reported. These included: 21 trisomy in Down's syndrome, Klinefelter's syndrome (47,XXY), Turner's syndrome (45,XO), and the Triple-X anomaly. In the same year the first case of translocation in man was detected. During the next 2 years, Patau's (trisomy 13) and Edward's (trisomy 18) syndromes, sex chromosomal aberrations, and many cases of translocations and deletions were discovered (see Turpin and Lejeune, 1969). Carr (1975) estimated that approximately 125 chromosomal abnormalities were detected between 1959 and 1970. For a discussion of the more common and clinically important chromosomal disorders, reference should be made to Bergsma (1973).

Until a few years ago, it was possible to recognize with certainty only four pairs of autosomal chromosomes (1, 2, 3 and 16) and sometimes the male Y-chromosome. However, the recent development of banding techniques now permits the differentiation of individual chromosomes as well as the precise localization of parts of chromosomes. Undoubtedly, the recognition and interpretation of even minor chromosomal changes should become possible following the mapping of the bands that characterize each chromosome (Carter, 1975; Robinson, 1976).

REFERENCES

Bergsma, D. (1973). *Birth Defects: Atlas and Compendium.* The National Foundation—March of Dimes. (Baltimore: The Williams and Wilkins Co)

Carr, D. H. (1975). Cytogenetics and the pathologist. In *Pathology Annual* (Ed. S. C. Sommers), Vol. 10, 93–144. (New York: Appleton-Century-Crofts)

Carter, C. O. (1975). Clinical genetics. In *Recent Advances in Pediatric Surgery* (Ed. A. W. Wilkinson), vol. 3, 1–10. (Edinburgh: Churchill Livingstone)

Ford, C. E. and Hamerton, J. L. (1956). The chromosomes of man. *Nature (London)*, **178**, 1020–1023.

Painter, T. S. (1923). The spermatogenesis of man. *J. Exp. Zool.*, **37**, 291–334

Robinson, J. A. (1976). Recent advances in cytogenetics and their relevance to medicine. *Proc. R. Soc. Med.*, **69**, 33–38

Turpin, R. and Lejeune, J. (1969). *Human Afflictions and Chromosomal Aberrations.* (Oxford: Pergamon Press)

von Hansemann, D. (1891). Über pathologische Mitosen. *Virchows Arch.*, **123**, 356 (cited in Turpin and Lejeune, 1969)

From J. H. Tjio and A. Levan (1956). Hereditas, **42,** *1–6. Copyright (1956).*
by kind permission of the authors and the Mendelian Society

THE CHROMOSOME NUMBER OF MAN

By *JOE HIN TJIO* and *ALBERT LEVAN*

ESTACION EXPERIMENTAL DE AULA DEI, ZARAGOZA, SPAIN, AND CANCER CHROMOSOME
LABORATORY, INSTITUTE OF GENETICS, LUND, SWEDEN

WHILE staying last summer at the Sloan-Kettering Institute, New York, one of us tried out some modifications of Hsu's technique (1952) on various human tissue cultures carried in serial *in vitro* cultivation at that institute. The results were promising inasmuch as some fairly satisfactory chromosome analyses were obtained in cultures both of tissues of normal origin and of tumours (LEVAN, 1956).

Later on both authors, working in cooperation at Lund, have tried still further to improve the technique. We had access to tissue cultures of human embryonic lung fibroblasts, grown in bovine amniotic fluid; these were very kindly supplied to us by Dr. RUNE GRUBB of the Virus Laboratory, Institute of Bacteriology, Lund. All cultures were primary explants taken from human embryos obtained after legal abortions. The embryos were 10—25 cm in length. The chromosomes were studied a few days after the *in vitro* explantation had been made.

In our opinion the hypotonic pre-treatment introduced by Hsu, although a very significant improvement especially for spreading the chromosomes, has a tendency to make the chromosome outlines somewhat blurred and vague. We consequently tried to abbreviate the hypotonic treatment to a minimum, hoping to induce the scattering of the chromosomes without unfavourable effects on the chromosome surface. Pre-treatment with hypotonic solution for only one or two minutes gave good results. In addition, we gave a colchicine dose to the culture medium 12—20 hours before fixation, making the medium 50×10^{-9} mol/l for the drug. The colchicine effected a considerable accumulation of mitoses and a varying degree of chromosome contraction. Fixation followed in 60 % acetic acid, twice exchanged in order to wash out the salts left from the culture medium and from the hypotonic solution that would otherwise have caused precipitation with the orcein. Ordinary squash preparations were made in 1 % acetic orcein. For chromosome counts the squashing was made very mild in order to keep the chromosomes in the metaphase groups. For idiogram studies a more thorough squashing was preferable. In many cases single cells were squashed under the microscope by a slight pressure of a needle. In such cases it was directly observed that no chromosomes escaped.

THE CHROMOSOME NUMBER

With the technique used exact counts could be made in a great number of cells. Figs. 1 *a* and *b* represent typical samples of the appearance of the chromosomes at early metaphase (*a*) and full metaphase (*b*), showing the ease with which the counting could be made. In Table 1 the numbers of counts made from the four embryos studied are recorded.

TABLE 1. *Number of exact chromosome counts made.*

Embryo No.	Number of cultures	Number of counts
1	5	15
2	10	98
3	3	119
4	4	29
Total	22	261

We were surprised to find that the chromosome number 46 predominated in the tissue cultures from all four embryos, only single cases deviating from this number. Lower numbers were frequent, of course, but always in cells that seemed damaged. These were consequently disregarded just as the solitary chromosomes and the groups with but a few chromosomes, which were frequent. In some doubtful cases the numbers 47 and 48 were counted (in four cases not included in the table). This may be due to one or two solitary chromosomes having been pressed into a 46-chromosome plate at the squashing. It is also possible that deviating numbers may originate through non-disjunction, thus representing a real chromosome number variation in the living tissue. This kind of variation will probably increase as a consequence of the change in environment for the tissue involved in the *in vitro* explantation. Hsu (1952) reports a certain degree of such variation in his primary cultures. Levan (1956), studying long-carried serial subcultures, found hypotriploid stemline numbers in two of them, and a near-diploid number in a third culture. In this culture one cell with 48 chromosomes was analysed. Naturally, at that time, this was thought to represent the normal diploid number.

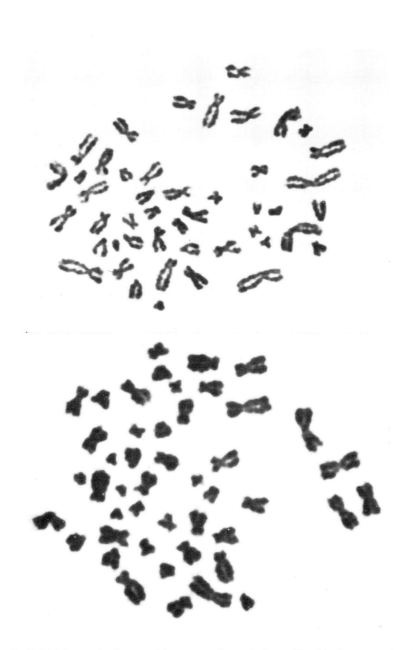

Fig. 1. Colchicine-metaphases of human embryonic lung fibroblasts grown *in vitro*.
a: early metaphase, *b*: full metaphase. The two cells are from embryos 2 and 3
(Table 1), respectively. — ×2300.

CHROMOSOME MORPHOLOGY

Some data on the chromosome morphology of the 46 human chromosomes will be communicated here. The detailed idiogram analysis will be postponed, however, until we are able to study individuals of known sex, the sex of the present embryos being unknown. The comparative study of germline chromosomes in spermatogonial mitoses constitutes an urgent supplement to the present work.

In Fig. 2 four cells are analysed ranging from late prophase (a) to late c-metaphase (d). The chromosomes of metaphases with moderate colchicine contraction vary in length between 1 and 8 μ (Fig. 2 b), but the entire range of variation of Fig. 2 is from 1 to 11 μ. The chromosome morphology is roughly concordant with the observations of earlier workers, as, for instance, the idiogram of Hsu (1952). The chromosomes may be divided into three groups: M chromosomes (median-submedian centromere; index long arm : short arm 1—1,9), S chromosomes (subterminal centromere; arm index 2—4,9), and T chromosomes (nearly terminal centromere; arm index 5 or more).

The M and S chromosomes are present in about equal numbers (twenty of each), while six T chromosomes are found. The classification of the three groups is arbitrary, of course, since gradual transitions of arm indices occur between the three groups. Certain submedian M chromosomes are hard to distinguish from some of the S chromosomes, and the most asymmetric S chromosomes approach the T group.

The chromosomes are easily arranged in pairs, but only certain of these pairs are individually distinguishable. Thus, the M chromosomes include the three longest pairs, which can always be identified. The two longest pairs are different: the second having a decidedly more asymmetric location of its centromere. The two or three smallest M pairs are also recognizable. Between the three longest and the three shortest pairs there are four intermediate pairs that cannot be individually recognized.

The S chromosomes are hardly identifiable, since they form a series of gradually decreasing length. The largest pair, however, is characteristic. Certain chromosomes were seen to have a small satellite on their short arms. Secondary constrictions, too, have been observed now and then, so that it may be hoped that the detailed morphologic study will lead to the identification of more chromosome pairs. The T chromosomes are recognizable; they constitute three pairs of middle-sized chromosomes. Unlike the mouse chromosomes, the human T chromosomes evidently have a small shorter arm.

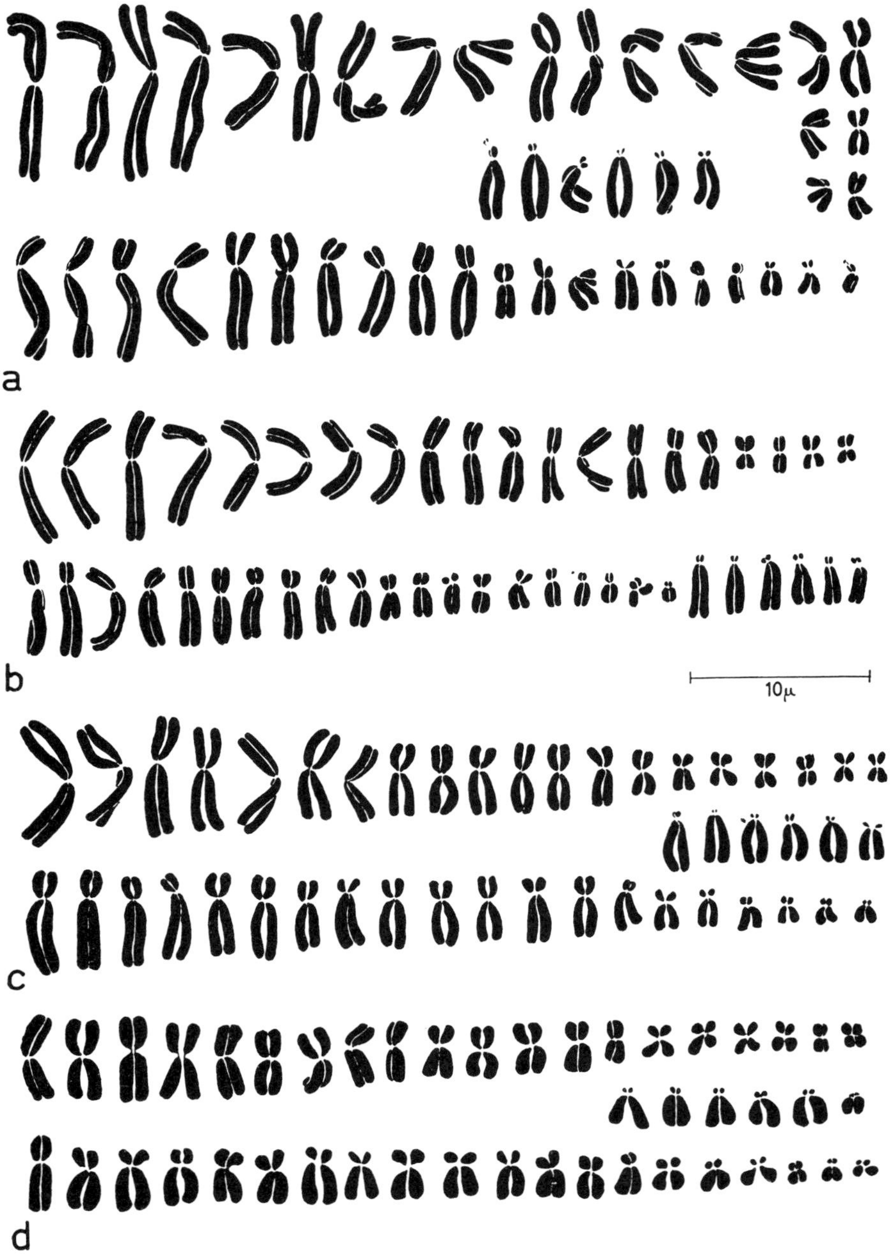

JOE HIN TJIO AND ALBERT LEVAN

Fig. 2. Four idiogram analyses of human embryonic lung fibroblasts grown *in vitro*. The chromosomes have been grouped in three classes: M (top row), S (bottom row), and T (in between, except in *b*, where T is at the end of the S row). Within each class the chromosomes have been roughly arranged in diminishing order of size. — ×2400.

CONCLUSION

The almost exclusive occurrence of the chromosome number 46 in one somatic tissue derived from four individual human embryos is a very unexpected finding. To assume a regular mechanism for the exclusion of two chromosomes from the idiogram at the formation of a certain tissue is unlikely, even if this assumption cannot be entirely dismissed at this stage of inquiry. Our experience from one somatic tissue in mice and rats, *viz.*, regenerating liver, speaks against this assumption. The exact diploid chromosome set was always found in regenerating liver.

After the conclusion had been drawn that the tissue studied by us had 46 as chromosome number, Dr. EVA HANSEN-MELANDER kindly informed us that during last spring she had studied, in cooperation with Drs. YNGVE MELANDER and STIG KULLANDER, the chromosomes of liver mitoses in aborted human embryos. This study, however, was temporarily discontinued because the workers were unable to find all the 48 human chromosomes in their material; as a matter of fact, the number 46 was repeatedly counted in their slides. We have seen photomicrographs of liver prophases from this study, clearly showing 46 chromosomes. These findings suggest that 46 may be the correct chromosome number for human liver tissue, too.

With previously used technique it has been extremely difficult to make counts in human material. Even with the great progress involved in HSU's method exact counts seem difficult, judging from the photomicrographs published (HSU, 1952 and elsewhere). For instance, we think that the excellent photomicrograph of HSU published in DARLINGTON's book (1953, facing p. 288) is more in agreement with the chromosome number 46 than 48, and the same is true of many of the photomicrographs of human chromosomes previously published.

Before a renewed, careful control has been made of the chromosome number in spermatogonial mitoses of man we do not wish to generalize our present findings into a statement that the chromosome number of man is $2n = 46$, but it is hard to avoid the conclusion that this would be the most natural explanation of our observations.

Acknowledgements. — We wish to express our sincere thanks to the Swedish Cancer Society for financial support of this investigation, and to Dr. RUNE GRUBB for supplying us with tissue cultures.

SUMMARY

The chromosomes were studied in primary tissue cultures of human lung fibroblasts explanted from four individual embryos. In all of them the chromosome number 46 was encountered, instead of the expected number 48. Since among 265 mitoses counted all except 4 showed the number 46, this number is characteristic of the tissue studied. The possible bearing of this result on the chromosome number of man is discussed.

Institute of Genetics, Lund, January 26, 1956.

Literature cited

DARLINGTON, C. D. 1953. The facts of life. — London, 467 pp.

HSU, T. C. 1952. Mammalian chromosomes *in vitro*. — The karyotype of man. — J. Hered. 43: 167—172.

LEVAN, A. 1956. Chromosome studies on some human tumors and tissues of normal origin, grown *in vivo* and *in vitro* at the Sloan-Kettering Institute. — Cancer (in the press).

PAPERS 14, 15 AND 16

14. Boué, J., Boué, A. and Lazar, P. (1975). Retrospective and prospective epidemiological studies of 1500 karyotyped spontaneous human abortions. *Teratology*, **12**, 11–26
15. Machin, G. A. (1974). Chromosome abnormality and perinatal death. *Lancet*, **i**, 549–551
16. Kim, H. J., Hsu, L. Y. F., Paciuc, S., Cristian, S., Quintana, A. and Hirschhorn, K. (1975). Cytogenetics of fetal wastage. *N. Engl. J. Med.*, **293**, 844–847

COMMENTARY

The high incidence of chromosomal aberrations in early spontaneous abortions has been demonstrated in many studies (Khudr, 1974; Boué *et al.*, 1975). These anomalies usually occur during meiosis, mostly as a result of non-disjunction, or at the time of fertilization (triploidy), or thereafter (tetraploidy or mosaicism).

Boué and her co-workers (Paper 14) estimated that approximately 50% of all zygotes are chromosomally abnormal. In a combined retrospective and prospective study of 1498 abortuses, all less than 12 weeks old, more than 60% had abnormal karyotypes. The frequency of chromosome abnormalities increased in cases of paternal exposure to irradiation and ovulation-inducing treatment in the mothers; no significant increase was observed after maternal irradiation. The use of oral contraceptives apparently had no effect on the incidence of chromosome abnormalities. In cases of maternal smoking, a high incidence (50%) of genetically normal embryos was aborted. There is definite indication from several recent studies (Boué *et al.*, 1975; McConnell and Carr, 1975) that more chromosomal abnormalities will likely be identified in abortuses using current banding techniques.

That chromosome aberrations are important etiological factors in perinatal death has been convincingly demonstrated by Machin (Paper 15). Chromosomal anomalies were found in 5·6% of 500 infants dying in the perinatal period; the incidence was 9% in the group of macerated stillbirth, 4% in fresh stillbirth, and 6% in neonates. Thirteen per cent of all infants with lethal malformations had abnormal karyotypes. In particular, a relatively high incidence of E trisomy was identified.

The incidence and types of chromosomal defects found in parents (50 couples) with a history of fetal wastage (more than two early abortions, stillbirth(s) or livebirth(s), or both of infants with multiple malformations) are discussed in Paper 16. The chromosomal changes observed included translocation, mosaicism, and breakage and re-arrangement, or both; these were highly related to the increased incidence of fetal wastage. It should be noted that the three cases of balanced translocation were detected only by banding techniques and would have been missed by conventional Giemsa staining.

REFERENCES

Boué, J. *et al.* (1975). Identification of C trisomies in human abortuses. *J. Med. Genet.*, **12**, 265–268

Khudr, G. (1974). Cytogenetics of habitual abortion. *Obstet. Gynecol. Surv.*, **29**, 299–310

McConnell, H. D. and Carr, D. H. (1975). Recent advances in the cytogenetic study of human spontaneous abortions. *Obstet. Gynecol.*, **45**, 547–552

From J. Boué et al. (1975). Teratology, **12,** 11–26. *Copyright* (1975),
by kind permission of the authors and the Wistar Institute Press

Retrospective and Prospective Epidemiological Studies of 1500 Karyotyped Spontaneous Human Abortions [1,2]

JOËLLE BOUÉ, ANDRÉ BOUÉ AND PHILIPPE LAZAR
*Centres d'Etudes de Biologie Prénatale, I.N.S.E.R.M., Groupe U. 73,
Château de Longchamp, 75016 Paris, and Unité de Recherches
Statistiques (I.N.S.E.R.M.), Institut Gustave Roussy,
94800 Villejuif, France*

ABSTRACT   Epidemiologic studies, retrospective and prospective, were done on 1500 abortions collected from 1966–1972. No secular or seasonal variations were observed. From the analysis of the relative frequencies of the different types of chromosome anomalies it is estimated that 1 out of every 2 conceptions has a chromosome anomaly. Maternal-age influence was found only for the autosomal trisomy group, mainly D and G trisomies. No effect of oral contraceptives was discovered. An increased frequency of chromosome anomalies occurred after ovulation-inducing therapy and after occupational exposure of the father to irradiation. No variations in the fertility rate and in the frequency of congenital malformations in births following abortions was noted. The incidence of recurring abortion was mainly influenced by the reproductive history of the couple before the karyotyped abortion.

Epidemiological studies of human chromosome anomalies have usually relied on case reports of malformed infants pooled from different sources to accumulate observations. The frequency of spontaneous abortions is about 15% of recognized pregnancies (Warburton and Fraser, '64); in 90% of the cases abortions occur during the first 4 months of gestation. Cytogenetic studies of abortuses have clearly demonstrated the important role of chromosome anomalies; epidemiological studies of early spontaneous abortions may contribute to a better understanding of consequences of chromosome anomalies on embryonic development and more generally on reproductive failure. The fact that many abortions occur shortly after conception facilitates the study of events surrounding fertilization; one laboratory is able to collect many observations in a relatively short time permitting a statistical analysis of the results, especially since parents are very cooperative in prospective studies of subsequent pregnancies. A cytogenetic survey of 1500 abortuses carried out in our laboratory from 1966–1972 provided the material for both the retrospective and prospective epidemiological analyses presented here.

MATERIAL AND METHODS

Specimens from spontaneous abortions were collected either in public hospitals or, more frequently, at home: a special flask was given to each patient when she consulted her obstetrician for a threatened abortion. Only abortions in which the embryo was less than 12 weeks old were studied. Tissue-culture and chromosome-preparation techniques were previously described (Boué et al., '67).

Retrospective study

At the time of the abortion (before the karyotype of the abortus was known) a questionnaire was completed by the parents. This questionnaire contains numerous questions concerning the medical histories of each parent, the gynecologic and obstetric history of the mother, and if feasible the circumstances surrounding conception (temperature curves, date of ovulation, dates of intercourse).

Prospective study

Two prospective studies were carried out: one in May 1971, the results of which have been published (Boué et al., '73), and a second in October 1972, in which a

Received Dec. 13, '74. Accepted May 7, '75.
[1] Presented as part of the symposium on methods of testing for teratogenicity and possibilities for the future, at The 14th Annual Meeting of the Teratology Society, July 7–10, 1974, University of British Columbia, Vancouver, B.C., Canada.
[2] Address for reprints: Dr. J. Boué, C.E.B.I.O.P., Château de Longchamp, 75016 Paris, France.

J. BOUÉ, A. BOUÉ AND P. LAZAR

questionnaire was sent to 1100 women who had previously had abortions karyotyped in our laboratory. The percentage of conceptions and of recurring abortions were calculated actuarially.

Analysis of the data

One of the most troublesome problems in such epidemiological studies is the fact that it is practically impossible to have a control group of normal pregnancies. Thus we had to compare abortuses having normal karyotypes with those of abnormal karyotypes. Chromosome analyses of 1498 abortuses less than 12 weeks old (postconception) showed 577 normal and 921 anomalous karyotypes (table 1).

In the "normal-karyotype" group were pooled different types of abortions: those due to nonzygotic factors (maternal, local or general, etc.); and those due to undetected zygotic factors. In about half of the specimens with normal karyotype pathologic examination revealed morphological anomalies comparable to those found in conceptuses with chromosome aberrations, implicating a zygotic cause. Certain structural chromosome anomalies (such as small deletions and pericentric inversions)

could not be detected by cytogenetic studies until recently, and gene defects must also be responsible for some developmental arrests.

The data were also analyzed according to the type of chromosome anomaly. The details of the "abnormal-karyotype" group (table 1) show that structural anomalies were observed in only 3.8%. Thus nearly all the aberrations were numerical and the results of errors at the time of gametogenesis (chromosome nondisjunctions at meiosis), at the time of fertilization (triploidy caused by digyny or dispermy), or during the first divisions of the fertilized ovum (tetraploidy or mosaicism).

It should be pointed out that any one type of chromosome anomaly may result from more than one possible mechanism. For example, trisomies may result from chromosome nondisjunction at meiosis either in male or female gametogenesis; triploidy may be produced by digyny, diandry, or dispermy; etc.

RESULTS

Retrospective study

Secular, seasonal, and geographical variations

The incidence of chromosome anomalies was relatively stable during the years studied. Table 2 shows the number of specimens per year that were karyotyped and the proportion of chromosome anomalies. During the first 2 years some induced abortions were undoubtedly included since the majority of abortions analyzed came from public hospitals, with relatively poor information about the parents. In the following

TABLE 1

Karyotypes of 1498 abortuses less than 12 weeks old

Karyotype	Abortuses	
	No.	%
Normal	577	38.52
Abnormal	921	61.48

Details of abnormal karyotypes

Monosomy	141	
45,X	140	15.30
45,G −	1	
Trisomy	479	
A +	12	
B +	6	
C +	86	
D +	109	52.00
E +	172	
F +	7	
G +	87	
Double Trisomy	16	1.73
Triploidy	183	
XXY	92	
XYY	7	19.86
XXX	57	
Unkaryotyped	27	
Tetraploidy	57	6.18
Translocations	35	3.80
Mosaicism	10	1.08

TABLE 2

Frequency of chromosomal anomalies in spontaneous abortions studied from 1965–1972

Year	No. of abortuses karyotyped	% Abnormal karyotype
1965–66	61	45.9
1967	84	50.0
1968	170	64.7
1969	264	62.5
1970	343	61.8
1971	362	62.5
1972	214	64.4
Total	1498	61.48

years efforts were made (a) to obtain specimens from abortions that occurred at home and (b) to have the specimens brought to the laboratory by a member of the patient's family. This change in collection technique accounts for the increase in frequency of anomalies since very few induced abortions were included and a great number of early specimens were obtained.

Figure 1 shows the relative frequency of the different types of chromosome anomalies (monosomy, trisomy, and triploidy) in relation to the month of fertilization. No significant difference was observed. The overall frequency of chromosome anomalies in various larger studies has ranged from 8% (Stenchever et al., '67) to 64% (Szulman, '65). It seems unlikely that these differences were linked to geographical factors. In fact these wide discrepancies probably mainly reflect variables involved in the collection of specimens (unknown number of induced abortions, different percentages of abortions in the first and second trimesters of pregnancy, etc.). Two recent studies, in Denmark (Therkelsen et al., '73) and Switzerland

(Kajii et al., '73), reported frequencies of 54.7 and 59% abnormal karyotypes, respectively, results in good agreement with ours.

Thus, there were no significant secular, seasonal, or geographical variations in the incidence of chromosome anomalies. In fact, possible seasonal or geographical variations would be difficult to demonstrate.

Even though cytogenetic analysis of abortuses represents an improvement over studies on liveborn infants, chromosome anomalies found in abortuses still represent only a part of the total that occur at fertilization.

Estimation of chromosome anomalies at the time of conception

In contrast with the variations in overall frequency the relative frequencies of different types of chromosome anomalies have been very similar in all surveys. Figure 2 shows the distribution of different karyotypes in 4 studies, done in Canada (Carr, '70), Denmark (Therkelsen et al., '73), France (Boué and Boué, '74), and Switzerland (Kajii et al., '73).

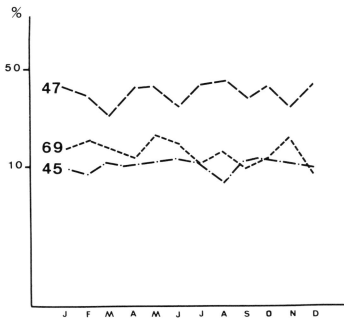

Fig. 1   Relative frequency of monosomies X, autosomal trisomies, and triploidies in abortuses, in relation to the month of fertilization.

J. BOUÉ, A. BOUÉ AND P. LAZAR

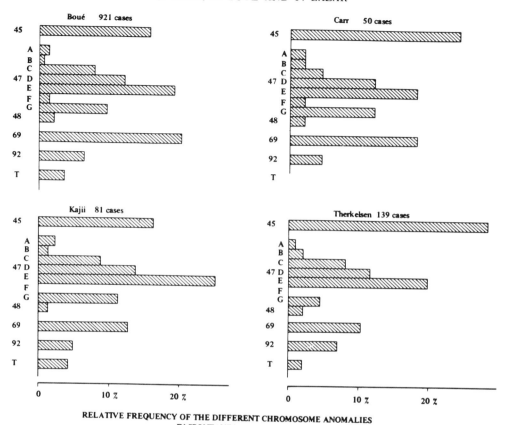

RELATIVE FREQUENCY OF THE DIFFERENT CHROMOSOME ANOMALIES
IN SPONTANEOUS ABORTIONS

Fig. 2 Relative frequency of the different types of chromosome anomalies in four studies: France, Canada, Switzerland, and Denmark.

Considering chromosome anomalies resulting from nondisjunction at the time of meiosis, it was noted that the monosomies were almost exclusively monosomy X, representing about 15% of the anomalies encountered. The relative frequency of the different autosomal trisomies varied; trisomy 16, identified by standard staining techniques, was the most frequent and accounted for about 15%. Identification of chromosomes by banding techniques confirmed the validity of these observations.

To account for the absence of autosomal monosomies and the low frequency of certain trisomies it has been suggested that these anomalies must lead to very early developmental arrest, most of the zygotes being eliminated before the pregnancy is recognized. This postulate is supported by morphological examination of zygotes with rare chromosome anomalies, which showed precocious developmental arrest, either complete absence of embryonic formation (blighted ovum) or malformed embryonic formation only a few millimeters long. The hypothesis of precocious elimination of zygotes with autosomal monosomies and certain autosomal trisomies has been experimentally confirmed (Gropp, '73) in mice containing translocations (Mus poschiavinus). If meiotic nondisjunction occurs with equal probability for each chromosome, an identical number of zygotes should be conceived with monosomy and trisomy for each chromosome pair, and thus the total number of monosomies and trisomies conceived can be estimated from the data for monosomy X and trisomy 16.

In general 15% of clinically recognized

pregnancies terminate in abortion (this figure is higher in prospective studies). Thus for every 1000 clinically recognized pregnancies there are 850 births and 150 spontaneous abortions. Of these 150 abortions about 100 (60%) have a chromosome anomaly. Among these 100 there are 15 with monosomy X and 15 with trisomy 16 on the average. This leads to an estimate of $15 \times 23 = 345$ monosomies and $15 \times 23 = 345$ trisomies, or a total of 690 anomalies resulting from meiotic nondisjunction. When the other anomalies are added to trisomies and monosomies the resulting figure for total chromosome anomalies conceived is quite closed to that of the 850 births at term, an estimate in agreement with those deduced from other observations on human beings (Hertig and Rock, '73; Pearson et al., '73). The figures, of course, are imprecise considering the data on which they are based, but they give an idea of the order of magnitude of the chromosome accidents that lead to reproductive failure: about 1 out of every 2 conceptions. Although this estimate may be valid for the population as a whole, for each couple the risk of conceiving zygotes with chromosome anomalies is extremely variable. These variations were revealed by the prospective studies of recurring abortions, the results of which will be presented below.

Maternal age

The first studies of karyotyped abortions showed that the mean maternal age of abortuses with chromosome anomalies is higher than of those with normal karyotypes; in the latter, maternal age is about the same as that of mothers of normal infants (Carr, '67; Arakaki and Waxman, '70; Lazar et al., '71). This seems to be in good agreement with the observations of increased maternal age in newborn trisomies. The age of mothers of children with Down syndrome is bimodally distributed, and Penrose and Smith ('66) showed that this distribution can be divided in 2 corresponding to 2 different classes of risk: class A, in which the risk is independant of maternal age, and class B, in which it is age-dependent.

All types of anomaly do not appear to be related to maternal age, however. In our study (table 3) no maternal-age influence was demonstrated for monosomy X, tri-

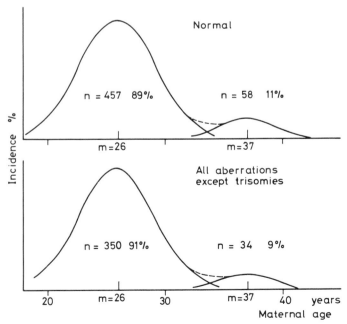

Fig. 3 Maternal-age distribution in abortions with normal karyotype, and in abortions with all chromosomal anomalies except trisomies. Hypothetical distribution in 2 classes. Reproduced by courtesy of Karger.

ploidy, tetraploidy, or translocation. In the case of monosomy X this agrees well with observations in Turner syndrome in which it was shown that about 74% of the patients have a maternal X chromosome (Fraser, '63). On the other hand, the studies of Pearson et al. ('73) showed that about 1% of spermatozoa with a normal haploid DNA complement have 2 Y chromosomes. It may be postulated that there are an equivalent number of spermatozoa with no sex chromosome.

An age influence was found only for the autosomal trisomy group, for which the mean maternal age was 31.3 years compared with 27.5 for the other categories (table 3). The large number of trisomies permitted a detailed analysis of maternal age (table 3). It is primarily the trisomies involving acrocentric chromosomes in which the influence of maternal age was marked; in double trisomies (with one exception) 1 or 2 acrocentric chromosomes were involved.

The maternal-age effect can be illustrated graphically: in each group of abortuses the observations were separated into 2 groups according to the classes described by Penrose and Smith ('66). Figure 3 shows the maternal-age distributions of abortuses with normal karyotypes and those with monosomy X, triploidy, tetraploidy, and translocation. The distributions were very

similar in the 2 populations. Class B observations represented around 10% and were linked to the incidence of the conceptions that are normally asymmetrically distributed, showing an excess in the older maternal-age group.

The maternal-age distributions of abortuses with autosomal trisomies (fig. 4) showed that class B included 37% of the cases. The maternal-age distributions for trisomy D and trisomy G showed more striking differences. That for trisomy G had a pattern very similar to the one described by Penrose and Smith ('66), who found that 60.2% of Down syndrome belongs to the age-dependent group (class B).

The striking agreement between the class A and class B curves for Down syndrome and for abortuses with trisomy G demonstrates that whether a *conceptus with trisomy G is spontaneously aborted or is delivered at term does not depend on the age of the mother.*

The marked influence of maternal age on trisomies of acrocentric chromosomes is in contrast with its minor influence on trisomies involving metacentric or telocentric chromosomes. This leads to speculation concerning possible causes of these nondisjunctions. The mechanism that seems to fit this selective action of aging best was proposed by Ford ('60) who implicates the nucleolus. The acrocentric chromosomes remain attached to the nucleolus throughout interphase; it is likely that its presence may interfere mechanically with chromosome pairing in the early meiotic prophase. Thus, if an aging factor interferes with the rapid breakdown of the nucleolus in the meiotic prophase of oogenesis, nondisjunction of the associated chromosome pair would be increased.

Paternal age

Table 3 also shows paternal ages in relation to the karyotypes of the abortuses. The figures are very similar to those for maternal age. To determine whether these results reflected the correlation between maternal and paternal ages or whether there was a paternal-age influence per se, a partial correlation was made. It showed a highly significant relation between trisomy and maternal age, $r = 0.20$, but no significance for paternal age, $r = 0.02$. The relation between the frequency of

TABLE 3

Parental ages of abortuses with different types of chromosome anomalies

Karyotype	Number	Parental age (year)	
		Mother	Father
		$\overline{V} \pm SE$	
Monosomy	134	27.6 ± 0.9	29.5 ± 1.1
Autosomal trisomy	448	31.3 ± 0.6	33.5 ± 0.7
Triploidy	167	27.4 ± 0.8	30.4 ± 1.0
Tetraploidy	53	26.8 ± 1.4	29.4 ± 1.7
Translocation	26	27.0 ± 2.3	28.0 ± 1.8
Normal	509	27.5 ± 0.4	30.6 ± 0.6
Details of autosomal trisomies			
47,A +	13	29.6 ± 2.2	31.4 ± 3.2
47,B +	7	33.4 ± 7.1	35.8 ± 11.2
47,C +	72	30.9 ± 1.7	33.0 ± 1.8
47,D +	92	32.5 ± 1.3	34.8 ± 1.6
47,E +	157	29.6 ± 0.9	32.4 ± 1.1
47,F +	8	30.1 ± 5.3	31.4 ± 6.7
47,G +	78	33.2 ± 1.4	35.2 ± 1.8
48	14	35.0 ± 6.1	39.4 ± 9.3

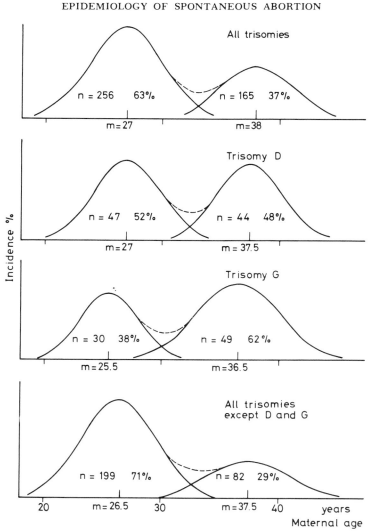

EPIDEMIOLOGY OF SPONTANEOUS ABORTION

Fig. 4 Maternal-age distribution in abortions with trisomies. Hypothetical distribution in 2 classes. Reproduced by courtesy of Karger.

trisomy and paternal age is thus explained by the correlation between the paternal and maternal ages, $r = 0.71$. Similar conclusions were reached by Lilienfeld ('69) for Down syndrome.

Chromosome nondisjunction in meiosis during spermatogenesis seems a frequent event as suspected by the observations of Pearson et al. ('73) on the frequency of spermatozoa with 2 chromosomes 1, or 2 chromosomes 9; implicating a high frequency of trisomic zygotes of paternal origin. The analysis of paternal age in tri-

somic abortuses did not demonstrate an age influence in this phenomenon.

Pregnancy order

The incidence of chromosome anomalies was similar regardless of whether the abortions occurred during the 1st, 2nd, or 3rd pregnancies (66, 64, and 62% respectively of 585 observations). Nor were differences observed in the proportions of the different types of chromosome anomalies. There was a slight increase in the frequency of chromosome anomalies starting with the 4th

J. BOUÉ, A. BOUÉ AND P. LAZAR

pregnancy but this may have been related to maternal age.

Delay in fertilization

Since the work of Witschi ('70) there has been a great deal of interest in the aging of gametes and delays between ovulation and fertilization. In addition to aging of oocytes as women grow older, whose effect seems to be limited to certain trisomies, other types of delay may be observed: aging of spermatozoa in the female genital tract, delay in release of mature oocytes (intrafollicular overripeness or preovulatory aging), and aging of ova released normally but fertilized late (intratubal overripeness or postovulatory aging). All 3 mechanisms are possible in human beings; the first and third are related to sexual activity and the second to anomalies in ovulation.

In our species it is extremely difficult to establish that a delay in fertilization involving aging of gametes occurs. Analysis of the questionnaires filled out by the parents at the time of the abortion offered some material for speculation.

Cases in which it was plausible to suppose that fertilization occurred at the time of ovulation were selected; the date of ovulation was usually estimated from temperature curves, and the couples had daily intercourse during this period or kept a record of the dates of intercourse. The mean intervals between the 1st day of the last menstrual period and the probable date of ovulation were 14.95 days for normal karyotypes, 15.0 days for trisomy, and 17.06 days for polyploidy (triploidy and tetraploidy). This significant increase in the frequency of polyploidy when ovulation occurred after the 14th day is illustrated in figure 5. The observations suggest that a delay in the presumed date of ovulation may play a role in the causation of polyploidy. This delay may reflect an anomaly of ovulation leading to intrafollicular overripeness.

It is difficult to demonstrate delay between ovulation and fertilization. Only those cases in which a temperature curve was available and in which the dates of intercourse seemed sufficiently reliable were selected for analysis. In 24 observa-

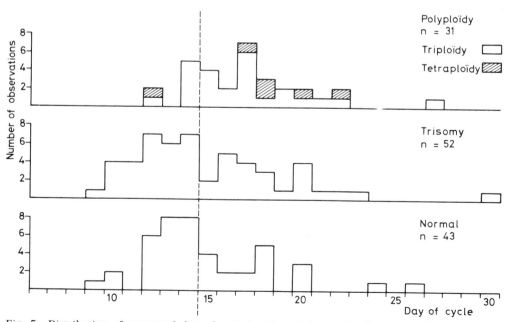

Fig. 5   Distribution of presumed day of ovulation in relation to the karyotype of the abortus. Reproduced by courtesy of Karger.

tions there were intervals of 2 days or more before and after the probable date of ovulation and the possible day of fertilization. Karyotypes of the abortuses were: 5 normal, 1 monosomy X, 11 autosomal trisomy, 6 triploidy, and 1 tetraploidy. The frequency of anomalies increased to 79% and there was an increased incidence of polyploidy. These results are not significant because of the small number of observations.

Drugs acting on ovulation

It has been suggested that drugs acting on ovulation might produce conditions favoring the occurrence of accidents leading to chromosome anomalies. Two types of therapy that are widely used were studied: (1) oral contraceptives, and (2) ovulation-inducing therapy.

Oral contraceptives. The analysis of 700 questionnaires completed at the time of abortion with information about contraceptive methods used permitted examination of the possible influence of ovulatory inhibition on the frequency of chromosome anomalies (Boué and Boué, '73a). Among these 700 observations 520 were selected in which conception followed ovulatory inhibition, either physiological or therapeutic: 180 after pregnancy with birth at term, 220 after pregnancy terminating in spontaneous abortion, and 120 after steroid contraceptives.

Table 4 gives the total frequency of chromosome anomalies according to the cause of ovulatory inhibition and according to the time elapsed between cessation of inhibition and conception. There was no significant difference. There was a slight difference in the frequencies of chromosome anomalies between the 3 groups of women that had ovulatory inhibition (either physiological or therapeutic) and those who never had inhibition. This difference, not significant, can be explained by the difference in age of the 2 groups of women (normal delivery: 30.46 years; spontaneous abortion: 30.13; oral contraceptives: 28.18; no ovulatory inhibition: 26.41). The relative frequencies of each type of chromosome anomaly were not different and in particular there was no significant increase in the frequency of triploidy (table 4).

TABLE 4

Chromosomal anomalies in abortuses from women that conceived after ovulation inhibition (physiological or therapeutic)

Type of ovulation inhibition	Normal delivery		Spontaneous abortion		Oral contraceptive		Controls	
Time elapsed before conception (months)	0–6	7–12	0–6	7–12	0–6	7–12	Ovulatory inhibition >12 months	No previous ovulatory inhibition
Karyotype of abortuses								
Normal	9	10	22	24	20	11	82	75
Monosomy	2	4	6	5	5	4	26	16
Trisomy	11	12	29	25	23	11	79	55
Triploidy	1 (12%)	6 (19%)	9 (16%)	10 (21%)	11 (20%)	2 (10%)	37 (19%)	22 (18%)
Tetraploidy	2	0	2	5	2	1	8	11
Translocation	0	0	1	0	2	0	1	1
Total abnormal	16 (64%)	22 (69%)	46 (67%)	46 (65%)	43 (68%)	18 (62%)	151 (65%)	105 (59%)
Total	25	32	68	70	63	29	233	180

J. BOUÉ, A. BOUÉ AND P. LAZAR

Detailed analysis of these results showed differences related to length of contraceptive treatment. The frequency of chromosome anomalies varied with the duration of contraceptive treatment, independently of the length of time between cessation of treatment and conception (table 5). The number of chromosome anomalies was higher when the duration of the therapy was short. The explanation for this phenomenom seems to be that we are dealing with 2 different populations of women: 1 group apparently took steroid contraceptives for a short time, either for therapeutic indications in fertility problems (1/3 of our observations) or because they did not tolerate the contraceptives well owing to their side effects. On the other hand, in the cases in which steroid-contraceptive treatment lasted 7 months or more the frequency of chromosome anomalies in abortuses was one of the lowest we have observed. The differences observed were not linked to the effects of steroid contraceptives but to the selection of groups of women in whom the risks of having conceptuses with chromosome aberrations were different.

Studies on spontaneous abortion material that attempted to detect the possible effects of steroid contraceptives on human gametes and zygotes were retrospective and extended over a long period, during which the drugs used varied in composition and concentration. In most investigations the oral contraceptives used were not even specified.

The contraceptives used by the women in our study were as follows: norethindrone acetate and ethynylestradiol (27 observations); lynestrenol and mestranol (25 observations); ethynodiol diacetate and mestranol (7 observations); others (8 different combinations) (1–5 observations per product). In two-thirds of the cases only 1 commercial product was used whereas in one-third of the cases 2 or more products were employed successively by the same woman. The duration of the contraceptive treatment was variable, ranging from very short to very long periods.

Despite these criticisms the general conclusion is that no increase in the frequency of chromosome anomalies was found in this study. Similar conclusions were drawn from other similar studies done in Europe in which the same types of oral contraceptives were used. These findings have also been confirmed by studies on newborn infants (Klinger et al., '73).

Ovulation-inducing therapy. During our study we received many specimens from pregnancies after ovulation-inducing therapy. Eighty-four abortions occurred in women that had been treated with human menopausal gonadotrophin (HMG) and human chorionic gonadotrophin (HCG), clomiphene citrate and HCG, or HCG alone. The frequency of chromosome aberrations in the abortuses was compared in 4 groups: group I, 47 abortions after therapy given in the cycle during which fertilization occurred; group II, 14 abortions after therapy given in the cycle before fertilization; group III, 23 abortions after therapy given 2 or more cycles before fertilization, and group IV, 1374 abortions in women that had not been treated with these drugs.

The results in groups I and II were similar (table 6); which agrees with the observation that these treatments are effective during 2 cycles. There was a significant difference ($\chi^2 = 4.9$) between groups I and II, and group III. The frequency of abnormal karyotypes in group III was similar to that in women that had never been treated for sterility (group IV). The results in groups I and II were similar whether therapy was given for amenorrhea or anovulation, or for recurrent abortion in women of normal fertility. The mean maternal age was the same in each group.

Parental exposure to irradiation

The radiation histories of both parents were classified under 2 headings: medical radiation (exposure to X-rays for investigation or for therapy); and occupational exposure to radiation (medical profession or

TABLE 5

Incidence of chromosome anomalies in abortuses in relation to the duration of oral contraceptive treatment

	Duration of oral contraception	
	0–6 months	> 6 months
Number of abortuses karyotyped	39	57
% Abnormal karyotype	87	56

EPIDEMIOLOGY OF SPONTANEOUS ABORTION

TABLE 6

*Frequency of chromosomal anomalies in abortuses from
pregnancies after ovulation stimulation*

Karyotype of abortus	Ovulation stimulation			Control group
	in the cycle of fertilization	1 cycle before fertilization	2 or more cycles before fertilization	no ovulation stimulation
Normal	8	2	9	546
Trisomy	23	7	9	441
Monosomy	3	1	2	134
Triploidy	10	2	3	167
Tetraploidy	3	2		49
Translocation				37
% Abnormal	83	86	61	60

TABLE 7

*Frequency of chromosomal anomalies in abortuses in relation to
professional exposure to radiation*

	Percentage of different karyotypes				
	Normal	Monosomy	Trisomy	Triploidy, tetraploidy	Total abnormal
Paternal exposure (60 cases)	22	15	38	25	78
Control (805 cases)	38	10	34	18	62
Maternal exposure (49 cases)	33	18	35	14	67
Control (829 cases)	37	10	35	18	63

atomic industry). No attempt was made to establish correlations with X-ray dose since it was difficult to obtain precise information. A significant increase in the frequency of chromosome anomalies was observed when the father was occupationally exposed to radiation (table 7).

Smoking habits

The analysis of the influence of cigarette smoking was based on the number of cigarettes smoked daily and whether smoke was inhaled. Table 8 shows that in younger mothers there is a significant difference: in the group of mothers that smoked and inhaled, 50% of the abortuses had a normal karyotype. This increase in abortuses with normal karyotype may be explained by an increase of the incidence of abortions of genetically normal embryos due to cigarette smoking.

Prospective study

Seven hundred and seventy-eight women answered a questionnaire sent in October

1972. The obstetric history taken following the karyotyping of the abortion was analyzed in terms of fertility, births, and abortions.

Fertility

Table 9 shows the proportion of women that conceived during the 4 years following a spontaneous abortion in relation to their age. Table 10 shows the fertility in relation to the karyotype of the abortus. No significant differences were observed between the different types of chromosome anomalies; maternal age was the only factor detected. The fertility of the women was generally high. Other studies (James, '63) reported an increased probability of pregnancy following an abortion.

Births at term

In response to the questionnaire 313 deliveries were reported: 106 after an abortus with normal karyotype, 25 after a monosomy, 117 after a trisomy, 44 after a triploidy, 13 after a tetraploidy, and 8 after

J. BOUÉ, A. BOUÉ AND P. LAZAR

TABLE 8

Frequency of chromosome anomalies in abortuses
in relation to maternal smoking

	No. of cases	% Chromosome anomalies
Maternal age <30		
Smoking and inhaling	101	50
Smoking without inhaling	72	62
No smoking	371	61
Maternal age >30		
Smoking and inhaling	38	71
Smoking without inhaling	39	67
No smoking	191	75

a translocation. Abnormal deliveries and infants with pathological problems are listed in table 11. No significant difference was noted from the general population. It may be of interest to report that 2 placenta previas followed a triploid abortus.

Spontaneous abortions

The prospective study clearly indicated that most of the abortions occurred during the first 3 months of gestation (77/85). This permitted an estimate of the abortion frequency in a large number of pregnancies and the inclusion of the pregnancies of more than 5 months in progress at the time of the study, giving a total of 516 pregnancies.

Table 12 shows the frequency of abortions in relation to maternal age and to the karyotype, euploid or aneuploid, of the abortus. First there was an increased frequency of abortion with advanced maternal age, but more interesting is the fact that the frequency of abortions was higher after an abortion with normal karyotype. This difference was found in the 2 age groups and is significant.

No significant differences were observed in relation to the different types of chromosome anomalies: the frequency of abortion in the pregnancy following a monosomy was 14.2%; a trisomy, 13.6%; a triploidy, 18.2%; and a tetraploidy, 12%.

The most striking differences in the frequency of abortions were related to the reproductive history of the couples before the karyotyped abortion (table 13). When the karyotyped abortion was the first obstetrical event for the couple the incidence of abortion in the following pregnancy was around 15% with no variation in maternal age and a slight increase in the normal-karyotype group. Significant differences were observed in the second group, which previously had only had full-term deliveries, with a good prognosis if there was an abnormal karyotype in the abortus. It may

TABLE 9

Fertility after a spontaneous abortion in relation to maternal
age at the time of the karyotyped abortus

Time of observation (years)	Maternal age			Total (778)
	<30 years (482)	31–40 years (214)	>40 years (32)	
1	54.5	42.0	9.5	48.5
2	74.7	61.0	19.6	67.7
3	83.3	66.3	19.6	75.1
4	87.3	73.0	19.6	80

TABLE 10

Fertility after a spontaneous abortion in relation to the karyotype of the abortus

Time of observation (years)	Karyotype of the abortus					
	Normal (249)	Monosomy (74)	Trisomy (269)	Triploidy (109)	Tetraploidy (36)	Translocation (19)
1	51.4	53.5	46.0	48.4	51.1	42.7
2	73.3	68.9	62.9	68.7	74.4	66.6
3	79.0	78.5	69.5	74.0	79.5	83.3
4	79.0	87.1	77.5	74.0	79.5	—

TABLE 11

Placenta previa	2	1 at 6 months; the infant died after a few days 1 at 38 weeks; normal infant
Stillbirth	3	1 anencephalus 1 obstetrical trauma (no malformation and normal karyotype) 1 death in utero at 7 months (no autopsy)
Congenital malformation	6	2 cardiac malformations 2 dislocations of the hip 1 clubfoot 1 umbilical hernia
Isoimmunization	2	normal babies after exchange transfusion
"Small for date" and premature	24	

TABLE 12

Frequency of recurring spontaneous abortion in relation to the karyotype of the previous abortus and to maternal age

Maternal age	Karyotype of the previous abortus	
	Normal	Abnormal
< 30 years (354)	21.1%	15.6%
> 30 years (135)	29.0%	18.6%
Total (489)	23%	16.5%

be postulated that maternal causes (incompetent cervix, etc.) are responsible for the high percentage of recurring abortion when the karyotype of the abortus is normal. Among women with previous abortions, with or without deliveries, the frequency of recurring abortion was generally high.

These results were established more precisely in 43 women that each had 2 consecutive spontaneous abortuses karyotyped (Boué and Boué, '73c). There were no correlations between the first and the second abnormal karyotype (table 14), and even in the group of trisomies the extra autosomes involved in 2 consecutive trisomies were different in most cases.

DISCUSSION

The few epidemiological studies that have been made of spontaneous abortions and their chromosome anomalies faced numerous methodological problems (Alberman, '73): no data could be obtained regarding the pregnancies of the mothers from whom the sample studied were derived (outcome of pregnancies with deliveries, true incidence of spontaneous abortions); abortions of primigravidas were underrepresented in all the surveys; and precise information about the reproductive history of the couples were difficult to obtain, being retrospective.

In addition technical aspects of such studies may influence the results: (a) methods of collecting specimens may affect (1) the incidence of induced abortions included in the sample and (2) the proportion of early spontaneous abortions; (b) the tissue cultures techniques influence the proportion of successfully cultured and karyotyped abortuses; and furthermore (c) the number and the quality of chromosome preparations analyzed for each specimen will likewise influence the frequency of chromosome anomalies detected. A study of in vitro growth characteristics, and of the in vitro lifespan of cell cultures initiated from aneuploid embryos, has shown that early-lethal chromosome anomalies (3.4 weeks of developmental age) are more difficult to grow than anomalies that permit longer development (5.7 weeks) (Boué et al., '75). The proportion of negative results may affect not only the abnormality rate but also the proportion of anomalies found. These problems must be considered when comparing the results of different surveys.

In our study some of the results are clear, namely the retrospective study showed differences in the relation of maternal age to the different types of chromosome anomalies. The maternal-age effect was restricted to a few anomalies, mainly to autosomal trisomy involving an acrocentric chromosome.

In the prospective study an important observation was the relation between the reproductive history and the risk of recurring abortion. This showed that couples take wide variations in risk of conceiving zygotes with numerical chromosome errors. With the exception of the maternal-age effect it was impossible to determine the relative importance of maternal or paternal factors or whether, in some cases,

J. BOUÉ, A. BOUÉ AND P. LAZAR

TABLE 13

Frequency of recurring spontaneous abortion in relation to the karyotype of the previous abortus, to reproductive history, and to maternal age

Reproductive history before the karyotyped abortus	Karyotype of the abortus studied	Frequency of recurring abortion		
			Maternal age	
		All ages	< 30 years	> 30 years
No obstetric events	Abnormal	13.3 (98)	13.3 (83)	13.3 (15)
	Normal	15.8 (46)	15.6 (40)	16.7 (6)
Delivery(ies) without spontaneous abortions	Abnormal	7.2 (70)	7.3 (41)	7.7 (26)
	Normal	24.3 (25)	19.2 (16)	33.3 (9)
Delivery(ies) with spontaneous abortions	Abnormal	24.5 (54)	23.0 (27)	24.0 (25)
	Normal	37.5 (24)	38.9 (18)	33.3 (6)
Abortion(s) only	Abnormal	22.1 (64)	14.3 (42)	41.5 (20)
	Normal	21.0 (39)	23.3 (31)	12.5 (8)

TABLE 14

Correlation between the karyotypes of 2 consecutive abortuses

Karyotype of first abortus		Karyotype of second abortus				
		Normal (12) [1]	Monosomy (2)	Trisomy (22)	Triploidy (5)	Translocation (2)
Normal	(15) [1]	7	1	5	2	
Monosomy	(4)	2		1	1	
Trisomy	(17)	2	1	13	1	
Triploidy	(5)	1		3	1	
Translocation	(2)					2

[1] ( ) number of observations.

abortions are related to the genotype of both parents.

Some of the results were only slightly significant, reflecting mainly the difficulties of conducting such studies. Concerning exposure to radiation the influence of paternal occupational exposure appears important; but no significant increase in chromosome anomalies was detected after maternal exposure to X-irradiation. Alberman et al. ('72) showed that mothers of abortuses with chromosome anomalies had been exposed to significantly more radiation than those of abortuses with normal chromosome constitution. In our study we were unable to collect enough information to try to evaluate the radiation doses received by the mothers.

The results concerning maternal smoking habits are in agreement with other studies of the effect of smoking on fetuses (Russell et al., '66; Schwartz et al., '72).

In the study of factors linked to delay at the time of fertilization an increase in the frequency of polyploidy was found. Likewise the increase of chromosome anomalies in abortuses after ovulation induction seems largely related to an increase of polyploidy. The high frequency of polyploidy after steroid-contraceptive treatment, noted by Carr ('70), was not observed in our study.

An analysis of certain factors did not show significant differences, but this may be inherent in this type of retrospective study. For instance, during our investigations it appeared that the incidence of triploid abortuses varied seasonally. Such variations were not shown upon analysis of the total data. If the results concerning the duration of the first part of the menstrual cycle are divided in 2 groups — conception occurring from April to September (warm season) and those occurring from

EPIDEMIOLOGY OF SPONTANEOUS ABORTION

TABLE 15

Seasonal influence on the presumed day of ovulation

| Karyotype of the abortus | Mean days of ovulation (after LMP) | |
| | Months of conception | |
	April–September	October–March
Normal	14.3	15.6
Trisomy	14.0	15.4
Polyploidy	15.5	18.3

October to March (cold season) — the difference observed in polyploidy is more impressive (table 15). It must be remembered that triploidy may result from different mechanisms: digyny, diandry, or dispermy, and a factor acting on one of these mechanisms may be obscured in an analysis of triploidy as a whole.

To clarify some of the factors influencing the incidence of chromosome anomalies it will be essential in the future to try to determine the origin of such anomalies as, for example, paternal or maternal origin in trisomy, the different mechanisms of triploidy, etc.

ACKNOWLEDGMENTS

These studies were supported by research grants from I.N.S.E.R.M. (Institut National de la Santé et de la Recherche Médicale), from D.G.R.S.T. (Délégation Générale à la Recherche Scientifique et Technique), and from private funds.

We are greatly indebted to Nicole Perraudin and Christiane Deluchat who provided fine technical assistance, to Mrs. S. Gueguen for her statistical work, to Susan Cure and Sam Berenberg for their assistance in writing the English text, and to Gisèle Robin who typed this manuscript many times.

LITERATURE CITED

Alberman, E. 1973 Epidemiology of spontaneous abortions and their chromosome constitution. In: Chromosomal Errors in Relation to Reproductive Failure. A. Boué and C. Thibault, eds. INSERM, Paris, pp. 305–316.
Alberman, E., P. E. Polani, J. A. F. Roberts, C. C. Spicer, M. Elliot, E. Armstrong, and R. K. Dhadial 1972 Parental X-irradiation and chromosome constitution in their spontaneously aborted foetuses. Ann. Hum. Genet., 36: 185–194.
Arakaki, D. T., and S. H. Waxman 1970 Effect of gestational and maternal age in early abortion. Obst. Gyn., 35: 264–269.

Boué, A., and J. G. Boué 1973a Etudes chromosomiques et anatomiques des grossesses suivant l'arrêt des contraceptifs. J. Gyn. Obst. Biol. Reprod., 2: 141–154.
——— 1974 Chromosome abnormalities and abortion. In: Physiology and Genetics of Reproduction. Vol. 2. F. M. Coutinho and F. Fuchs, eds. Plenum, New York, pp. 317–339.
Boué, J. G., and A. Boué 1973b Increased frequency of chromosomal anomalies in abortions after induced ovulation. Lancet, 1: 679–680.
——— 1973c Chromosomal analysis of two consecutive abortuses in 43 women. Humangenetik, 19: 275–280.
Boué, A., J. G. Boué, S. Cure, C. Deluchat and N. Perraudin 1975 In vitro cultivation of cells from aneuploid human embryos, initiation of cell lines and longevity of the cultures. In Vitro, in press.
Boué, J. G., A. Boué, and P. Lazar 1967 Les aberrations chromosomiques dans les avortements. Ann. Genet., 10: 179–187.
——— 1974 The epidemiology of human spontaneous abortions with chromosomal anomalies. In: Biology and Pathology of Aging Gametes. R. J. Blandau, ed. Karger, Basel, pp. 330–348.
Boué, J. G., A. Boué, P. Lazar, and S. Gueguen 1973 Outcome of pregnancies following a spontaneous abortion with chromosomal anomalies. Am. J. Obst. Gyn., 116: 806–842.
Carr, D. H. 1967 Chromosome anomalies as a cause of spontaneous abortion. Am. J. Obst. Gyn., 97: 283–293.
——— 1970 Chromosome studies in selected spontaneous abortions. 1. Conception after oral contraceptives. Can. Med. Ass. J., 103: 343–348.
Ford, C. E. 1960 Chromosomal abnormality and congenital malformation. In: CIBA Foundation Symposium on Congenital Malformations. G. E. W. Wolstenholme and C. M. O'Connor, eds. Churchill, London, pp. 32–47.
Fraser, G. R. 1963 Parental origin of the sex chromosomes in the XO and XXY karyotypes in man. Ann. Hum. Genet., 26: 297.
Gropp, A. 1974 Fetal mortality due to aneuploidy and irregular meiotic segregation in the mouse. In: Chromosomal Errors in Relation to Reproductive Failure. A. Boué and C. Thibault, eds. INSERM, Paris, pp. 255–269.
Hertig, A. T., and J. Rock 1973 Searching for early fertilized human ova. Gyn. Inv., 4: 121–139.
James, W. H. 1963 Note towards an epidemiology of spontaneous abortion. Am. J. Hum. Genet., 15: 223–240.
Kajii, T., K. Ohama, N. Nükawa, A. Ferrier, and S. Avirachan 1973 Banding analysis of chromosomal karyotypes in spontaneous abortion. Am. J. Hum. Genet., 25: 539–547.
Klinger, H. P., H. W. Kava, M. Glasser, and A. Kallenberg 1973 Cytogenetic, anthropometric and developmental studies of postcontraceptive reproduction in man. An interim report In: Chromosomal Errors in Relation to Reproductive Failure. A. Boué and C. Thibault, eds. INSERM, Paris, pp. 371–389.
Lilienfeld, A. M. 1969 Epidemiology of Mongolism. Johns Hopkins Press, Baltimore.
Pearson, P. L., J. P. M. Geraldts, and I. H. Pawlowitzki 1974 Chromosomal studies on hu-

J. BOUÉ, A. BOUÉ AND P. LAZAR

man male gametes. In: Chromosomal Errors in Relation to Reproductive Failure. A. Boué and C. Thibault, eds. INSERM, Paris, pp. 219–229.

Penrose, L. S., and G. F. Smith 1966 Down's Anomaly. Churchill, London.

Russel, S. C., R. Taylor, and R. N. Madison 1966 Some effects of smoking on pregnancy. J. Obst. Gyn. Br. Comm., 73: 742.

Schwartz, D., J. Goujard, M. Kaminski, and C. Rumeau = Rouquette 1972 Smoking and pregnancy. Results of a prospective study of 6989 women. Rev. Eur. Etud., 17: 867–874.

Stenchever, M. A., J. M. Hempel, and M. N. MacIntyre 1967 Cytogenetics of spontaneously aborted human fetuses. Obst. Gyn., 30: 683–691.

Szulman, A. E. 1965 Chromosomal aberrations in spontaneous human abortions. New Eng. J. Med., 272: 811–818.

Therkelsen, A. J., N. Grunnet, T. Hjort, O. Myhre Jensen, J. Jonasson, J. G. Lauritsen, J. Lindsten, and B. Petersen 1974 Studies on spontaneous abortions. In: Chromosomal Errors in Relation to Reproductive Failure. A. Boué and C. Thibault, eds. INSERM, Paris, pp. 81–93.

Warburton, D., and F. C. Fraser 1964 Spontaneous abortion risks in man: data from reproduction histories collected in a medical genetic unit. Am. J. Hum. Genet., 16: 1–25.

Witschi, E. 1970 Teratogenetic effects from overripeness of the egg. In: Congenital Malformations. Excerpta Med. Int. Cong. Ser. No. 204, Amsterdam, pp. 157–169.

From G. A. Machin (1974). Lancet, i, 549–551. Copyright (1974), by kind permission of the author and The Lancet Ltd

CHROMOSOME ABNORMALITY AND PERINATAL DEATH

G. A. MACHIN

Paediatric Research Unit, Guy's Hospital Medical School, London SE1 *

Summary   A survey of the chromosome constitution of unselected necropsied infants dying in hospital in the perinatal period was carried out in South and East London over a period of two years and nine months. Chromosome results were obtained from 500 of the 726 infants examined. There were 28 infants with chromosome abnormalities, accounting for 9% of macerated stillbirths, 4% of fresh stillbirths, and 6% of early neonatal deaths for which results were obtained. Chromosome abnormalities were found in 13% of infants with lethal malformations and 2·5% of infants dying from other causes. The incidence of E18-trisomy in this survey indicates that this abnormality is more common at birth than is generally accepted. It is suggested that a chromosome analysis should be an integral part of the perinatal necropsy.

INTRODUCTION

IN the early phases of pregnancy wastage (pre-implantation loss and spontaneous abortion), at least 35% of fetuses are chromosomally abnormal.[1-5] By contrast, the frequency of chromosomal abnormalities in liveborn infants is only 0·5%.[6-12] Information is not available regarding the incidence and types of chromosome abnormalities to be found in the later phase of pregnancy wastage (perinatal death).

MATERIALS AND METHODS

From September, 1970, to May, 1973, a survey of 726 unselected hospital perinatal necropsies was carried out in a continuous geographical area of east, south-east,

* Present address: Department of Pathology, Royal Hospital for Sick Children, Edinburgh EH9 1LF.

and south-central London. Tissues were taken for culture and chromosome analysis in all but 3 cases (in which chromosome analysis on peripheral leucocytes had been done in life). Gonad was the tissue of choice in neonatal deaths; placental amnion was used in macerated stillbirths, while both gonad and amnion were used from fresh stillbirths. After transport to the laboratory in culture medium, tissues were set up as explants in 30 ml. Falcon flasks and cultured in medium 199 with 20% human serum at pH 7·2 (Hepes buffer). Routine methods were used for processing cultures through to chromosome preparations. For each specimen at least 10 cells were counted and analysed. Suitable metaphases were photographed and karyotyped in all cases. G and Q banded chromosome preparations were made where indicated, using modifications of published methods.[13,14]

RESULTS

The frequency of chromosome abnormality was 5·6% (table I). Although results were obtained from only 18% of macerated stillbirths, the chromosome abnormality rate was the highest in that group. As expected, most chromosomal abnormalities were found in malformed infants (table II). Nevertheless, of infants dying from causes other than malformation,

TABLE I—CHROMOSOME RESULTS BY TIME OF DEATH

Time of death	Total	Chromosome results	Chromosome abnormality
Antepartum (macerated stillbirth)	185	34 (18%)	3 (9%)
Intrapartum (fresh stillbirth)	160	122 (76%)	5 (4·1%)
Early neonatal	381	344 (90%)	20 (5·8%)
Total	726	500 (69%)	28 (5·6%)

TABLE II—CHROMOSOME RESULTS BY PRIMARY NECROPSY FINDINGS

Primary necropsy finding	No. of infants	Chromosome result	Chromosome abnormality
Lethal malformation (stillbirths and neonatal deaths)	173	142	19 (13·4%)
Antepartum stillbirth ..	154	27	2 (7%)
Intrapartum anoxia and/or trauma	181	145	1
Prematurity-associated disease	135	124	4 (3·2%)
Infection	45	39	2 (5%)
Other	38	23	0
Total	726	500	28 (5·6%)

2·5% were chromosomally abnormal.

Table III lists the individual chromosome abnormalities; E-trisomy was the most common abnormality, and E-trisomic males exceeded females. While G-trisomy was generally diagnosed clinically, the D and E trisomic infants, all of whom were lethally malformed, were seldom recognised as such. 6 infants had chromosomal translocations, and 2 others had structural abnormalities that may have represented unbalanced translocations.

Table IV demonstrates a seasonal variation in the occurrence of chromosomal abnormalities. Two-thirds of the infants with chromosome abnormalities were born in the period April to July. All the infants with E-trisomy were born between the months of March and July inclusive, and this pattern was repeated in the three consecutive years.

The effect of maternal age on the chromosome abnormality rate is shown in table v. The chromosomally abnormal infants born to women over forty years of age were all trisomic.

DISCUSSION

The frequency of chromosome abnormality among infants dying in the perinatal period was intermediate between that found in spontaneous abortions and in

TABLE III—CHROMOSOME RESULTS

Chromosome results	No.	Suspected clinically	Lethal malformation
46,XY	280	0	61
46,XX	208	0	62
47,XX, +21	3*	3	1
47,XX, +18	3*,†	1	3
47,XY, +18	5*	1	5
47,XX, +13	2*	0	2
47,XY, +13	1	0	1
47,XX, +t(21q21q)	1	1	1
45,XY,t(13q21q)	1	0	0
45,XY,t(14q15q)pat ..	1	0	0
46,XX, −13, +t(13q21q) ..	1	0	0
46,XX,t(12;17) (q24;q21)mat	1*	0	1
46,XX, −21, +t(16p21p)mat	1	0	1
45,X	1	1	1
47,XXY	2†	0	0
46,XY/47,XXY	1†	0	0
47,XYY	1	0	1
69,XXY	1	0	1
46,XX,Gp −	1	0	0
46,XX,15p + ...	1	0	1

* Fresh stillbirths (5).
† Macerated stillbirths (3)
The remainder (20) were in early neonatal deaths.

TABLE IV—SEASONAL VARIATION IN CHROMOSOMALLY ABNORMAL NECROPSIES

	Jan.	Feb.	March	April	May	June	July	Aug.	Sept.	Oct.	Nov.	Dec.
Chromosome results	49	31	57	53	58	36	43	43	30	39	37	24
Chromosome abnormality ..	1	1	2	5	4	5	4	2	1	1	0	2
E-trisomy ..	0	0	2	2	1	2	1	0	0	0	0	0

TABLE V—MATERNAL-AGE DISTRIBUTION OF CHROMOSOME ABNORMALITIES

—	Maternal age (yr.)						
	< 20	20–24	25–29	30–39	≥ 40	Total	Not known
Karyotyped infants ..	75	124	113	81	14	407	93*
Chromosomally abnormal ..	1	6	9	7	5	28	0

* The proportion in each of the maternal-age groups accords well with the figures for all births in 1971, according to the Registrar General.[15]

unselected liveborn infants. While it might be expected that a substantial proportion of the malformed infants would be chromosomally abnormal, the rate of 2·5% in infants dying from causes other than malformation was five times that found in surveys of unselected liveborn infants.[6–12] The types of chromosome abnormality resembled those found in liveborn infants rather than in aborted fetuses, but the phenotypic expression was often difficult to recognise; D and E trisomic infants in particular showed multiple lethal malformations which tended to obscure the clinical diagnosis because they were more severe than those found in infants surviving the early neonatal period.[16]

Although the yield of chromosome results was low in macerated stillbirths, a 9% frequency of chromosome abnormality indicates that this group of perinatal deaths is especially worthy of investigation for chromosome constitution. Other work indicates that 2·7% of stillborn infants have sex-chromatin abnormalities.[17]

There was a high incidence of E-trisomy in this series. According to the surveys of unselected liveborn infants,[6–12] the incidence of E-trisomy is 1 in 10,000, although a better estimate may be 1 in 5000.[18] Since 13% of E-trisomic infants have been reported to die in the first week of life,[16,19] early neonatal death with E-trisomy may be expected to have an incidence of 1 in 38,000 to 1 in 77,000 livebirths. It was not possible to ascertain the exact number of live births from which the 344 karyotyped early neonatal deaths in this survey were derived, but the early-neonatal death-rate in Greater London in 1971 was 9·9 per 1000 live births[15]; thus, the 344 karyotyped infants dying in the first week may be considered to have

been derived from 34,400 live births. By this calculation, 5 to 10 times the expected number of E-trisomic infants were found in this series. When the 3 stillborn E-trisomics are considered, the discrepancy becomes even greater.

This finding accords with other reports[20–23] that a larger number of E-trisomic infants is born than had been observed in large surveys.[6–12] The frequency sometimes approaches that for G-trisomy, and this view is confirmed by the chromosome constitution of fetuses aborted after antenatal diagnosis on the grounds of risk for maternal-age-dependent autosomal trisomy.[24] The observation of an increased frequency of E-trisomy at birth[20–23] has been attributed either to a genuinely increased incidence or to temporal clustering. The present survey, over a period of nearly three years, supports both views, since all the E-trisomic infants were born in the months of March to July inclusive; this is a peak period for the birth of chromosomally abnormal infants that has also been reported by others.[18,25] However, one series of E-trisomic infants had a peak incidence for births in June to November.[16]

The sex ratio is disturbed in most series of E-trisomics.[16,19] This has been attributed to the earlier death of affected males, and the findings of the present survey support this view.

The maternal-age effect was striking. Chromosome abnormality was found in roughly a third of infants dying in the perinatal period where the maternal age exceeded forty years. It is possible that younger mothers of all primary trisomic infants have an increased risk of trisomy in subsequent pregnancies.[26] All parents who came for genetic advice on this subject were offered antenatal chromosome diagnosis in any subsequent pregnancy.

Of the eight infants with presumed or proven chromosome translocations (both balanced and unbalanced), only five families were studied in detail. In three cases, a parent carried the chromosomal abnormality in a balanced form. So far, one couple has had two subsequent pregnancies. One was terminated because antenatal diagnosis revealed an unbalanced translocation in the fetus; the second went to term because the fetus was shown to be chromosomally normal.

Chromosome abnormalities are most commonly found among malformed infants, macerated stillbirths, and perinatal deaths where the maternal age exceeds forty years. The present results indicate that chromosome analysis on all infants dying in the perinatal period would contribute considerably towards a further understanding of ætiology, and sometimes provide a useful indication for preventive action in future pregnancies.

This work was carried out with grants from the Medical Research Council and the Research Fund of the University of London. I thank Prof. P. E. Polani, F.R.S., for guidance and discussion of this work, and Mr J. A. Crolla for technical assistance. The cooperation and interest of pathologists, obstetricians, and pædiatricians is also gratefully acknowledged.

REFERENCES

1. Carr, D. H. *Am. J. Obstet. Gynec.* 1967, **97**, 283.
2. Boué, J. G., Boué, A. *Presse méd.* 1970, **78**, 635.
3. Dhadial, R. K., Machin, A. M., Tait, S. M. *Lancet*, 1970, ii, 20.
4. Stenchever, M. A., Hempel, J. M., MacIntyre, M. N. *Obstet. Gynec.* 1967, **30**, 683.
5. Arakaki, D. T., Waxman, S. H. *J. med. Genet.* 1970, 7, 118.
6. Sergovich, F., Valentine, G. H., Chen, A. T. L., Kinch, R. A. H., Smout, M. S. *New Engl. J. Med.* 1969, **280**, 851.
7. Court Brown, W. M., Smith, P. G. *Br. med. Bull.* 1969, **25**, 74.
8. Ratcliffe, S. G., Stewart, A. L., Melville, M. M., Jacobs, P. A., Keay, A. J. *Lancet*, 1970, i, 121.
9. Gerald, P. S., Walzer, S. *in* Human Population Cyto-genetics (edited by P. A. Jacobs, W. H. Price, and P. Law); p. 143. Edinburgh, 1970.
10. Turner, J. H., Wald, N. *ibid.* p. 153.
11. Lubs, H. A., Ruddle, F. H. *ibid.* p. 119.
12. Hamerton, J. L., Ray, M., Abbott, J., Williamson, C., Ducasse, G. C. *Can. med. Ass. J.* 1972, **106**, 776.
13. Seabright, M. *Chromosoma*, 1972, **36**, 204.
14. Caspersson, T., Lomakka, G., Zech, L. *Hereditas*, 1971, **67**, 89.
15. Registrar General's Statistical Review of England and Wales for the year 1971. H.M. Stationery Office.
16. Taylor, A. I. *J. med. Genet.* 1968, **5**, 227.
17. Bochkov, N. P., Antoschina, M. M., Stonova, N. S. *Cytologia*, 1966, **8**, 215.
18. Conen, P. E., Erkman, B. *Am. J. hum. Genet.* 1966, **18**, 387.
19. Weber, W. W. *ibid.* 1967, **19**, 369.
20. Kardon, N., Hsu, L. Y., Beratis, N., Hirschhorn, K. *Lancet*, 1970, ii, 782.
21. Shapiro, L. R. *ibid.* p. 1035.
22. Anderson, N. G., Smithurst, B., Regius, Mary, Walsh, S. *ibid.* p. 1085.
23. Cohen, M. M. *ibid.* 1971, i, 1017.
24. Polani, P. E., Benson, P. F. *Guy's Hosp. Rep.* (in the press).
25. Robinson, A., Good, W. B., Puck, T. T., Harris, J. S. *Am. J. hum. Genet.* 1969, **21**, 466.
26. Boué, J., Boué, A. *Humangenetik*, 1973, **19**, 275.

CYTOGENETICS OF FETAL WASTAGE

Hyon J. Kim, M.D., Lillian Y.F. Hsu, M.D., Sophie Paciuc, B.S.,
Steluta Cristian, B.S., Alicia Quintana, M.D.,
and Kurt Hirschhorn, M.D.

Abstract A consecutive series of 50 couples with a history of fetal wastage were studied cytogenetically with current banding technics. Fetal wastage was defined as occurring in couples who had more than two early abortions, stillbirth(s) or livebirth(s) or both of infants with multiple congenital anomalies. Three women were found to be balanced reciprocal translocation carriers; all translocations were not detectable by the conventional method but were demonstrable by current banding technics. In addition to the translocation carriers, one woman was found to be a mosaic for 45,X/46,XX/47,XXX. Four of the parents showed increased mitotic instability or chromosome breakage and rearrangement, or both. Parental chromosome abnormalities may therefore account for fetal wastage in between 6 and 16 per cent (or about one in 10) of couples having such a history. Such couples, if identified, can potentially benefit by prenatal monitoring of future pregnancies. (N Engl J Med 293:844-847, 1975)

CYTOGENETIC studies have shown that numerical and structural chromosome aberrations are important etiologic factors in spontaneous abortion, in stillbirth and in livebirths of infants with multiple anomalies. A number of studies on spontaneous abortuses have demonstrated that a substantial proportion of such abortuses are chromosomally abnormal.[1] Recently, Kajii et al. (1973)[2] reported that 82 of 152, or 54 per cent, of products of spontaneous abortions successfully cultured had chromosome anomalies. Most of the anomalies consisted of de novo events occurring in the course of meiosis or in early mitotic division, but some of these chromosomal aberrations could be traced to parental balanced translocations resulting in an unbalanced gamete.

In 1962, Schmid[3] presented the results of chromosome analysis in couples with a history of two or more spontaneous abortions. There have been 10 major cytogenetic studies of couples with fetal wastage in the literature. In 1971, Carr[1] reviewed these studies and found 25 persons who were considered to have karyotypes with variant chromosomes and 11 who had abnormal karyotypes out of the 664 people whose chromosomes were studied. One was mosaic for 45,X/46,XX and 10 were translocation car-

From the Division of Medical Genetics, Department of Pediatrics, Mount Sinai School of Medicine, 100th Street and Fifth Ave., New York, NY 10029, where reprint requests should be addressed to Dr. Kim.

Supported by grants (GM-19443 and HD-02552) from the U.S. Public Health Service and a Medical Service Grant from the National Foundation (C-155) (Drs. Hsu and Hirschhorn are career scientists of the Health Research Council of the City of New York [LYFH, I-761; KH, I-513]). Dr. Quintana was a visiting fellow from the University of Barcelona.

riers. He concluded that the occurrence of 10 translocation carriers among 664 people with a history of fetal wastage was about 12 times higher than the occurrence of translocations in the newborn population,[4] which is a noteworthy increase.

The past few years have seen great advances in human genetics owing to the discovery of several technics permitting accurate recognition of each chromosome and its parts. The application of these technics has already led to more accurate identification of several chromosomal abnormalities.[5] Before the development of the current banding technics, only numerical aberrations and obvious deletions or unequal translocations were identified. It seemed quite probable that many translocations involving exchanged pieces of approximately the same length, and therefore undetectable by ordinary staining, would be detected by the new technics. To determine the frequency and types of chromosome aberrations in couples with fetal wastage we used current banding technics.

MATERIALS AND METHODS

From July, 1972, to January, 1975, we studied a consecutive series of 50 couples with a history of two or more spontaneous abortions, stillbirth (or stillbirths) or livebirth (livebirths), or both, with multiple congenital anomalies (Table 1). Most of the couples were referred by obstetricians after other known causes of fetal wastage (such as pelvic abnormality, endocrinopathy, diabetes, and blood-group incompatibility) were ruled out.

Table 1. Classification of 50 Couples with Fetal Wastage.

HISTORY OF FETAL WASTAGE	NO. OF COUPLES
Spontaneous 1st-trimester abortion (s) + stillbirth or livebirth with multiple congenital anomalies (or both)	16
>2 spontaneous abortions, with or without normal offspring	34

Slides were prepared from peripheral blood cultures by a modification of the method of Moorhead et al.[6] for conventional karyotype analysis with Giemsa stain. Both the quinacrine fluorescent method[7] and a modified trypsin G-banding method[5] were employed for further identification of chromosomes. Twenty good metaphases were counted for each subject, and three of the better metaphases were photographed to prepare karyotypes. If numerical variation was found in the first 20 cells, a total of 50 metaphase cells were counted and analyzed. Regardless of the findings in the conventional karyotypes, all cases were studied with technics using Q or G banding or both.

RESULTS

Banded karyotypes were analyzed to search for structural variation. Results of cytogenetic studies were divided into three groups as shown in Table 2.

Group A

In this group 92 subjects (44 females and 48 males) were found to have normal karyotypes. Although a number (24 per cent of subjects studied) of polymorphisms (e.g., 1qh+, 9qh+, 9qh−, Ds+, Gs+, Yq+, Yq−) were found, these are generally considered to be normal vari

Table 2. Results of the Cytogenetic Study of 50 Couples with Fetal Wastage.

GROUP	NO. OF SUBJECTS	RESULT
A	92	Normal karyotype
B	4	Mitotic instability or an increased chromosome breakage & rearrangement (or both)
C	4	Abnormal karyotypes: Mosaicism — 1 case (Case 5, 45, X/46,XX/47,XXX) Balanced translocation — 3 cases (Case 6, 46,XX,t[17;19] [q23;p13], Case 7, 46,XX,t[4;11] [q25;q13], & Case 8, 46,XX,t[13;22] [q22;q12]).

ants,[8] with a frequency recently estimated to be about 26 to 29 per cent.[9,10] Two subjects were found to carry small pericentric inversions of chromosome 9, inv 9 (p+q−), which is also thought to be a normal variant[11] although its potential effect has not been fully evaluated.

Group B

Four subjects demonstrated mitotic instability or an increase in chromosome breakage (or both). The family of Case 1 was studied because of one early abortion and a still-born infant with multiple congenital anomalies. Chromosome analysis of cultured peripheral leukocytes from the husband revealed that 16 per cent of the metaphase cells had chromosome breakage in a C-group chromosome. Q-banding demonstrated that the chromosomes involved in the breakage were all No. 10 and that the breakage point was always 10q24.[12] The normal value in our laboratory for chromosome breakage is between 0 and 4 per cent. A second peripheral blood culture showed 8 per cent of the metaphase cells with abnormal findings: one cell with a breakage in 10q24, one cell with a pericentric inversion of No. 4, one cell with an extra acrocentric chromosome and a tri-radial rearrangement figure and one cell that was triploid (69, XYY). Subsequent skin fibroblast cultures showed that 10 per cent of the cells had chromosome breakage involving different groups of chromosomes. During this study the patient's wife was pregnant. Amniocentesis showed a normal female karyotype; a normal female infant was delivered. In Case 2 mosaicism of type 46,XY/47,XYY was found, and skin fibroblast culture showed 6 per cent chromosome breakage. His wife had three spontaneous abortions and a trisomy 21. Case 3, a female, had had four early abortions. The karyotype showed 46,XX with a No. 1 chromosome that had an extended heterochromatic area (1qh+). In addition to this polymorphism, she had mitotic instability in 8 per cent of cultured peripheral leukocytes (one cell with 46,XX,r(1), one cell with 47,XXX, one cell with 47,XX,+21, and one cell with 47,XX, +D[?15]). Case 4, a female, had had two spontaneous first-trimester abortions. Ten per cent of the cultured peripheral leukocytes showed abnormal karyotypes: three cells had 47,XX,+16, one cell had 46,XX, r(1) and one cell had 47,XX, with a ring chromosome or a fragment.

Group C

This group had abnormal karyotypes probably responsible for increased fetal wastage. Case 5, a female, (45,X/46,XX/47,XXX) had a history of infertility, one stillbirth, and two first-trimester abortions. Three women were identified as balanced translocation carriers. In two out of these three cases, regular karyotypes were considered normal and translocations were recognized only with banding karyotypes. Case 6, a female, came to us for genetic counseling because of a first-trimester abortion and a stillbirth with multiple congenital anomalies. The couple had been married for six years, and the wife was taking oral contraceptive pills for the first four years. They did not have any problems in conceiving. The wife's conventional karyotype revealed a normal female constitution. However, a G-banding study showed a balanced translocation involving a No. 17 and a No. 19 chromosome. The distal band of the long arm of a No. 17 was translocated to the short arm of a No. 19 chromosome. Without banding patterns, it is easy to misinterpret the 17q− as the 19 and the 19p+ as the 17 chromosome (Fig. 1a). Case 7's (a female) first pregnancy resulted in a male infant with multiple congenital anomalies who died at six weeks of age. She then gave birth to two phenotypically normal sons.

Her fourth pregnancy resulted in a spontaneous first-trimester abortion. Two years later (at the age of 32 years) she gave birth to a daughter with trisomy-21 Down's syndrome. Banded karyotypes demonstrated a balanced translocation involving chromosomes No. 4 and 11, with the two exchanged chromosome segments identical in size (Fig. 1b). Therefore, although this translocation was also not detectable by a conventional karyotype, the different banding patterns of the exchanged segments made it possible to identify the abnormality. Both her phenotypically normal sons also revealed the balanced reciprocal translocation identical to the one found in the mother. Case 8, a female, was ascertained through an abnormal infant with multiple anomalies. She had a first-trimester spontaneous abortion in addition to the abnormal offspring. Her conventional karyotype showed an apparently normal female karyotype. A reciprocal translocation, involving a No. 13 and a No. 22 chromosome, was identified by both Q and G banding (Fig. 1c). The male infant was found to have 47 chromosomes with an extra acrocentric chromosome of a size close to that of the G group that was identified as the smaller of the two translocation chromosomes as found in his mother, der (22),t(13;22) (q22;q12)mat.[12] The clinical features and subsequent autopsy findings showed a combination of both trisomy-13 and trisomy-22 syndromes.

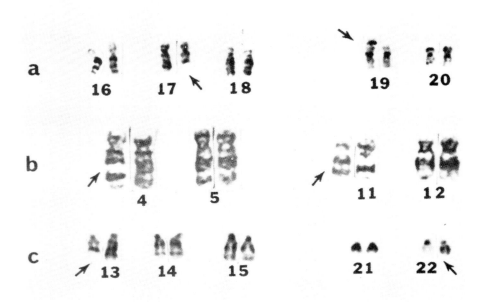

Figure 1. Partial Giemsa Banding Karyotypes of Three Patients with Balanced Reciprocal Translocations (Arrows Indicate the Translocation Chromosomes): Case 6 (a) — 46,XX,t(17;19) (q23;p13); Case 7 (b) — 46,XX,t (4;11) (q25;q13); and Case 8 (c) — 46,XX,t(13;22)(q22;q12).

Discussion

Earlier cytogenetic studies in our laboratory, using only conventionally stained karyotypes, yielded three numerical chromosome aberrations (two mosaics for 45,X/46,XX/47,XXX,[13] one mosaic for 46,XY/47,XY, + D and one obvious structural rearrangement, 46,XX, inv 2 [p+q−]),[14] in 53 parents, including 24 couples and five single parents with fetal wastage. In 1972, Lucas, Wallace and Hirschhorn reported chromosome abnormalities in 42 families with recurrent abortions and estimated, from a review of the literature, that one in 26 couples with fetal wastage carry a balanced translocation. They predicted that the frequency of translocations among such couples would be even higher if banding technics were used in future studies. Our present investigation, in which 50 couples were studied with both conventional and banding technics, revealed three balanced translocations (one in 16 couples). In fact, all three structural rearrangements were considered to be normal by conventional staining but were demonstrated to be balanced translocations in banded karyotypes. All three balanced translocations were found in the group of couples who had at least one stillbirth or a live-born infant with multiple congenital anomalies in addition to earlier spontaneous abortions. Although carriers of balanced translocations are usually phenotypically normal, the chance for such persons to produce chromosomally abnormal gametes is high, owing to unbalanced segregation and nondisjunction of the involved chromosomes,[15] as in our Case 8. If such an abnormal gamete is fertilized, it will result in either a non-viable or a malformed fetus. Furthermore, carriers of balanced translocations have an apparently increased risk of meiotic nondisjunction of other chromosomes, leading to a trisomic offspring,[15-20] as also seen in our Case 7.

Persons showing increased mitotic instability (mosaicism) or chromosome breakage and rearrangement, or both, require additional study. It is necessary to determine whether there is any causal relation between these findings and abnormal embryogenesis, or meiotic events leading to fetal wastage.

Couples with fetal wastage, particularly in families with a history of at least one abnormal offspring in addition to repeated spontaneous abortions, would be studied with the new banding technics for precise chromosome identification. Identification of abnormal karyotype in such cases allows for more precise genetic counseling. It also permits these couples to have subsequent pregnancies monitored by amniocentesis, and provides them either with reassurance or with the option to terminate a pregnancy with an unbalanced chromosome constitution.

References

1. Carr DH: Chromosomes and abortion. Adv Hum Genet 2:201-257, 1971
2. Kajii T, Ohama K, Niikawa N, et al: Banding analysis of abnormal karyotypes in spontaneous abortion. Am J Hum Genet 25:539-547, 1973
3. Schmid W: A familial chromosome abnormality associated with repeated abortions. Cytogenetics 1:199-209, 1962
4. Jacobs PA: Chromosome mutations: frequency at birth in humans. Humangenetik 16:137-140, 1972
5. Hirschhorn K, Lucas M, Wallace I: Precise identification of various chromosomal abnormalities. Ann Hum Genet 36:375-379, 1973
6. Moorhead PS, Nowell PC, Mellman WJ, et al: Chromosome preparations of leukocytes cultured from human peripheral blood. Exp Cell Res 20:613-616, 1960
7. Breg ER: Quinacrine fluorescence for identifying metaphase chromosomes, with special reference to photomicrography. Stain Technol 47:87-93, 1972
8. Court Brown WM, Buckton KE, Jacobs PA, et al: Chromosome studies on adults, Eugenics Laboratory Memoirs 42. London, Cambridge University Press, 1966
9. Mikelsaar AVN, Tüür SJ, Käosaar ME: Human karyotype polymorphism. I. Routine and fluorescence investigation of chromosomes in a normal adult population. Humangenetik 20:89-101, 1973
10. Holbek S, Friedrich U, Lauritsen JG, et al: Marker chromosomes in parents of spontaneous abortuses. Humangenetik 25:61-64, 1974
11. Madan K, Bobrow M: Structural variation in chromosome No 9. Ann Genet (Paris) 17:(2)81-86, 1974
12. Paris Conference (1971): standardization in human cytogenetics. Birth Defects 8(7), 1972
13. Hsu LYF, Garcia FP, Grossman D, et al: Fetal wastage and maternal mosaicism. Obstet Gynecol 40:98-103, 1972
14. Hsu LYF, Barcinski M, Shapiro LR, et al: Parental chromosomal aberrations associated with multiple abortions and an abnormal infant. Obstet Gynecol 36:723-730, 1970
15. Lucas M, Wallace I, Hirschhorn K: Recurrent abortions and chromosome abnormalities. J Obstet Gynecol Br Commonw 79:1119-1127, 1972
16. Hamerton JL, Giannelli F, Carter CO: A family showing transmission of a D/D reciprocal translocation and a case of regular 21-trisomic Down's syndrome. Cytogenetics 2:194-207, 1963
17. Palmer CG, Conneally PM, Christian JC: Translocation of D chromosomes in two families: t(13q 14q) and t(13q 14q) + (13p 14p). J Med Genet 6:166-173, 1963
18. Subrt I, Prchlíková H: Double chromosomal aberration trisomy G and the balanced translocation t(3p−;17q+). Humangenetik 8:111-114, 1969
19. Forabosco A, Dutrillaux B, Toni G, et al: Enfant trisomique 21 libre et translocation t(14q22p) maternelle. Ann Genet (Paris) 16:57-59, 1973
20. Tenconi R, Baccichetti C, Dussini N, et al: Familial translocation t(6:18) (q16:q23) with free trisomy 21. Ann Genet (Paris) 17:275-277, 1974

PAPERS 17 AND 18

COMMENTARY

The fertilizing capacity of the ovum and spermatozoa in the female genital tract extends to about 24 and 72 hours respectively. Fertilization occurs predominantly within these periods in normal embryonic development. Blandau (1954) and Lanman (1968a, b) have reviewed the consequences of ageing of the gametes before fertilization, although much of this information is derived from animal studies. Loss of fertilizing capacity and chromosomal aberrations are usual findings in this condition.

In Paper 17, Guerrero and Rojas (1975) present substantial clinical evidence indicating that ageing of human gametes before fertilization results in an increased frequency of spontaneous abortions. Boué *et al.* (see Paper 14) reported that more than 60% of all abortions were associated with chromosomal abnormalities. The high incidence of spontaneous abortions detected by Guerrero and Rojas may very well represent nature's rejection of abnormal embryos. This interesting hypothesis is discussed by Roberts and Lowe in Paper 18. These authors postulate that prenatal losses may be the 'rule rather than the exception, with the implication that in the world of early embryos, malformations may be the norm rather than the exception'.

REFERENCES

Blandau, R. J. (1954). The effects on development when eggs and sperm are aged before fertilization. *Ann. N.Y. Acad. Sci.*, **57**, 526–530

Lanman, J. T. (1968a). Delays during reproduction and their effects on the embryo and fetus. I. Aging of sperm. *N. Engl. J. Med*, **278**, 993–999

Lanman, J. T. (1968b). Delays during reproduction and their effects on the embryo and fetus. II. Aging of eggs. *N. Engl. J. Med.*, **278**, 1047–1054

*From R. Guerrero and O. I. Rojas (1975). N. Engl. J. Med., **293**, 573–575. Copyright (1975), by kind permission of the authors and the Massachusetts Medical Society*

SPONTANEOUS ABORTION AND AGING OF HUMAN OVA AND SPERMATOZOA

Rodrigo Guerrero V., M.D., Dr.P.H., and Oscar I. Rojas, M.D.

Abstract   To test the hypothesis that aging of human gametes within the genital tract increases the chance of abortion, we measured the probabilities of abortion after insemination on a given day of the menstrual cycle in relation to the day of the shift in the basal body temperature in 965 patients. Cases came from family-planning and sterility clinics where basal body temperature and coital records are kept routinely. The probability of abortion diminished significantly (P < 0.001) as the shift in temperature was approached and then increased to its highest point (24 per cent) three days later.

Animal experiments have shown that aging of both spermatozoa and ova before fertilization is accompanied by higher probabilities of abortion. Present evidence indicates that this higher prevalence is also true for human beings. (N Engl J Med 293:573-575, 1975)

THE effects on development when eggs and sperm are aged before fertilization have been reviewed by Blandau[1] and more recently by Lanman.[2,3] In general it can be said that, in the animal species studied, aging of spermatozoa in the female genital tract is accompanied by a gradual decrease in the fertilizing capacity. This decrease in fertility has not been reported to be accompanied by an increased frequency of abnormalities with the exception of the hen. Aging of spermatozoa in the male genital tract is typically accompanied by a declining fertility without resulting defects in the offspring. Tesh and Glover[4] reported, however, that rabbit spermatozoa aged in the epididymis also led to pre-implantation and post-implantation losses and some malformations. Scarce and indirect evidence exists for human beings.

Aging of the ovum is conveniently separated into intrafollicular aging (preovulatory over-ripeness), when the ovum is retained in the follicle beyond the normal time, and intratubal aging (postovulatory over-ripeness), when the ovum is shed at the normal time but fertilization occurs late. Mikamo[5] has described well the teratogenic effects of preovulatory over-ripeness in laboratory-bred xenopus. Butcher and Fugo[6,7] have induced preovulatory over-ripeness and shown an increased frequency of chromosome defects in the rat. Typically, postovulatory over-ripeness, in the species studied, has been found to be associated with an increased proportion of sterile insemina-tions, a decrease in litter size and an increase in polyspermy, abortions and chromosomal anomalies.

The effects of certain kinds of delays occurring near the time of fertilization may have particular relevance in the human being because coital activity is not restricted to times of estrus or of coitus-induced ovulation as in many animals.[2,8] The human ovum seems to be unprotected against late fertilizations, and it has been suggested that women using the "rhythm method" may be especially at risk for this problem.[9-11] There are reports suggesting that fertilization late in the menstrual cycle may lead to abortions[12,13] and malformations.[14-16] The similarities of the anatomic and chromosomal anomalies found in human spontaneous abortions to those found in laboratory animals led Mikamo[17] to postulate fertilization of over-ripe ova (probably intrafollicular over-ripeness) as a cause of abortion. In a previous paper we submitted the hypothesis, based on empirical evidence, that aging of human gametes was associated with a higher risk of abortion.[18] The present paper confirms this finding with additional data.

Basal body temperature is a simple and reliable test for ovulation and is routinely used in infertility clinics and family-planning clinics using the rhythm method. Basal body temperature has shown to correlate well with ovulation,[19,20] and although some variation is known to occur,[21] it is generally accepted that ovulation takes place one or two days before the rise in temperature.

METHODS

A total of 1980 basal-body-temperature conception charts were analyzed for this study; 1125 came from rhythm family-planning

Address reprint requests to Dr. Guerrero at the Universidad del Valle, Apartado Aéreo 2188, Cali, Colombia, South America.

Supported by a grant (M 73.133) from the Population Council.

clinics, and 855 from sterility clinics. A detailed description of the collection of cases has been presented elsewhere.[22] Cases of artificial insemination were not included in this analysis. Each case was blindly coded for the following items:

Day of Temperature Shift

To define the day of the thermal shift, a line was drawn from left to right across the basal-body-temperature chart, just above the preovulatory readings (excluding temporary elevations presumably due to illness or other episodic factors). The day before the temperature rose to stay above that line was called day of the shift or Day 0. Days before Day 0 were counted with a minus sign, and those after with a plus sign. No attempt was made to relate changes in basal body temperature to ovulation, but although difficult to quantify, ovulation is believed to have a constant relation to the day of the shift.

Responsible Insemination

Any single insemination occurring during the fertile period thus determined was considered responsible for the pregnancy. If more than one insemination had taken place during this period the responsible inseminations could not be determined except when they were located on the same side of the shift. In this case, the one closest to it was assumed to be responsible. If there were no inseminations in this period, the limits of the fertile period were expanded to Days −10 and +3, and the same rules were followed. If there were no inseminations in these days the case was discarded. Only three cases fell in this latter category.

After discarding the cases in which a responsible insemination could not be determined 965 cases remained, of which 890 corresponded to term deliveries and 75 to spontaneous abortions. We determined the probability of abortion for each day in relation to the temperature shift by dividing the number of abortions on that day by the number of abortions plus term deliveries for the same day. Conceptions occurring to the right of the temperature shift (Days +1, +2 and +3) would be more likely to have resulted from over-ripe ova. Conceptions resulting from inseminations on the left side of the shift (Days −3, −4, −5, etc.) probably resulted from aged spermatozoa, whereas those from Days −2, −1 and 0 would normally be expected to come from fresh spermatozoa.

RESULTS

Table 1 summarizes the results. The overall probability of abortion was 7.8 per cent. The lowest corresponded to Day −2 (3.2 per cent), and the highest to Day +3 (24 per cent). A declining trend in the probability of abortion was found from days −9 to day 0 and then a sharp increase until Day +3 (Fig. 1).

The statistical significance was measured by using the chi-square test for linear trends described by Armitage.[23] Because of the biologic assumptions made above, two separate trends were calculated from Days −9 to Day 0 and Day +1 to Day +3. Both analyses showed highly significant results: 13.4 (with 1 degree of freedom), $P < 0.001$, for the first group; and 10.1 (with 1 degree of freedom), $P < 0.01$, for the second. These tests indicate that results were unlikely to be due to chance. The results were not altered when cases from infertility clinics were excluded; the probabilities of abortion remained very similar. An analysis of the data by country of origin was attempted. Despite the reduced number of cases in some studies, the probability of abortion for Day +3 was above 25 per cent in cases from France, Mauritius and Canada. In the Colombian cases there was only one pregnancy on that day, and it resulted in a term delivery.

The percentage distribution of term deliveries and

Table 1. Probability of Abortion for Given Days of Insemination in Relation to the Temperature Shift.

DAY OF INSEMINATION	ABORTIONS	TERM DELIVERIES	ABORTIONS + DELIVERIES	PROBABILITY OF ABORTION (%)
−9	1	8	9	11.1*
−8	1	13	14	7.1
−7	6	25	31	19.3
−6	3	38	41	7.3
−5	5	42	47	10.6
−4	9	67	76	11.8
−3	6	102	108	5.5
−2	4	122	126	3.2
−1	14	186	200	7.0
0	10	124	134	7.5
+1	6	104	110	5.5†
+2	4	40	44	9.1
+3	6	19	25	24.0
Totals	75	890	965	7.8

*Chi-square linear trend (Days −9 to 0) = 13.4 (with 1 degree of freedom), P < 0.001.
†Chi-square linear trend (Days +1 to +3) = 10.1 (with 1 degree of freedom), P < 0.01.

abortions in relation to the day of the thermal shift is presented in Figure 2. As expected, there was an excess of abortions from Days −3 to −9 and +2 and +3.

The day in the menstrual cycle on which the thermal shift occurred showed no significant difference (mean abortions, 17.465 vs. mean term, 16.672), although the variance of abortion for the distribution was significantly larger than for the term deliveries.

DISCUSSION

The possibility of faulty records must always be borne in mind. In this study we do not believe that they were a serious source of error or bias since, in both infertility and family-planning clinics, basal-body-temperature readings and sexual activity are recorded routinely. The effect of faulty memory is thus minimized. Deceptive records (e.g., not recording sexual activity during the fertile period in an attempt to attribute the failure to the method) should be equally distributed among term deliveries and abortions, and it is difficult to see how they can explain our findings.

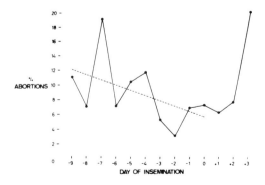

Figure 1. Probability of Abortion According to the Day of Insemination in Relation to the Day of the Thermal Shift in Basal Body Temperature.

The dotted line represents a regression line fitted with the data from Days −9 to 0. Observe the high probability for Day +3.

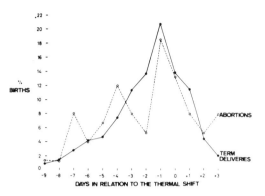

Figure 2. Percentage Distribution of Term Deliveries and Abortions According to the Day of Insemination in Relation to the Day of the Thermal Shift in Basal Body Temperature.

Observe the excess of abortions for days to the left of Day −4 and to the right of Day +2. These pregnancies correspond to aged sperm and aged ova respectively.

These results strongly suggest that aging of human spermatozoa in the female genital tract is associated with an increased frequency of spontaneous abortions. The objection can still be made that a pregnancy produced by an insemination on Day −6 does not necessarily mean that the spermatozoa were aged six days before fertilization, since ovulation may have taken place before the thermal shift. But if we assume that ovulation tends to occur around the shift, on the average, these spermatozoa would be older. The most striking finding was the high probability of abortion found for Day +3. There is ample evidence that conception is very unlikely to occur on that day.[24,25] Yet it must be remembered that the method for collecting cases in the present study lent itself to the inclusion of such cases even if they were of rare occurrence.

Marshall,[26] using a method similar to ours, could not find an association between aging spermatozoa and abortions or congenital malformations in 81 pregnancies. His numbers were too small to detect the trend that we found.

Failures with the rhythm method may be more likely to end in spontaneous abortion. This effect may be particularly true of the calendar rhythm method, which affords only very inexact knowledge of the time of ovulation. Symptothermic rhythm, especially if sexual activity is restricted to the postovulatory phase, has a minimum chance of problems because sexual activity is initiated when the risk of conception is extremely low.

Aneuploidy is a frequently described chromosome abnormality in association with post-ovulatory over-ripeness in animals.[27,28] Mikamo[17] has shown that human abortions have an appreciable number of aneuploidies. Nondisjunction anomalies have been described in intrafollicular over-ripeness.[5-7] The association of trisomies with post-ovulatory over-ripeness is not clear from animal experiments. It is likely that post-ovulatory aging of human ova leads to aneuploidies and less probably to non-disjunction anomalies. Our data suggest that post-ovula-

tory aging of human ova also leads to post-implantation losses.

Conceptions occurring from the extreme ends of the temperature shift are more likely to be aborted, as we show here. The preponderance of males for those cases[22] would explain the high sex ratio for human abortions that has frequently been found.[29,30]

REFERENCES

1. Blandau RJ: The effects on development when eggs and sperm are aged before fertilization. Ann NY Acad Sci 57:526-530, 1954
2. Lanman JT: Delays during reproduction and their effects on the embryo and fetus. I. Aging of sperm. N Engl J Med 278:993-999, 1968
3. *Idem:* Delays during reproduction and their effects on the embryo and fetus. II. Aging of eggs. N Engl J Med 278:1047-1054, 1968
4. Tesh JM, Glover TD: Influence of aging of rabbit spermatozoa on fertilization and prenatal development. J Reprod Fertil 12:414-415, 1966
5. Mikamo K: Intrafollicular overripeness and teratologic development Cytogenetics 7:212-233, 1968
6. Fugo NW, Butcher RL: Overripeness and the mammalian ova. I. Overripeness and early embryonic development. Fertil Steril 17:804-814, 1966
7. Butcher RL, Fugo NW: Overripeness and the mammalian ova. II. Delayed ovulation and chromosome anomalies. Fertil Steril 18:297-302, 1967
8. Critical viability of human sperms and oocytes. N Engl J Med 278:1121-1122, 1968
9. Welch JP: Down's syndrome and human behaviour. Nature 219:506, 1968
10. Jongbloet PH: Mental and Physical Handicaps in Connection with Overripeness Ovopathy. Leiden, HE Stenfert Kroese, 1971, pp 22-46
11. Witschi E: Natural control of fertility. Fertil Steril 19:1-14, 1968
12. Hertig AT: Morphologic criteria of the time of ovulation in the human being, Human Ovulation. Edited by CS Keefer. Boston, Little, Brown and Company, 1965, pp 75-83
13. Boué JG, Cohen J, Henry-Suchet J, et al: Étude clinique et biologique de 16 cas d'avortments spontanés par aberration chromosomique. Presse Med 76:1717-1720, 1968
14. Jongbloet PH: Mental and Physical Handicaps in Connection with Overripeness Ovopathy. Leiden, HE Stenfert Kroese, 1971, pp 6-21
15. Ingalls TH, Bazemore MK: Prenatal events antedating the birth of thoracopagus twins. Arch Environ Health 19:358-364, 1969
16. Ingalls TH: Maternal health and mongolism. Lancet 2:213-215, 1972
17. Mikamo K: Anatomic and chromosomal anomalies in spontaneous abortion. Am J Obstet Gynecol 106:243-254, 1970
18. Guerrero R, Lanctot CA: Aging of fertilizing gametes and spontaneous abortion: effect of the day of ovulation and the time of insemination. Am J Obstet Gynecol 107:263-267, 1970
19. Buxton CL, Engle ET: Time of ovulation: a correlation between the basal temperature, the appearance of the endometrium, and the appearance of the ovary. Am J Obstet Gynecol 60:539-551, 1950
20. Siegler SL, Siegler AM: Evaluation of basal body temperature. Fertil Steril 2:287-301, 1951
21. Abarbanel AR: Transvaginal pelvioscopy: further studies in infertility, Proceedings of the Second World Congress on Fertility and Sterility. Vol. 1. Edited by G Tesauro. Naples, Institute of Clinical Obstetrics and Gynecology, University of Naples, 1956, pp 1140-1159
22. Guerrero R: Association of the type and time of insemination within the menstrual cycle with the human sex ratio at birth. N Engl J Med 291:1056-1059, 1974
23. Armitage P: Statistical Methods in Medical research. New York, John Wiley and Sons, 1971, p 271
24. Döring GK: Über die Zuverlässigkeit der Temperaturmethode zur Empfängnisverhütung. Dtsch Med Wochenschr 92:1055-1061, 1967
25. Marshall J: A field trial of the basal-body-temperature method of regulating births. Lancet 2:8-10, 1968
26. *Idem:* Congenital defects and the age of spermatozoa. Int J Fertil 13:110-120, 1968
27. Vickers AD: Delayed fertilization and chromosomal anomalies in mouse embryos. J Reprod Fertil 20:69-76, 1969
28. Yamamoto M, Ingalls TH: Delayed fertilization and chromosome anomalies in the hamster embryo. Science 176:518-521, 1972
29. Strandskov HH, Bisaccia H: The sex ratio of human stillbirths at each month of uterogestation and at conception. Am J Phys Anthropol 7:131-143, 1949
30. Stevenson AC: Observation on the results of pregnancies in women resident in Belfast. III. Sex ratio with particular reference to nuclear sexing of chorionic villi of abortions. Ann Hum Genet 23:415-420, 1959

From C. J. Roberts and C. R. Lowe (1975). Lancet, **i**, 498–499. *Copyright* (1975), *by kind permission of the authors and The Lancet Ltd*

WHERE HAVE ALL THE CONCEPTIONS GONE?

C. J. ROBERTS   C. R. LOWE

Department of Social and Occupational Medicine, Welsh National School of Medicine, Cardiff CF4 4XN

THE frequency with which congenital malformations occur varies considerably from country to country and, within countries, from area to area and social class to social class. For example, neural-tube malformations are five times commoner in England and Wales than in Japan[1] and nearly three times commoner in the coalmining valleys of South Wales than along its coastal plain[2]: in Scotland they are three times commoner in infants born into social class v than in infants born into social classes i and ii.[1] From these and similar observations it has been inferred that environmental teratogens must be at work, but in making such an inference few research workers stop to consider what relation, if any, the prevalence of malformations at birth bears to their incidence at the time they are laid down—early in the first trimester of pregnancy.

It has been claimed that the prevalence of anencephalus and severe spina bifida will be reduced by 90% when screening for the presence of high levels of alpha-fetoprotein early in pregnancy followed by therapeutic abortion[3] becomes the accepted practice. The notion of controlling the problem of severe malformation at birth by early recognition and abortion is so good and so simple that one wonders why Nature did not think of it first. We believe she did. There is now good evidence that product rejection by way of implantation failure and spontaneous abortion is her principal method of quality control.

Evidence is accumulating that prenatal elimination may perhaps be the rule rather than the exception, with the implication that, in the world of early embryos, malformation may be the norm rather than the exception. In 1956 Hertig and others[4] published the results of examining 34 fertilised ova in the first 17 days of development, recovered after hysterectomy performed on 210 women of proven fertility. Of these 34 very early embryos, 10 were grossly abnormal and would have been lost early in pregnancy, perhaps even before the women themselves had realised that they were pregnant. If we relate this observation to the observation that at least a third of fetuses lost early in pregnancy are chromosomally abnormal,[5,6] we can only conclude that around half of all post-implantation conceptions are aborted.

In table I some speculative arithmetic of our own supports this conclusion. Indeed, it suggests that in England and Wales married women aged 20–29 may on a conservative estimate abort 78% of their conceptions. Animal studies, which allow a more systematic investigation of this difficult problem, have shown detectable prenatal losses ranging from 15 to 60% in domestic cattle, sheep, and pigs and in wild forms such as stoats, rats, squirrels, and rabbits.[7]

In a very large series of surgical abortions

TABLE I—ESTIMATED FETAL LOSS (MARRIED WOMEN AGED 20–29 IN ENGLAND AND WALES, 1971)

—	No. in millions
Married women aged 20–29	2·437
Annual acts of coitus (assuming a mean of twice a week)	253·448
Annual acts of unprotected coitus (assuming one in four is unprotected)	63·362
Unprotected acts occurring within 48-hour period around ovulation (i.e., 1/14) ..	4·526
Assume one in two of these results in fertilisation[4] ..	2·263
Actual number of infants (live and stillborn) born to these women	0·505
Estimated loss (2·263−0·505)	1·758
Percentage loss $\left(\dfrac{1·758}{2·263} \times 100\right)$	78%

TABLE II—PREVALENCE OF CERTAIN EXTERNAL MALFORMATIONS IN 3000 EMBRYOS AND FETUSES COMPARED WITH PREVALENCE AT BIRTH*

Type of malformation	Prevalence per 1000		"Wastage" (%)
	Abortions	Births	
Neural tube	13·1	1·0	92
Cleft lip and palate	21·4	2·7	87
Polydactyly	9·0	0·9	90
Cyclopia and cebocephaly ..	6·2	0·1	98

* Derived from Nishimura.[8]

Nishimura [8] has reported a prevalence of neural-tube malformation of 13 per 1000 (table II). This is ten times greater than their prevalence at birth, which in Japan is very low (a little over 1 per 1000), and suggests that perhaps 90% of all neural-tube malformations in that country are lost early in pregnancy. A study of 3418 fetuses (974 spontaneous abortions and 2444 hysterotomies) undertaken at the tissue bank at the Royal Marsden Hospital, London,[9] showed malformations to be some three times as frequent in spontaneously aborted fetuses as in fetuses from artificially interrupted pregnancies.

A high frequency of chromosomal abnormality has been stressed by Nishimura,[8] whose data suggest that between 25 and 30% of all spontaneous abortions have chromosomal aberrations, and by Machin,[10] who found in a survey of unselected necropsied perinatal deaths in hospital that 9% of macerated stillbirths, 4% of fresh stillbirths, and 6% of early neonatal deaths had chromosome abnormalities.

In our study of neural-tube malformation-rates in all the infants born in South Wales over the three-year period 1964–66,[11] we have been able to relate those rates to the frequency with which the women reported previous spontaneous abortions.[12] Women who gave birth to a malformed infant reported slightly but not consistently higher previous spontaneous-abortion rates than women who gave birth to infants without neural-tube defects. With remarkable consistency, however, both types of women at each parity reported lower abortion-rates in the coal-mining valleys than in the rest of South Wales. This difference was confirmed for manual workers' and non-manual workers' wives separately, and for all parities. It seems clear that the mining valleys, with their high neural-tube malformation-rates, have lower spontaneous-abortion rates than the rest of South Wales, with its lower malformation-rates. The difference between the abortion-rates was not large (13·0% in the mining valleys compared with 14·9% in the rest of South Wales); but if Nishimura's data on the incidence of neural-tube malformations in abortions are accepted as reliable (i.e., 90% are lost), these are enough to explain the almost three-fold difference in the prevalence at birth of neural-tube malformations between the valleys and the coastal plain. The inference is that the environmental factors at work in South Wales are not directly teratogenic but in some way change the uterine environment so that more

abnormal fetuses remain in the uterus until the 28th week of pregnancy—i.e., abortion of malformed fetuses is the factor of overriding importance in the determination of area differences in the prevalence of neural-tube malformations at birth.

Notwithstanding the great advances in electron microscopy, the biologist of today in his study of genetic defects is in much the same position as an Egyptian astronomer exploring the secrets of the universe with the naked eye. As knowledge and techniques improve, many abortions which now pass for normal will almost certainly be reclassified as defective. This may well mean that our own estimates of a 78% early fetal loss could prove to be too low.

DISCUSSION

Austin [7] has this to say about prenatal fetal wastage:

" Accumulating evidence suggests that prenatal elimination is in the main an important and valuable provision of Nature. The fact is becoming increasingly clear that a large proportion of resorbed or aborted embryos and fetuses are abnormal, and that their summary disposal is in the best interests of the race. Probably this represents the main way in which disadvantageous features from gene mutation are prevented from being incorporated into the overall hereditary pattern. Indeed if we must grieve over pregnancy losses it should be rather because so many products of anomalous development will succeed in evading this act of natural selection."

What, then, are the implications of changing the conceptual framework within which we consider the relation between prevalence of abnormalities at birth and their incidence early in pregnancy? They are probably not unlike the implications of the discovery that the earth was round, not flat. For most people life went on much the same except that what was regarded as a serious problem—what happened to ships when they disappeared over the horizon—was no longer a problem, and therefore ceased to be a source of worry. The only people whose lives were immediately affected by the change of viewpoint were savants fruitlessly searching for a solution to a non-existent problem and university lecturers who had based their teaching programmes on a false premise. In the long term, however, the discovery that the earth was round had a profound effect on the history of the human race.

Let us consider some of the implications of accepting that about three-quarters of all human conceptions are aborted, most of them because they are abnormal. It seems likely that inferences about causal environmental teratogens and genetic mechanisms now drawn from the study of the prevalence of congenital defects at birth have been based on false premises. The notion that genetic mutations resulting in life-threatening abnormalities are rare may have to be replaced by the notion that they are very common. Infertile women, the cause of whose infertility is unknown or put down to deficiencies of ovarian or uterine function, may in fact be a group at high risk for gene mutation. If Nature resorts to abortion to maintain genetic stability by discarding as many as 3 in every 4 conceptions, it will be difficult for anti-abortionists to oppose abortion on moral and ethical grounds. In the long term society may come to regard abortion as a natural function responsible for control not only of quantity but also of quality, and the moral, ethical, and legal rights of the embryo, the fetus, and the mother will be very different from those which now seem to apply. Biologists may well seek to supplement artificially the natural process of elimination; geneticists may have to undergo some reorientation in respect of their views about the ætiology of life-threatening malformations; and epidemiologists may have to concede that further investment in the search for controllable environmental teratogens will yield negligible dividends.

REFERENCES

1. Lowe, C. R. *Br. med. J.* 1972, ii, 515.
2. Richards, I. D. G., Roberts, C. J., Lloyd, S. *Br. J. prev. soc. Med.* 1972, **26**, 89.
3. *Lancet*, 1974, i, 907.
4. Hertig, A. T., Rock, J., Adams, E. C. *Am. J. Anat.* 1956, **98**, 435.
5. Dhadial, R. K., Machin, A. M., Tait, S. M. *Lancet*, 1970, ii, 20.
6. Araki, D. T., Workman, S. H. *J. med. Genet.* 1970, **7**, 118.
7. Austin, C. R. *in* Reproduction in Mammals (edited by C. R. Austin and R. V. Short); vol. II, p. 134. London, 1972.
8. Nishimura, H. *in* Proceedings of the Third International Conference on Congenital Malformations (edited by F. C. Fraser and A. McKusick). Amsterdam, 1970.
9. Gal, I. *Humangenetik*, 1973, **20**, 367.
10. Machin, G. A. *Lancet*, 1974, i, 549.
11. Richards, I. D. G., Lowe, C. R. *Br. J. prev. soc. Med.* 1971, **25**, 59.
12. Roberts, C. J., Lloyd, S. *Br. med. J.* 1973, iv, 20.

PAPER 19

19. Carter, C. O. (1969). Genetics of common disorders. *Br. Med. Bull.*, **25**, 52–57

COMMENTARY

Paper 19 is included because of the novelty of the hypothesis proposed to explain some of the common congenital malformations. The multifactorial threshold hypothesis depends on genetic predisposition and assumes an interaction between polygenic inheritance with intrauterine environmental factors. In most cases, however, very little is known about the actual mechanisms involved. Prevention of the common congenital defects should therefore become possible if couples genetically at risk could be protected from the triggering environmental factors. For this reason, individual gene loci and the environmental factors involved need to be identified (Carter, 1976).

The validity of this model has recently been questioned by Melnick and Shields (1976) who suggested 'allelic restriction' as an alternative model to account for the more common congenital malformations, in particular those occurring with a high frequency in the population and with relatively few families 'showing an atypical type of vertical transmission'.

REFERENCES

Carter, C. O. (1976). Genetics of common congenital malformations in man. *Proc. R. Soc. Med.*, **69**, 38–48
Melnick, M. and Shields, E. D. (1976). Allelic restriction: a biological alternative to multifactorial inheritance. *Lancet*, **i**, 176–179

From C. O. Carter (1969). Br. Med. Bull., *25*, 52–57. *Copyright* (1969),
by kind permission of the author and the British Council

GENETICS OF COMMON DISORDERS

C. O. CARTER M.A. D.M. F.R.C.P.

Medical Research Council
Clinical Genetics Research Unit
Institute of Child Health
The Hospital for Sick Children, London

Genetic and part-genetic disorders may be subdivided into those determined by chromosome abnormality; those determined by mutant genes of large effect; those determined by maternal–foetal incompatibility; and those determined or partly determined by extremes of "normal" variation caused by alleles at many gene loci.

The incidence at birth of conditions due to chromosome abnormalities depends essentially on the mutation rate and the intra-uterine mortality of those affected. These conditions are nearly all severe, or at any rate substantially reduce reproductive fitness, and so there are few second-generation cases. Such disorders are not uncommon at conception and, since major chromosome anomalies are present in about 1 in 4 spontaneous abortions, it may be estimated that about 1 in 25 conceptions is affected by such a major chromosome abnormality. Because of this high intra-uterine loss, only a minority of conditions due to chromosome anomalies have an incidence of the order of 1 in 1,000 or more at birth. This minority includes Down's syndrome and the sex-chromosome anomalies, Klinefelter's syndrome and the XXX syndrome.

Single-gene-determined conditions, if at all serious, are also likely to have their incidence largely determined by the mutation rate at the gene locus concerned. Gene mutation rates are known to be low; few, if any, are higher than 1 in 10,000. Therefore of the individual conditions caused in this way, if serious, almost all have an incidence of less than 1 in 10,000. Milder single-gene conditions may have a high incidence; there is reasonable evidence, for example, that Dupuytren's contracture, which has a population incidence of almost 1 in 6, is a dominant condition (Ling, 1963). The few serious single-gene-determined conditions that have incidences of more than 1 in 1,000 are those where there is heterozygote advantage. A proved example is sickle-cell anaemia, where the heterozygote advantage is in resistance to malaria; and a probable example is congenital microcytosis. In Britain the commonest serious single-gene-determined disorder is cystic fibrosis of the pancreas, which has a population incidence in this country of the order of 1 in 2,000 (Pugh & Pickup, 1967; Hall & Simpkiss, 1968).

Mother–child incompatibility is also a mechanism which could give conditions with an incidence of more than 1 in 1,000,

as it does with haemolytic disease of the newborn. Recently and remarkably it has been shown that sensitization of the rhesus-negative mother by the rhesus-positive child is largely preventable (Clarke, 1968).

The genetic element in most common disorders, however, is neither chromosome abnormality nor mutant gene of large effect, but very probably an underlying polygenically[1] determined and continuously distributed genetic predisposition with a threshold beyond which individuals are at risk. Conditions determined in this way may be persistently common even if those affected have a low reproductive fitness, provided that there is also selection against extreme deviants for the genetic predisposition in the direction opposite to that of those affected with the disorder.

The hypothesis of polygenic inheritance has been made more plausible in recent years by the discovery of polymorphism at many gene loci—that is to say that, at many gene loci, allelic genes are present with frequencies that cannot be readily explained by mutation (Harris, 1966; Lewontin, 1967). It is almost inevitable with such polymorphism that variation for any character which is not a direct product of gene action will have a continuous distribution that is polygenically determined. It is also very probable that, where many genes are concerned, the phenotypic expression of some at least of them will vary with differences in the environment.

1.   Polygenic Variation: Continuous and Discontinuous

Polygenic inheritance is best established for characters showing continuous variation, such as stature, intelligence or blood pressure. Here, however, extremes in normal variation will not always be regarded as disease. The very short and the very tall probably have reduced physical and physiological efficiency, but are not considered to have any disease. Individual types of dwarfism are recognized as diseases, but here, as in achondroplasia or the severest forms of spondylo-epiphysial dysplasia, inheritance is due to single genes. As regards intelligence, the label of mental retardation is given to the subnormal and this label has social relevance, but is artificial; and, once again, when pathology is present the abnormality is usually determined by a single gene or by environmental factors. In the case of blood pressure, the label hypertension is given for extreme deviations to the right of the distribution; such a label has clinical and prognostic significance, but again is artificial except where this hypertension is secondary to renal or other abnormality (Hamilton, Pickering, Roberts & Sowry, 1954), or where there is (as some have argued, Platt (1959)) evidence that the hypertension is due to a single-gene effect.

In recent years, however, it has become apparent that some discontinuous traits that are clearly pathological appear likely to be inherited as the result of a polygenic predisposition and a threshold beyond which individuals are at risk. Environmental factors also play a part in the aetiology of almost all these conditions. More than 30 years ago, Wright (1934) showed that polydactyly in the guinea-pig was probably inherited in this way. He concluded that alleles at least 4 gene loci were involved.

---

[1] Such genetic predisposition has been called "polygenic" or "multifactorial". I prefer to use the term "polygenic" with reference to the genetic predisposition and the term "multifactorial" to include environmental as well as the genetic factors. The term polygenic is not intended to imply the existence of any special class of genes called polygenes.

GENETICS OF COMMON DISORDERS *C. O. Carter*

2. Common Congenital Malformations

Examples of common conditions that appear to be determined in this way are provided by those congenital malformations that have an incidence at birth of at least 1 in 1,000. These are now the predominant cause of stillbirth and of infant mortality. The common malformations in Britain are listed in Table I, with their approximate incidence per 1,000 total births and their sex ratio. There is, however, much racial and geographical variation in the incidence of congenital malformations (Stevenson, Johnston, Stewart & Golding, 1966).

TABLE I. Malformations with incidences of at least 1 in 1,000 total births

Malformations	Incidence/1,000	Sex ratio (male : female)
Down's syndrome	2	1.0
Cleft lip ($\pm$ cleft palate)	1	1.8
Pyloric stenosis	3	5.0
Talipes equinovarus	3	2.0
Congenital hip dislocation	1	0.15
Spina bifida cystica	2.5	0.8
Anencephaly	2	0.4
Congenital heart defects	4	1.0

Down's syndrome is a case apart, being determined by a chromosome abnormality. The genetics of the other conditions have much in common and their family patterns strongly suggest polygenic inheritance interacting with environmental factors.

The best family data available are those for cleft lip and palate, since reliable family histories are fairly easy to obtain, and almost all cases come to operation, so that the affection in relatives is readily documented. Three large-scale studies are available, from Denmark (Fogh-Andersen, 1942), Utah (Woolf, Woolf & Broadbent, 1963) and from London (J. A. F. Roberts, A. Buck and C. O. Carter, personal communication, 1968). The London study was in particular designed to provide information on offspring of index patients. The findings are shown in Table II.

This family pattern is not easily interpreted as being due to single-gene inheritance. Recessive inheritance is made unlikely by the close resemblance of the proportion of sibs and of children affected. Dominant inheritance is made unlikely by the sharp fall in the proportion affected as one passes from monozygotic co-twins to first-degree relatives (represented by

TABLE II. Proportion of relatives affected in three large family studies of cleft lip (with or without cleft palate)

Relatives	Denmark (%)	Utah, USA (%)	London (%)	Incidence relative to that of the general population
First-degree relatives				
Sibs	4.9	4.6	3.2	× 40
Children	—	4.3	3.0	× 35
Second-degree relatives				
Aunts and uncles	0.8	0.7	0.6	× 7
Nephews and nieces	—	0.8	0.7	× 7
Third-degree relatives				
First cousins	0.3	0.4	0.2	× 3

FIG. I. Model for polygenic inheritance of cleft lip, with, or without, cleft palate

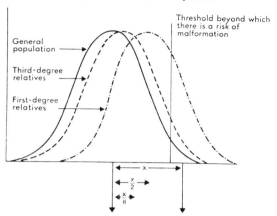

x: deviation of mean of malformed individuals from the population mean

sibs and children) and again as one passes from first- to second- (represented by aunts and uncles, and nephews and nieces) to third-degree relatives (represented by first cousins). With dominant inheritance one may expect a reduction by about 0.5 with each of these steps, since the proportion of relatives sharing the dominant gene with index patients is unity for monozygotic co-twins, 0.5 for first-degree, 0.25 for second-degree and 0.125 for third-degree relatives. (Few patients would be affected as the result of a fresh mutation, since on the hypothesis of dominant inheritance it must be assumed that the manifestation rate is low.)

The findings, however, are very much those that one would expect with polygenic inheritance with a threshold beyond which there is a risk of malformation (see fig. 1). The distribution of the polygenic predisposition for the general population will on an appropriate scale be Normal,[2] and this is illustrated by the continuous curve in the diagram. First-degree relatives will have a curve of distribution about a mean approximately half-way between that of the general population and the index patients beyond the threshold. This will bring a substantial proportion of them beyond the threshold, and so at risk of developing the malformations. Second-degree relatives would have a distribution about a mean shifted to the right by approximately one-quarter of the distance between the mean of the general population and the index patients. Third-degree relatives would have a distribution about the mean approximately one-eighth of the distance from the population mean towards that of the index patients. This representation is over simplified. The distribution in relatives would not be Normal on the scale which gives Normality in the general population (Edwards, cited by Falconer, 1967); the variance in relatives would probably be rather less than in the general population; the manifestation rate would probably increase as the geno-

---

[2] The capital letter N here and elsewhere in this paper refers to observations whose statistical variation is describable by the Normal (Gaussian) Distribution Function.—ED.

GENETICS OF COMMON DISORDERS *C. O. Carter*

TABLE III. Family patterns for some common congenital malformations

	Cleft lip with or without cleft palate	Talipes equinovarus	Congenital dislocation of hip (males only)	Congenital pyloric stenosis (females only)	Spina bifida and anencephaly
General population	0.001	0.001	0.002	0.005	0.008
Monozygotic twins	× 400	× 300	× 200	× 80	—
First-degree relatives	× 40	× 25	× 25	× 10	× 7
Second-degree relatives	× 7	× 5	× 3	× 5	—
Third-degree relatives	× 3	× 2	× 2	× 1.5	—

type deviates further beyond the threshold; but the errors introduced are not large.

On this simple hypothesis, assuming that 3 in 1,000 of the population are beyond the threshold and that one of the three is clinically affected (giving an incidence of 1 in 1,000), the proportion beyond the threshold of first-, and second- and third-degree relatives respectively would be approximately × 30, × 8 and × 3 that of the general population. This fits well with the findings for cleft lip and palate.

Similar, but less complete, data are available for other congenital malformations: for example, pyloric stenosis (C. O. Carter and K. A. Evans, personal communication, 1968), talipes equinovarus (Wynne-Davies, 1964), congenital dislocation of the hip (Record & Edwards, 1958; C. O. Carter and J. A. Wilkinson, unpublished work, 1968), spina bifida cystica and anencephaly (Record & McKeown, 1950; Williamson, 1965; Carter, David & Laurence, 1968), and these are summarized in Table III, the data for spina bifida being those of Carter *et al.* (1968). The least complete data for relatives other than sibs are those for anencephaly and spina bifida, where family history is least reliable and documentation, for example for stillbirths, is difficult for second- and third-degree relatives.

Modern family studies of specific congenital heart malformations are only just becoming available (Zoethout, Bonham Carter & Carter, 1964; Nora, McNamara & Fraser, 1967; Emanuel, Nichols, Anders, Moores & Somerville, 1968; E. M. Williamson, personal communication, 1968; Wilkins, 1969). These and older studies based on questionnaires (Lamy, de Grouchy & Schweisguth, 1957; Campbell, 1965) indicate recurrence risks to later sibs of between 1% and 3%. For example, Nora *et al.* (1967) found the risk of similar defect in the sibs of patients with atrial septal defect (ostium secundum type) to be a little over 3% and E. M. Williamson (personal communication, 1968) found a proportion of a little over 3% affected in both sibs and children. The population incidence of atrial septal defect is estimated to be about 0.5 per 1,000 births, so that first-degree relatives have about 60 times the population incidence.

3. Tests for Polygenic Hypothesis

Family patterns determined by polygenic inheritance have several other features which may be used to test the hypothesis (see Penrose, 1953; Edwards, 1960; Carter, 1961b, 1964; Newcombe, 1964; Vogel & Krüger, 1967).

i. The risks in relatives compared with those of the general population would be expected to be absolutely greater, but proportionately less, as the population incidence of the malformations increases; this is well seen in Table II. For example, assuming the higher population incidence, 2/1,000

beyond the threshold, and again a manifestation rate of those at risk of 1 in 3, which would be appropriate for congenital dislocation of the hip in females, the expected relative risks for first-, second- and third-degree relatives would be × 25, × 6 and × 2.5. This is similar to the ratios actually observed. Assuming a still higher population incidence, 5/1,000, and again a manifestation ratio of 1 in 3, which would be appropriate in males for infantile pyloric stenosis, the relative incidences would be × 12, × 4 and × 2, which are again in good agreement with those actually found.

As the proportion of the population at risk rises, the decline in the proportion affected as one passes from first- to second- to third-degree relatives becomes progressively less useful in distinguishing polygenic from dominant inheritance. This test would be more useful for neural-tube malformations in a low-incidence area such as Japan than in the United Kingdom.

ii. In contrast to the usual situation with single genes, in polygenic inheritance the risk to relatives will vary from family to family. Therefore the risk will be increased where there are already two affected in a family. This is seen, for example, with anencephaly and spina bifida, where the risk to later offspring is about twice as great for mothers who have already had two affected children, compared with those who already have had one such child (Carter & Roberts, 1967). In contrast, with a recessive condition such as cystic fibrosis of the pancreas the risk remains 1 in 4 whether the mother has already had one, two or even three affected children. Again, with cleft lip, where parent and one child is already affected the risk to subsequent children rises from 3–4% to over 10% (Fogh-Andersen, 1942). With pyloric stenosis also there are indications of a substantial rise in the risk where one parent and a child is already affected.

iii. With polygenic inheritance one would expect that the more severe degrees of malformation would carry a relatively higher risk to relatives. This is seen, for example, with cleft lip. When combining the Danish data of Fogh-Andersen and the London data (J. A. F. Roberts, A. Buck and C. O. Carter, personal communication, 1968), the risk to subsequent sibs after a child with unilateral cleft lip is about 2.5%, but after bilateral cleft lip and palate is nearly 6%. Similarly with aganglionic megacolon (Hirschsprung's disease) the risk to sibs increases with the length of the aganglionic segment (Bodian & Carter, 1963).

iv. An extension of the test of increasing risk with increasing severity is provided by the malformations in which the sex ratio deviates markedly from unity. Patients of the more rarely affected sex will tend to be more extreme deviants from the population mean and so the risk to their relatives will be correspondingly higher (Carter, 1961a). In pyloric stenosis the ratio is 5 males to 1 female and the proportion affected among relatives of girl index patients is more than three times higher than amongst the relatives of affected boys. This is best seen in the offspring of index patients, and the data (C. O. Carter and K. A. Evans, personal communication, 1968) are summarized in Table IV.

v. An increase in parental consanguinity is also to be expected with polygenic inheritance, since a consanguineous marriage is a form of assortative marriage. For common conditions the small increase in parental consanguinity

GENETICS OF COMMON DISORDERS *C. O. Carter*

TABLE IV. Proportion of those affected among children of patients with pyloric stenosis

	Affected, and total, children of patients with pyloric stenosis	
	Sons	Daughters
330 boy index patients	19 : 346 (5.5 %)	8 : 337 (2.4 %)
239 girl index patients	20 : 103 (19.4 %)	7 : 96 (7.3 %)

expected, a 50–100% increase, is little less than that expected for recessive conditions, though with rare conditions recessive inheritance implies much higher consanguinity rates.

4. Common Diseases

Family data on the common diseases of adult life have not on the whole been collected as extensively as for congenital malformations, and such studies involve difficulties in definition, diagnosis, and correction for the unexpired risk of developing the disease, which hardly arise with congenital malformations. Nevertheless the family patterns in several instances appear similar to those for the common malformations and examples are provided by the major psychoses, early-onset ischaemic heart disease, rheumatoid arthritis, ankylosing spondylitis and diabetes mellitus.

Major psychoses. The data on schizophrenia and manic depressive psychosis (Stenstedt, 1952; Kallmann, 1953; Ödegård, 1963; Winokur & Pitts, 1965) suggest that for these two major types of psychosis, the risk to first-degree relatives is of the order of 10–15%. In comparison each has a life-time population risk of 5–10/1,000. In the case of schizophrenia this risk to children applies even when they have been separated from the schizophrenic parent at birth (Heston, 1966). The risk to sibs appears to be about doubled when one parent is also affected (Winokur & Pitts, 1965). The proportion of monozygotic co-twins of index patients also affected is of the order of 50%. Both the family data and the twin data show that the polygenic predisposition tends to be specific for one or other major type of psychosis and not for both. The reproductive fitness of the patients, especially of schizophrenics, is reduced. It has been plausibly argued for schizophrenia (Irving, Gottesman & Shields, 1967) that this and other findings are more consistent with polygenic than single-gene-determined inheritance. The same arguments apply with equal strength for manic depressive psychosis.

Ischaemic heart disease. The studies of Gertler & White (1954), Rose (1964) and Suri, Singh & Tandon (1966) suggested that the first-degree relatives of patients with ischaemic heart disease had only about 2.5 times the risk of a control population of dying of ischaemic heart disease. However, a more elaborate analysis (Slack & Evans, 1966) has shown that, for unselected patients with early-onset ischaemic heart disease ("early onset" being defined as before the age of 55 years in men and 65 years in women), deaths in first-degree relatives were on average about 6 times the expected number in the general population. It is known that, in a small proportion of cases, such a disease is associated with a single-gene-determined condition, "pure hypercholesterolaemia" (Epstein, Block, Hand & Francis,

1959; Nevin & Slack, 1968). These cases, however, are not sufficiently common to contribute much of the familial concentration for unselected patients (Slack & Evans, 1966). For the years under consideration the risk of death from early-onset ischaemic heart disease in the general population is about 15/1,000 in males and 10/1,000 in females, so that the sixfold increase in first-degree relatives is compatible with a polygenic element in the—no doubt multifactorial—aetiology of ischaemic heart disease.

Rheumatoid arthritis. Family data for rheumatoid arthritis are available from a number of surveys (Miall, 1955; Lawrence & Ball, 1958; de Blécourt, Polman & de Blécourt-Meindersma, 1961), as also are data for ankylosing spondylitis (Stecher, 1957; de Blécourt et al. 1961; Emery & Lawrence, 1967). For rheumatoid arthritis, with a population incidence of perhaps 20–30/1,000, Lawrence and Ball found an increase of close to fourfold in first-degree relatives, and the results from the other two studies are comparable. For the rarer condition, ankylosing spondylitis, the risks in relatives compared to those in the general population are understandably higher. The population incidence in north-east Europe is of the order of 2/1,000 in men and 0.4/1,000 in women. In the 1961 survey of de Blécourt et al., based on 74 male and 26 female index patients, the incidence in relation to that of the general population was × 35, × 10 and × 3 the population incidence in first-, second- and third-degree male relatives and about × 100 the population incidence in first-degree female relatives. The situation appears similar to that with pyloric stenosis, but a full comparison cannot be made because the relatives were not subdivided according to sex of index patient. Recently Emery & Lawrence (1967) have reported a further family study in which approximately 7% of first-degree male and 2% of first-degree female relatives were affected with clinical ankylosing spondylitis, i.e., approximately × 35 and × 50 the incidence in the general population of that sex. These authors make the point that the best genetic hypothesis to explain the finding is a polygenic one, and they apply Falconer's techniques (see section 5) to estimate "heritability".

Diabetes mellitus. The early studies of the family histories of patients with diabetes mellitus were interpreted as indicating that the condition was determined by a single gene, some regarding the condition as a dominant and others as a recessive one. Pincus & White (1934) suggested that diabetes was a recessive condition. Harris (1949) suggested that those patients with early onset (before the age of 40 years) were homozygotes and those with later onset were heterozygotes for the gene responsible. Lamy, Frézal & de Grouchy (1957) put forward an essentially similar hypothesis: that patients with severe diabetes, whether of early or late onset, were homozygotes and milder cases were heterozygotes. Later, however, they preferred a hypothesis closer to polygenic inheritance (Lamy, Frézal & Rey, 1961). Single-gene inheritance is perhaps an attractive idea when the abnormality is suspected to be in a single plasma protein. Single-gene determination, however, has never seemed plausible to clinicians. The absence of any clear dividing line between normal and abnormal blood-sugar curves, the change in the renal threshold for glucose and the change in blood-sugar curve with increasing age, the absence of any suggestion of bimodality in the sugar-tolerance curves of either controls or the first-degree relatives of diabetics (see, e.g., Thompson, 1965), the obvious importance of environmental factors (especially diet) in the cases of late onset, all suggest that, if a single gene were concerned, its manifestation

GENETICS OF COMMON DISORDERS *C. O. Carter*

must be much influenced by other genetic and by environmental factors.

Recessive inheritance is, in fact, made unlikely by the consistent finding that the incidence of diabetes in parents and children (when corrections have been made for age) is as high as in sibs. Dominant inheritance is made unlikely by the finding that the risks to sibs of diabetic patients is more than twice as high when one parent is also diabetic as when neither parent is diabetic (Harris, 1949; Steinberg & Wilder, 1952; Thompson & Watson, 1952). When both parents are diabetics the risk is further increased; thus Cooke, Fitzgerald, Malins & Pyke (1966) found that 7 in 57 (12%) children of couples with diabetes of onset before the age of 40 are diabetic.

Polygenic inheritance is compatible with the family findings, though it may well be that the factors concerned with early-onset severe diabetes are different from those in late-onset mild diabetes. The population incidence in the survey of the family history of diabetes made by a working party in Birmingham (College of General Practitioners, 1965) is shown in Table V below, by age-group compared with the incidence in siblings. The age distribution in siblings is not shown, but it is assumed to be similar to that in the index patients. Similar ratios are seen in the study of Simpson (1964), in which the age distribution of the sibs, but not the index patients, is given.

TABLE V. The relative incidence of known diabetes in sibs of diabetics and in the comparable general population

(Data from College of General Practitioners (1965))

Age-group (years)	Population incidence per 1,000	Relative incidences in sibs of diabetics
0–29	2	× 24
30–49	4	× 6
50–69	13	× 2.4
70–80	21	× 1.5

5. Correlation between Relatives and Heritability

Falconer (1965) has shown that it is possible to estimate the regression of relatives on index patients (or correlation of relatives and index patients) for the liability to disease (liability including both genetic and environmental predisposing factors) for threshold characters, if it be assumed that the genetic element in the liability is polygenic. The information needed is the incidence of the condition in the general population and the incidence in particular types of relatives. Assuming that the liability is normally distributed (and as the scale is an arbitrary one it may be assumed to be such that the distribution will be Normal), from the incidence in the general population the deviation of the threshold from the population mean may be estimated, also the mean deviation of affected individuals. Further, Falconer (1965) has noted that, with due reservations, it is then possible to make estimates of the heritability of the condition in the sense of the proportion of the variance of the liability which is determined by additive genetic variance. For example, for a condition where the variation in liability is entirely determined by additive genetic variance, and so heritability is 100%, the regression of first-degree relatives on index patients would be 0.5, for second-degree relatives 0.25, and for third-degree relatives 0.125. This corresponds to the

number of genes that the relatives are likely to have in common with the index patients. When the regressions are less, the estimated heritability is correspondingly reduced below 100%. Any difference in the variance in the general population and the relatives does not affect this estimate of regression (Smith, cited by Falconer, 1967).

Using Falconer's procedure on cleft lip and palate, and taking the figures shown in Table II, the regression of first-degree relatives on the index patients would be 0.38, for second-degree 0.19, and for third-degree 0.084, implying heritabilities of 76%, 76% and 67%. The incidence in monozygotic twins, based on only small and perhaps unrepresentative series, also suggests a heritability of the order of 80%.

Estimates of heritability from sib regressions will be too high if non-additive genetic variance (due to dominance or epistasis) is present; however, this is not the case with regression of child on index patient. Perhaps more important in human material, the estimates of heritability will be too high if there is similarity of relatives due to the environmental differences within families being less than those between families. The greatest effect of this source of error will be on the regression for monozygotic co-twins, then for sibs, then for children and least perhaps for second- and third-degree relatives. In the case of cleft lip, however, estimates are similar for all types of relatives.

On the same principle, estimation of regression coefficients for first-degree relatives for some of the other common conditions considered above are: pyloric stenosis, males only, 0.3 (heritability about 60%), females only, 0.45 (heritability about 90%); talipes equinovarus, 0.3 (heritability about 60%); congenital dislocation of the hip, females only, 0.35 (heritability about 70%); spina bifida cystica, 0.3 (heritability about 60%). For the major psychoses, a population incidence of 1% and a risk for first-degree relatives of 10% implies a regression coefficient of about 0.4 and a heritability of about 80%. For early-onset ischaemic heart disease, a population risk of about 1% and a sixfold increase in first-degree relatives implies a coefficient of 0.3 and a heritability of about 60%. For rheumatoid arthritis, the findings of Lawrence & Ball (1958) imply a regression of about 0.35 and a heritability of about 70%. For ankylosing spondylitis, a regression of 0.4 for males implies a heritability of about 80%. For diabetes mellitus, a regression of about 0.35 implies a heritability of about 70% for cases with onset before the age of 30 years, but a regression of 0.15 implies a heritability of only about 30% for cases with onset of the condition after the age of 50–70 years.

While these estimates of heritability are to be considered as upper limits of the true heritability, they do indicate that the genetic component of all these common diseases, if polygenic, may be a substantial one.

6. Conclusions

The investigation of the genetics of common disorders should not stop at the stage of the polygenic hypothesis. There is a need to discover the individual gene loci involved. In the case of duodenal ulcer, the *ABO* locus and the secretor locus are known to be involved, but they account for only about 3% of the increased risk to sibs (Roberts, 1965). There is also need to discover the mechanisms by which genetic predisposition acts, the nature of the additional environmental factors, and the way these interact with the genetic predisposition. Some success has been achieved in these last aims, for example, with congenital dislocation of the hip (Carter & Wilkinson, 1964). Much too is known of the additional environmental factors concerned in the aetiology of ischaemic heart disease.

Where the heritability of a condition is high, however, it implies that ultimate prevention will usually, though not necessarily, depend on special environmental prophylaxis for

those known to be genetically predisposed, rather than on measures of prophylaxis applied to the whole population. Further, where inheritance is polygenic it is unlikely, in contrast to the situation with single-gene-determined diseases, that a search for a single biochemical abnormality underlying the condition will be profitable (Vogel & Krüger, 1967).

REFERENCES

Blécourt, J. J. de, Polman, A. & Blécourt-Meindersma, T. de (1961) *Ann. rheum. Dis.* **20**, 215

Bodian, M. & Carter, C. O. (1963) *Ann. hum. Genet.* **26**, 261

Campbell, M. (1965) *Br. med. J.* **2**, 895

Carter, C. O. (1961a) *Br. med. Bull.* **17**, 251

Carter, C. O. (1961b) In: Jones, F. Avery, ed. *Clinical aspects of genetics. (Proceedings of a conference held in London at the Royal College of Physicians of London, 17–18 March 1961)*, p. 30. Pitman Medical, London

Carter, C. O. (1964) In: *Second International Conference on Congenital Malformations*, p. 306. International Medical Congress, New York

Carter, C. O., David, P. A, & Laurence, K. M. (1968) *J. med. Genet.* **5**, 81

Carter, C. O. & Roberts, J. A. F. (1967) *Lancet*, **1**, 306

Carter, C. O. & Wilkinson, J. A. (1964) *Clin. Orthop.* **33**, 119

Clarke, C. A. (1968) *Lancet*, **2**, 1

College of General Practitioners (1965) *Br. med. J.* **1**, 960

Cooke, A. M., Fitzgerald, M. G., Malins, J. M. & Pyke, D. A. (1966) *Br. med. J.* **2**, 674

Edwards, J. H. (1960) *Acta genet. Statist. med.* **10**, 63

Emanuel, R., Nichols, J., Anders, J. M., Moores, E. C. & Somerville, J. (1968) *Br. Heart J.* **30**, 645

Emery, A. E. H. & Lawrence, J. S. (1967) *J. med. Genet.* **4**, 239

Epstein, F. H., Block, W. D., Hand, E. A. & Francis, T., jr (1959) *Am. J. Med.* **26**, 39

Falconer, D. S. (1965) *Ann. hum. Genet.* **29**, 51

Falconer, D. S. (1967) *Ann. hum. Genet.* **31**, 1

Fogh Andersen, P. (1942) *The inheritance of harelip and cleft palate.* (Op. Domo Biol. hered. hum., Kbh., vol. 4.) Arnold Busck, Copenhagen

Gertler, M. M. & White, P. D. (1954) *Coronary heart disease in young adults: a multidisciplinary study.* Harvard University Press, Cambridge, Mass.

Hall, B. D. & Simpkiss, M. J. (1968) *J. med. Genet.* **5**, 262

Hamilton, M., Pickering, G. W., Roberts, J. A. F. & Sowry, G. S. C. (1954) *Clin. Sci.* **13**, 273

Harris, H. (1949) *Ann. Eugen.* **14**, 293

Harris, H. (1966) *Proc. R. Soc. B*, **164**, 298

Heston, L. L. (1966) *Br. J. Psychiat.* **112**, 819

Irving, I., Gottesman, I. I. & Shields, J. (1967) *Proc. natn. Acad. Sci. U.S.A.* **58**, 199

Kallmann, F. J. (1953) *Heredity in health and mental disorder.* Norton, New York

Lamy, M., Frézal, J. & Grouchy, J. de (1957) *Revue fr. Etud. clin. biol.* **2**, 907

Lamy, M., Frézal, J. & Rey, J. (1961) *Journées ann. Diabet. Hôtel Dieu*, **2**, 5

Lamy, M., Grouchy, J. de & Schweisguth, O. (1957) *Am. J. hum. Genet.* **9**, 17

Lawrence, J. S. & Ball, J. (1958) *Ann. rheum. Dis.* **17**, 160

Lewontin, R. C. (1967) *Am. J. hum. Genet.* **19**, 681

Ling, R. S. M. (1963) *J. Bone Jt Surg.* **45B**, 709

Miall, W. E. (1955) *Ann. rheum. Dis.* **14**, 150

Nevin, N. C. & Slack, J. (1968) *J. med. Genet.* **5**, 9

Newcombe, H. B. (1964) Discussion in: *Second International Conference on Congenital Malformations*, p. 345. International Medical Congress, New York

Nora, J. J., McNamara, D. G. & Fraser, F. C. (1967) *Circulation*, **35**, 448

Ödegård, Ö. (1963) *Acta psychiat. scand.* Suppl. No. 169, p. 94

Penrose, L. S. (1953) *Acta genet. Statist. med.* **4**, 257

Pincus, G. & White, P. (1934) *Am. J. med. Sci.* **188**, 782

Platt, R. (1959) *Lancet*, **2**, 55

Pugh, R. J. & Pickup, J. D. (1967) *Archs Dis. Childh.* **42**, 544

Record, R. G. & Edwards, J. H. (1958) *Br. J. prev. soc. Med.* **12**, 8

Record, R. G. & McKeown, T. (1950) *Br. J. soc. Med.* **4**, 217

Roberts, J. A. F. (1965) In: Neel, J. V., Shaw, M. W. & Schull, W. J., ed. *Genetics and the epidemiology of chronic diseases*, p. 77. (Publ. Hlth Serv. Publs, Wash. No. 1163.) U.S. Government Printing Office, Washington, D.C.

Rose, G. (1964) *Br. J. prev. soc. Med.* **18**, 75

Simpson, N. E. (1964) *Diabetes*, **13**, 462

Slack, J. & Evans, K. A. (1966) *J. med. Genet.* **3**, 239

Stecher, R. M. (1957) *Heredity in joint diseases.* (Documenta rheum. No. 12.) Geigy, Basle

Steinberg, A. G. & Wilder, R. M. (1952) *Am. J. hum. Genet.* **4**, 113

Stenstedt, A. (1952) *Acta psychiat. neurol. scand.* Suppl. No. 79

Stevenson, A. C., Johnston, H. A., Stewart, M. I. P. & Golding, D. R. (1966) *Congenital malformations: a report of a study of series of consecutive births in 24 centres.* (Suppl. to *Bull. Wld Hlth Org.* 1966, **34**)

Suri, V. P., Singh, D. & Tandon, O. P. (1966) *Indian J. med. Sci.* **20**, 321

Thompson, G. S. (1965) *J. med. Genet.* **2**, 221

Thompson, M. W. & Watson, E. M. (1952) *Diabetes*, **1**, 268

Vogel, F. & Krüger, J. (1967) In: Crow, J. F. & Neel, J. V., ed. *Proc. III int. Congr. hum. Genet., Chicago, Illinois, September 5–10, 1966*, p. 437. Johns Hopkins Press, Baltimore, Md

Wilkins, J. L. (1969) *J. med. Genet.* (In press)

Williamson, E. M. (1965) *J. med. Genet.* **2**, 161

Winokur, G. & Pitts, F. N. (1965) *J. psychiat. Res.* **3**, 113

Woolf, C. M., Woolf, R. M. & Broadbent, T. R. (1963) *Am. J. hum. Genet.* **15**, 209

Wright, S. (1934) *Genetics, Princeton*, **19**, 537

Wynne-Davies, R. (1964) *J. Bone Jt Surg.* **46B**, 445

Zoethout, H. E., Carter, R. E. Bonham & Carter, C. O. (1964) *J. med. Genet.* **1**, 2

PAPER 20

20. Shephard, D. A. E. (1975). Genetic hazards to man from environmental agents. *Can. Med. Assoc. J.*, **112**, 1460–1465

COMMENTARY

Paper 20 is a brief review of some of the issues raised at an international symposium on genetic hazards from environmental agents, in particular chemicals. Attention is directed to the problems of environmental contamination by potential mutagens, the relationship between mutagenesis and teratogenesis, detection of mutagens by laboratory and epidemiological studies and public health policy relating to protection of the population against these hazards.

From D. A. E. Shephard (1975). Can. Med. Assoc. J., **112**, 1460–1465. *Copyright* (1975), *by kind permission of the author and the Canadian Medical Association*

Genetic hazards to man from environmental agents

By David A.E. Shephard, FRCP [C]

"Genes are important." This seemingly simplistic statement was one side of a coin tossed many times during a recent international symposium on genetic hazards to man from environmental agents.* The other side of the coin: many of the myriad chemicals in our environment induce genetic mutations, and mutations, more often than not, are harmful rather than beneficial. Moreover, if, as many geneticists believe, our genes are our most treasured heritage, any deterioration in the quality of our genes can only lead to a deterioration in the quality of our lives. This, in essence, is the price society must pay for convenience living: for convenience foods, convenience domestic and industrial goods, convenience drugs, indeed, for the convenience of our very way of life, so dependant on the whole chemical environment. Is the price worth paying, in view of the risks involved?

Consider:

● An appreciable proportion of hospital admissions reflect genetic disabilities.

● There are more than 1500 inherited diseases with a simple mode of mendelian inheritance that are primarily caused by point mutations.

● Among clinically recognizable spontaneous abortions more than 35% are associated with chromosomal aberrations.

● Among 10 000 newborns there is a mean of 50 babies with a chromosomal anomaly, and in approximately 37 of these the anomaly is due to a new chromosome or a genome mutation.

● On the basis of the frequency of chromosomal aberrations among abortuses and newborns we can conclude that at least 7% of all human zygotes manifest chromosomal anomalies.

*International symposium: genetic hazards to man from environmental agents. Ottawa, May 26-28, 1975. Cosponsored by health protection branch of Department of National Health and Welfare; the Genetics Society of Canada; and the International Association of Environmental Mutagen Societies. One of a series of international symposia organized to mark the centenary of health protection in Canada.

Reprint requests to: Dr. D. Shephard, Box 8650, CMA House, Ottawa K1G 0G8.

● A large number of chemicals in daily use have been recognized as being mutagens — a growing number of them are mutagenic in mammals *in vivo* and some of them in man.

This fundamental question — how to balance the benefits of useful chemicals against the risks of their use — was implicit throughout this symposium, which brought together scientists from the United States, Mexico, Great Britain, Germany, Sweden, Italy and the host country, Canada. The overt purpose of the symposium was twofold: to permit scientists to exchange information and ideas about the genetic hazards of the sea of chemicals that surrounds us and to create a basis for decision-making that is essentially political — how to protect the public from undesirable exposure to environmental chemicals in particular. But a covert purpose was just as important: to make the public aware of the hazards that concern the scientific community now and will concern scientists increasingly for the rest of our lives. We have ignored these hazards for too long. Action based on understanding of the scientific evidence is overdue, for the problems that face us today will undoubtedly become ever more complex during the remaining years of this century. This report is a discussion of the important issues raised during the Ottawa symposium.

The recognition of mutagenesis by chemicals is comparatively recent; it was just over 30 years ago when C. Auerbach (Great Britain), a much revered participant at the symposium, showed that mustard gas damaged chromosomes. More and more chemicals thereafter were found to be mutagenic, but the magnitude of the problem was not realized until the 1950s. Then, as C. Ramel (Sweden) pointed out, methyl mercury pollution resulted not only in clinically evident tissue damage but also, both in animals and in man, in an increased incidence of chromosome breakage and aneuploidy in lymphocytes.

More recently another widespread industrial chemical, vinyl chloride, has focused our attention on environmental hazards. Now, vinyl chloride is not only mutagenic but carcinogenic as well, so

that the threat becomes a double one. As another symposium participant, B. Ames (USA), has shown, carcinogens are in fact mutagens, so that there is a close link between mutagenicity and carcinogenicity. Furthermore, as several participants reminded those attending the symposium, at least 80% of cancers are environmental in origin — hence the emphasis on carcinogenicity as well as mutagenicity of environmental agents.

But we must go further; as H. Kalter (USA) told the participants, there is also a close relationship between teratogens and mutagens. The relations between teratogens and mutagens are not easy to distinguish but we must learn about the complexity of such relations so that we can control complexities we recognize. For a start we can identify environmental agents that are teratogenic (Tables I and II); then, identification is the basis for action against what is now a triple threat. One basic problem, then, is that environmental agents, particularly chemicals, produce a complexity of hazards; any new environmental agent therefore must now be examined, at the very least, from three points of view — carcinogenicity, teratogenicity and (common to these two) mutagenicity.

Yet underlying this problem is a deeper one: in dealing with the numerous hazards in our environment, man seems too often to be one jump behind. No sooner had a *virus*, rubella, been identified as causing congenital malformations and attention directed to the search for viruses, than a *drug*, thalidomide, was belatedly recognized as inducing birth defects. Then, after we switched to a closer look at relatively simple drug-lesion relationships, we had to face a much more subtle relationship: the time-expanding, generation-separating effect of a drug like diethylstilbestrol (DES). Astonishingly, this drug given to a pregnant mother can cause clear-cell vaginal cancer *years later* in the mother's daughter, a point well emphasized by D.T. Janerich (USA).

What is the lesson? Where at all possible, we must avoid mutagens. As J.W. Drake (USA) has emphasized, chemicals and environmental agents induce mutations through a wide variety of mechanisms; therefore, it is most likely that generalized schemes to protect the public against mutagens will be programs aimed at preventing exposure entirely.

Recognition of mutagens

Not surprisingly, therefore, much of the symposium was devoted to a consideration of how we can avoid mutagens. Two approaches are useful: mutagenicity testing,* and epidemiologic studies.

Mutagenicity tests were mentioned by many speakers, but particularly useful were the contributions of F.J. de Serres (USA) and of Ames. de Serres reminded his audience that mutagens can be found among a wide variety of commonly used chemicals including food additives, cosmetics (e.g. hair dyes), household agents, pesticides, industrial chemicals and drugs. Such a large number of potentially harmful environmental chemicals — and many have not yet even been recognized as harmful — means that a particular approach to testing is needed. Tests on whole animals have limitations with respect to sensitivity, time and money. Hence, the value of short-term tests using microbial assay systems: these offer a practical solution to the problem of testing hundreds of chemicals rapidly and inexpensively. This approach amounts to one of screening. Such short-term tests have been developed in particular by Ames, who uses a test incorporating histidine mutants of *Salmonella typhimurium* and rat (or human) liver microsomes. Such tests are recommended for the screening of food additives, drugs and chemicals to which humans are at present exposed and for the routine screening of all new chemicals to which humans are likely to be exposed. Compounds giving a positive test result for mutagenicity should be considered potentially hazardous and then scrutinized for benefit, risk and the need for further testing by other, more time-consuming methods — part of a three-tier system proposed by B. Bridges (Great Britain). Many other tests are being developed for screening, and their interest to physicians lies in their rationale — preventive, rather than curative, medicine. As de Serres advocated, "short-term tests should most properly be considered assays for *potential* mutagenic activity in man and as a highly efficient mechanism both for screening large numbers of environmental agents and for establishing priorities for further

testing in higher organisms." Man needs, more than ever, to keep his wits about him, and tests such as those of Ames help him do so.

W.O. Rohrborn (Germany) took a slightly different approach to testing. First, a variety of host-mediated assay systems would be used. Substances found mutagenic in such qualitative studies and of no benefit (or replaceable by nonmutagenic compounds having the same degree of benefit) should be either banned from the marketplace or at least declared potentially hazardous. Those found to be mutagenic but not replaceable should then be tested quantitatively in mammalian systems (preferably mammals whose systems are as similar as possible to man's). In the case of drugs, for example, mutagenicity testing would be an inherent part of initial investigations and would be continued during the first clinical trials.

The other method of recognizing mutagens is epidemiologic. Of particular value here were the contributions of J.R. Miller (Canada) and Janerich. Miller pointed out that until perfect animal tests are available and until such time as no harmful agents pass through the defence walls of the placenta, "we are obligated to devote our time to the monitoring of newborns (and ideally, fetuses and embryos) for the presence of agents which might damage many hundreds or thousands of conceptuses." Various monitoring systems are in use, in different countries, including Canada, where, by 1974, data from five provinces were being entered into the system.

The value of such surveillance systems is indicated by the observation that the Swedish system if it had been in operation in 1963 would have identified thalidomide-induced abnormalities.

Janerich, in addition to referring to the value of epidemiologic studies in ascertaining the relationship between maternally administered DES and the occurrence of vaginal cancer in female offspring, stressed the contributions epidemiologists can make to identification of those environmental agents that are mutagenic. He used as an example a recent report on the study of a cohort of 257 polyvinyl chloride workers. Even so, as Miller observed, astute clinical observations are frequently the initial clues to mutagenicity (whether carcinogens or teratogens are involved), and good clinical medicine remains paramount in the recognition of clinically important mutagens.

Protecting the public

Scientists from the United States, Great Britain, Sweden and Germany

discussed national strategies dealing with the next phase: protecting the public from exposure to environmental chemicals. Most relevant to Canada was the contribution of Ramel, perhaps because of some similarities in social, political and legislative areas in the two countries. In particular, Canadian legislation, one hopes, will follow Swedish practice.

The central Swedish law is a 1973 act concerning products that are hazardous to health and to the environment. Two items are of particular interest: first, any manufacturer, importer or vendor of chemical products is responsible for preventing ill effects from such products; second, authorities are empowered to intervene even on the mere suspicion that a chemical product is toxic. In other words, the burden of uncertainty as to the hazard of any product does not rest on the the public but on those who manufacture, import or sell it. Moreover, a manufacturer, importer or vendor must supply the authorities with all such information relating to each product as is necessary in assessing the dangers the product presents to the public health or to the environment. A products control board decides what tests are required to assess chemicals for hazards, and in particular a scientific reference group advises on mutagenicity testing. The importance of such a group is reflected in the realization that the carcinogenicity of vinyl chloride could have been detected by simple mutagenicity tests. As yet, however, there are no legislative requirements for mutagenicity testing.

In Canada, legislation for the regulation of environmental chemicals is being prepared. Currently, there is no legal requirement for mutagenicity testing, although different branches of the Department of National Health and Welfare are, on their own initiative, testing various environmental chemicals for mutagenicity as well as carcinogenicity. One of the department's representatives, J.A. Abbatt, presented a useful and well-reasoned political viewpoint. In "the present state of ignorance," Abbatt said, "decisions must be based on the best available scientific evidence" (much of which was presented at the Ottawa symposium). Yet this, in the "less than perfect conditions" of the real world, is not enough. In balancing the benefits of environmental chemicals against their risks, it is up to society to decide what degree of risk is acceptable in achieving the degree of benefit desired. In short, the people, through their elected representatives, must express what they want. But, at the same time, the public must be protected and they must be informed.

---

*The Testing of Chemicals for Mutagenicity, Carcinogenicity and Teratogenicity, Ottawa, 1975, Department of National Health & Welfare.

Human exposure: how much?

The final session of the symposium was designed to take up this last point: to enable "authorities" to inform the public how much exposure is too much. F.C. Fraser (Canada) mused that this question was almost impossible to answer unless we were to say "less than an excess but more than not enough". C.R. Scriver (Canada) emphasized the view that a single guideline will not suffice, for every one is at some specific risk for a specific hazard, and there are wide individual variations related to genetic makeup. A certain exposure is too much for some but not too much for others. Other participants spoke more seriously on the vexing question of whether there is a threshold below which there is no damage, but this question, not surprisingly, was never fully answered.

Bridges, however, made a telling point: at the level of DNA in the cell (the ultimate target of environmental agents) if there is mutagen, then some form of reaction is likely. J.A. Heddle (Canada) summarized this part of the symposium when he commented that the essential problem is estimating the amount of harm done by environmental agents. He advocated taking a safe position, as far as dose and effect are concerned; that is, a dose-response curve should be regarded as being linear. Realistically, however, we have far to go in knowing where we stand.

But there is much we do know, and this symposium particularly directed the attention of its participants to separating fact from hypothesis. The fact is that many environmental chemicals are potentially mutagenic; therefore they are potentially dangerous. This symposium, which the health protection branch of DNH&W hosted, will expand our awareness of this fact. It will also point the direction in which medical thinking should be orientated — a direction consistent with that of the 1974 working paper, "A New Perspective on the Health of Canadians". As Scriver pointed out, this document conceives the environment as being an important element in health care considerations. The constructive and enlightening Ottawa symposium supported in particular the entirely reasonable view expressed in "New Perspective" that "future improvement in the level of health of Canadians lies mainly in improving the environment..." as well as in "moderating self-imposed risks and adding to our knowledge of human biology". From this viewpoint, therefore, this international symposium on genetic hazards to man from environmental agents was highly successful; it was, in my opinion, topical, enlightening, constructive and in tune with the future course of medical practice and with the good of society as a whole. ■

Table II—Nonchemical mammalian teratogens

Type	Examples
Infectious agents	Rubella, H-1 rat, and blue tongue viruses
Trauma	Amniocentesis, uterine clamping, immobilization
Temperature extremes	Hypo- and hyperthermia
Gas-level extremes	Hypo- and hyperoxia
Dietary imbalance	Vitamin (A, B_2, B_6, etc.), calorie deficiency
	Mineral and trace element deficiency
	Vitamin excess (A, D)
Immunological	Antibodies against various tissue
Miscellaneous	Delayed fertilization, dehydration, ultrasound

Table I—Some drugs and other chemicals shown to be teratogenic in one or more species of laboratory mammal

Type	Examples
Salicylates	Aspirin, oil of wintergreen
Certain alkaloids	Caffeine, nicotine, colchicine
Tranquillizers	Meprobamate, chlorpromazine, reserpine
Antihistamines	Buclizine, meclizine, cyclizine
Antibiotics	Chloramphenicol, streptonigrin, penicillin
Hypoglycemics	Carbutamide, tolbutamide, hypoglycins
Steroid hormones	Triamcinolone, cortisone, testosterone
Alkylating agents	Busulfan, chlorambucil, cyclophosphamide, TEM
Antimalarials	Chloroquine, quinacrine, pyrimethamine
Anesthetics	Halothane, urethane, nitrous oxide, pentobarbital
Antimetabolites	Folic acid, purine and pyrimidine analogues
Solvents	Benzene, dimethylsulfoxide, propylene glycol
Pesticides	2, 4, 5-T, carbaryl, captan, folpet
Industrial effluents	Some compounds of Hg, Pb, As, Li, Cd
Miscellaneous	Trypan blue, triparanol, acetazolamide etc.

Source: Wilson's Environment and Birth defects

PART V

ENVIRONMENTAL INFLUENCES AND CONGENITAL ABNORMALITIES

PAPER 21

21. Hale, F. (1933). Pigs born without eye balls. *J. Hered.*, **24**, 105–106

COMMENTARY

That developmental defects could experimentally be induced in amphibian and avian embryos has been known for a very long time. In mammals, however, this is a more recent development, having been achieved only at the turn of the present century. The exogenous agents used for producing fetal abnormalities were radiation and nutritional imbalances.

von Hippel (1906, 1907) detected ocular anomalies in the offspring of rabbits following maternal irradiation. Low birth weight and fetal resorptions, but no congenital malformations, were reported in cases of maternal malnutrition (Jackson, 1925). In 1933, Hale reported that pregnant sows, given a diet deficient in vitamin A, produced offspring without eyeballs. For the first time, a relatively simple experimental approach was used for inducing abnormal development in a mammal. It demonstrated 'the marked effect that a (nutritional) deficiency may have in disturbance of the internal factors that control the mechanism of development'.

Hale's observation marks the modern beginnings of experimental teratology. It has pioneered numerous studies which have led to the development of animal models suitable for the experimental investigation of birth defects. A wide spectrum of environmental factors, including nutritional imbalances, drugs and chemicals, and irradiation, have been shown to be teratogenic in many species of laboratory animals. Because investigations of this nature are neither ethical nor justifiable in pregnant women, teratological studies in subhuman mammals will continue to provide valuable information, not only for predicting possible harmful effects on the human fetus, but also in determining the underlying mechanisms operating at various phases of prenatal development.

Only a few cases of human fetal malformations have been reported in association with maternal nutritional imbalances. With specific reference to vitamin A, congenital anomalies have been detected in maternal vitamin A deficiency (Sarma, 1959) and hypervitaminosis A (Bernhardt and Dorsey, 1974). In severe maternal vitamin A deficiency, the infant was born prematurely with microcephaly and anophthalmia; in the infant born to the mother with hypervitaminosis A, urinary tract anomalies were present.

These observations are supported by numerous experimental studies in many species of animals; their full implications, however, are difficult to assess at the present time.

REFERENCES

Bernhardt, I. B. and Dorsey, D. J. (1974). Hypervitaminosis A and congenital renal anomalies in a human infant. *Obstet. Gynecol.*, **43**, 750–755

Jackson, C. M. (1925). *Effects of Inanition and Malnutrition upon Growth and Structure.* (Philadelphia: P. Blakiston's Son & Co.)

Sarma, V. (1959). Maternal vitamin A deficiency and fetal microcephaly and anophthalmia. *Obstet. Gynecol.*, **13**, 299–301

von Hippel, E. (1906). Mikrophthalmus und Colobom. Bericht über die 33. Versammlung der ophthalmologischen Gesellschaft in Heidelberg, p. 293

von Hippel, E. (1907). Über experimentelle Erzeugung von angeborenen Star bei Kaninchen nebst Bemerkungen über gleichzeitig beobachteten Mikrophthalmus und Lidcolobom. *Arch. Ophthalmol.*, **65**, 326–360

From F. Hale (1933). *J. Hered.*, **24,** 105–106. *Copyright* (1933), *by kind permission of the author and the American Genetic Association*

PIGS BORN WITHOUT EYE BALLS

Fred Hale

Texas Agricultural Experiment Station, College Station, Texas

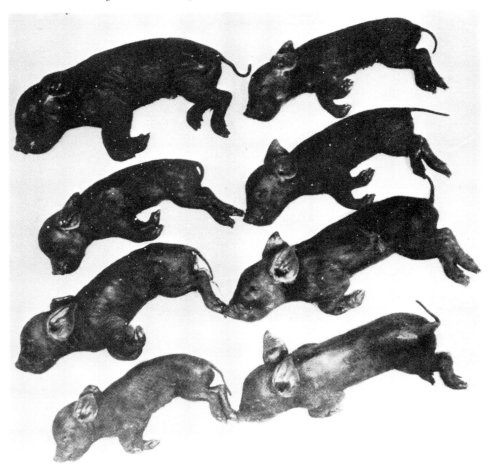

A LITTER OF EYELESS PIGS

Figure 7

Progeny of normal Duroc-Jersey sow all showing complete absence of eye balls. Since both the parents were normal-eyed it is practically certain that this defect is not hereditary. It is rather to be taken as an example of the profound effect that vitamin deficiency may have upon development.

A REGISTERED Duroc-Jersey gilt receiving a ration deficient in Vitamin *A* at the Texas Agricultural Experiment Station, farrowed on March 29, 1932, eleven pigs, all of which were born without eye balls. Ten of the pigs were alive at birth, one lived four days, one lived three hours, while the others died within five minutes after birth. The gestation period for the litter was 111 days, and their average birth weight before nursing was 1 pound 14 ounces. This gilt was placed on the vitamin *A* deficient ra-

The Journal of Heredity

tion when four months of age, and was bred 160 days later. She was kept in a pen with a concrete floor, and was fed in a self-feeder. Thirty days after being bred, she became too weak to get up. Cod liver oil was then supplied in daily doses of two ounces for 20 consecutive days. The gilt gained enough strength to move about the pen and eat regularly five days after she was started on the cod liver oil. After 20 days, the cod liver oil was given every other day for one week, after which it was discontinued, as the gilt appeared to be strong and had a good appetite. Forty-six ounces of cod liver oil were given in all. The litter of pigs was farrowed 53 days after discontinuing the cod liver oil.

Hereditary eye defects have been noted in rabbits by Guyer,* and there is also an "eyeless" recessive character in Drosophila, but a litter of eyeless pigs has not previously been noted.

Since both the sire and dam of this litter of pigs had normal eyes, this defect, if hereditary, would have to be the result of a recessive factor, and in which case both sire and dam must have been heterozygous.

Assuming that both sire and dam were heterozygous for a single factor, the chance that all of the eleven pigs in the litter would be homozygous recessive for this character are only one in approximately four million.

Further evidence that this defect is not hereditary is furnished by one litter of eleven and one litter of eight pigs with normal eyes, sired by the same boar but farrowed by different sows.

While the cause of this abnormality has not been fully determined, and the study is being continued, evidence points to a vitamin A deficiency as the causal factor. The condition is illustrative of the marked effect that a deficiency may have in the disturbance of the internal factors that control the mechanism of development.

---

*GUYER, M. F. 1924) "Further Studies on Inheritance of Eye Defects Induced in Rabbits," *Jour. Exp. Zool.*, 38:449-474.

PAPERS 22, 23 AND 24

22. Gregg, N. M. (1941). Congenital cataract following German measles in the mother. *Trans. Ophthalmol. Soc. Aust.*, **3**, 35–46
23. Blattner, R. J. (1974). The role of viruses in congenital defects. *Am. J. Dis. Child.*, **128**, 781–786
24. Desmonts, G. and Couvreur, J. (1974). Congenital toxoplasmosis. A prospective study of 378 pregnancies. *N. Engl. J. Med..*, **290**, 1110–1116

COMMENTARY

Few studies have been of such fundamental importance to our understanding of the causes of abnormal development in man as the paper by the late Sir Norman Gregg, an Australian ophthalmologist. He reported an 'unusual number of cases of congenital cataract' and other anomalies, including microphthalmia and cardiac defects, in the offspring of mothers who had contracted rubella in early pregnancy during a severe epidemic of German measles. His findings were based on a retrospective study of 78 children with congenital cataract, of which 68 revealed a definite history of maternal rubella infection (Paper 22).

The impact of Gregg's original discovery has been considerable. Not only was an infectious agent incriminated in the aetiology of human birth defects, but the concrete evidence he presented also convincingly demonstrated the susceptibility of the human embryo to its immediate environment. Thus, for the first time the role of environmental influences in the aetiology of human malformations was clearly demonstrated.

Much is now known about the problem of intrauterine infection, and other viruses which may harm the fetus have been identified (see Paper 23). Because congenital rubella represents the most important viral cause of fetal damage it has received more attention than any other forms of intrauterine infections. Although many problems still remain unsettled, significant advances have been made in the general area of diagnosis and prevention of this condition.

It would be inappropriate to deal here with the vast literature relating to rubella infection during pregnancy. Reference should be made to the following reviews: Giles (1973), Harris (1974), and Marshall (1975).

Certain maternal infections are real risks to the fetus. Apart from rubella virus, it is now known that cytomegalovirus, herpes simplex virus, *Treponema pallidum* (syphilis), leptospires, and *Toxoplasma gondii* (Paper 24) may also cause fetal abnormalities. Congenital cytomegalic inclusion disease contributes up to 2% of infant mortality and is associated with malformations of the brain (microcephalus and hydrocephalus) and eyes (chorioretinitis and blindness), hepatosplenomegaly, and mental retardation. Maternal infection of the genital area with type II herpes virus produces congenital abnormalities resembling those induced by cytomegalovirus. Placental transfer of the intracellular parasite *Toxoplasma gondii* may lead to brain damage and ocular abnormalities in the fetus. Wasting of fetal tissues, meningitis, hydrocephalus, deformed teeth, mental retardation, and deafness have been observed in the offspring of mothers with syphilis. Fetal abnormalities have been reported in association with mumps, echovirus, influenza, varicella, vaccinia, coxsackie viruses, and hepatitis. These viruses are suspected to be teratogenic in man, but the available evidence is not sufficient (Dudgeon, 1976; Harris, 1974; Krugman and Gershon, 1975).

REFERENCES

Dudgeon, J. A. (1976). Infective causes of human malformations. *Br. Med. Bull.*, **32**, 77–83

Giles, P. F. H. (1973). Rubella and the obstetrician—a review of recent advances. *Aust. N.Z. J. Obstet. Gynaecol.*, **13**, 77–91

Harris, R. E. (1974). Viral teratogenesis: a review with experimental and clinical perspectives. *Am. J. Obstet. Gynecol.*, **119**, 996–1008

Krugman, S. and Gershon, A. A. (1975). *Infections of the Fetus and the Newborn Infant.* (New York: Alan R. Liss, Inc)

Marshall, W. C. (1975). Effects of rubella virus on the human fetus. *Proc. R. Soc. Med.*, **68**, 369–371

From N. M. Gregg (1941). Trans. Ophthalmol. Soc. Aust., **3**, 35–46. *Copyright* (1941),
by kind permission of the author and the Australasian Medical Publishing Co. Ltd

CONGENITAL CATARACT FOLLOWING GERMAN MEASLES IN THE MOTHER

By N. McAlister Gregg,
Sydney

In the first half of the year, 1941, an unusual number of cases of congenital cataract made their appearance in Sydney. Cases of similar type, which appeared during the same period, have since been reported from widely separated parts of Australia. Their frequency, unusual characteristics and wide distribution warranted closer investigation, and this report is an attempt to bring to notice some of the more important features of what might almost be regarded as a mild epidemic.

I am indebted to many of my colleagues in New South Wales, Victoria and Queensland for particulars of very many of the cases reviewed. These, for the most part, conform very closely to the general features noted in my own series of cases on which the following description is based. The total number of cases included in this review is seventy-eight. My own cases total thirteen, and in addition I have seen seven others included in my colleagues' lists.

General Description and Special Features.

The first striking factor is that the cataracts, usually bilateral, were obvious from birth as dense white opacities completely occupying the pupillary area. Most of the babies were of small size, ill nourished and difficult to feed, with the result that many of them came under the care of the pædiatrician before being seen by the ophthalmic surgeon. Many of them were found to be suffering from a congenital defect of the heart—a fact which, as will be explained later, has adversely affected full investigation of the condition of the lens and in some cases the treatment. The pupillary reaction to light was weak and sluggish; in some cases the irides had a somewhat atrophic appearance. This was more noticeable after mydriasis when the pupillary border appeared as a flat dark band seemingly devoid of any iris stroma.

Full mydriasis was difficult to obtain; in my experience it varied from one-half to three-quarters of the normal; moreover, an unusual number of the patients showed intolerance to atropine. In a large proportion of the cases one was forced to rely upon repeated instillations of homatropine to maintain the mydriasis.

Cataract.—In the undilated condition of the pupil the opacities filled the entire area. After dilatation the opacities appeared densely white—sometimes quite pearly—in the central area with a small, apparently clear, zone between this and the pupillary border of the iris. Closer examination revealed in this zone a less dense opacity of smoky appearance, and outside this only a narrow ring through which a red reflex could be obtained.

The cataractous process seemed to have involved all but the outermost layers of the lens, and was considered to have begun early in the life of the embryo. Generally the cataract was symmetrically situated, but in a few cases it was somewhat excentric—in these there was some sparing of more of the fibres in the lower portion of the peripheral zone. Although the general appearance was much the same in all cases, two main types were noticed in the character of the cataract. In one the contrast between the larger dense white central area and the smaller cloudy more peripheral zone was very marked. In the other the density of the cataract was more uniform throughout and occupied an intermediate stage between that of the two portions of the other type. This distinction has been confirmed by the immediate results of operation. When needling was undertaken in cases of the first group, the dense white central portion was difficult to divide and sometimes separated off as a firm white disk. In others the whole lens seemed to be pushed away by the needle. Subsequent absorption in this group was delayed.

In the second type discission was easier to perform and absorption regular and uniformly progressive. In one case under my care both these types were present, the first type in the right eye and the second type in the left eye. In my opinion these variations and those described by other observers are not essentially different from each other, and the apparent differences are due merely to a variation in intensity and duration of action of the same noxious factor.

The appearance of the cataract does not, in my opinion, exactly correspond to any of the large number of morphological types of congenital and developmental lenticular opacities that have been described. I do not wish to add to what Duke Elder[1] has described as "the confusion which has arisen from the enthusiasm of various observers in the multiplication of types which differ but little in their essential pathology and vary only in their shape and position". I shall, therefore, merely describe the cataract as subtotal. Other descriptions by my colleagues in notes on their cases have been: central nuclear, complete, discoid, nuclear plus, anterior polar, dense central with riders, complete pearly, mature, and total lamellar. In sixteen cases of the whole series reviewed the cataract was unilateral.

Vision.—In all cases the response to light was good; the babies appeared to follow readily any movement of the light stimulus.

Nystagmus.—In the very young patients nystagmus was not noted, but in older babies or in cases in which treatment had to be delayed it was present. The movements were of a coarse, jerky, purposeless nature rather than a true nystagmus. It was a searching movement of the eyeballs and indicated the absence of any development of fixation. In my own cases it was always present if treatment had been delayed beyond the age of three months. In one case, in which the parents deferred operation in order to try some other form of treatment of which they had been informed, it developed before they consented to operation. In another case it developed after operation during the process of absorption. This development during the waiting period before operation has been noticed by other observers.

Variations.—One case in my series was particularly interesting. The baby was referred to me at the age of three weeks with a diagnosis of bilateral keratitis. The corneæ were quite white at birth and both parents had been subjected to a Wassermann test with negative results. At examination I noted a peculiar corneal haze, denser in the centre than in the periphery. The iris was just visible through this haze in the peripheral zone. The tension was normal and there was no inflammation. I advised reexamination under anæsthesia. This was done two weeks later. By this time the corneæ had cleared and the typical white cataracts were seen in the pupillary areas. This baby subsequently became very ill and it was only a few weeks ago that I was able to operate. At operation mydriasis was fuller than usual in these cases and the cataracts were the largest observed in this series.

Two other cases with similar corneal involvement have been noted—namely, by A. Odillo Maher and H. E. Robinson. Involvement was unilateral in Maher's and bilateral in Robinson's case. In these cases there had apparently been some temporary interference with the nutrition of the cornea. Maher's case is also interesting in that the mother developed cataract during pregnancy at the age of twenty-seven. This is the only instance throughout the series of any familial history of cataract.

In another case, reported by S. R. Gerstman, there was "bilateral subluxation of the lenses, mature cataracts, accompanied by arachnodactyly and large fontanelle. Hip regions appeared normal."

Other complications reported have been cleft palate, one; congenital stenosis of naso-lachrymal duct, three; *calcaneus rarus*, one; although it is not certain whether these are above the average incidence in any group of infants of similar numbers.

Monocular Cases.—The monocular cases merit special consideration. Sixteen of these have been reported, and in ten of them definite microphthalmia has been described.

In one of my cases—there were three in all—the cataract was noted by the mother only when the child was seven weeks old, though she stated that it may have been present before that date. The affected eye was definitely microphthalmic, and examination of the other eye under mydriasis revealed a large pale area with some scattered pigmentation in the lower half of the fundus suggestive of a coloboma.

In another case the mother gave a history that both eyes were said to have had conjuncti-vitis at birth. This inflammation, she stated, cleared up under treatment in three weeks, and then two weeks later she noticed a white mass in the left pupil. Conceding the accuracy of these histories, I have no doubt that the cataracts were present at birth in the central portion of the lens and that it was the final opacification of the more peripheral fibres which made them apparent. In all other cases the cataracts have been apparent from birth.

Reporting her case of left-sided monocular cataract, Dr. Aileen Mitchell wrote:

No difference was noticed in the size of the eyes when the child was seven weeks old; when the child was aged four months there was microphthalmia of the left eye. The mother said the eye had got small. Diameter of the right cornea was about 11 millimetres, of the left cornea 8·5 milli-metres. Nystagmus, which was not present at the first examination, had developed and was coarse in nature with roving movements of the eyeballs. The fundus of the right eye appeared pale, and some scattered irregular shaped spots of pigment were observed.

L. Stanton Cook described one case, monocular central opacity of the lens, and writes: "It would appear that this cataract is a developmental defect rather than a toxic type." As the baby also had the typical congenital defect of the heart, I feel that this is open to question.

The accompanying microphthalmia, definitely noted in 66% of cases, suggests an inhibi-tory effect on the development of the eye generally. In an autopsy performed in a monocular case at the Royal Alexandra Hospital for Children the following measurements were recorded: Left eye (affected), antero-posterior diameter, 1·6 centimetres; transverse diameter, 1·5 centi-metres. Right eye (unaffected), these measurements were respectively 1·8 centimetres and 1·9 centimetres. It was also noted that the left cornea was smaller than the right in proportion to the general variation in size of the eyes.

Microphthalmia.—Microphthalmia is present so frequently (66%) in the cases of monocu-lar cataract that closer attention to the size of the eyes in the binocular cases is advisable. Is it not possible that both eyes may be smaller than normal, and that this feature may be un-noticed because it is bilateral? Further information on this aspect can be obtained from measurements at autopsies and by observation of the subsequent growth of the eyes in the living infants. In this respect the following measurements obtained at autopsies in other cases at Royal Alexandra Hospital for Children are interesting:

B.S., *ætatis* five months. Right eye: antero-posterior diameter, 1·5 centimetres; transverse, 1·7 centimetres. Left eye: antero-posterior diameter, 1·4 centimetres; transverse, 1·7 centimetres.

M.M., *ætatis* three months. Right eye: antero-posterior diameter, 1·5 centimetres; transverse, 1·5 centimetres. Left eye: antero-posterior diameter, 1·6 centimetres; transverse, 1·6 centimetres.

M.O's., *ætatis* five and a half months. Both eyes: antero-posterior diameter, 1·6 centimetres; transverse, 1·8 centimetres.

J. Maude described one case as "bilateral microphthalmos, right eye smaller". According to Scammon and Armstrong,[2] the average measurements of the eyeball at birth are: sagittal diameter, 17·6 millimetres; transverse diameter, 17·1 millimetres; vertical diameter, 16·5 millimetres. Post-natal growth is very small in the first six months, but they stated that it is most probable that the figures for this period are too low because of the inclusion of premature cases.

By comparison with these average measurements of the normal eye at birth the figures quoted above show a definite diminution in the antero-posterior diameter and a reversal of the normal relationship between the respective lengths of the antero-posterior and transverse diameters.

In the cases under consideration here it must be remembered that many of the babies are generally undersized, so that any estimation of the size of the eyes must be considered in relation to the general size and body weight of the baby.

Heart.—As previously mentioned, an extremely high percentage of these babies had a congenital defect of the heart. I am indebted to Dr. Margaret Harper for the following description of eight cases seen by her:

All these babies were seen because of difficulty in feeding and failure to thrive. They all had symptoms suggesting a cardiac defect such as difficulty in taking the breast; they had to be fed in their cots by bottle and some by gavage. They were all in the acyanotic or potentially cyanotic groups of cardiac defects. None was cyanotic. There was a harsh systolic murmur over the base of the heart and down the sternum in all. Some had a thrill. All had signs suggesting the continuance of a fœtal condition or of a malformation of the heart.

In my own series this condition was present in all but one case. In the whole series it has been present in forty-four cases; in eleven cases there is no record of the cardiac condition in ten cases it has been recorded as normal or apparently normal; in four cases in which the condition was not reported upon, the babies died and death was sudden; in another the baby was "ill nourished"; and in three cases the report was "no defect noted".

Autopsy in three cases at the Royal Alexandra Hospital for Children revealed a wide patency of the *ductus arteriosus*, and I understand that in autopsies performed elsewhere a similar condition has been found. The reports on the cardiac condition from autopsies in three cases at the Royal Alexandra Hospital for Children are as follows:

M.O'S.: There was hypertrophy of the ventricular muscle; the left measured 0·9 centimetre and the right 0·5 centimetre. A few petechial hæmorrhages were detected on the surface of the myocardium. The endocardium and valves were normal and all the septa intact. The *ductus arteriosus*, however, was widely patent.

B.S.: There was no free fluid in the pericardial sac. The heart was enlarged, with particular hypertrophy of the right ventricle. Right ventricle measured 0·7 centimetre and the left 0·8 centimetre. There were a few petechial hæmorrhages visible on the surface of the myocardium and one fairly large "milk spot". The membranous portion of the interventricular septum was patent. The *foramen ovale* was not completely occluded, although it appeared to have been functionally closed. The heart valves and great vessels were normal, but the *ductus arteriosus* was widely patent.

P.F.: The right heart was somewhat dilated. The right ventricle wall was 0·35 centimetre in its thickest part. The left ventricle wall was 0·5 centimetre in its thickest part. All valves were normal. No septal defect was present. Vessels were normal except for a wide patency of the *ductus arteriosus*.

Additional Findings.—In one case at the Royal Alexandra Hospital for Children there were several additional findings worth record here.

Both lungs had a considerable degree of hypostatic congestion at the bases. Throughout the remainder of the lungs there were a very large number of hæmorrhagic spots, some of which were confluent and covered considerable areas. Hæmorrhagic spots were detected on the inner surface of the pericardium and on the surface of the myocardium. In addition, the visceral pericardium over the upper anterior aspect of the left ventricle bore a "milk spot". The right kidney was situated in such a position that the ureter entered the pelvis on the lateral side of the kidney after coursing across its anterior surface. The right kidney consisted of two distinct lobes, the upper one about twice as large as the lower. Each lobe had its own separate pelvis, and the ureter divided outside the kidney into two branches, one to each lobe. Both ovaries were cystic. The uterus was bicornuate in type.

Another complication noted in a few cases was the development of a dry scaly eczematous condition, involving the face, scalp and limbs, which was very resistant to treatment.

Sex.—Thirty-three of the patients were males, thirty-five were females. In the remaining ten cases the reports did not specify the sex of the child.

Deaths.—In this series of cases fifteen deaths have been recorded. Details are not available in all cases of the mode or cause of death, but broncho-pneumonia has been noted in several. In three cases within my own knowledge there has been a sudden rise of temperature up to 105° F. or even 106° F., accompanied by extreme distress, and death has followed within twenty-four hours.

Intolerance to Atropine.—Intolerance to atropine has been a noticeable feature of the cases in my own series and in no single instance has it been possible to continue its administration throughout the treatment. It most cases, even after one or two instillations, the baby has exhibited considerable constitutional disturbance with pyrexia, restlessness and irritability, and the difficulty of feeding has been intensified. In one case in which two instillations were made over a period of twenty-four hours, the temperature rose to 105° F. Homatropine, 2%, was substituted and the temperature returned to normal, and was not subsequently elevated. Other observers have noted the same intolerance to atropine.

ÆTIOLOGY

Although one was struck with the unusual appearance of the cataracts in the first few cases, it was only when other similar cases continued to appear that serious thought was given to their causation.

The remarkable similarity of the opacities in the lens, the frequency of an accompanying affection of the heart and the widespread geographical incidence of the cases suggested that there was some common factor in the production of the diseased condition, and suggested it was the result of some constitutional condition of toxic or infective nature rather than of a purely development defect.

The question arose whether this factor could have been some disease or infection occurring in the mother during pregnancy which had then interfered with the developing cells of the lens. By a calculation from the date of the birth of the baby it was estimated that the early period of pregnancy corresponded with the period of maximum intensity of the very widespread and severe epidemic in 1940 of the so-called German measles.

Special attention was accordingly paid to the history of the health of the mothers during pregnancy, and in each new case it was found that the mother had suffered from that disease early in her pregnancy, most frequently in the first or second month. In some cases she had not at that time yet realized that she was pregnant.

The investigation was then repeated in the early cases in which such a history had not been sought, and again the history of early "German measles" infection was definite. Moreover, in all these cases the health of the mother during the remainder of the pregnancy was described as good.

As the constant involvement of the central nuclear fibres in the cataractous process suggested an early incidence of the noxious factor, it was considered that a possible solution of the problem had been obtained. Confirmation for this theory was therefore sought from any of my colleagues who had seen lesions of this type, and they kindly agreed to assist me by inquiry into the health of the mothers during pregnancy. The result of their inquiries confirmed the amazing frequency of the "German measles" infection.

"Congenital cataract may be due to a maldevelopment, a physical or chemical element acting on the developing lens, or inflammation during the embryonic or fœtal period."[3]

Duke Elder[4] stated: "The ætiology of these opacities depends upon some disturbances of the development of the lens, but what the actual disturbance may be, or the precise method of its action, is a matter of considerable doubt in most cases."

From his anatomical studies Jaensch[5] (1924) concluded that an intra-uterine inflammation was a frequent cause of a total opacity of the lens. Toxic influences also may play a part in the production of opacities, and it is conceivable, writes Duke Elder,[6] that toxic or infective processes in the mother may cause a derangement in the lens of the fœtus, or that similar causes, error of feeding and nutrition or acute exanthemata in the infant, may have a similar effect.

Ida Mann[7] has stated that the exanthemata, measles, mumps, smallpox, chickenpox, scarlet fever *et cetera*, are all known to be transmissible transplacentally.

Whatever the disturbing factor may be, it is fair to assume that the earlier it acts, the more will the central portion of the lens be likely to suffer.

In the developing lens, in the 26-millimetre stage of the embryo, the original central primitive fibres, elongations of the cells of the posterior wall, have completed their growth. Then begins the development of the secondary lens fibres from the cells in the equatorial region. All subsequent growth in the lens is from these equatorial cells, which give rise to successive layers of new lens fibres, these fibres enveloping and compressing the central fibres. With the development of these fibres comes the appearance of the suturing which eventually takes on the typical "Y" pattern of the fœtal nucleus.

In the cases under review the cataractous process has involved these early fibres. Can we not fairly assume that the morbid influence began early? As successive layers of fibres were also affected, until the greater part of the lens became involved, this noxious factor must also have persisted in diminishing strength until finally with its disappearance some normal fibres were formed.

Just how and where this disturbance took place I cannot say. Much more histological evidence than is at present available will have to be obtained before any suggestions can be made. However, if we allow the possibility that the lens may be affected by infective processes in the mother, and if we find the same infection occurring at approximately the same early period in the pregnancy in almost all the cases, and if we then find that the babies of these mothers have cataracts of a more or less uniform type which involve the fibres formed at that period, then I think it is reasonable to assume that the occurrence cannot be a mere coincidence, but that there must be some definite connexion between that infection and the morbid condition of the lens.

Although it is rare, cases of the exanthemata have been seen in the newborn baby. Ballantyne[8] noted twenty recorded examples of fœtal measles up to 1893; whilst up to 1902 not more than twenty well authenticated cases of scarlet fever in the fœtus had been recorded, varicella *in utero* was not unknown.

The remarkable frequency of the accompanying congenital defect of the heart and the apparent constancy in type of this defect seem to me to indicate a common causative factor. Could this not be some toxic or infective process resulting in a partial arrest of development?

INCIDENCE OF GERMAN MEASLES IN THIS SERIES

In all but ten cases in this series the history of "German measles" infection is present. In two of these ten cases the report is negative for measles; in one there was "history of kidney trouble"; in two others the report is definitely "history not asked for"; in the remaining five causes the report is "no history of measles" or "not known". It is interesting to note that the majority of these were cases occurring in 1940 or early in 1941 before the theory of a possible association between "German measles" and the congenital cataracts was promulgated.

Amongst the cases that have come under my own notice in only one is the history negative. In this case the mother stated that she was kept so busy looking after her ten children that she could not recollect any details of her own health beyond the fact that she was ill at about the sixth week of pregnancy when one of the other children died suddenly from whooping cough. Even though she was ill, she was unable to go to bed during the last month before the baby was born one month before full term. In the vast majority of the cases infection occurred either in the first or second month of pregnancy. In a few cases it was during the third month, and in one it is reported as a severe attack occurring three months before pregnancy.

This maternal infection occurred in July or August, 1940, in the majority of cases; in the minority of cases outside this period the date of infection ranged from December, 1939, to January, 1941.

Out of thirty-five cases in which the record is available, the affected baby was the first child in twenty-six instances; in three others it was a second child; whilst in the six remaining cases the baby was the third, fourth, fifth, seventh, eighth and tenth child respectively. I believe that these figures, with the noticeably high incidence in the children of *primiparæ*, afford confirmatory evidence of the close association between congenital cataract in the baby and the maternal infection. For it was this young adult group, to which these *primiparæ* belong, which was particularly affected by this epidemic of "German measles".

GEOGRAPHICAL DISTRIBUTION

Although the majority of the cases reported came from the suburban districts of Sydney and Melbourne, others were from widely separated country towns in New South Wales and Victoria, and eight were from Queensland distributed between Brisbane, Rockhampton and Ipswich.

NATURE OF EPIDEMIC

Within my own experience I have not previously seen German measles of such severity and accompanied by such severe complications as occurred during this epidemic in 1940. The swelling of the glands of the neck, the sore throat, the involvement of the wrist and ankle joints and the general constitutional disturbance were all very pronounced. The average stay in hospital of patients treated at the Prince Henry Hospital was eight days as against four days in previous years.

The peak period of the epidemic from returns at this hopsital was from mid-June to early August.

Running concurrently with this epidemic were the epidemics of sore throat known as the Ingleburn throat or Puckapunyal throat *et cetera*, deriving its name from the military camp with which it was associated. These epidemics started in the camps and spread to the civilian population. Could they not have been streptococcal in origin and is it not possible that the rash diagnosed as "German measles" may have been, in some cases, a toxic erythema accompanying a streptococcal infection?

In this respect it is interesting to note that the rash occurring in this so-called "German measles" epidemic has been described to me by physicians as macular, morbilliform, scarlatiniform and toxic erythematous; in other words, it was pleomorphic. I have also been informed by two physicians that they have at present an unusual number of young adult patients suffering from arthritis and other rheumatic conditions, and these patients all have a history of "German measles" last year. Because "German measles" is not a notifiable disease it is impossible to obtain any details of the epidemic from the health authorities, but from my own observations and inquiries I have formed the opinion that the 1940 "German measles" epidemic differed greatly from the ordinary virus infection bearing that name.

MANAGEMENT

From the purely ocular standpoint the essential consideration is the same as in cases of the ordinary lamellar type of cataract—to permit sufficient light stimulus to reach the retina so that fixation may be developed. In this respect the time factor is of the utmost importance. If the stimulus is insufficient or delayed, nystagmus will result.

The special considerations in this series are: (*a*) the marked density and large size of the opacity; (*b*) the difficulty in obtaining mydriasis, so that the transparent area for entrance of light is minimal; (*c*) the high frequency of intolerance to atropine.

These factors compel us to operate at the earliest possible moment. In my opinion the only contraindication to early interference is the general state of health of the baby. In many cases this has been so bad that physicians have refused to give an anæsthetic until some improvement has been obtained in the general condition. So frequently has nystagmus been observed to develop during this waiting period that I am convinced that some risk is justified in order to operate at the earliest possible moment, particularly as later experience has shown that the babies take the short anæsthetic required more easily than had been anticipated.

When operation has to be deferred it is essential to maintain the fullest possible degree of mydriasis, by atropine if tolerated. If atropine cannot be employed, then repeated instillation of homatropine must be substituted for it.

The value of early operation is well illustrated by one case reported by E. Temple Smith in which he performed discission on a baby aged three weeks. Clear pupils resulted and there has been no sign of nystagmus developing.

Operation

Discission has frequently proved more difficult than usual. The anterior chamber is particularly shallow, and in many cases the very dense central portion of the lens has proved very resistant to the needle. Sometimes it has separated off as a firm disk, in others the whole lens has tended to move away from the point of the needle, and one has obtained the impression that it would have been possible to perform an ordinary extraction. In other cases, on the other hand, discission has been straightforward and easy.

Results of Operation.—Absorption has been slower than that of the ordinary lamellar cataracts. I have not yet had an opportunity to examine the fundi of any patient after absorption of the lens matter, but I propose to do so in as many cases as possible under general anæsthesia. Careful search will be made for any other defects. The unhealthy appearance of the iris in some cases suggests that there may be possibly some changes in the choroid, particularly since the patients in the monocular cases are so frequently microphthalmic.

PROGNOSIS

It is difficult to forecast the future for these unfortunate babies. We cannot at this stage be sure that there are not other defects present which are not evident now but which may show up as development proceeds. The cardiac condition also tends to make the prognosis doubtful. One baby which had survived two operations some months ago, suddenly died quite recently at the age of seven months. The possibility of the appearance of neurotropic manifestations at a later date will be kept in mind. The prognosis for vision depends on the presence or absence of nystagmus and, of course, on the condition of the retina and choroid.

I look forward to further improvements in contact glass development, for herein lies the greatest possibility for help in the future.

If we agree that these cases are the result of infection of the mother by "German measles", what can we do to prevent a repetition of the tragedy in any future epidemic? Is the mass of modern research into the causation of senile cataract going to be helpful by the discovery of some remedy which could be given to the mother to inhibit the formation of opacity in the developing lens of the embryo?

In the present state of our knowledge the only sure treatment available is that of prophylaxis. We must recognize and teach the potential dangers of such an epidemic or, I think, any other exanthem, and do all in our power to prevent its spread and particularly to guard the young married woman from the risk of infection.

As to confirmation of the theory of causation put forward in this paper, I suggest that the following line of investigation may be helpful. In all prenatal clinics and maternity hospitals very careful histories should be taken and recorded of exposure of the mother to infection of any kind during the entire period of pregnancy.

ACKNOWLEDGEMENTS

I wish to thank all those colleagues, too numerous to mention, for the reports they have furnished me of their cases and for their permission to include them in this review.

I am also indebted to Dr. J. Ringland Anderson for his help with the literature on the subject; to Dr. Margaret Harper for her report on the cardiac condition; to Dr. B. Van Someren, of the New South Wales Government Health Department, for placing the records of his department at my disposal, and particularly to the sisters in charge of several of the baby health centres for the excellent reports they so kindly furnished; to Dr. Douglas Reye for his reports on the autopsies; and to Professor Harold Dew for his timely and helpful criticism on the presentation of this paper.

REFERENCES

[1] W. Stewart Duke Elder: "Text Book of Ophthalmology", Volume ii, page 1364.

[2] Richard E. Scammon and Ellery N. Armstrong: "On the Growth of the Human Eyeball and Optic Nerve", *Journal of Comparative Neurology*, Volume xxxviii, 1924–1925, page 165.

[3] Daniel B. Kirby: "The Eye and its Diseases", edited by C. Berens, 1936, page 577.

[4] W. Stewart Duke Elder: *Loco citato*, page 1365.

[5] P. A. Jaensch: "*Anatomische Untersuchungen eines angeborenen Totalstars*", *Archiv für Ophthalmologie*, Volume cxv, 1924, page 81.

[6] W. Stewart Duke Elder: *Loco citato*, page 1366.

[7] Ida Mann: "Developmental Abnormalities of the Eye", 1937, page 18.

[8] J. W. Ballantyne: "Manual of Antenatal Pathology and Hygiene", 1902, Part 1, page 196.

D. R. GAWLER (Perth) referred to a child with this disease. It was seen when four months old and was ill nourished and suffering from impetigo. It showed intolerance to atropine and mydriasis was poor. The cataracts were nuclear and bilateral. The irides were blue and atrophic around the pupil. The Wassermann test applied to blood and cerebro-spinal fluid produced no reaction. No inquiry was made regarding maternal German measles. D. R. Gawler needled one eye and found the cortex and nucleus resistant. The cortex flaked off the anterior surface. There was little reaction to the needling. There was no epidemic of German measles in the district during the early months of pregnancy, but the mother said that there was another child in the town similarly affected. D. R. Gawler had no particular theories, but there might have been an endocrine deficiency, possibly involving the parathyreoids.

ARCHIE S. ANDERSON (Melbourne) had seen a few cases of this type and in every instance the mother had had German measles during the second month of pregnancy. He congratulated N. McA. Gregg on his striking and original inquiry.

G. H. BARHAM BLACK (Adelaide) said that he had seen one case in which monocular cataract and nystagmus were present. The mother had German measles six weeks after the last menstrual period. No inquiry had been made into the child's heart condition. The epidemic of German measles had occurred about the same time as in other States. There had been a number of severe cases. A soldier had died of encephalitis at Renmark. In South Australia an investigation had been made of streptococcal infections of the throat, but no streptococci had been found. Volunteers had submitted to inoculations from "camp" throat infections, but the results were inconclusive.

A. W. O'OMBRAIN (Newcastle) had seen four patients, two of whom had heart disease. He asked why the infection was described as "so-called German measles". One mother had German measles three months before pregnancy.

A. L. TOSTEVIN (Adelaide) spoke of a case he had seen. The mother, aged twenty-eight years, had had good health during pregnancy except for German measles at three months. There was no evidence of any abnormality of the child's heart. The mother noticed, when the child was six weeks old, that it could not see. He needled the eyes at three months. One cataract absorbed quickly, but the other, which was difficult, did not absorb well and the eye converged. Nystagmus did not develop. He preserbed +10 dioptre spheres and the child could apparently see reasonably well. The pupil did not dilate sufficiently well to allow of fundus examination. The eyes looked small and the irides were atrophic. He considered that N. McA. Gregg's contribution was very important and offered his congratulations.

W. M. C. MACDONALD (Sydney) added his compliments and stated that he had performed needling in some cases. One patient so treated had obtained a good result, but yet had developed nystagmus. In some of the others needling was difficult and the results were indifferent. It would be interesting to watch further developments. In all his cases there were heart conditions, and this showed how widespread was the involvement. The patients were all weakly.

LEONARD J. C. MITCHELL (Melbourne) asked whether there was more in the new syndrome than a mysterious association with German measles. He considered it a matter for continued research by internists in order to discover the unknown factor at work in this most remarkable series of cases. He congratulated Dr. Gregg, and said he thought that this series of cases would be epoch-making.

N. McA. GREGG, in reply, said he did not want to be dogmatic by claiming that it had been established the cataracts were due solely to the "German measles". However, the evidence afforded by the cases under review was so striking that he was convinced that there was a very close relationship between the two conditions, particularly because in the very large majority of cases the pregnancy had been normal except for the "German measles" infection. He considered that it was quite likely that similar cases may have been missed in previous years either from casual history-taking or from failure to ascribe any importance to an exanthem affecting the mother so early in her pregnancy. He quoted the case of one mother with an affected child who was informed by another mother that her boy, who was born with cataracts, had died suddenly from disease of the heart at the age of seven, and that during this pregnancy she had had German measles. For the past five months he had asked the mother of every healthy young baby he had contacted whether she had been affected by "German measles" during the pregnancy and in no single case had there been any infection.

In regard to the few cases in the series in which there was no history of "German measles", he considered it quite likely that the infection had been slight and overlooked. He quoted Professor Dew as saying that in every virus epidemic some cases were subclinical. In reply to A. W. D'Ombrain, he said he had used the term "so-called German measles" because he believed this epidemic was different from the usual mild epidemics of this infection. The severity of the symptoms, the variability in the character of the rash and the frequency of rheumatic sequelæ in the victims seemed to him to support this view. He felt it was virus *plus*. He congratulated A. L. Tostevin on prescribing glasses for his patient at such an early age. He regretted he had been unable to make a slit lamp examination in his cases, but considered he was not justified in subjecting the babies to an anæsthetic for the length of time necessary to make such examination. In answer to L. J. C. Mitchell he said that in the more recent cases he had operated on both eyes at once, as this involved only one anæsthetic.

He informed G. H. Barham Black that he had operated on one child with a monocular cataract. He mentioned that in those cases in which the weight of the baby at birth was known, the average weight was five pounds.

From R. J. Blattner (1974). Am. J. Dis. Child., **128**, 781–786. *Copyright* (1974),
by kind permission of the author and the American Medical Association

The Role of Viruses in Congenital Defects

Russell J. Blattner, MD

The rubella-induced congenital defects have, hopefully, been curtailed through the years of study that culminated in the rubella vaccination program. For other teratogenic viruses, such control is not yet in sight. Moreover, continued study of virus infections indicates an expanding role for cytomegalovirus and possibly other viruses in causing enormous damage to the health of unborn children. The social and economic drain on society of these damaged children cannot be accurately assessed. The cost of institutional care and special education facilities for children born with congenital rubella during 1964 and 1965 has been estimated to be approximately $920 million. In addition, the emotional burden to the family and to the affected individual, as well as problems of society in assisting with the social adjustment of the individuals, cannot be evaluated.

In 1941, Gregg[1] made the epoch-making discovery that rubella infection, acquired by the mother during gestation, caused congenital defects in the offspring. Soon after,

Accepted for publication June 17, 1974.
From the Department of Pediatrics, Baylor College of Medicine; and Texas Children's Hospital, Houston.
Read as the Abraham Jacobi Award Address before the 123rd annual convention of the American Medical Association, Chicago, June 25, 1974.
Reprint requests to Department of Pediatrics, Baylor College of Medicine, 1200 Moursund Ave, Houston, TX 77025 (Dr. Blattner).

our group began seeking methods for studying the mechanisms involved in the production of defects by viruses. The rubella virus had not been isolated at that time and, in fact, was not to be isolated for another 21 years. Therefore, other available viruses had to be used in the early investigations.

The studies in placental-type animals were hindered by the considerable chance of selecting a virus that did not have teratogenic potential and by the possibility that affected embryos would be lost through death and resorption before birth or sacrifice of the animals for study. It seemed logical, therefore, that the chick embryo, which was easy to observe through a window placed over an opening in the shell, was the first experimental model in which specific teratogenic defects were demonstrated.

Hamburger and Habel[2] were the first to study the effects of viruses in chick embryos. Using type A influenza virus, they found twists of the axis, retarded amniotic development, and a flattening of the encephalon due to tissue damage that allowed the ventricular fluid to escape; they did not, however, report defects in specific organs of the embryo.

To my knowledge, our laboratory was the first to report specific defects in developing organs of the chick embryo following a virus infection.[3] Using Newcastle disease virus (NDV), a virus specifically infectious for chickens, we were able to demonstrate retarded development, small size, or complete absence of such organs as the lens and auditory vesicle. Further studies showed that mumps virus[4] produced cataract, general growth retardation, and defects of feathering and that type A influenza virus[5,6] produced brain defects and myeloschisis (an open neural plate believed to be the basic anomaly of myelomeningocele), as well as defects of lens and auditory anlage similar to those of NDV.

In subsequent studies, using NDV,[7-9] mumps virus,[10] and influenza virus,[11] we were able to record important observations concerning the teratogenic potential of viruses. It was shown that viruses share properties in common with other teratogenic agents, ie, the greatest damage occurs to organs when they are in critical stages of differentiation and development. In addition, these studies showed the following results:

1. The defects occurred only in the presence of fully infective virus and were, in some cases, directly related to necrosis of infected cells in the affected primordium; in other cases, the defects appeared to result from inhibition of growth of specific tissues.

2. If embryos were inoculated after certain critical stages of development had passed, the defects no longer occurred.

3. Each virus produced a slightly different syndrome of defects, and the effects of various viruses on the same organ showed a wide range of differences.

4. At least one of the viruses studied (NDV) was able to replicate in most embryonic tissues to which it had access but showed a substantial preference for tissues that were in early stages of rapid growth and differentiation.

5. Gross defective development was more likely to occur if there was a high concentration of virus in the inoculum initially reaching the embryo.

Rubella

Although many clinical investigations were carried out in the years following Gregg's initial observations, rubella was, for a long time, the only virus that appeared to be teratogenic for humans. Furthermore, there had been little additional information available to increase our understanding of the role of viruses in human teratology. In 1962, however, the rubella virus was isolated by Parkman et al[12] and by Weller and Neva.[13] Serologic techniques for demonstrating the infection in the mother and the fetus later became available. These events occurred fortuitously before the worldwide rubella epidemic of 1964 and 1965 when 20,000 to 30,000 infants were born with the congenital rubella syndrome. Studies of these children greatly increased our understanding of gestational virus infections and further information is still being accumulated. Particularly useful is the new information regarding fetal immune responses. Although maternal IgG antibody begins to enter the fetal circulation around the third month, no maternal antibody of the IgM type crosses the placental barrier. It was learned, however, that the fetus, if directly exposed to infection, can respond by producing both IgG and IgM. The IgM often increases to high levels. Thus, elevated levels of IgM in the newborn period is suggestive of intrauterine infection. Positive identification of infection can be made if specific antibody to the infectious agent is found in the IgM serum fraction of the infant.

During this period, a collaborative study group at Baylor College of Medicine and its affiliated hospitals (conducted at the Clinical Research Center, Texas Children's Hospital, Houston) was organized to study many newborns exposed in utero to the rubella infection. It soon became apparent that, in addition to the classical picture of cataract, heart defects, deafness, and mental retardation, these infants showed other findings that had been largely overlooked in previous years. The phrase, "expanded rubella syndrome," was coined[14] to apply to these findings, which included thrombocytopenic purpura, hemolytic anemia, hepatosplenomegaly, necrotizing myocarditis, pneumonitis, and long bone lesions.[15] Central nervous system (CNS) abnormalities that were observed included neurosensory impairment, chronic meningitis, encephalitis, and, more rarely, microcephaly. Infants with the expanded rubella syndrome were often acutely ill and the mortality was significant. The most unexpected finding was that virus was still present in many tissues and body secretions[16] and could be repeatedly isolated, especially from the spinal fluid and nasopharynx, for long periods of time, even in the presence of circulating specific antibodies.[17] It could occasionally be isolated from the urine of infants up to 10 weeks of age. Thereafter, it became evident that congenital rubella is an active, contagious disease with multisystem involvement and a wide range of clinical expression.

As this dynamic, developing clinical picture unfolded, evidence of the more subtle effects of rubella were recognized. Many children were found who showed restlessness, instability, auditory imperception, motor defects, learning disability, language delay, and behavioral disorders.

Desmond and associates at the Leopold L. Meyer Center for Developmental Pediatrics at Texas Children's Hospital found that eight of 64 congenital rubella children studied exhibited behavior patterns highly associated with autism, ie, mannerisms, ritualistic patterns associated with sensory loss, etc. It was their opinion that these fitted the pattern of behavior associated with autism.[18] Later, Chess[19] noted the surmise of Desmond et al and stated that, in a group of 243 patients, she had found 10 with autistic syndrome, 8 with partial syndrome, and 18 who demonstrated behavior suggestive of autism. This is a high incidence, since the greatest incidence of autism in control studies is 4.5/10,000.

Cytomegalovirus (CMV)

An understanding of the role of CMV in human congenital defects is slowly evolving. This infection, usually asymptomatic in older persons, was originally considered to be of little importance to humans. Recently, however, infectious mononucleosis-like illness in adults has been associated with CMV. The CMV-infected cell is characteristic, containing great amounts of cytoplasm and one or two intranuclear inclusions and occasional cytoplasmic inclusions. It attracted the attention of investigators who found it first in salivary glands. Later it was found in many organs of 15% to 20% of young children at the time of autopsy, regardless of the cause of death. After isolation of the virus by Smith in 1956,[20] it became established that the cytomegalic inclusion disease acquired in utero can cause brain damage associated with mental retardation, periventricular calcification, auditory defects, microcephaly, and chorioretinitis. Although CMV is the most common congenital virus infection (0.5% to 1.0% of all infants excrete virus), it is only now that we are beginning to appreciate the serious implications of this widespread congenital infection. Manifestations in congenitally infected infants may range from a severe, rapidly fatal illness to a relatively mild disease with transient symptoms. Findings may include purpura, respiratory illness, jaundice, hepatosplenomegaly, CNS symptoms,

small size for gestational age, feeding difficulties, or general failure to thrive. It should be emphasized, however, that many infants who excrete virus are asymptomatic at birth. Follow-up studies of infected infants are beginning to indicate that CMV may be the most important cause of virus-induced mental impairment.[21,22] It has been estimated that every year a minimum of 5,000 infants will be born with some degree of brain damage associated with CMV infection in the United States and in England and Wales, and that 200 to 600 children yearly are born with brain damage due to CMV. This may be compared to an estimated 1,300 cases of mongolism. In a recent study of 18 children with subclinical CMV,[23] the whole group showed a trend toward subnormal intelligence in follow-up studies, although only two showed definite mental and social disability. In this study, some degree of sensorineural hearing loss occurred in nine of 16 patients, although only four showed a frank auditory handicap. From this and other studies, hearing impairment has also emerged as an important finding in congenital CMV infection.

Ocular disease following CMV infection first became evident through observation of chorioretinitis in approximately 25% of the infants who showed severe infection. The true incidence of ocular disease is not known. However, as noted by H. M. Hittner, MD (written communication, June 1974), of 15 infants with CMV infection examined in our department, seven had substantial morphological changes of the retina or optic nerves. In three, unilateral coloboma of the optic nerve head was observed; this had not, to our knowledge, been previously reported following CMV. In two, unilateral optic neuritis was verified. Two other infants were observed to have chorioretinitis. Inflammation of the conjunctiva, cornea, and ciliary body, as well as retinal pseudocolobomas, retinal hemor-

rhages, and perivascular exudates, have been reported by others.

Prolonged excretion of the virus in congenital CMV has been verified, and damage may continue after birth. The CMV is widespread in the population as an endemic infection. Since it is generally asymptomatic in adults, it is difficult to relate the time of infection during gestation with the defects produced. It has been suggested that the most serious damage to the fetus is noted when the maternal infection occurs during the first six months of gestation and that primary maternal infections are more apt to cause fetal wastage or severe damage. It is noteworthy that congenital infection in siblings from consecutive pregnancies can occur, although it may be rare. In one instance in which the siblings were born three years apart, the first child showed growth retardation and psychomotor retardation, as well as other symptoms of CMV infection, whereas the second child was asymptomatic.[24]

The importance of the role of CMV in congenital disease continues to expand as more information becomes available. Continuing prospective-type studies are needed to verify the type and extent of damage that will eventually be recognized as the infected individual grows and matures.

Herpesvirus Hominis (HVH)

Herpesvirus hominis infection of the cervix is widespread in women and may sometimes be asymptomatic. The infection can be transmitted to the fetus during gestation, but most cases observed in the newborn period are acquired by passage of the infant through the infected birth canal of the mother. Infection of the newborn, however, appears to be relatively rare. One estimate indicates about one case occurs in 7,500 births,[25] but it is believed that many cases may not be diagnosed even though less than 5% are asymptomatic. Slightly more than half of the infected newborns will have skin manifestations, such as vesicles or bullous lesions. Others may show various symptoms, such as conjunctivitis followed by keratitis, episodes of cyanosis, seizures, bleeding from the gastrointestinal tract, fever, vomiting, feeding difficulties, irritability, and lethargy. Disseminated infection may occur and can be fatal.

Gestational HVH infections associated with developmental defects of the offspring have been reported in only six cases thus far.[25-30] Isolation of the virus in five of the cases and failure to find CMV or toxoplasmosis in three of the six suggest that HVH may be the cause of the defects. Microcephaly, periventricular calcification, and microphthalmia were prominent features of the cases described. Chorioretinitis has also been observed in these and in other unpublished cases. In one case, a patent ductus arteriosus and shortened digits were described.[28] The majority of cases of herpes infection in the newborn are due to the genital type (type 2) virus, but the oral (type 1) can also infect the newborn and can occasionally be isolated from genital infections of the mother. In one of the congenitally infected infants, type 1 virus was isolated. An ascending infection from the maternal cervix has been suspected as a possible route of infection of the fetus. Morphological evidence (chorioamnionitis) of ascending infection from the maternal cervix has recently been published for one case[30] in which developmental defects occurred.

Varicella-Zoster Virus

From recent reports[31] and a review of the literature (A. P. Williamson, unpublished data), it appears certain that congenital anomalies can, rarely, follow varicella-zoster infection during the early months of pregnancy. The defects may evidently occur whether the maternal clinical symptoms appear in the form of chicken pox or herpes-zoster. The most convincing evidence that the defects are due to the varicella-zoster infection consists in the obsevation of five cases showing strikingly similar patterns of hypoplasia of limbs, digits, and other areas of the trunk or body in association with skin lesions or scars characteristic of varicella-zoster infection. The scars were often prominent on (but were not confined to) the skin of the defective part. Club foot also occurred in three of the cases.

A tabulation of defects in 11 cases from the literature indicates that the eye may be the most commonly affected organ (A. P. Williamson, unpublished data). Ocular effects, including cataract, microphthalmus, Horner syndrome, anisocoria, optic atrophy, nystagmus, and chorioretinitis, were seen in nine of the infants. Brain damage was observed in seven of the cases. Hypoplasia of specific areas of limbs and trunk was seen in five cases.

Other Viruses

Other viruses have been suspected of causing congenital defects in the human. These include mumps, Coxsackievirus B, infectious hepatitis, influenza, echovirus 7, and adenovirus. It is likely that some will be convincingly implicated in future studies. Mumps virus has long been suspected of causing endocardial fibroelastosis, but its role in the cause of this condition has been controversial. Our studies in chick embryos have shown that mumps virus causes cataract and general growth inhibition (much like that caused by rubella and CMV). Studies by St. Geme et al,[32] in chick embryos, have also shown that mumps causes delay in maturation of some immunoglobulins and reduced weight of brain and heart in the newly hatched chick. These workers also recently showed that mumps virus can be recovered from the placentas of seronegative pregnant women following vaccination with attenuated mumps virus.[33] Coxsackievirus may be acquired in utero, and there is statistical evidence suggesting that the B group, especially, may be a cause of congenital heart disease in humans.[33] Infectious hepatitis may be suspect.[34] Some children with congenital defects have harbored the Australia antigen in their blood at birth, and some of the mothers have shown evidence of hepatitis. Influenza has been studied for its teratogenic potential in humans, but no consistent evidence of defects has been found in the various reports. It is hoped that continued, well-planned, prospective-type studies, as well as careful attention to individual cases, wherever the conceptus is suspected of being exposed to an infectious agent will clarify the role of other viruses in the cause of human congenital defects.

Influences and Mechanisms Involved in Production of Defects

As information has accumulated about the teratogenic viruses, it has become increasingly clear that we are dealing with a very complex situation in which the outcome for the conceptus depends on the interaction of many factors. While the same organs may be affected by different viruses at the same stages of development, the specific tissue affinities and biological characteristics of different viruses may cause a wide range of effects on these organs. The maternal immune status is, of course, of paramount importance, but there is also evidence to indicate that women are more susceptible to infection during pregnancy than at other times and that this susceptibility increases as gestation progresses. Thus, primary exposure to virus infection may be particularly hazardous and the chances of developing infection from secondary exposure may be increased. In addition, there is the chance of activation of a latent maternal virus infection such as can occur with herpesvirus hominis and varicella-zoster virus and probably also with CMV. The possibility of iatrogenic infection through maternal or fetal transfusion should also be kept in mind.

Morphological evidence of placental infections has been verified for both rubella and CMV, and transplacental transmission is probably the most common means of access of virus to the fetus. There is evidence suggesting that ascending infections from cervical lesions and from virus in cervical secretions may also occur. Herpesvirus hominis, CMV, and rubella virus have each been isolated from the cervix of infected women. In cases of ascending infection, the virus would very likely be released into the amniotic fluid where, in early stages of development, the organs developing from the ectodermal tissues (encephalon, neural tube, eye, lens, auditory vesicles, visceral arch epithelium, limb bud epithelium, etc) would be primarily involved. Fetal viremia, on the other hand, would bring about a more disseminated infection.

Thus, the outcome for the individual exposed to prenatal virus infection may be influenced by such variables as the maternal immune status, the particular virus in question, different strains of the same virus, variation in susceptibility of the maternal or fetal host, the developmental stage at which infection occurs, the amount of virus reaching the embryo, the route of access of the infection to the fetus, and probably many other presently unknown factors.

In the human there is still little definitive information to explain the mechanisms by which defective development occurs. Some viruses such as measles, variola, vaccinia, and poliomyelitis do not usually cause congenital defects but tend to produce abortion or acute disease in the neonate, with clinical findings similar to those in the older age group. It has been presumed that abortion results from death due to widespread necrosis in the fetus, but it is known that abortion may also occur from side effects of the maternal illness, for instance, from fever, toxins, or placental changes. The teratogenic viruses, on the other hand, appear to be types that cause relatively mild or chronic infections in both prenatal and postnatal hosts. The teratogenic viruses do not fall into any specific group according to the physical and chemical characteristic by which they are classified. Rubella (RNA virus), for instance, belongs to the togavirus group, is intermediate in size, and replicates in the cytoplasm. It is of interest that all three of the other known human teratogenic viruses belong to the herpesvirus group (DNA viruses). These are of relatively large size and they replicate in the nucleus.

It has been suggested in the case of rubella that the slowing of mitosis and shortened life span of infected cells that have been observed in vitro may account for the small size of the virus-infected newborns and the defective development of specific organs in vivo. In chick embryos infected with type A influenza virus, it was observed by Robertson et al[11] that the volume of brain tissue and the number of cells were consistently less than in control embryos, and it was concluded that the virus infection resulted in inhibition of the growth of the brain primordium. Examination of clinical material from human conceptuses infected with rubella has also indicated that the cell size is normal but the number of cells is decreased.[37] It has been proposed, on the other hand, that some congenital defects may occur secondarily to disseminated vascular lesions that might cause varying degrees of hypoxia or inadequate supply of nutrients in the organs supplied by the affected blood vessels.[38] Chromosomal injury has been considered but no definite evidence in support of this hypothesis has been presented. It seems likely that death of cells or inhibition of mitosis through damage to infected cells plays a part and may be a mechanism in the unique defects seen in association with specific viruses. Vascular lesions leading to ischemic necrosis and possibly to growth inhibition are also a complicating factor.

Methods of Prevention

The only practical method of prevention of congenital defects appears to be vaccination of women well in advance of conception. Women should avoid pregnancy for at least two months following vaccination and three months would be a safer interval. The ideal method would be to vaccinate girls during the premenarcheal period. The rubella vaccine is the only vaccine against a human teratogenic virus that has been licensed for use. The antibody titers have not declined appreciably in the years since the vaccine has been in use, but there is evidence that the herd immunity concept, which has worked well with the smallpox and poliomyelitis vaccination programs, may not be effective in eradicating rubella from the community. In spite of vaccination of large segments of the population, sporadic outbreaks of rubella still occur. The vaccines that are now in use do appear to be effective, however, in protecting individuals with a minimum of side effects, although the immunity is not as solid as that acquired with the wild-type virus infection. It is also not known to what extent the attenuated rubella vaccine strains may be teratogenic for the fetus in case of inadvertent vaccination of pregnant women. Rubella virus has occasionally been isolated from the conceptus in cases of inadvertent vaccination of pregnant women, and in one case there was evidence of a lens cataract from which rubella virus was isolated.[39] It is of interest that vaccination in this case had taken place seven weeks prior to conception.

Establishment of a vaccine for CMV has recently been attempted through subcutaneous inoculation of a tissue-culture-adapted strain of CMV.[40] Although preliminary tests of this vaccine in volunteers were successful in stimulating antibody production without causing important immediate side effects, these studies are still in very preliminary stages.

References

1. Gregg NM: Congenital cataract following German measles in the mother. *Trans Ophthalmol Soc Aust* 3:35-46, 1941.

2. Hamburger V, Habel K: Teratogenic and lethal effects of influenza-A and mumps virus on early chick embryos. *Proc Soc Exp Biol Med* 66:608-617, 1947.

3. Blattner RJ, Williamson AP: Developmental abnormalities in the chick embryo following infection with Newcastle disease virus. *Proc Soc Exp Biol Med* 77:619-621, 1951.

4. Williamson AP, Blattner RJ, Simonsen L: Cataracts following mumps virus in early chick embryos. *Proc Soc Exp Biol Med* 96:224-228, 1957.

5. Williamson AP, Simonsen L, Blattner RJ: Specific organ defects in early chick embryos following inoculation with influenza-A virus. *Proc Soc Exp Biol Med* 92:334-337, 1956.

6. Robertson GG, Williamson AP, Blattner RJ: Origin of myeloschisis in chick embryos infected with influenza-A virus. *Yale J Biol Med* 32:449-463, 1960.

7. Williamson AP, Blattner RJ, Simonsen L: Mechanism of the teratogenic action of Newcastle disease virus in the chick embryo. *J Immunol* 76:275-280, 1956.

8. Williamson AP, Blattner RJ, Robertson GG: The relationship of viral antigen to virus-induced defects in chick embryos: Newcastle disease virus. *Dev Biol* 12:498-519, 1965.

9. Robertson GG, Williamson AP, Blattner RJ: A study of abnormalities in early chick embryos inoculated with Newcastle disease virus. *J Exp Zool* 129:5-44, 1956.

10. Robertson GG, Williamson AP, Blattner RJ: Origin and development of lens cataracts in mumps-infected chick embryos. *Am J Anat* 115:473-485, 1964.

11. Robertson GG, DeBandi HO, Williamson AP, et al: Brain abnormalities in early chick embryos infected with influenza-A virus. *Anat Rec* 158:1-9, 1967.

12. Parkman PD, Buescher EL, Artenstein MS: Recovery of rubella from army recruits. *Proc Soc Exp Biol Med* 111:225-230, 1962.

13. Weller TH, Neva FA: Propagation in tissue culture of cytopathic agents from patients with rubella-like illness. *Proc Soc Exp Biol Med* 111:215-225, 1962.

14. Members of the Baylor Rubella Study Group: Rubella: Epidemic in retrospect. *Hosp Prac* 2(3):27-35, 1967.

15. Rudolph AJ, Yow MD, Phillips CA, et al: Transplacental rubella infection in newly born infants. *JAMA* 191:843-845, 1965.

16. Alford CA, Neva FA, Weller JH: Virologic and serologic studies on human products of conception after maternal rubella. *N Engl J Med* 271:1275-1281, 1964.

17. Bellanti JA, Artenstein MS, Olson LC, et al: Congenital rubella: Clinicopathologic, virologic, and immunologic studies. *Am J Dis Child* 110:464-472, 1965.

18. Desmond MM, Wilson GS, Verniaud WM, et al: The early growth and development of infants with congenital rubella. *Adv Teratol* 4:39-63, 1970.

19. Chess S: Autism in children with congenital rubella. *J Autism Child Schizo* 1:33-47, 1971.

20. Smith MG: The propagation in tissue culture of a cytopathogenic virus from human salivary gland virus (SGV) disease. *Proc Soc Exp Biol Med* 92:424-430, 1956.

21. Melish ME, Hanshaw JB: Congenital cytomegalovirus infection: Developmental progress of infants detected by routine screening. *Am J Dis Child* 126:190-194, 1973.

22. Stern H, Tucker SM: Prospective study of cytomegalovirus infection in pregnancy. *Br Med J* 11:268-270, 1973.

23. Reynolds D, Stagno S, Stubbs K, et al: Inapparent congenital cytomegalovirus infection with elevated cord IgM levels: Relation to auditory and mental deficiency. *N Engl J Med* 290:291-296, 1974.

24. Stagno S, Reynolds DW, Lakeman A, et al: Congenital cytomegalovirus infection: Consecutive occurrence due to viruses with similar antigenic composition. *Pediatrics* 52:788-794, 1973.

25. Nahmias AJ, Alford CA, Korones SB: Infection of the newborn with herpesvirus hominis. *Adv Pediatr* 17:185-226, 1970.

26. Schaffer AJ: *Diseases of the Newborn*, ed 2. Philadelphia, WB Saunders Co, 1965, pp 733-734.

27. South MA, Thompkins WAF, Morris CR, et al: Congenital malformations of the central nervous system associated with genital (type 2) herpesvirus. *J Pediatr* 75:13-18, 1969.

28. Montgomery JR, Flanders RW, Yow MD: Congenital anomalies and herpesvirus infection. *Am J Dis Child* 126:364-366, 1973.

29. Florman AL, Gershon AA, Blackett PR, et al: Intrauterine infection with herpes simplex virus: Resultant congenital malformations. *JAMA* 225:129-132, 1973.

30. Altshuler G: Pathogenesis of congenital herpesvirus infection: Case report including a description of the placenta. *Am J Dis Child* 127:427-429, 1974.

31. Srabstein J, Morris N, Larke R, et al: Is there a congenital varicella syndrome? *J Pediatr* 2:239-243, 1974.

32. St Geme JW Jr, Davis CWC, Peralta HJ, et al: The biologic perturbations of persistent embryonic mumps virus infection. *Pediatr Res* 7:541-552, 1973.

33. Yamauchi T, Wilson C, St Geme JW Jr: Transmission of live attenuated mumps virus to the human placenta. *N Engl J Med* 290:710-712, 1974.

34. Brown GC: Maternal virus infection and congenital anomalies: A prospective study. *Arch Environ Health* 21:362-365, 1970.

35. Marshall WC, Dudgeon JA: Australia antigen in a child with congenital malformations and in his mother. *Am J Dis Child* 123:378-379, 1972.

36. Rawls WE, Melnick JL: Rubella virus carrier cultures derived from congenitally infected infants. *J Exp Med* 123:795-816, 1966.

37. Naeye RL, Blanc W: Pathogenesis of congenital rubella. *JAMA* 194:1277-1283, 1965.

38. Singer DB, Rudolph AJ, Rosenberg HS, et al: Pathology of the congenital rubella syndrome. *J Pediatr* 71:665-675, 1967.

39. Fleet WF Jr, Benz EW Jr, Karzon DT, et al: Fetal consequences of maternal rubella immunization. *JAMA* 227:621-627, 1974.

40. Elek SD, Stern H: Development of a vaccine against mental retardation caused by cytomegalovirus infection in utero. *Lancet* 1:1-5, 1974.

From G. Desmonts and J. Couvreur (1974). N. Engl. J. Med., **290,** 1110–1116.
Copyright (1974), *by kind permission of the authors and the Massachusetts Medical Society*

CONGENITAL TOXOPLASMOSIS A Prospective Study of 378 Pregnancies

Georges Desmonts, M.D., and Jacques Couvreur, M.D.

Abstract Of 378 pregnant women with high initial toxoplasma antibody titers or seroconversion during pregnancy, 183 acquired the infection during pregnancy, a rate of 6.3 per 100 pregnancies. There were 11 abortions; seven infants were stillborn or died. Toxoplasmosis occurred in 59 of the non-aborted offspring. Among these, two died, and seven had severe disease with cerebral and ocular involvement. Of the remaining 50, 11 had mild, and 39 had subclinical illness. Severe disease was noted only when maternal infections were acquired during the first two trimesters. Later acquisition resulted in subclinical or no fetal infections. Parasites were isolated from the placentas of 25 per cent of those who acquired toxoplasma during pregnancy. Treatment with spiramycin during pregnancy reduced the overall frequency of the fetal infections but not of overt disease. Mothers with antibodies before they became pregnant had no infected infants. (N Engl J Med 290:1110-1116, 1974)

THE demonstration of *Toxoplasma gondii* in the brain of a newborn infant with encephalomyelitis by Wolf, Cowen and Paige[1] precipitated interest in defining the clinical characteristics of this congenital infection, whose relative frequencies have been described from various countries.[2-9] Such data are usually collected from retrospective studies, but only prospective studies can provide the information required for the definition of fetal risks. To make possible such definition, surveys for identifying and studying women who acquire toxoplasmosis during pregnancy have been conducted in this laboratory for about 15 years. Thanks to these surveys, the probability of transmission to the fetuses and the consequent effects on them can be estimated. Although several preliminary reports already have been published,[10-14] the overall results, including additional data, are summarized here.

MATERIALS AND METHODS

Serologic

The Sabin–Feldman dye test,[15] as modified in this laboratory,[16] was used for all serologic determinations. Since 1968 we have recorded such antibody titers as relative to a standard positive serum in International Units (IU) per milliliter.[17] Although this method permits accurate comparisons between the serum specimens of one subject, in the present study the paired serum samples of a given patient were always examined in the same test. The lowest serum dilution routinely examined was 1:10. A positive reaction at this level approximates a titer of 2 IU per milliliter. Serums with less than 2 IU per milliliter were recorded as negative. The titers of mothers of infants with congenital toxoplasmosis usually are ⩾1:1000, and may run from 300 to 3000 IU per milliliter. Before the 1968 standardization, titers ⩾1:1000 were considered strongly positive. Since then, titers of 300 IU per milliliter or more have been included in this category.

Additional serologic methods that we have employed included complement fixation and indirect hemagglutination.[18,19] The immunoglobulin M fluorescent-antibody test[20-22] was added after its introduction several years ago, but the number of cases studied with it was not large enough to warrant a separate discussion.

From the Laboratoire Central de Microbiologie and the Policlinique Consultation, Hôpital Saint Vincent de Paul, the Service de Pédiatrie, Hôpital Trousseau, Paris, and the Services de Protection Maternelle et Infantile de la Caisse de Sécurité Sociale de la Région Parisienne (address reprint requests to Dr. Desmonts, Institut de Puericulture, 26 Blvd. Brune, Paris 14, France).

Supported in part by the Institut National de la Santé et de la Recherche Médicale, Paris, France, the World Health Organization, Geneva, Switzerland, the National Institutes of Health (grant E-2235), Bethesda, Maryland, and the Fondation pour la Recherche Médicale Française, Paris, France.

Parasitologic

For parasite isolations, material was injected intraperitoneally into toxoplasma-free laboratory-reared mice. Peritoneal exudate, if present, was examined on the seventh day for toxoplasma trophozoites. Surviving animals were bled after six weeks for the Sabin–Feldman dye test. Impression smears of the brains of seropositive mice were examined for toxoplasma cysts.

When available, lymph-node tissues obtained from mothers by needle biopsies were inoculated into mice. Placentas, blood and cerebrospinal fluids from living infants and brain, liver, spleen and myocardium in fatal cases were also inoculated. Tissues were digested before inoculation as described by Remington, Melton and Jacobs[23] except that trypsin replaced pepsin. (Only encysted parasites survive pepsin digestion.) After mincing, 100 g of tissue was incubated at 37°C for two hours with trypsin (2.5 g per 1000 ml of buffered saline, pH 7.2) and antibiotics. This sample was centrifuged, the supernatant fluid discarded, and the sediment washed three times with buffered saline to remove excess enzyme. The sediment was resuspended in buffered saline with antibiotics and inoculated into 10 mice, which were studied as usual and observed for six weeks.

Study Population

Women included in the various surveys generally resided in Paris and its suburbs. Many were North African Moslems, Spaniards or Portuguese who had immigrated into the area. Those in the initial surveys were mainly of low socioeconomic status, but as the study progressed, the participants became more diversified.

Screening Procedure

Although some pregnant women were referred for serologic studies because of lymphadenopathy, either current or previous, most cases were identified through systematic serologic screening tests. In the first survey[10,11] serum specimens obtained during pregnancy were stored frozen and tested months or years later along with another specimen obtained at delivery. In other surveys, specimens taken at the first prenatal examination (usually at the end of the second month, but sometimes later) were tested promptly. Such women, if antibody negative, were re-examined for seroconversion during the sixth or seventh month and again at delivery. Those whose initial serum specimens had high antibody titers (dye test ⩾1:1000, or ⩾300 IU per milliliter) or IgM antibodies also were retained in the study.

Treatment

Spiramycin, a macrolide antibiotic derived from *Streptomyces ambofaciens,* with antibacterial activity comparable to that of erythromycin, is active against toxoplasma as demonstrated in animal experiments.[24,25] It produces high tissue concentrations, particularly in the placenta,[26] and has been used widely in Europe for about 15 years without demonstrable harmful effects on fetal development. Consequently, this antibiotic was selected as an alternative for the pyrimethamine-sulfonamide combination that was often used in the treatment of acquired toxoplasmosis but could not be given during pregnancy because of its hematologic and possible teratogenic effects.

Daily oral doses of 2 to 3 g of spiramycin were administered in four divided doses for three weeks. Such courses arbitrarily were repeated at two-week intervals up to delivery. Only women who completed at least one such course were considered "treated."

Offspring

The demonstration of toxoplasma after animal inoculation was considered diagnostic in children who failed to survive. Those who were born alive were subsequently observed for evidence of congenital toxoplasmosis with repeated clinical and serologic examinations, skull x-ray films and funduscopic examinations. Electroencephalograms and spinal-fluid studies generally were performed when congenital infections were confirmed. Because of the possible appearance of chorioretinitis months or even years after birth, particular attention was paid to the fundi by repeated examinations.

Since most children appeared clinically normal, their classification as well, or suffering from subclinical toxoplasmosis, depended chiefly on serologic findings. Each child at birth had a high antibody titer similar to that of its mother. Infants whose initial dye-test titers decreased steadily to negative between the sixth and ninth months were concluded to have passively transferred antibodies and not to have been congenitally infected. Other infants without clinical toxoplasmosis but with dye-test titers that remained high or rose were considered to have had subclinical infections. This diagnosis was often supported by the isolation of parasites from either blood or placental tissue.

Treatment of Children

In the initial survey children were not treated during the neonatal period. Since maternal serums were not tested for some months or even years after delivery, the children had not been examined for congenital toxoplasmosis. In later surveys infants were treated with pyrimethamine and sulfonamide or spiramycin (or both) as soon as congenital toxoplasmosis was suspected or proved.

RESULTS

Pregnant Women

The incidence of toxoplasma infections in pregnant women in this study, as determined from the follow-up of those who were initially seronegative, was 6.3 per 100 per year. The incidence of acquired toxoplasmosis among pregnant women in the area was estimated to be nearly 10 per 1000 per year.

High antibody titers (dye-test titer $\geqslant 1{:}1000$ or $\geqslant 300$ IU per milliliter) or seroconversion was detected in 520 pregnant women. For 142 of these, no information about the outcome of the pregnancy was obtainable, so that only data from the other 378 (73 per cent) are considered here in detail. These cases were classified as follows:

Group 1. The 183 (48 per cent) women whose infections were acquired during the observed pregnancy (Table 1).

Group 2. The remaining 195 (52 per cent) women included those whose toxoplasmosis had been acquired before they became pregnant and those whose infection dates in relation to conception were unknown (Table 2).

Placenta Studies

Placental tissue from 201 (53 per cent) of the pregnant women was inoculated into mice. Toxoplasmas were isolated from 25 per cent of women in Group 1 and from only three mothers (2 per cent) in Group 2

Table 1. Data in Women whose Toxoplasmosis Was Acquired during Pregnancy (Group 1).

FINDING	NO. OF CASES
Seroconversion*	121 (66%)
Lymphadenopathy with rising antibody titer	21 (11%)
Lymphadenopathy with elevated, not rising, antibody titer	24 (13%)
Rising antibody titer only (no illness)	17 (9%)
Totals	183 (100%)

*Negative to positive for antibodies, with or without illness.

(Table 3). Both of the latter had had subclinical infections as evidenced by high, stable antibody titers, but since their initial serum specimens were obtained at the end of the sixth month of pregnancy, their infections could have been acquired during the first four months or before conception. The fluorescent-antibody test in one of these two cases was positive, suggesting that infection had recently been acquired.

There was a close correlation between positive placental isolations and congenital infection since the children involved usually had serologic or parasitologic evidence of toxoplasmosis. Conversely, only three infections were noted among children whose placentas were parasite negative. In one, much of the placental sediment was lost. The second was an asymptomatic child but had a strongly positive dye test. However, he was not bled until he was two years old. Thus, even though rare in this age group, acquired toxoplasmosis could not be ruled out. In the third case parasitemia was demonstrated, in a newborn infant, but the inoculation of placental tissue paradoxically yielded negative results.

Congenital Toxoplasmosis

Of the 378 pregnancies, 11 (3 per cent) ended in abortion, seven in Group 1 and four in Group 2 (Table 4). Seven other offspring either were stillborn or died shortly after birth. Post-mortem examinations were performed on three of these infants, and parasites were isolated from the tissues of two of them. Histologic findings correlated positively with the diagnosis. No parasites were isolated from the placenta of the third, so that congenital toxoplasmosis was considered unlikely and the case was included with the noninfected. Parasites were isolated from the blood or cerebrospinal

Table 2. Data in Women with Toxoplasmosis Acquired but Infection of Undetermined Date or Occuring before Conception (Group 2).

TOXOPLASMOSIS	NO. OF CASES
Clinical, diagnosed:	
Before pregnancy	15 (8%)
Around conception time	14 (7%)
Subclinical:	
High, stable antibody titer	150 (77%)
Seroconversion between preceding delivery & 3d mo of study pregnancy	16 (8%)
Total	195 (100%)

Table 3. Toxoplasma Isolations from Placentas of Women with High* Antibody Titers.

Period in Which Maternal Toxoplasmosis Acquired	Placentas			
	Total		Positive†	
	no.	%	no.	%
During pregnancy (Group 1)	96	48	24	25
Before pregnancy or unknown (Group 2)	105	52	2‡	2
Totals	201	100	26	13

*Dye test ≥ 1:1000 or ≥ 300 IU/ml.   †Toxoplasma demonstrated in mice.
‡Infection acquired during 1st 4 mo of, or before, pregnancy.

fluid of seven of the 360 live offspring. The remainder were classified according to the clinical and serologic data.

After the 11 aborted cases were excluded, the 367 remaining offspring were classified as either definitely infected congenitally or possibly so, or (by far the largest category) excluded on other counts. The breakdown then became as follows: definitely infected congenitally, 59 (16 per cent); possibly so infected, 15 (4 per cent); and excluded, 293 (78 per cent). In the last group, diagnosis of congenital toxoplasmosis had to be ruled out because of negative clinical and parasitologic findings (one stillbirth) and because of post-partum disappearance of antibodies. Several of these babies were not tested repeatedly because babies that appear normal are not always brought back for re-examination.

Table 4 also summarizes the outcomes of the 378 pregnancies according to the previously defined groups of the mothers. In Group 2 (infection date undetermined or before the pregnancy) congenital infections were ruled out in 94 per cent of the offspring. There were two unusual exceptions, one a neonatal death and the other a survivor with severe cerebral damage. Parasitologic examination of the placenta of the former was negative whereas neither the clinical features nor the serologic findings in the second were consistent with the diagnosis of congenital toxoplasmosis. Subclinical infections were diagnosed in four children (2 per cent), but since their serums were collected late, acquired infections could not be excluded. Congenital toxoplasmosis with ocular involvement only was proved in four cases (2 per cent) in this group. Two of

the mothers had had high but not rising titers shortly before delivery, and the other two were first examined during the sixth month. It was concluded that in these cases infection was acquired before the fourth month in two, and prior to the seventh in the others. In contrast, 30 per cent of the children in Group 1 (infection acquired during pregnancy) had definite but usually subclinical congenital toxoplasmosis.

Among the factors that might affect the fetuses of newly infected mothers, two appeared to be most important: the stage of pregnancy when maternal infection was acquired, and treatment of mothers during the pregnancy. After pregnancies that ended in abortion were excluded, the remaining 176 cases in Group 1 were analyzed along with the four cases from Group 2 in which congenital infections were demonstrated in the offspring.

These 180 women were divided according to the trimester in which infection probably had occurred (Table 5). For 27, the data were insufficient for such a classification. Because of the design of the serologic survey system employed, "first-trimester" infections were acquired mainly during the third month. Severe congenital toxoplasmosis with either neonatal death or brain and ocular involvement was seen only in the offspring of mothers who had acquired their infections during the first or second trimester of pregnancy. Third-trimester acquisitions more often resulted in subclinical infections.

The effect of spiramycin treatment on the outcomes of these pregnancies was estimated by analysis of the 98 (54 per cent) who had been "treated" (Table 6). Both "definite" and "possible" cases of congenital toxoplasmosis were significantly ($p < 0.001$ by chi square) more frequent among the untreated (63 per cent) than among the treated (26 per cent), but each group just as frequently had clinically apparent disease, 11 per cent.

Discussion

The prevalence of toxoplasma infections is very high in women of childbearing age in the Paris area, 84 per cent having antibodies.[10-12] The proportion of seropositive women increases with age but varies with meat-cooking habits and ethnic origin; 90 per cent of French women have antibodies, but this decreases to 70 per cent for Spanish, Portuguese and North African women and to 50 per cent for those of Vietnamese ori-

Table 4. Outcomes of 378 Pregnancies with High Maternal Toxoplasma Dye-Test Titers* at Delivery.

Maternal Toxoplasmosis Acquired			Abortions		Diagnosis of Congenital Toxoplasmosis					
					Definite		Possible		Excluded	
group†	no.	%	no.	%	no.	%	no.	%	no.	%
1	183	48	7	4	55	30	11‡	6	110	60
2	195	52	4	2	4	2	4‡	2	183§	94
Totals	378	100	11¶	3	59	16	15	4	293	78

*≥1:1000 or ≥ 300 IU/ml.   †Group 1, acquired during pregnancy; Group 2, acquired before pregnancy or time unknown.
‡Neonatal deaths. Fetus lost for examination, 4 cases (Group 1). Initial examinations at 14-45 mo: Group 1, 7, & Group 2, 4.
§1 neonatal death & 1 infant with psychomotor retardation (neither related to congenital toxoplasmosis).   ¶6 induced: Group 1, 4; Group 2, 2.

Table 5. Outcomes of 180 Pregnancies According to Trimester in Which Maternal Toxoplasmosis Was Acquired.

Maternal Toxoplasmosis Acquired			Diagnosis of Congenital Toxoplasmosis											
			DEFINITE						POSSIBLE				EXCLUDED	
TRIMESTER	total		total		clinical		subclinical		total		subclinical			
	no.	%	no.	%	no.	%	no.	%	no.	%	no.	%	no.	%
1st	30	17	5	17	4	13	1	3	1	3	0	0	24	80
2d	84	47	20	24	11	13	9	11	5	6	3	4	59	70
3d	39	22	24	62	2	5	22	56	2	5	2	5	13	33
Undetermined	27	15	10	37	3	11	7	26	3	11	2	7	14	52
Totals	180	100	59*	33	20	11	39	22	11†	6	7	4	110	61

*2 neonatal deaths.   †4 neonatal deaths.

gin. Thus, Paris is a favorable place in which to study maternal toxoplasmosis and its effects on the fetus. The number of exposed susceptible persons is rather small, but the incidence of infection is comparatively high.[27-30]

Support for the clinical diagnosis of acquired toxoplasmosis most often was provided by lymph-node enlargement, which, as in previous reports,[31-33] most frequently involved the posterior cervical chains. Such nodes are often bilateral, painful at onset and nonsuppurating and seem to occur two to four weeks after infection. Thus, a woman with recently swollen, painful and nonsuppurating cervical lymph nodes may be suspected of having acquired toxoplasmosis within the preceding few weeks. Corroboration usually depends on suitable serologic evidence.

Seroconversion offered the best proof of recent toxoplasma infection, even helping to determine its date. A noteworthy rise in antibody titer was considered evidence for both occurrence and timing of the infection. As a rule, dye-test titers reach their maximum within two months and remain elevated for five to six months or even for years. Consequently, a definite rise between paired serum samples obtained at three-week intervals indicates that infection probably was acquired within two months or less of the initial sample. A high, stable titer generally indicates that the infection was acquired more than two months previously. The infection might even date back years.

Women with high but not increasing antibody titers detected during serologic surveys most probably were infected before pregnancy since the elevated antibody titer was usually observed in the initial serum in the first trimester. When such a sample was obtained later (fourth to eighth month), the acquisition of infection early in pregnancy could not be excluded. Occasionally, the date of infection could be ascertained more closely if the mother had been studied in an immediately preceding pregnancy and if seroconversion occurred between the previous delivery and the first serum in the present pregnancy (Table 2).

Abortion

Toxoplasmosis has been said to be a cause of abortion.[34-35] The 378 pregnancies classified in Table 4 showed 11 (3 per cent) abortions, six induced for fear that congenital effects might result from toxoplasmosis. The timing of the initial samples for the serologic surveys performed in this study was such as to make the detection of abortions due to toxoplasmosis unlikely since the screening serums usually were those collected at the end of the second or during the third month of pregnancy for routine serologic tests for syphilis. Among the 14 women in whom toxoplasmic lymphadenopathy was diagnosed around conception time (Table 2) and was still present during the first months of pregnancy, there was only one spontaneous abortion. Even if it can be assumed that this abortion resulted from the toxoplasmosis, this infection remains an infrequent cause of such events.

Neonatal Deaths

Although six of the seven stillbirths or deaths shortly after birth occurred in offspring of Group 1 mothers,

Table 6. Outcomes of 180 Pregnancies in Which Maternal Toxoplasmosis Was Acquired, According to Spiramycin Treatment.

Group			Diagnosis of Congenital Toxoplasmosis											
			DEFINITE						POSSIBLE				EXCLUDED	
	total		total		clinical		subclinical		total		subclinical			
	no.	%	no.	%	no.	%	no.	%	no.	%	no.	%	no.	%
Spiramycin treated*	98	54	22	22	11	50	11	50	2	2	1	50	74	76
Untreated	82	46	37†	45	9	24	28	76	9	11	6	67	36	44
Totals	180	100	59	33	20	11	39	22	11‡	6	7	4	110	61

*Spiramycin, 2 g/day for at least 1 3-wk course.   †2 neonatal deaths.   ‡4 neonatal deaths.

only one was from among Group 2, and it could be ruled out as congenital toxoplasmosis. In contrast, two of the six Group 1 cases were available for study and tissue inoculation; both fetuses had generalized toxoplasmosis. Because the remaining four fetuses could not be examined, they were considered to be "possible" but not proved cases of congenital toxoplasmosis. This assumption is not unreasonable since four neonatal deaths (2.9 per cent) is more than would normally be expected.

Acute or Chronic Maternal Infections

It is generally believed that congenital toxoplasmosis results from acute but often subclinical maternal infections acquired during pregnancy. The report by Sabin et al.[36] has often been confirmed by others. On this basis, such mothers cannot produce children with congenital toxoplasmosis in subsequent pregnancies. Toxoplasma have been demonstrated in the progeny of several pregnancies in chronically infected mice,[37] and it has been suggested that similar events are possible in human beings.[38] Because of the importance of this question in the pathogenesis of congenital toxoplasmosis, the data from the present study were analyzed for ths purpose.

Clinical, serologic or parasitologic evidence of congenital toxoplasmosis was sought in the products of pregnancies in women who, from their high antibody titers, were at some risk of giving birth to affected children. These data disclosed a difference between the two groups of women. Maternal infections definitely or probably acquired during pregnancy (Group 1) most frequently led to infection of the offspring. Among 59 definite cases of congenital toxoplasmosis observed in these surveys, 55 (93 per cent) were born to mothers from this group. Conversely, congenital toxoplasmosis was infrequent or questionable when maternal infections were not definitely acquired during the pregnancy (Group 2). Only four mothers in the latter group gave birth to children with congenital toxoplasmosis, and since they had their initial serologic examinations late in pregnancy, it is uncertain whether they acquired their infections before conception or during the first half of the pregnancy. Unfortunately, all children with subclinical infection in Group 2 were examined more than one year after birth, so that postnatal acquisitions could not be excluded.

Overall, there was not one definitely proved case of congenital toxoplasmosis in a child born to a mother infected before she became pregnant. This observation agrees with the statement by Sabin et al.,[36] "The chief practical benefit to be derived from a specific diagnosis of congenital toxoplasmosis is the good prognosis for subsequent children," which is true for any maternal infection whether or not it resulted in congenital disease, so long as it occurred before the current pregnancy. The same conclusion applies to maternal infections acquired just before conception. Since exceptions to this rule, if they do occur, must be rare, congenital toxoplasmosis could be eradicated if acute infections were prevented in pregnant women.

Placental Parasites

Parasites were isolated from 25 per cent of the placentas in the cases in which maternal toxoplasmosis was acquired during pregnancy. The offspring in these positive cases also were infected. The demonstration of toxoplasma cysts on microscopical examination of the placenta has been reported[39,40] and was confirmed in several cases in this study. Unfortunately, the procedure takes time and is usually negative. Mouse inoculation of placental tissue after tryptic digestion appears to be a more effective method for demonstrating parasites in this organ from suspect cases. These experiences suggest that inoculation with placental tissue is useful for the diagnosis of congenital toxoplasmosis and might be performed when suggestive serologic findings have been obtained before delivery.

Infection in Offspring

Maternal toxoplasmosis acquired during pregnancy does not necessarily result in congenital infection, let alone disease. In the present study (Table 5), fetal infections were noted only in 33 per cent (39 per cent if the additional 6 per cent "possible" cases are included), in close agreement with the 44 per cent transmission in 18 mothers reported by Kräubig.[41] The important finding is that more than half the offspring remained free of infection. Even when it occurred, it more often resulted in subclinical or mild, rather than overt, severe disease.

The well known broad clinical spectrum of congenital toxoplasmosis is illustrated in our series. Among the 59 infected infants, injury was severe (systemic involvement with either stillbirth or death shortly after birth, or survival with serious cerebral damage) in nine (15 per cent). The 11 (19 per cent) with mild disease appeared normal at birth, and congenital toxoplasmosis would have been overlooked in most except for the findings, principally ophthalmologic, during their systematic follow-up examinations.

In some, the recognition of the first clinical finding, usually chorioretinitis, was delayed until several weeks or months after birth, illustrating an often reported observation in congenital toxoplasmosis. There are numerous clinical reports of children with congenital toxoplasmosis diagnosed on clinical grounds who appeared quite normal for some months before overt disease was recognized.[40,42-44] The prospective observation of children born to mothers with toxoplasmosis acquired during pregnancy may provide stronger supporting evidence for the diagnosis since abnormalities are more carefully sought during systematic follow-up examinations. The antibody titer of one infant who appeared to be normal despite thorough examinations during the first few weeks and so was not treated, rose at four months of age, suggesting infection. Re-examination of this still healthy-appearing infant then revealed both chorioretinitis and cerebral calcifications. Two infants had normal fundi on repeated examinations, but at seven months chorioretinitis was discovered; mental retardation was recognized in one of them at one year of age. A fourth, considered to have been infected subclinically, was found to have a retinal scar in his second year. Cases such as these, along with other observations, suggest that the diagnosis of subclinical infection should be delayed until after a prolonged follow-up observation.

We considered the risk of subsequent appearance of injury to the retina and brain to be important enough to require the systematic treatment of any child suspected of congenital toxoplasmosis even when it was subclinical. Consequently, the majority of the infants studied were treated after delivery, thus possibly reducing the number with overt disease.

Maternal Toxoplasmosis and Gestational Stage

The importance of the stage of gestation in the child's fate was stressed long ago. In 1958 Feldman, in an analysis of four cases previously reported by others, stated that "infections acquired just before, and soon after, onset of pregnancy (onset of lymphadenopathy) may not result in congenital infections even though viable parasites persist in the nodes. However, infections that disseminate to the lymph nodes of the mother after the third month of pregnancy may also spread to the fetus."[45] This hypothesis is confirmed by the present data, for not a single case of congenital toxoplasmosis was observed when maternal toxoplasmosis was acquired either before or around the beginning of pregnancy. Such cases were included in previous reports along with those acquired during the course of the pregnancy.[10-12] Since their review led us to conclude that their consequences resembled those acquired before the pregnancy, they were included in Group 2.

When mothers infected after the beginning of pregnancy (between the second month and delivery) are considered, it is evident that the outcome of the pregnancy is largely determined by the stage in which the maternal infection was acquired. Fetal death or severe disease occurred only as the result of toxoplasma acquisitions from the second to the sixth month. In this group, subclinical infections were relatively infrequent. On the other hand, subclinical infections were usual among babies born to mothers infected during the third trimester. Thus, congenital infections with toxoplasma can be separated into two groups: congenital infections with disease resulting mainly from maternal infections during the second to the sixth month; and infections without disease, more usually after maternal infections acquired during the third trimester.

Maternal Treatment during Pregnancy

Cases of congenital toxoplasmosis were fewer among the offspring of mothers treated with spiramycin than of untreated mothers. The number of "possible" infect-

ed children was smaller in the treated group, but overall, 76 per cent of children born to treated mothers were normal, as opposed to 44 per cent among the untreated. Although this difference is highly significant ($p < 0.001$), the untreated mothers do not represent a good control group for several reasons. Among first-trimester women, 24 were treated, and only six untreated, but in the third trimester, 10 were treated, and 29 were untreated. Thus, more infections occurred earlier among the treated than among the untreated, a fact that of itself might have led to fewer congenital infections. Nevertheless, congenital infections were less frequent among the treated in each trimester of pregnancy. Consequently, one could assume that the decrease in fetal infections not only reflects bias in the selection of cases but is due to treatment as well.

Spiramycin is said not to cross the placental barrier freely, so that its administration would be unlikely to cure an already infected fetus. The apparent therapeutic benefits might better be accounted for by action of the antibiotic within the placenta. This assumption might explain why the number of infected offspring was markedly decreased in the treated group, whereas the proportion with clinical disease remained unmodified (11 per cent in each).

The experience reported here indicates that the diagnosis of maternally acquired toxoplasmosis during pregnancy should not suggest a hopeless prognosis for the child. Without any maternal treatment, healthy, uninfected infants were born to 44 per cent. This figure increased to 76 per cent when the mothers were treated with spiramycin during the pregnancy. Clinical disease was noted in only 20 (11 per cent) of the infants in these 180 pregnancies during which toxoplasmosis was acquired by their mothers. Thus, 89 per cent of their offspring were unaffected.

We are indebted to Dr. Weill-Spire, formerly chief physician of "Service de Protection Maternelle et Infantile de la Caisse de Sécurité Social de la Région Parisienne," to Professor M. Lelong for advice, to Drs. Hazeman and Seror, who provided most of the specimens for systematic serologic studies, to the obstetricians and pediatricians who referred their patients for study and generously supplied their historical data, to Dr. Rumeau Rouquette (Unité Statistique of INSERM) for aid with the statistical analysis of the data, and to Dr. Harry A. Feldman for advice and support during this study and for a critical review of the manuscript.

REFERENCES

1. Wolf A, Cowen D, Paige BH: Toxoplasmic encephalomyelitis. III. A new case of granulomatous encephalomyelitis due to a protozoon. Am J Pathol 15:657-694, 1939
2. Feldman HA, Miller LT: Congenital human toxoplasmosis. Ann NY Acad Sci 64:180-184, 1956
3. Eichenwald H: A study of congenital toxoplasmosis with particular emphasis on clinical manifestations, sequellae and therapy, Human Toxoplasmosis. Edited by JC Siim. Copenhagen, Ejnar Munksgaard, 1960, pp 41-49
4. De Roever-Bonnet H: Congenital toxoplasmosis. Trop Geogr Med 13:27-41, 1961
5. Hedenström G, Huldt G, Lagercrantz R: Toxoplasmosis in children: a study of 83 Swedish cases. Acta Paediatr 50:304-312, 1961
6. Couvreur J, Desmonts G: Congenital and maternal toxoplasmosis: a review of 300 congenital cases. Dev Med Child Neurol 4:519-530, 1962
7. Thalhammer O: Die angeborene Toxoplasmose, Toxoplasmose; Prak-

tische Fragen und Ergebnisse. Edited by H Kirchhoff, H Kraubig. Stuttgart, Georg Thieme Verlag, 1966, pp 151-173
8. Miller MJ, Seaman E, Remington JS: The clinical spectrum of congenital toxoplasmosis: problems in recognition. J Pediatr 70:714-723, 1967
9. Bamatter F: The differential diagnosis of connatal toxoplasmosis, Toxoplasmosis. Edited by D Hentsch. Bern, Hans Huber Publishers, 1971, pp 97-109
10. Desmonts G, Couvreur J, Ben Rachid M-S: Le toxoplasme, la mère et l'enfant. Arch Fr Pediatr 22:1183-1200, 1965
11. Desmonts G, Couvreur J: Toxoplasmose congénitale, 21éme Congrés des Pédiatres de Langue Française. Édité par l'Éxpansion Scientifique Française. Paris, 1967, pp 450-488
12. Colloque sur la toxoplasmose de la femme enceinte et al prévention de la toxoplasmose congénitale. Monographie du Lyon Médical. Lyon, Specia ed. 1970
13. Couvreur J: Prospective study of acquired toxoplasmosis in pregnant women with a special reference to the outcome of the foetus. Toxoplasmosis. Edited by D Hentsch. Bern, Hans Huber Publishers, 1971, pp 119-135
14. Desmonts G, Couvreur J: Toxoplasmosis in pregnancy and its transmission to the fetus. Bull NY Acad Med 50:146-159, 1974
15. Sabin AB, Feldman HA: Dyes as microchemical indicators of a new immunity phenomenon affecting a protozoon parasite (toxoplasma). Science 108:660-663, 1948
16. Desmonts G: Sur la technique de l'épreuve de lyse des toxoplasmes: réaction de Sabin et Feldman. Sem Hop Paris 31:193-198, 1955
17. Comité OMS d'experts de la Standarization Biologique: 20ème rapport (Série de rapports techniques No 384:18), Geneva, Organisation Mondiale de la Santé, 1968
18. Jacobs L, Lunde MN: A hemagglutination test for toxoplasmosis. J Parasitol 43:308-314, 1957
19. Ben Rachid M-S, Ferrero G, Desmonts G: Résultats de la réaction d'hémagglutination dans la toxoplasmose humaine. Arch Inst Pasteur Tunis 44:391-400, 1967
20. Remington JS, Miller MJ, Brownlee I: IgM antibodies in acute toxoplasmosis I. Diagnostic significance in congenital cases and a method for their rapid demonstration. Pediatrics 41:1082-1091, 1968
21. *Idem:* IgM antibodies in acute toxoplasmosis: prevalence and significance in acquired cases. J Lab Clin Med 71:855-866, 1968
22. Desmonts G, Couvreur J, Colin J, et al: Vers un diagnostic précoce de la toxoplasmose aiguë: étude critique du test de Remington. Nouv Presse Med 1:339-362, 1972
23. Remington JS, Melton ML, Jacobs L: Chronic toxoplasma infection in the uterus. J Lab Clin Med 56:879-883, 1960
24. Garin J-P, Eyles DE: Le traitement de la toxoplasmose expérimentale de la souris par la spiramycine. Presse Med 66:957-958, 1958
25. Mas Bakal P, In 'tveld N: Postponed spiramycin treatment of acute toxoplasmosis in white mice. Trop Geogr Med 17:254-260, 1965
26. Garin J-P, Pellerat J, Maillard M, et al: Bases théoriques de la prévention par la spiramycine de la toxoplasmose congénitale chez la femme enceinte. Presse Med 76:2266, 1968

27. Lamb GA, Feldman HA: Risk in acquiring *toxoplasma* antibodies: a study of 37 "normal" families. JAMA 206:1305-1306, 1968
28. Warren KS, Dingle JH: A study of illness in a group of Cleveland families. XXII. Antibodies to *Toxoplasma gondii* in 40 families observed for ten years. N Engl J Med 274:993-997, 1966
29. Ruoss CF, Bourne GL: Toxoplasmosis in pregnancy. J Obstet Gynaecol Br Commonw 779:1115-1118, 1972
30. Feldman HA: Toxoplasmosis. N Engl J Med 279:1370-1375, 1431-1437, 1968
31. Gard S, Magnusson JH: A glandular form of toxoplasmosis in connection with pregnancy. Acta Med Scand 141:59-64, 1951
32. Siim JC: Clinical and diagnostic aspects of human acquired toxoplasmosis. Human Toxoplasmosis. Edited by JC Siim. Copenhagen, Ejnar Munksgaard, 1960, pp 53-79
33. Lelong M, Bernard J, Desmonts G, et al: La toxoplasmose acquise (étude de 227 observations). Arch Fr Pediatr 17:281-331, 1960
34. Frenkel JK: Toxoplasmosis. Comparative Aspects of Reproductive Failure. Edited by K Benirschke. New York, Springer Verlag, 1967, pp 296-321
35. Remington JS: Toxoplasma and chronic abortion. Obstet Gynecol 24:155-156, 1964
36. Sabin AB, Eichenwald H, Feldman HA, et al: Present status of clinical manifestations of toxoplasmosis in man: indications and provisions for routine serologic diagnosis. JAMA 150:1063-1069, 1952
37. Beverley JKA: Congenital transmission of toxoplasmosis through successive generations of mice. Nature (Lond) 183:1348-1349, 1959
38. Langer H: Repeated congenital infection with *Toxoplasma gondii*. Obstet Gynecol 21:318-329, 1963
39. Beckett RS, Flynn FJ Jr: Toxoplasmosis: report of two new cases, with a classification and a demonstration of the organisms in the human placenta. N Engl J Med 249:345-350, 1953
40. Glasser L, Delta BG: Congenital toxoplasmosis with placental infection in monozygotic twins. Pediatrics 35:276-283, 1965
41. Kräubig H: Präventive Behandlung der konnatalen Toxoplasmose. Toxoplasmose-Praktische Fragen und Ergebnisse. Edited by H Kirchhof, H Kräubig. Stuttgart, Georg Thieme Verlag, 1966, pp 104-122
42. Couvreur J, Desmonts G: Les poussées évolutives tardives de la toxoplasmose congénitale. Cahiers Coll Med 5:752-758, 1964
43. Ribierre M, Couvreur J, Canetti J: Les hydrocéphalies par sténose de l'aqueduc de Sylvius dans la toxoplasmose congénitale. Arch Fr Pediatr 27:501-510, 1970
44. Alford CA Jr, Foft JW, Blankenship WJ, et al: Subclinical central nervous system disease of neonates: a prospective study of infants born with increased levels of IgM. J Pediatr 75:1167-1178, 1969
45. Feldman HA: Toxoplasmosis. Pediatrics 22:559-574, 1958

BACKGROUND READING

References 21 and 30
Remington JS: Toxoplasmosis, Obstetric and Perinatal Infections. Edited by D Charles, M Finland. Philadelphia, Lea and Febiger, 1973, pp 27-74

PAPER 25

25. Thiersch, J. B. (1952). Therapeutic abortions with a folic acid antagonist, 4-amino-pteroylglutamic acid (4-amino P.G.A.) administered by the oral route. *Am. J. Obstet. Gynecol.*, **63**, 1298–1304. (Extract)

COMMENTARY

This was the first report of birth defects caused by a drug in humans. The folic acid antagonists are potent cytotoxic agents, producing their cellular effects by inhibiting thymidine synthesis. Aminterin (4-amino P.G.A.) was found to be useful for the treatment of Hodgkin's disease and certain other malignancies. It is seldom used therapeutically at the present time.

Following previous observations that small doses of aminopterin injected into pregnant rats and mice caused fetal death and resorptions, Thiersch (1952) administered this substance orally to 12 pregnant women during early gestation for the purpose of inducing therapeutic abortion. Ten cases resulted in spontaneous abortion of dead fetuses; in the remaining two mothers, live malformed fetuses were recovered surgically. Three of the fetuses showed multiple anomalies, including growth retardation, anencephaly, hydrocephaly, meningoencephalocele, cleft palate with cleft lip, and skull defects. Similar findings were reported in several cases of attempted illegal abortion involving folate antagonists.

Most cytotoxic agents used in cancer treatment and for immunosuppression are now known to be teratogenic in man (Connors, 1975). These substances included methotrexate, mercaptopurine, azathioprine, and cyclophosphamide; their administration to pregnant women, particularly during the first trimester of pregnancy, is contraindicated.

In the early sixties there was an unparalleled surge of interest in the causes and prevention of birth defects. The hideous damage done to unborn children by the use of the sedative thalidomide during early pregnancy focused attention on the potential hazards of other drugs and environmental factors in pregnant women. This tragedy and its far-reaching consequences are considered in the papers immediately following.

REFERENCES

Conners, T. A. (1975). Cytotoxic agents in teratological research. In C. L. Berry and D. E. Poswills (eds.). *Teratology: Trends and Applications*, pp. 49–79 (New York: Springer Verlag)

From J. B. Thiersch (1952). Am. J. Obstet. Gynecol., **63**, 1298–1304. *Copyright* (1952), *by kind permission of the author and the C. V. Mosby Company, St Louis, Mich., USA*

THERAPEUTIC ABORTIONS WITH A FOLIC ACID ANTAGONIST, 4-AMINOPTEROYLGLUTAMIC ACID (4-AMINO P. G. A.) ADMINISTERED BY THE ORAL ROUTE

JOHN B. THIERSCH, M.D., SEATTLE, WASH.

(From the Department of Pathology, University of Washington Medical School)

Summary and Conclusions

1. Oral doses of 6 to 12 mg. 4-amino P. G. A. induced fetal death in the first trimester of pregnancy followed by spontaneous delivery of the products of conception in 10 out of 12 cases treated.

2. The doses lethal to the embryos had only a slight and transitory depressing effect on the hemoglobin and white blood counts of the mothers.

3. In three instances, a second course of the drug was given needlessly because of persistent positive "pregnancy tests."

4. The lesions found in the younger fetuses were depression of hematopoiesis, necrosis of the liver, adrenals, and intestinal epithelia.

5. In three older fetuses the drug failed to produce immediate death, but apparently induced malformations of the cranium. One of these fetuses died later and was delivered spontaneously. The other two were alive when surgically removed.

6. The study shows that usage of the drug to induce abortions should in the absence of reliable pregnancy tests be limited to patients in whom surgical intervention is possible to avoid malformations.

7. The action of the drug is regarded as entirely "antifolic," indicating the importance of folic acid in the early embryonic life.

8. The probable role of a folic acid deficiency in certain spontaneous abortions, in the development of malformations, and the importance of folic acid in seasonal breeding in some species is suggested by this study.

PAPERS 26, 27, 28 AND 29

26. Lenz, W. (1961). Diskussionsbemerkung von Privatdozent Dr. W. Lenz, Hamburg, zu dem Vortrag von R. A. Pfeiffer und K. Kosenow: Zur Frage der exogenen Entstehung schwerer Extremitätenmissbildungen. *Tagung der Rheinisch-Westfälischen Kinderärztevereinigung in Düsseldorf.* (Extract)
27. McBride, W. G. (1961). Thalidomide and congenital abnormalities. *Lancet*, **ii**, 1358
28. Lenz, W. (1962). Thalidomide and congenital abnormalities. *Lancet*, **i**, 45
29. Lenz, W. and Knapp, K. (1962). Foetal malformations due to thalidomide. *Ger. Med. Mthly*, **7**, 253–258

COMMENTARY

Thalidomide, a derivative of glutamic acid, was discovered in Germany and first marketed in 1956. The drug was well tolerated and considered to be safe, animal studies having demonstrated that it was non-toxic. The oral LD_{50} in mice was 5 g/kg, and large doses consumed by man produced no acute toxic effects. Peripheral neuritis was reported in a small number of isolated cases, but this was attributed to large doses of the substance ingested over prolonged periods of several months. Thalidomide was therefore considered the ideal sedative and hypnotic agent. It found ready acceptance and was widely used for the treatment of a variety of conditions, including emesis gravidarum, anxiety, headache, migraine, and arthritis.

In November 1961, Lenz, contributing to a discussion on the striking increase of severe limb malformations in West Germany, expressed the opinion that these congenital defects might be associated with the use of a specific drug during pregnancy. By then, he had already informed the manufacturing firm of the possible harmful effects of this substance, based on his personal clinical observations (Paper 26).

Independently of Lenz, McBride in a letter to the *Lancet* reported that he had seen a high incidence (20%) of infants with severe multiple malformations, born to mothers who had ingested thalidomide during pregnancy (Paper 27). Lenz responded to McBride's communication, indicating that he had seen 52 similar cases (Paper 28). Thalidomide was withdrawn from the German market on November 24th, 1961. However, by then at least 2000 children were born in West Germany alone with thalidomide-induced deformities.

Lenz and Knapp (Paper 29), in a carefully documented study, reviewed the clinical material from several countries relating to the thalidomide embryopathy. A causal relationship between the use of thalidomide during pregnancy and the rare limb malformations was convincingly demonstrated. Indeed, that the malformations observed could have been a chance occurrence was estimated to be less than 1 : 1000 million. They also reported that the critical period of development, during which the conceptus is susceptible to the teratogenic action of thalidomide, extends from day 27 to day 40 after conception. In all studies reviewed, the pattern of congenital malformations observed was the same, thus providing the first clinical evidence in support of a common aetiological factor for these abnormalities.

Thalidomide has been intensively investigated in laboratory animals. It is now considered to be a classic teratogenic agent. Surprisingly, it is difficult to induce the thalidomide-pattern of malformations in most common laboratory animals. Furthermore, very little is known about the teratological mechanism of action of this substance, despite the numerous studies which have been carried out. Certain species of primates and rabbits are sensitive to the action of thalidomide; the rat and mouse, which are routinely used in teratological screening of drugs, proved to be insensitive. There is no satisfactory explanation for the chemical and species specificity of thalidomide. Heine *et al.* (1964) in duced malformations, similar to those observed in humans, in New Zealand white rabbits following oral treatment with both thalidomide and carbon tetrachloride (temporary hepatic damage). The teratogenicity of thalidomide in the rabbits was correlated to a high concentration of the substance in serum and in various tissues, and a reduced concentration of ATP-activated glutamine (Heine, 1966). For a discussion of other biochemical studies relating to possible mechanisms of thalidomide action, reference should be made to the paper by Schumacher *et al.* (1972). Recently, McCredie and McBride (1973) have suggested that the limb deformities caused by thalidomide are secondary to an embryonic sensory peripheral neuropathy, and that the primary action of thalidomide is on the neural crest and its derivatives. This hypothesis is of considerable interest and undoubtedly represents a fruitful area for further investigation.

Between 6000 and 8000 children were crippled by thalidomide. In recent years, this has led to several litigation cases seeking compensation for damages caused by the drug. The legal rights of the unborn child and compensation for injuries received before birth are now questioned and widely debated as problems of immediate importance. By far, however, the hideous deformities produced by thalidomide had its greatest impact on public opinion, both medical and lay, because of the moral and ethical implications. It gave impetus to a renewal of interest in the causes and pathogenesis of congenital abnormalities, leading to intensified research in this field. The thalidomide tragedy alerted pregnant women and physicians to the potential hazards of normally non-toxic drugs during pregnancy. Furthermore, the need for reliable teratological screening procedures became most evident. In most countries, legislation now makes it mandatory that all drugs developed for clinical use must be tested for possible teratogenicity.

Despite the thalidomide tragedy and the known teratogenic hazard of certain other substances (see Paper 36), the consumption of drugs by pregnant women is surprisingly high and still increasing. It has been estimated that only 2–3% of all cases of congenital malformations are directly attributable to drugs. Nevertheless, their involvement in the aetiology and pathogenesis of developmental defects may be greater as a result of their combination or interaction with other factors, genetic or environmental (Wilson, 1973).

REFERENCES

Heine, W. (1966). Thalidomid-Embryopathie im Tierversuch (III). *Z. Kinderheilkd.*, **96**, 141–146

Heine, W., Kirchmair, H., Fiedler, M., and Stuewe, W. (1964). Thalidomid-Embryopathie im Tierversuch (I). *Z. Kinderheilkd.*, **91**, 213–221

McCredie, J. and McBride, W. G. (1973). Some congenital abnormalities: possibly due to embryonic peripheral neuropathy. *Clin. Radiol.*, **24**, 204–211

Schumacher, H. J., Terapane, J., Jordan, R. L. and Wilson, J. G. (1972). The teratogenic activity of a thalidomide analogue, EM_{12}, in rabbits, rats, and monkeys. *Teratology*, **5**, 233–240

Wilson, J. G. (1973). Present status of drugs as teratogens in man. *Teratology*, **7**, 3–16

Diskussionsbemerkung von Privatdozent Dr. W. Lenz, Hamburg, zu dem Vortrag von R. A. Pfeiffer und K. Kosenow: Zur Frage der exogenen Entstehung schwerer Extremitätenmißbildungen

Tagung der Rheinisch - Westfalischen Kinderärztevereinigung
in Düsseldorf am 19. 11. 1961

Discussion contribution by Dr. W. Lenz, Hamburg, on the lecture by R. A. Pfeiffer and K. Kosenow 'On The Exogenous Origin of Malformations of The Extremities'

Meeting of the Association of Paediatricians in Rhineland-Westphalia,
Dusseldorf, Nov. 19, 1961

Since early November 1961 we have been taking more detailed histories of the new type of malformation of the extremities. Initially we had thought that reasonably complete histories could be obtained by spending 1 to 2 hours on each case and using a carefully planned 3-page questionnaire. After some histories had been taken, we had to check the data on medication in the first few months of pregnancy. This time, specific questions were asked, and it was possible in some cases to supplement the histories originally taken. However, that was not enough. Further information was yielded by inspecting the contents of medicine cupboards in the mothers' homes. Again, this was not enough. An attempt was made to supplement the data by questioning the practitioners who had treated the mothers during their pregnancies. This procedure appears to have produced fairly complete medication histories. Fourteen mothers of children with severe malformations of the extremities had taken a certain substance in early pregnancy. With three other mothers there was a probability that they had taken the same substance at that time, while they had certainly taken it at a different time. One mother had taken a chemically similar substance with similar indication. In three cases detailed research failed to produce any evidence that the substance had been taken. Each of these three mothers had been treated by three different doctors in early pregnancy. One mother stated that her doctor had visited her and had produced some tablets wrapped in cellophane from his coat pocket. It was impossible to determine what these tablets had been. Two of the three mothers had been treated by the same doctor. For various reasons these three negative histories cannot with certainty be considered complete. Shorter histories on the basis of specific questions, taken from 20 mothers of healthy children up to 2 years, showed that the substance had been taken only in one case, towards the end of the pregnancy. There is nothing to prove an aetiological relationship between the intake of the substance and the appearance of malformations. From a scientific point of view it would therefore be premature to discuss this. However, it is conceivable that a relationship might exist. I feel that it is my human and civic duty not to conceal my observations. In view of the tremendous human, psychological, legal and financial implications, I have discussed the matter with a paediatrician and pharmagologist, and subsequently informed the manufacturers of my observations and of my personal opinion that the drug should be taken off the market immediately and not marketed again until its harmlessness has been proved. We have tried to take many aspects into consideration, but have been able to devote full attention to only some of them in our research. The same attention should be devoted also to other factors. I wonder whether our present investigations are being carried on with sufficient intensity. Every month by which the elucidation of this phenomenon is delayed will mean the births of maybe 50 to 100 terribly mutilated children.

DECEMBER 16, 1961   THE LANCET

Letters to the Editor

THALIDOMIDE AND CONGENITAL ABNORMALITIES

SIR,—Congenital abnormalities are present in approximately 1·5% of babies. In recent months I have observed that the incidence of multiple severe abnormalities in babies delivered of women who were given the drug thalidomide (' Distaval ') during pregnancy, as an antiemetic or as a sedative, to be almost 20%.

These abnormalities are present in structures developed from mesenchyme—i.e., the bones and musculature of the gut. Bony development seems to be affected in a very striking manner, resulting in polydactyly, syndactyly, and failure of development of long bones (abnormally short femora and radii).

Have any of your readers seen similar abnormalities in babies delivered of women who have taken this drug during pregnancy?

Hurstville, New South Wales.   **W. G. McBRIDE.**

₀ In our issue of Dec. 2 we included a statement from the Distillers Company (Biochemicals) Ltd. referring to " reports from two overseas sources possibly associating thalidomide (' Distaval ') with harmful effects on the fœtus in early pregnancy ". Pending further investigation, the company decided to withdraw from the market all its preparations containing thalidomide.—ED.L.

JANUARY 6, 1962   THE LANCET

THALIDOMIDE AND CONGENITAL ABNORMALITIES

SIR,—Dr. McBride (Dec. 16) describes congenital abnormalities in babies delivered of women who have taken thalidomide. I have seen 52 malformed infants whose mothers had taken ' Contergan ' in early pregnancy, and I understand that contergan is a synonym of thalidomide, others being ' Distaral,' ' Softenon ', ' Neurosedyn ', ' Isomin ', ' Kedavon ', ' Telargan ', and ' Sedalis '.

Since I discussed the possible ætiological role of contergan in human malformations at a conference on Nov. 18, 1961, I have received letters from many places in the German Federal Republic, as well as from Belgium, England, and Sweden, reporting 115 additional cases in which this drug was thought to be the cause.

Though these malformations are variable, they are of a rather specific nature. It is usually possible to infer from the type of the abnormalities alone whether contergan has been taken. Typical of a contergan history are defects of the arms (amelia, atypical phocomelia with absence of the thumbs and sometimes of other fingers as well, aplasia of the radius, defects of the long bones of the legs, especially the femora and tibiæ, absence of the auricles, hæmangiomata of the nose and the upper lip [wine-spot variety], atresia of the œsophagus, the duodenum, or the anus, cardiac anomalies, and aplasia of the gallbladder and of the appendix).

Judging from case histories of more than 300 women who have borne normal infants, and of whom none had taken contergan between the 4th and the 8th week after conception, the risk to a fœtus of a mother taking contergan during this period may be definitely higher than 20%. I venture the estimate that at least 2000, possibly more than 3000, " contergan " babies have been born in Western Germany since 1959.

Universitäts-Kinderklinik,
Hamburg-Eppendorf, Germany.   **W. LENZ.**

From W. Lenz and K. Knapp (1962), Ger. Med. Mthly., 7, 253–258. *Copyright* (1962),
by kind permission of the authors and Georg Thieme Verlag, Stuttgart, Germany

GERMAN MEDICAL MONTHLY

ENGLISH LANGUAGE EDITION OF THE DEUTSCHE MEDIZINISCHE WOCHENSCHRIFT

Vol. VII   Stuttgart, August 1962   No. 8

ORIGINAL ARTICLES

From the Paediatric Department (Director: Prof. K. H. Schäfer), University of Hamburg

Foetal Malformations Due to Thalidomide[1]

W. Lenz and K. Knapp

At a meeting of the German Paediatric Society at Kassel in October 1960, Kosenow and Pfeiffer (5) presented the photographs and X-ray films of two infants showing aplasia of the thumbs, the radii and the tibiae, duodenal stenosis and capillary haemangiomas of the upper lip. In addition, one of the infants had aplasia of the femur. Wiedemann (14, 15), less than a year later, once again drew the attention of the medical profession to the incidence of similar malformations which had assumed frightening and almost epidemic proportions since 1959. He recognized variations in the manifestations of the new syndrome: in some cases all limbs were missing; in others apparently only the thumbs and radii were absent; and in a number of cases there were associated malformations of the heart, kidneys and intestinal tract. In the discussion which arose at a meeting on 18th November 1961, one of us (W. L.) expressed the opinion that the drug thalidomide was under suspicion as a possible aetiological factor, for it appeared in 17 of 20 maternal records. Because of this suspicion the manufacturers withdrew the preparation known as Contergan®[*] (thalidomide) and all other preparations containing thalidomide from the market on 25th November 1961.

Our subsequent studies have shown that the damaging effect of thalidomide on the embryo was confined to a critical phase of about 14 days. Prospective mothers who have taken this preparation during pregnancy at times other than this brief period therefore have no cause for anxiety.

Case Material

We divided the cases that came to our knowledge into two groups. The first group of 129 cases included those studied by us at the Paediatric Clinic, University of Hamburg, and those reported to us from other clinics in Hamburg, Brunswick and Stade. The criterion for inclusion in this group was the presence of the typical foetal malformations, regardless of whether or not the mother had taken thalidomide. In 90 of these cases the mother had certainly or very probably taken thalidomide; in 22 there was no definite evidence of thalidomide intake; and in 17 cases the information obtainable was incomplete.

The second group comprised 203 cases that had been reported to us because of maternal thalidomide intake. The majority of cases reported to us by letters were from West Germany, but there were also isolated cases from Egypt, Belgium, Brazil, England, Israel, Sweden, Switzerland and the U.S.A. In addition we included series of cases with typical malformations and a history of thalidomide intake, reported to us by a number of medical practitioners.

Incidence of Malformations

In 13 maternity hospitals in Hamburg during the years 1960 and 1961 there were 27 with the new type of malformation out of 15,776 infants born. If this figure was representative for West Germany as a whole, the total number of infants born with these malformations would be between 2,000 and 3,000. The incidence in Northrhine-Westphalia was actually higher. In a few of the smaller cities several per cent of all newborn infants were apparently affected. On the other hand, the incidence in Schleswig-Holstein and Bavaria was apparently much lower. Various data of 212,000 births during the years 1930 to 1958 were available for comparison: delivery room books and obstetric records from eight maternity hospitals in Hamburg, and the birth records of domiciliary deliveries from four health centres. During this period no increase in the incidence of malformations of the limbs was noted. On the other hand, there was no increase in the incidence of spina bifida, anencephaly or cleft lip and palate among the 15,776 infants born during the years 1960 and 1961.

A review of the 148 cases of congenital deformities of the limbs seen in the Orthopaedic Clinic of the University of Münster during the years 1948 to 1961 showed that the number of cases of amelia (absence of limb or limbs), peromelia (malformation of limb or limbs) and cleft hands and feet had remained approximately constant. However, there was an incidence of cases of phocomelia (absence of proximal portion of limb or limbs) since 1958: there was one case each per year in 1948, 1951, 1956 and 1957; three cases in 1958 and again in 1959; 27 cases in 1960 and 65 cases in 1961 (4). Wiedemann's findings (14, 15) supported these observations: of his cases from Krefeld two were born in 1960 and 11 in 1961, and of those from Kiel two were born in 1959, another two in 1960 and 14 in 1961. Table I shows the dates of birth

---

[1] Abridged translation of the article in the Dtsch. med. Wschr. 87 (1962), 1232.

[*] Other trade-names: Distaval, Softenon. It is contained in K 17, Noctosediv, Valgis and others.

201

Lenz, Knapp: Foetal Malformations Due to Thalidomide   Germ. med. Monthly, Vol. VII

of our own cases: their distribution suggests that the cases observed in various geographical areas were part of the same "epidemic".

Table I. Dates of birth of children with the new type of malformation.

Born		History of maternal thalidomide intake			
Year	Half	Positive[1]	Positive[2] (by letter)	Negative[3]	In-complete[4]
1959	1.	0	0	0	0
	2.	1	1	1	1
1960	1.	3	7	1	1
	2.	15	24	3	7
1961	1.	28	49	6	5
	2.	28	106	10	3
1962	1.	15	14	1	0
Totals		90	201	22	17

[1] Definitely proven or highly probable intake of thalidomide. The cases of malformation in this series were included before an enquiry was made into whether or not thalidomide had been ingested.
[2] From written communications of the presence of foetal malformations believed to have followed thalidomide intake.
[3] Cases in which no definite or unequivocal history of thalidomide intake was obtainable. These included cases in which the intake of thalidomide was believed to have occurred only at times other than the critical period, and cases in which the nature of the sedatives taken could not be recalled.
[4] Cases with insufficient information. Only those cases with obvious large gaps in the histories or those altogether without histories were included. Among the cases listed as "negative" there were a few with some gaps in their histories.

Nature of the Malformations*

The first aspect to attract attention was the increase in the number of major malformations of the limbs. At the same time a number of lesser malformations, such as hypoplasia of the thumb or thenar eminence, syndactyly between hypoplastic thumb and index finger, and triphalangia of the thumb, were seen more frequently. Malformations such as anotia, bowel stenosis and atresia appeared to be increasing in incidence not only in association with the limb malformations but also independently of them. The association between these various manifestations was illustrated by the findings in one pair of binovular twins: the boy had a typical phocomelia of the arms and the girl had anal atresia and duodenal stenosis. The mother had taken thalidomide during the early part of pregnancy.

The incidence of the various types of malformation and the combinations in which they occurred were practically identical in the two groups of cases studied: the first group collected without prior knowledge as to maternal thalidomide intake (although this was subsequently found to have occurred), and the second group consisting of cases reported to us because of maternal thalidomide intake.

The only likely explanation of these observations was that thalidomide was in fact the one common aetiological factor in all these cases.

Moreover, the internal malformations which accompanied the malformations of the extremities were of the same nature in the cases reported to us by letter as in our own group of cases. These malformations are set out in Table III from which we have omitted those malformations usually only discovered

* Cf. Figs. 1—4 on p. 265.

Table II. Details of malformations.

Parts affected	History of maternal thalidomide intake			
	Positive	Positive (by letter)	Negative	In-complete
	%	%	%	%
Arms	54.5	50.6	54.6	50.0
Arms and legs	22.2	29.6	31.8	22.2
Arms, legs and ears	2.2	3.4	4.5	—
Arms and ears	7.8	4.9	4.5	5.6
Ears	7.8	6.9	—	22.2
Legs	1.1	2.0	4.5	—
Other organs or parts[1]	4.4	2.5	—	—
Numbers	90	203[2]	22	18

[1] One atrial septal defect and multicystic kidneys; one right multicystic kidney, left renal aplasia, and aplasia of the left Fallopian tube and the left uterine horn; one multicystic kidneys; one anal stenosis and right hydronephrosis; one cervical fistula; one congenital malformation of the heart; one choanal atresia; one anal atresia. In addition, we received letters reporting one case each of cleft lip and palate, spina bifida, and osteogenesis imperfecta. In these three cases the time of the thalidomide intake could not be determined. The taking of thalidomide in these cases was probably a coincidence.
[2] These cases only partly correspond to cases in the same column in Table I, because in some cases the date of birth was not available and in others no exact description of the type of malformation was provided.
Arms: amelia, phocomelia, defects of the radius and/or thumb, triphalangia of the thumb.
Legs: amelia, phocomelia, tibial aplasia, marked shortening, polydactyly of the feet. Talipes, pes adductus and subluxation of the hip were not included.
Ears: complete or almost complete anotia. Lesser deformities of the outer ear were not included.

Table III. Associated malformations in cases of thalidomide induced foetal damage.

Nature of malformation	History of maternal thalidomide intake			
	Positive	Positive (by letter)	Negative	In-complete
Spastic pyloric hypertrophy	2	2	—	—
Duodenal stenosis	3	4	—	—
Duodenal atresia	3	2	—	1
Cardiac anomaly	17	13	2	2
Anophthalmia, microphthalmia	6	3	1	—
Anal atresia	3	4	—	1
Choanal atresia	1	1	—	—

(The conditions listed in Table II under "other organs or parts" are not included here)

at autopsy as the parents would probably have had no knowledge of them (aplasia of the gallbladder, appendix, one kidney, the middle lobe of the right lung).

The malformations following maternal thalidomide intake reported from Australia (McBride [6]), Brazil (Diefenthaeler, personal communication), England (1, 2, 3, 10, 11, 12, 13) and Sweden, all showed the same characteristic features.

The Critical Period of Thalidomide Intake in Relation to the Development of Malformations

In 86 cases dated prescription forms, medical records of early pregnancy, or other documentation of the exact dates of thalidomide intake were available. Certain errors may, however, have crept into these data for various reasons: memory may have been deceptive; the stated date of conception may have been erroneous; prescriptions did not show when the drugs were taken; and not every tablet of sedative taken would have been recorded in the case notes.

In our own group of cases the "critical period" of thalidomide intake extended from the 37th to the 50th day after the first day of the last menstrual period; in the few cases in which the exact date of conception was available the critical period ranged from the 27th to the 33rd day after conception. Comparison of the dates of thalidomide intake and the various deformities associated with these showed that a relatively early intake was associated predominantly with serious damage to the arms, and a relatively late intake with only minor malformations. Thus, one infant (Case 61 07 23), whose mother had taken the first tablet of Contergan® (thalidomide) on the 50th day after menstruation, had triphalangia of the thumbs as the only malformation. In another case (61 06 15) maternal thalidomide intake from the 38th to the 42nd days after menstruation had been followed by amelia of the left arm and phocomelia of the right arm. In all cases studied by us in which the exact date of conception was known the malformations were of a very serious nature. Presumably therefore these did not include any cases in which medication was started relatively late.

In the group of cases reported to us by letters the critical period was apparently of slightly longer duration but corresponded fairly closely with that in our own cases. It started practically on the same day but lasted a little longer.

Thalidomide intake occurring for the first time after the 54th day was certainly exceptional. In all cases in which the only dates available were those of the last menstrual period, the dates were consistent with a critical period of thalidomide intake between the 27th and 40th days after conception.

Thalidomide Intake during Pregnancy Without Foetal Malformations

Since November 1961 we have asked numerous obstetricians, paediatricians and general practitioners to tell us about mothers who had taken thalidomide during pregnancy and had been delivered of infants without malformations. This request was also made through the "Deutsche Medizinische Wochenschrift" and was reprinted in one of the daily newspapers. In this way we collected reports of 139 mothers who had taken thalidomide during pregnancy without the infants showing evidence of thalidomide damage. In Table IV we have set out details of those mothers who had taken thalidomide before, during or shortly after what we regard as the critical period.

Assessment of the Risk Involved in Thalidomide Intake During Pregnancy

Our data did not lend themselves to an analysis of the risk involved in taking thalidomide during what we have described as the "critical period". McBride (6) reported that almost 20% of mothers who had taken thalidomide to combat nausea or as a sedative during pregnancy gave birth to infants with malformations.

Arguments to Support the Aetiological Relationship between Maternal Thalidomide Intake and Foetal Malformations

1. The characteristic foetal malformations were observed after the introduction of thalidomide preparations wherever they were used fairly extensively. In countries such as France, Spain, the U.S.A. and East Germany, where thalidomide was unknown, no increase in malformations of this nature was observed.

2. In a series of 122 typical cases of foetal malformations our studies showed that 90 mothers had taken thalidomide during the early months of pregnancy. On the other hand, amongst 188 mothers who gave births to healthy children during the years 1960 to 1962, there were only seven who were reported to us as having taken thalidomide during pregnancy: in five this was taken at some time other than during the critical period and in two the exact time of thalidomide intake could not be ascertained. The difference between 80.4% and 1.1% amounts to 79.3 ± 3.8%, i.e. 21 times the standard deviation. The probability that the relationship between thalidomide and the malformations is due to chance is thus less than 1 : 1,000 million. Confirmation of our figures has been provided by independent observations of the incidence of maternal thalidomide intake in children born with the new type of malformation and in healthy children at various centres in Bonn, Bremen, Duisburg, Freiburg, Hannover, Cologne, Lübeck, Ludwigshafen and Münster.

3. Seven cases were reported to us from four maternity clinics in which the mother disclosed before delivery that she had taken thalidomide during early pregnancy. In six of these

Table IV. Maternal thalidomide intake during the first trimester of pregnancy without subsequent foetal malformations.

Number	Thalidomide intake — time and amount	Remarks
(62 01 26)	17th—23rd days p. m.[1] 1 tablet Contergan® forte daily	
(62 04 02)	14th day p. conc.[2] 1½ tabs.	
(61 02 14)	22nd—31st days and 34th day p.m. 1 tab. Contergan® forte daily	Also a few tablets occasionally later, but exact time not available
(61 03 26)	36th and 37th days p.m. ½ tab. Contergan® fort. each day	Infant had subluxation of hip, as did its older sister
(62 03 30)	37th—43rd days p.m. (= 24th—30th days p. conc.) 1 teaspoonful Contergan® liq. daily	Slight malformation of ears
(61 09 24)	41st—56th days p. m. (= 27th—42nd days p. conc.) 1 teaspoonful Contergan® liq. daily	Slight malformation of ears, coccygeal dimple
Mal.	On and after 51st day p.m. Contergan®	
(61 12 10)	52nd—112th days p. m. Contergan®	
4 cases:	Started between 61st and 69th days p.m.	
3 cases:	Started between 70th and 79th days p.m.	
3 cases:	Started between 80th and 89th days p.m.	

[1] p.m. = after the first day of the last menstrual period.
[2] p. conc. = after the date of conception.

For the article by Lenz, Knapp (p. 253—258)

Foetal Malformations Due to Thalidomide

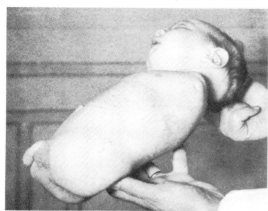

Fig. 1. Case 61 11 01. The mother had taken 100 mg. of thalidomide daily between the 44th and 50th days after the first day of the last menstrual period. The infant died at the age of one and a half months of an infection with hyperpyrexia.

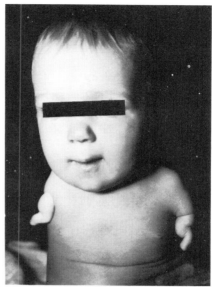

Fig. 2. Case 61 05 07. The mother had purchased twenty 100 mg. tablets of thalidomide on the 20th day after the onset of the last period.

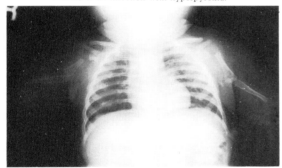

Abb. 3a

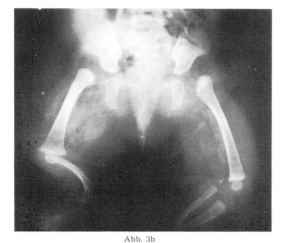

Abb. 3b

Fig. 3 a and b. Case 61 06 09. Thalidomide was prescribed on the 39th day after the onset of the last period.

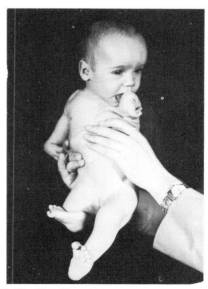

Fig. 4. Thalidomide tablets of 100 mg. were prescribed on the 36th day after the last menstrual period.

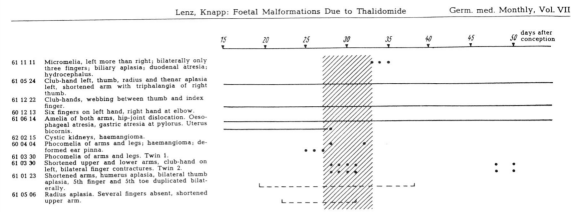

Fig. 5 a. Time of thalidomide intake and congenital anomalies in personal cases (days after conception)

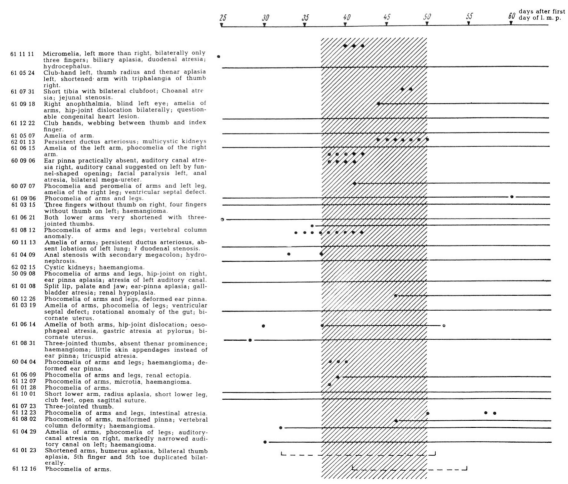

Fig. 5 b. Time of thalidomide intake and type of congenital anomalies in the personally investigated cases (time after beginning of last menstrual period [l. m. p.]). 61 01 03: Polydactyly present in the mother's family

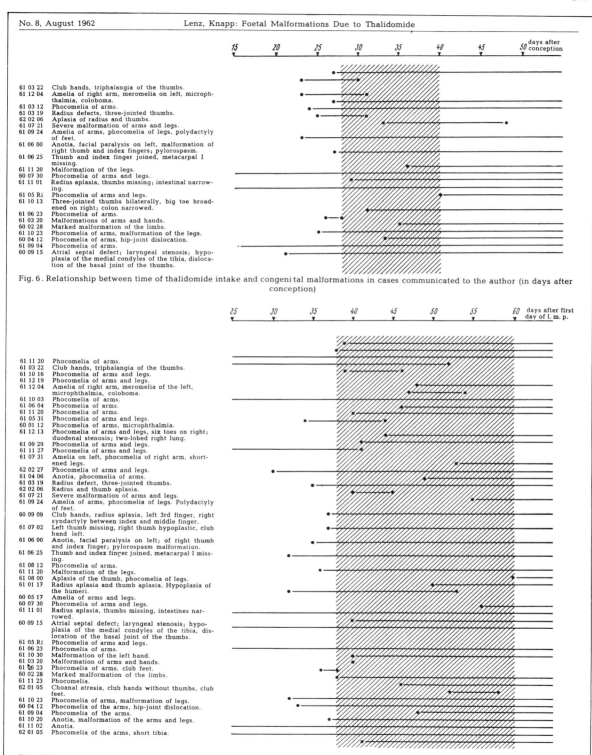

Fig. 6. Relationship between time of thalidomide intake and congenital malformations in cases communicated to the author (in days after conception)

Fig. 6 b. Relationship between of thalidomide intake and congenital malformations in the cases communicated to the author (time in days after last menstrual period [l. m. p.]

seven cases the infants subsequently showed the characteristic malformations.

4. Even to-day the thalidomide cases constitute but a small fraction of all malformations. If it were assumed that there was no causal relationship between thalidomide intake and the malformations, and if it were suggested that the various deformities were reported to us just because the mother happened to have taken thalidomide, then one would have expected the types of malformation encountered to be representative of all types of malformation found in the newborn. However, the 48 cases reported to us by letters with exact dates were exclusively malformations characteristically seen after maternal thalidomide intake.

5. The close time relationship between the maternal thalidomide intake and the phase of foetal development of the affected part clearly support the hypothesis of a causal relationship.

6. It is expected that the last of the thalidomide-induced malformations will be seen in infants born before the end of July 1962, i.e. within eight months of the withdrawal of the drug from the market. If, as expected, these malformations do in fact cease to occur the last reasonable doubt about the role played by thalidomide will have been removed.

Typical Cases of Malformation Without Maternal Thalidomide Intake

In 22 cases we were unable to obtain any definite evidence of thalidomide intake during the critical period. In seven of these cases the history was incomplete. We have included these amongst the thalidomide-negative cases as there were a few cases included amongst the thalidomide-positive group with comparable gaps in their histories. Had we not followed this procedure, the groups would not have been comparable. In the negative cases, despite our very thorough and repeated questioning, no other possible noxious factor could be found. On the whole we thought it improbable that these malformations were attributable to some hitherto unknown factor and inclined to the view that even the negative cases were likely to have taken thalidomide. Amongst 100 women from whom we took very careful histories we did not find a single one of whom we could have said "with certainty" that she had not taken thalidomide. Similarly, from the type of information supplied in the thalidomide-negative cases, we were unable to exclude thalidomide intake during early pregnancy with absolute certainty.

Summary

A greatly increased incidence of certain congenital anomalies, particularly phocomelia, was noted in 1961 in many parts of Germany and other countries. In Hamburg the incidence of such congenital anomalies was 0.17% of all newborns while that of other types of congenital anomalies had not changed.

Retrospective enquiry has shown that most mothers of children with the newly observed types of embryopathy (phocomelia) had taken thalidomide or thalidomide-containing drugs during the early months of pregnancy. In half of the cases only the arms have been involved, in a quarter of the cases arms and legs, while absence of ears occurred in one-sixth of the cases.

The critical phase of toxic thalidomide action has been found to be between the 27th and 40th day after conception.

Various, mutually independent, statistical analyses leave no reasonable doubt that thalidomide is the cause of the described congenital anomalies. There has been no evidence of other aetiological factors, even contributory ones.

Acknowledgements

This paper could not have been written without the kind and active support of some 100 general practitioners, obstetricians, paediatricians and government medical officers. We gratefully acknowledge the help unstintingly given by Drs. Dannenbaum (Brunswick) and Karte (Ludwigshafen), Prof. Kirchhoff (Göttingen), Dr. Loeser (Minden), Prof. Nitsch (Hanover), Prof. Schubert (Hamburg) and Dr. Wessolowski (Stade) and their associates, to all of whom we are especially indebted. Our investigation was greatly facilitated by the excellent co-operation of parents who, in their anxiety to have the cause of their children's misfortunes brought to light, spared no effort in the support they gave to this investigation.

References

(1) Burley, D. M.: Lancet 1962/I, 271.
(2) Devitt, R. E. F., S. Kenny: Lancet 1962/I, 430.
(3) Ferguson, A. W.: Lancet 1962/I, 691.
(4) Hepp, O.: Med. Klin. 57 (1962), 419.
(5) Kosenow, W., R. A. Pfeiffer: Mikromelie, Haemangiom und Duodenalstenose. Scient. exhibit, No. 39. 59th Meeting of the Dtsch. Ges. f. Kinderheilk. Kassel, 26.—28. September (1960).
(6) McBride, W. G.: Lancet 1961/II, 1358.
(7) Martius, H.: Lehrbuch der Geburtshilfe. 2nd ed. (Stuttgart 1952).
(8) Petersen, C. R.: Med. Welt (1962), 753.
(9) Pfeiffer, R. A., W. Kosenow: Münch. med. Wschr. 104 (1962), 68.
(10) Rogerson, G.: Lancet 1962/I, 691.
(11) Russell, C. S., M. D. Mekichan: Lancet 1962/I, 429.
(12) Speirs, A. L.: Lancet 1962/I, 303.
(13) Stabler, F.: Lancet 1962/I, 591.
(14) Wiedemann, H.-R.: Med. Welt (1961), 1863.
(15) Wiedemann, H.-R., K. Aeissen: Med. Mschr. 15 (1961), 816.

(Authors' address: Prof. Dr. W. Lenz; Dr. K. Knapp, Universitäts-Kinderklinik, Martinistr. 52, Hamburg-Eppendorf, Germany)

PAPERS 30, 31 AND 32

30. Grunwaldt, E. and Bates, T. (1957). Nonadrenal female pseudohermaphrodism after administration of testosterone to mother during pregnancy. *Pediatrics*, **20**, 503–505
31. Wilkins, L. (1960) Masculinization of female fetus due to use of orally given progestins. *J. Am. Med. Assoc.*, **172**, 1028–1032
32. Herbst, A. L., Ulfelder, H. and Poskanzer, D. C. (1971). Adenocarcinoma of the vagina. Association of maternal stilbestrol therapy with tumor appearance in young women. *N. Engl. J. Med.*, **284**, 878–881

COMMENTARY

Sex development in the fetus is complex. At fertilization, the genetic sex of the offspring is determined, but this does not become evident until the 12th week of fetal development when the external genitalia reveal distinct sexual characteristics. Differentiation of the testes from the indifferent gonads is controlled by the Y-chromosome, and the establishment of the male external genitalia is dependent on male hormones, produced by the fetal testes.

Unlike the male, the female genital system develops independently of specific hormonal influences. However, an excess of male hormones during this critical stage of development may readily lead to masculinization of the female genitalia. In contrast, feminization of the male fetus has been associated with a deficiency of male hormones. True hermaphroditism is a rare condition and is caused by a derangement in sexual determination, whereas pseudohermaphroditism is not uncommon and usually results from increased androgen secretion, e.g. in congenital virilizing adrenal hyperplasia (Moore, 1974).

Grunwaldt and Bates (Paper 30) reported the first case of masculinization of the female fetus caused by exogenous testosterone. Large doses of the androgen had been administered to the mother from the 7th to 15th week of pregnancy. Masculinization of female fetuses following maternal treatment with progestogens was reported by Wilkins; in Paper 31 a detailed analysis of 70 such cases, caused by administration of synthetic progestins to the mothers, is preser Since these early observations, there have been umerous reports confirming that androgenic steroids, estrogens and progestogens can produce masculinization of the female infant. It would appear that the fetus is susceptible to the virilizing effects of these substances during the first 5 months of pregnancy, but hypertrophy of the clitoris may result from exposure later in pregnancy.

Progestational compounds are still used for preventing threatened and habitual abortion. In these cases, it is likely that large doses reach the embryo. Hormonal pregnancy tests also expose the embryo to significant levels of progesterone or a combination product of androgen and estrogen. Oral contraceptives contain progestogen and estrogen, or progestogen alone. These substances are perhaps the most widely and consistently used drugs by females of child-bearing age and their unintentional use during an unsuspected pregnancy is not uncommon.

How safe are sex steroids during pregnancy? In several recent studies congenital malformations have been found in association with hormonal pregnancy tests and oral contraceptives. In contrast, other investigations have indicated that there is no substantial evidence to believe that these substances are teratogenic in humans (see Tuchmann-Duplessis, 1973; Oakley Jr, 1973; Editorial: *Lancet*, 1974; Nora and Nora, 1975; Smithells, 1976). Clearly, carefully planned prospective studies are required to resolve the controversy. As an interim solution, Nora and Nora (1975) have rightly advocated that hormonal pregnancy tests should be discontinued, and that oral contraceptives should be used only when a pregnancy has been ruled out with certainty.

The paper by Herbst and his colleagues (Paper 32) that vaginal adenocarcinomas have developed in adolescent girls many years after diethylstilbestrol (DES), a non-steroidal estrogenic compound, had been given to their mothers during pregnancy is of considerable importance and has wider implications. For the first time, attention has been drawn to the carcinogenic action of drugs on the human fetus and to the prenatal origin of certain cancers, as well as to the long-term postnatal effects of any drug even in the absence of recognizable developmental abnormalities at birth.

The association between DES and vaginal adenosis and adenocarcinoma in young adolescent girls is now well documented. It has been estimated that between 10 000 and 16 000 female infants born each year between 1960 and 1970 were exposed to DES. In less than 0·1% of these women is there a risk of developing adenocarcinoma, but 30% may eventually show pathological changes in the cervix and vagina. Maternal treatment with DES or some related chemical substance occurred before the first 18 weeks of gestation in 85% of the cases reviewed. Whether the fetus developed the lesions depended on the time of exposure to the carcinogen. The mechanisms of these possible teratogenic effects are not understood. (Ulfelder, 1973, 1976).

REFERENCES

Editorial (1974). Are sex hormones teratogenic? *Lancet*, **ii**, 1489–1490

Moore, K. L. (1974). Sex determination. Normal and abnormal sexual development. *J. Obstet. Gynecol. Nursing*, **3**, 61–69

Nora, A. H. and Nora, J. J. (1975). A syndrome of multiple congenital anomalies associated with teratogenic exposure. *Arch. Environ. Health*, **30**, 17–21

Oakley Jr., G. P. (1973). Hormonal pregnancy tests and congenital malformations. *Lancet*, **ii**, 256–257

Smithells, R. W. (1976). Environmental teratogens in man. *Br. Med. Bull.*, **32**, 27–33

Tuchmann-Duplessis, H. (1973). Teratogenic screening methods and their application to contraceptive products. *Meeting on Pharmacological Models to Assess Toxicity and Side Effects of Fertility Regulating Agents Geneva*, pp. 203–223

Ulfelder, H. (1973). Stilbestrol, adenosis, and adenocarcinoma. *Am. J. Obstet. Gynecol.*, **117**, 794–800

Ulfedler, H. (1976). DES—Transplacental teratogen—and possibly also carcinogen. *Teratology*, **13**, 101–104

From E. Grunwaldt and T. Bates (1957). Pediatrics, **20**, 503–505. *Copyright* (1957), *by kind permission of the authors and the American Academy of Pediatrics*

NONADRENAL FEMALE PSEUDOHERMAPHRODISM AFTER ADMINISTRATION OF TESTOSTERONE TO MOTHER DURING PREGNANCY Report of a Case

By Edgar Grunwaldt, M.D., and Talcott Bates, M.D.

Department of Pediatrics, University of California Hospital, San Francisco

THE DIAGNOSIS of nonadrenal female pseudohermaphrodism should be based on the following criteria: (1) the external genitalia should show hypertrophy of the clitoris and some degree of labial fusion; (2) in infants, measurement of 17-ketosteroids or pregnanetriol should be performed to rule out the adrenogenital syndrome; in older patients this syndrome can be ruled out clinically by the lack of precocious puberty and progressive masculinization; (3) laparotomy should reveal a female internal genital apparatus, and (4) adequate biopsies of both gonads should show normal ovaries, excluding the possibility of ovotestes and true hermaphrodism.

The subject of pseudohermaphrodism is adequately covered by Wilkins *et al.*[1] in a recent article in which 12 cases[2-11] of nonadrenal female pseudohermaphrodism are mentioned; however, not all of these meet the four conditions described above. There are two cases[11, 12] in the literature in which pseudohermaphrodism followed the occurrence of masculinizing tumors (arrhenoblastoma) during pregnancy, but no mention was found of a case in which testosterone had been administered to the mother.

CASE REPORT

History

This infant was the first born of a 28-year-old white woman who consulted her obstetrician because of nausea and vomiting 10 weeks after the onset of the last menstrual period. On that day 100 mg of testosterone propionate was administered intramuscularly, and 10 mg of methyl testosterone three times a day was prescribed. Three days later another 100 mg of testosterone propionate was administered. She had taken 30 mg of testosterone by mouth daily for 51 days when administration was discontinued because of deepening voice.

Pregnancy terminated uneventfully and she was delivered of a 3.4 kg infant who had cyanosis and bradycardia of short duration. The baby seemed to have undescended testes and a very small penis from which there was some white, mucoid discharge on the second and third days of life. A urologist was consulted and he agreed with the obstetrician and attending pediatrician that the infant was probably male.

The infant thrived but at the age of 6 months there had been no significant growth of the "penis" and no erections. As there was still some question about the sex, the child was referred to the University of California Hospital for further studies.

Physical Findings

The infant was 65 cm long and weighed 8.1 kg. The external genitalia consisted of two skin folds with scrotal rugae but no palpable testes, and a phallus 1.5 cm long with a tight prepuce which could not be retracted to reveal a glans (Fig. 1). Palpation of the shaft of the phallus revealed a small amount of firm tissue. The infant urinated with a good stream through the tip of the phallus. On rectal examination a small midline structure could be palpated and this was thought to represent a uterus. The remainder of the physical examination was within normal limits.

Laboratory Findings

Blood count and urinalysis were normal. The rate of excretion of 17-ketosteroids was 0.3 mg in 24 hours, a normal value indicating no excess of adrenal androgen. Roentgenograms showed normal bone age. An excretory urogram was normal.

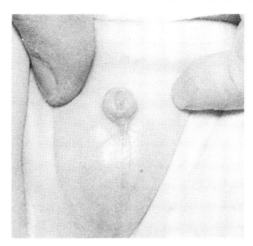

FIG. 1. External genitalia.

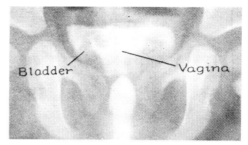

FIG. 2. Roentgenogram of bladder and vagina after the introduction of radiopaque material into the urogenital sinus.

Course

Exploratory laparotomy revealed the presence of normal uterus, tubes and ovaries. Two biopsies taken from each ovary showed normal ovarian tissue. A skin biopsy taken at the time of operation showed a female chromatin pattern. Attempts to visualize the urogenital sinus and the relation of the structures therein with a cystoscope failed because the instrument could be introduced only a very short distance. It was impossible to pass a catheter into the bladder, an obstruction being met about 4 cm from the tip of the phallus. However, dye introduced at this point filled the bladder and the vagina (Fig. 2).

The consulting gynecologist felt that definitive surgery on the external genitalia should be deferred until the infant was older, when plastic repair would be easier.

As the result of these studies the infant's sex of rearing was changed to female.

DISCUSSION

The large doses of testosterone started at approximately the seventh or eighth week of gestation and continued for 51 days, a time when the genital tract is in its formative stages, could well have produced the malformations described. This view is substantiated by the experiments of Greene et al.,[13] who produced similar malformations in rats by administering androgens to pregnant females.

The two cases[11, 12] that occurred in association with arrhenoblastoma in the mother are similar to that reported here except for the endogenous source of the androgens.

While no definite conclusions can be reached on the basis of these three cases, the evidence is suggestive enough to indicate the need for caution in using sex hormones during the first trimester of pregnancy.

REFERENCES

1. Wilkins, L., Grumbach, M. M., Van Wyck, J. J., Shephard, T. H., and Papadatos, C.: Hermaphroditism: Classification, diagnosis, selection of sex and treatment. PEDIATRICS, 16:287, 1955.
2. Chanis, D.: Some aspects of hermaphroditism. J. Urol., 47:508, 1942.
3. Haynes, E., Thomas, H. P., and Wheeler, M. S.: Pseudohermaphroditism with psychosis. M. Rec., 154:307, 1941.
4. Money, J., Hampson, J. G., and Hampson, J. L.: An examination of some basic sexual concepts: The evidence of human hermaphroditism. Bull. Johns Hopkins Hosp., 97:301, 1955.
5. Cotte, G.: Plastic operations for sexual ambiguity. J. Mt. Sinai Hosp., 14:170, 1947.
6. Atkinson, W., and Masson, J. G.: Pseudo-hermaphrodism. S. Clin. North America, 14:573, 1934.
7. Wilkins, L.: The Diagnosis and Treatment of Endocrine Disorders in Childhood and Adolescence, 1st Ed. Springfield, Thomas, 1950, p. 270.
8. Howard, F. S., and Hinman, F.: Female pseudohermaphroditism with supplementary phallic urethra: Report of 2

ARTICLES

cases. J. Urol., **65**:439, 1951.

9. Perloff, W., Conger, K. B., and Levy, L. M.: Female pseudohermaphrodism: A description of 2 unusual cases. J. Clin. Endocrinol., **13**:783, 1953.

10. Papadatos, C., and Klein, R.: Nonadrenal female pseudohermaphroditism. J. Pediat., **45**:662, 1954.

11. Brentnall, C. P.: A case of arrhenoblastoma complicating pregnancy. J. Obst. & Gynaec. Brit. Emp., **52**:235, 1945.

12. Felicissimo Paula Xavier, J., and Abreu Junqueira, M.: Sobre un caso de arrhenoblastoma do ovario e gravidez topica simultanea. Virilisação da gestante e do feto feminino. Rev. Gyn e Obst., **1**: 356, 1938.

13. Greene, R. R., Burrill, M. W., and Ivy, A. C.: Experimental intersexuality. The effect of antenatal androgens on sexual development of female rats. Am. J. Anat., **65**:415, 1939.

SUMMARIO IN INTERLINGUA

Nonadrenal Pseudohermaphroditismo Feminin Post Administration de Testosterona Durante le Pregnantia

Le diagnose de nonadrenal pseudohermaphroditismo feminin debe esser basate super le sequente criterios: Le genitales externe debe monstrar hypertrophia del clitoris e un certe grado de fusion labial. In infantes, determinationes de 17-cetosteroides o de pregnanetriol debe esser obtenite pro excluder le possibilitate del syndrome adrenogenital. In subjectos de etates plus avantiate, le exclusion de iste syndrome pote esser basate super le constatation clinic que il ha ni pubertate precoce ni masculinisation progressive. Laparotomia debe revelar le presentia de interne organos feminin. Adequate biopsias de ambe gonades debe demonstrar ovarious normal e justificar le exclusion del possibilitate de ovotestes e hermaphroditismo genuin.

Es presentate un caso que şatisface iste criterios. Le matre del patiente, un infante de 6 menses de etate, habeva recipite un total de 1, 5 g de testosterona durante le prime trimestre de su pregnantia.

Le occurrentia de duo previe casos in que le matres suffreva le effectos masculinisante de arrhenoblastoma, insimul con le constatation experimental que androgenos pote effectuar tal anormalitates, justifica le recommendation que le administration de hormones mascule durante le prime semestre del pregnantia deberea esser tractate con alte grados de circumspection.

From L. Wilkins (1960). J. Am. Med. Assoc., **172**, 1028–1032. *Copyright* (1960),
by kind permission of the author and the American Medical Association

MASCULINIZATION OF FEMALE FETUS DUE TO USE
OF ORALLY GIVEN PROGESTINS

Lawson Wilkins, M.D., Baltimore

Female pseudohermaphroditism due to congenital virilizing adrenal hyperplasia is a well-known condition.[1] The abnormality of sex differentiation is confined to partial masculinization of the external genitalia, while the ovaries are normal and the genital ducts are differentiated along the normal female pattern, forming vagina, uterus, and fallopian tubes. Embryonic masculinization of the external genitalia results in an enlarged phallus, which may or may not be associated with varying degrees of fusion of the labioscrotal folds. If little or no fusion occurs, separate vaginal and urethral orifices are visible. Fusion results in the formation of a urogenital sinus whose opening is either funnel-shaped or slit-like or in the form of a small meatus at the base or even on the shaft or tip of the phallus. Such a female infant may be readily mistaken for a hypospadic male or even a normal male infant with simple cryptorchism.

Fetal masculinization of the external genitalia with identical anatomic findings occurs also in females who do not have any adrenal abnormality. Unlike patients with the adrenogenital syndrome, these infants do not have elevated levels of urinary 17-ketosteroids and, as they grow older, they do not show progressive virilization with precocious growth of sexual hair and accelerated growth and osseous development. At puberty normal feminization, with menstruation and ovulation, occurs.

The diagnosis of female pseudohermaphroditism not due to adrenal abnormality depends on demonstration in the buccal smear of the "chromatin-positive" type of nuclei which are found in normal females[2] and on the finding of normal levels of 17-ketosteroids in the urine. When a urogenital sinus is present, it is generally advisable to perform a urethroscopic examination to demonstrate the communicating vagina and to observe the cervix.

A markedly masculinized female infant is readily mistaken for a hypospadic male or for a normal male with simple cryptorchism. This congenital condition is sometimes caused by virilizing adrenal hyperplasia, but data here presented show that it has also frequently resulted from administration of progestins to mothers in treating habitual or threatened abortion. Seventy cases of fetal masculinization of female infants associated with the oral administration of progestins to their mothers are analyzed. Thirty-one followed the use of 17-α-ethinyltestosterone, and 35 followed the use of 17-α-ethinyl-19-nortestosterone. In 25 cases the mothers were given estrogens with the progestins in order that the estrogen might offset the virilizing effect of the progestin, but the evidence showed that the estrogens did not prevent fetal masculinization. These data do not argue against the use of progesterone, for the progestins concerned in all cases were synthetic.

With high degrees of masculinization it may be advisable to perform an exploratory laparotomy to exclude the possibility of true hermaphroditism with mixed testes and ovaries, which is an exceedingly rare condition.

In 1958 my colleagues and I[2b] reported 17 instances of nonadrenal female pseudohermaphroditism, 12 of which occurred in infants born of mothers who, because of habitual or threatened abortions, had received 17-α-ethinyltestosterone (ethisterone, pregneninolone), a synthetic, orally given progestin, during gestation. This compound has

From the Division of Pediatric Endocrinology, Department of Pediatrics, Johns Hopkins University School of Medicine.

been used for about 15 years under such trade names as Progestoral, Pranone, and Lutocylol. In this paper warning was given that a newer progestin, 17-a-ethinyl-19-nortestosterone, marketed as Norlutin, might have even greater masculinizing effects on the fetus.

Report of Cases

Seventy cases of fetal masculinization of female infants associated with the oral administration of progestins to their mothers are presented. All of these cases fulfilled the diagnostic criteria discussed above. Twenty-three of these patients were studied by myself in the pediatric endocrine clinic of the Harriet Lane Home. Seventeen cases were

plasia of the prepuce. In general, the degree of hypertrophy was considerably less than that usually seen in cases of congenital virilizing hyperplasia of the adrenal. In some cases the organ was not sufficiently conspicuous to make amputation advisable. Some of the infants having high degrees of labioscrotal fusion (for designation of the degrees of fusion see footnotes to tables 1 and 2) had been mistaken for males at birth and had been raised as such. With both 17-a-ethinyltestosterone and Norlutin, fusions occurred only when administration of the drug was begun before the 12th week of gestation. Phallic enlargement can result when androgenic activity is exerted over a sufficient period at any time during fetal or postnatal life.

TABLE 1.—*Masculinized Females Whose Mothers Received 17-a-ethinyltestosterone (Ethisterone) During Gestation*

Observer	Case Identification	Birth, Yr.	Age Studied	Phallus	Fusion*	17-a-Ethinyltestosterone Daily Dose, Mg.	Period of Gestation, Wk.	Other Steroids	Maternal Virilization†
Wilkins	1	1957	1 day	+	++++	200	4-22	17-a-hydroxprogesterone, 1 dose	...
	2	1955	2 day	++	+++	50-200	4-35	Progesterone, 25-50 mg./day	...
	3	1955	15 mo.	+	+++	150-200	6-39	Progesterone, 100 mg. for 4 days	...
	4	1957	1 day	+	+++	200	4-26	17-a-hydroxprogesterone, 250 mg./wk.	...
	5	1957	4½ mo.	++	+++	200	8-39	...	...
	6	1959	1½ mo.	+	+++	60	3-26	...	...
	7	1958	4¾ yr.	++	++	30	10-22	Diethylstilbestrol, 100 mg.	...
	8	1957	7 day	+	++	40	5-39	Diethylstilbestrol, 30 mg.	...
	9	1952	4¾ yr.	++	+	100-80	4-39	Diethylstilbestrol, 40-120 mg.	...
	10	1953	3¼ yr.	++	+	30	8-26	...	...
	11	1950	7 day	++	+	30	10-39	Ethinylestradiol, 0.1 mg.	...
	12	1957	2 yr.	+	+	40	6-35	Diethylstilbestrol, unknown	...
	13	1950	7 yr.	++	0	...	6-30	Diethylstilbestrol, unknown	...
	14	1954	2 yr.	++	0	40	5-39	Diethylstilbestrol, unknown	...
	15	1953	4 yr.	+	0	20-40	7-39	Diethylstilbestrol, 100 mg.	...
	16	1953	7 yr.	++	0	30	8-35	...	...
	17	1952	6 yr.	++	0	60	14-35	...	...
	18	1958	1½ mo.	+	0	20	16-8	...	
Grumbach and others[3]	H.N.	1953	3 yr.	++	+++	200	2-22	Diethylstilbestrol, 5-75 mg.	...
	S.H.	1954	4 yr.	++	+++	200-250	4-33	...	
	D.F.	1951	8 yr.	++	+++	...	7-38	...	V
	B.N.	1957	Stillbirth	++	++++	30	11-15	...	
	S.S.	1958	10 mo.	+	+++	100-50	4-36	...	
	D.McC.	1950	5 yr.	++	++	30	6-32	...	
	L.W.	1952	5 yr.	++	0	50	8-12	...	
	B.S.	1958	1 day	+	0	45	16-28	...	A H
Bongiovanni and Eberlein	1	...	...	++	+++	10	1-28	Progesterone, 50-100 mg./wk.	...
	2	...	...	++	0	30-10	14-35	Conjugated equine estrogens (Premarin), 5 mg.	
	3	1958	2½ mo.	++	+++	100-200	10-39	...	
	4	1959	2 mo.	++	+++	50-100	6-39	Diethylstilbestrol, 25-50 mg.	...
Foxworthy		1957	...	++	0	40	4-17	Ethinylestradiol, 0.04 mg.	...
Hayles and Nolan[5]	2	1953	3 yr.	+	0	20-60	4-37	Conjugated equine estrogens, 2.5 mg.	...
Reilly and others[6]	7	1957	1 day	+	0	120-240	18-39	...	...
Moncrieff[4]	2	1957	9 day	++	++	60	6-39	Ethinylestradiol, 0.06 mg.	...

* Labioscrotal fusion: ++++ urogenital sinus opening on shaft or tip of phallus; +++ urogenital sinus with small meatus at base of phallus; ++ urogenital sinus with slit-like or funnel-shaped orifice; + slight posterior fusion, separate vaginal and urethal orifices.
† Maternal virilization: V = deepening of voice; H = hirsutism of face; A = acne; C = clitoral enlargement.

reported on by Grumbach and co-authors,[3] and one case each by Moncrieff,[4] Hayles and Nolan,[5] and Reilly and co-authors.[6] Jacobson[7] observed 17 cases in his obstetric practice. The rest of the cases were brought to my attention by other colleagues. In visiting various clinics throughout the United States I have heard of many more cases, but I do not have sufficiently accurate data to include them in this study.

Table 1 lists 34 cases associated with the use of 17-a-ethinyltestosterone. Table 2 shows 35 cases in which Norlutin, 17-a-ethinyl-19-nortestosterone, had been given and one case in which Enovid (norethynodrel and ethinylestradiol 3-methyl ether) had been used. The phallic enlargement, designated "+" or "++" (tables 1 and 2), consisted of hypertrophy of the corpus and glans and was not merely hyper-

The 34 cases of masculinization associated with administration of 17-a-ethinyltestosterone were observed in infants born between the years 1950 and 1959; the 36 infants whose mothers had been given Norlutin or Enovid were all born in 1958 and 1959. Although the daily doses of 17-a-ethinyltestosterone ranged from 20 to 250 mg., seven of the mothers had received 100 to 250 mg. daily. The doses of Norlutin ranged from 10 to 40 mg. per day, and high degrees of masculinization were observed with doses as small as 15 mg. daily. It is of particular interest that Jacobson[7] found that of 53 female infants born to mothers to whom he had given Norlutin in doses between 10 and 40 mg. per day, 17 showed masculinization, some in high degrees. Two mothers who had received 17-a-ethinyltestosterone, three who had received Norlutin, and one who had received Enovid showed mild androgenic manifestations, such as deepening of the voice, facial hair, and acne, which disappeared after the termination of pregnancy.

These findings indicate that (1) high degrees of masculinization occur with much smaller doses of Norlutin than of 17-a-ethinyltestosterone and (2) there has been a higher incidence of masculinized infants born to mothers who have received Norlutin than to those given 17-a-ethinyltestosterone.

Mode of Action

As shown in table 3, in 70 of 101 cases of nonadrenal female pseudohermaphroditism reported the mother had received one of the orally given progestins during gestation and in 15 cases testosterone or one of its androgenic derivatives. The probable mode of action of the orally given synthetic progestins has been discussed in previous communications.[8]

patients whose mothers received two or three of these same pills daily (6 or 9 mg. of methyltestosterone).

17-a-ethinyltestosterone, Norlutin, and Enovid are chemically similar to 17-methyltestosterone, since all have the 17-OH group in the beta position. 17-a-ethinyltestosterone has been shown to have androgenic effects in animals. In 1942 Courrier and Jost [10] reported that its administration to pregnant rabbits caused masculinization of the female fetus. This was confirmed in 1947 by Jost [11] in additional experiments. Recently, Revesz and co-workers [12] have brought about fetal masculinization by administration of 0.5 mg. of Norlutin daily and of 0.25 mg. of medroxyprogesterone (6-methyl-17-acetoxy-progesterone) to pregnant rats, although daily doses of 200 mg. of progesterone had no masculinizing effects. It would seem that both 17-a-ethinyltestosterone and Norlutin, and probably Enovid, are androgenic. Norlutin seems to be much more andro-

TABLE 2.—*Masculinized Females Whose Mothers Received Norlutin (17-a-ethinyl-19-nortestosterone) or Enovid (Norethynodrel and Ethinylestadriol 3-methyl Ether) During Gestation*

					Drugs Given			
					Norlutin			
Observer	Case Identification	Birth, Yr.	Age Studied	Phallus	Fusion*	Daily Dose, Mg.	Period of Gestation, Wk.	Other Steroids	Maternal Virilization†
Wilkins	1	1958	5 day	+	+++	5-20	6-30	...	...
	2	1958	12 mo.	+	+++	20-35	3-39	...	...
	3	1958	1 day	++	+	15	10-30	...	...
	4	1958	3½ mo.	++	-/-	10	7-35	Diethylstilbestrol	...
	5	1958	6 mo.	++	0	30-20	15-39	...	...
Grumbach and others[3]	A.R.	1958	4 day	+	+++	40-20	7-27	...	...
	S.B.	1959	1 day	++	+++	15- 5	8-29	Diethylstilbestrol, 75 mg.	...
	B.W.	1958	1 day	++	+++	10-15	7-29	Diethylstilbestrol, 25-175 mg.	V H
	S.B.1	1959	13 day	+	+++	15-40-20	5-35	Conjugated equine estrogens	V H
	B.B.	1959	6 day	+	++	15	7-24	...	...
	G.L.	1957	4 day	++	+	15- 5	10-36	...	...
	T.J.	1959	2 mo.	++	-/-	40-20	6-28	...	...
	D.W.	1958	2 day	++	0	10	15-31	17-a-hydroxyprogesterone, 250-500 mg./wk.	V
	S.M.	1957	5 mo.	++	0	10	19-28	Diethylstilbestrol	...
Bongiovanni	1	1958	...	+	++	10-15	1-39	Diethylstilbestrol, 75-100 mg.	...
	1	1958	...	+	+	10-20	10-39	Diethylstilbestrol, 25 mg.	...
D. W. Smith	1	1958	...	++	0	20	14-33	Progesterone (IM), 50 mg.	...
Valentine	1	1958	...	+	0	10	5-39	...	...
Jacobson	17 of 53 masculinized female infants born to mothers receiving Norlutin 10-40 mg./day.								
Grumbach	1	1958	1¼ mo.	++	++	Enovid, 10 mg.	6-38	...	V H A

* Labioscrotal fusion: ++++ urogenital sinus opening on shaft or tip of phallus; +++ urogenital sinus with small meatus at base of phallus; ++ single slit-like or funnel-shaped orifice; + slight posterior fusion, separate vaginal and urethral orifices.
† Maternal virilization: V = deepening of voice; H = hirsutism of face; A = acne; C = clitoral enlargement.

It has been demonstrated that testosterone and its known androgenic analogs, when administered to pregnant animals, can bring about masculinization of the fetus; in addition, 14 cases of fetal masculinization due to administration of these drugs to pregnant women have been reported.[9] It is probable that fetal masculinization may result from doses so small that they do not cause androgenic manifestations in the mothers or in normal adults. This may be due to increased sensitivity of the fetal end-organs or to impairment of the degradation and disposal of these steroids by the fetus. We have studied a highly virilized female infant from Vancouver, British Columbia, whose mother, from the 8th to the 39th week of pregnancy, had received one pill daily containing only 3 mg. of 17-methyltestosterone and 0.01 mg. of 17-ethinylestradiol. Moncrieff [4] has reported on two

genic than 17-a-ethinyltestosterone. Even though bioassays may show that these compounds are relatively weak in terms of their androgenic effects on adults, they are sufficiently potent when they cross the placenta to masculinize the relatively sensitive end-organs of the developing fetus. It is no longer necessary to assume that the mothers who give birth to masculinized females metabolize these steroids abnormally. The fact that not all the offspring of mothers who received these drugs during gestation are affected may be due to differences in placental transmission or fetal sensitivity.

The question whether estrogens and progesterone can play a role in fetal masculinization has been raised. It will be noted that in 16 of our cases in which 17-a-ethinyltestosterone was given and in 9 in which Norlutin was used, the mothers received in addition either diethylstilbestrol (Stilbestrol), conjugated equine estrogens (Premarin), or 17-a-hydroxyprogesterone caproate. In some cases the diethylstilbestrol was given in very large doses. These substances certainly did not prevent fetal masculinization. Bongiovanni and co-authors,[13] reported on four masculinized female infants whose mothers had received diethylstilbestrol in doses of 5 to 75 mg. per day. In a previous communication we [2b] reported on two cases in which the mothers had been given only progesterone intramuscularly, over short periods of time, in doses which did not seem excessive. In addition, we have now observed four masculinized female infants whose mothers had received no medication of any kind, and there are similar cases in the literature.

There is no evidence that masculinization of the fetus is due to a direct androgenic action of progesterone itself.[12] Jost [14] recently restudied purified progesterone and could demonstrate no androgenic activity. One may postulate, however, that mothers of masculinized infants who have received no treatment and those treated with progesterone may metabolize either endogenous or exogenous progesterone abnormally to form androgens, since progesterone may be a precursor of both androgens and corticosteroids. The mothers who received diethylstilbestrol alone may belong to this group of abnormal progesterone metabolizers. On the other hand, Bongiovanni and co-workers' [13] suggestion that diethylstilbestrol may stimulate the fetal adrenal to increase the output of androgens cannot be refuted. Further work needs to be done in this field.

Comment

I am not qualified to discuss the debatable efficacy of progestational steroids or estrogenic compounds in the prevention of abortions. If they are valuable and necessary, the ones which are least likely to cause fetal masculinization should be used. There is no excuse for giving a known androgenic steroid, such as methyltestosterone, even in small doses. There is no valid reason to blame the administration of progesterone, the natural hormone of pregnancy, for the masculinization of female infants, although occasionally there may be a mother who metabolizes progesterone abnormally. On the other hand, the synthetic progestins given orally are not natural hormones of the body and have weakly androgenic as well as progestational action. During the past year or two, Norlutin has caused fetal masculinization with sufficient frequency to preclude its use or advertisement as a safe hormone to be taken during pregnancy. Although the older compound 17-a-ethinyltestosterone has caused masculinization comparatively infrequently, it should also be considered potentially hazardous to the fetus.

It is most important for the obstetrician, pediatrician, and family physician to recognize that nonadrenal female pseudohermaphroditism does occur, especially when mothers have been treated with the orally given synthetic progestins under discussion. These infants can readily be mistaken for males. If they are raised as males, the physician will be greatly embarrassed when they feminize and menstruate at puberty. Whenever the external genitalia have an ambiguous appearance or when an infant appears to be a hypospadic male or even a normal male with impalpable testes, the possibility of female pseudohermaphroditism should be considered and excluded. The nuclear chromatin pattern of the buccal smear should be studied.[2a] If it is chromatin-positive, the urinary 17-ketosteroid levels should be measured, to determine whether or not virilizing adrenal hyperplasia is present. Nonadrenal female pseudohermaphrodites should always be raised as girls. One can reassure the parents that they will develop as normal girls and mature into normal, fertile women. No hormonal therapy is required. If there is no labioscrotal fusion, no surgical correction is necessary unless the

TABLE 3.—*Nonadrenal Masculinization of Female Infants*

	Number of Infants Masculinized				
Drug Given Mother	Studied by Wilkins	Studied by Others	Total	Daily Dose, Mg.	Mothers Virilized
Ethinyltestosterone	18	16	34	20-200	2
Norlutin	5	30	35	10-40	3
Enovid	0	1	1	10	1
Testosterone and known androgens	1	14*	15	3-10	+(?)
Progesterone (IM)	2	0	2	50-100(?)	...
Diethylstilbestrol	0	4†	4	5-75	...
None	4	6‡	10	...	2
Total :.................	30	71	101		

* Grumbach and Ducharme.[3]
† Bongiovanni and others.[13]
‡ Wilkins and others.[2b]

phallus is so large that its removal seems advisable for cosmetic or psychological reasons. Labioscrotal fusion, when present, should be corrected by an operation such as that described by Jones [15] in early infancy or certainly before the age of 2 or 3 years.

This study was supported by a grant from the National Institutes of Health, Bethesda, Md.

References

1. Wilkins, L.: Diagnosis and Treatment of Endocrine Disorders in Childhood and Adolescence, ed. 2, Springfield, Ill. Charles C Thomas, Publisher, 1957, chap. 16.

2. (*a*) Grumbach, M. M., and Barr, M. L.: Cytologic Tests of Chromosomal Sex in Relation to Sexual Abnormalities in Man, Recent Prog. Hormone Research **14**:255-334, 1958. (*b*) Wilkins, L.; Jones, H. W., Jr.; Holman, G. H.; and Stempfel, R. S., Jr.: Masculinization of Female Fetus Associated with Administration of Oral and Intramuscular Progestins During Gestation: Non-adrenal Female Pseudohermaphrodism, J. Clin. Endocrinol. **18**:559-585 (June) 1958.

3. Grumbach, M. M.; Ducharme, J. R.; and Moloshok, R. E.: On Fetal Masculinizing Action of Certain Oral Progestins, J. Clin. Endocrinol. **19**:1369-1380 (Nov.) 1959.

4. Moncrieff, A.: Non-adrenal Female Pseudohermaphroditism Associated with Hormonal Administration in Pregnancy, Lancet **2**:267-268 (Aug. 2) 1958.

5. Hayles, A. B., and Nolan, R. B.: Masculinization of Female Fetus, Possibly Related to Administration of Progesterone During Pregnancy: Report of Two Cases, Proc. Staff Meet. Mayo Clin. **33:**200-203 (April 16) 1958.

6. Reilly, W. A.; Hinman, F., Jr.; Pickering, D. E.; and Crane, J. T.: Phallic Urethra in Female Pseudohermaphroditism, A. M. A. J. Dis. Child. **95** (pt. 1)**:**9-17 (Jan.) 1958.

7. Jacobson, B. D.: Personal communication to the author.

8. (a) Wilkins, L.: Masculinization of Female Fetus Due to Use of Certain Synthetic Oral Progestins during Pregnancy, Arch. Anat. Microsc. et Morph. Exper., to be published. (b) Wilkins and Others.[2b] (c) Grumbach and others.[3]

9. Grumbach, M. M., and Ducharme, J. R.: Effects of Androgens on Fetal Sexual Development: Androgen-induced Female Pseudohermaphroditism, Fertil. & Steril., to be published.

10. Courrier, R., and Jost, A.: Intersexualité foetale provoquée par la Prégnèninolone au cours de la grossesse, Compt. rend. Soc. de biol. **136:**395-396 (June 13) 1942.

11. Jost, A.: Recherches sur la differenciation sexuelle de l'embryon de lapin: 2. Action des androgénes de synthese sur l'histogenèse genitale, Arch. Anat. Microsc. et Morph. Exper. **36:**242-270, 1947.

12. Revesz, C.; Chappel, C. I.; and Gaudry, R.: Masculinization of Female Fetuses in Rat by Progestational Compounds, Endocrinology **66:**140-143 (Jan.) 1960.

13. Bongiovanni, A. M.; DiGeorge, A. M.; and Grumbach, M. M.: Masculinization of Female Infant Associated with Estrogenic Therapy Alone During Gestation: Four Cases, J. Clin. Endocrinol. **19:**1004-1011 (Aug.) 1959.

14. Jost, A.: Personal communication to the author.

15. Jones, H. W., Jr., and Wilkins, L.: Genital Anomalies Associated with Prenatal Exposure to Progestogens, Fertil. & Steril., to be published.

From A. L. Herbst et al. (1971). N. Engl. J. Med., **284**, 878–881. *Copyright* (1971),
by kind permission of the authors and the Massachusetts Medical Society

ADENOCARCINOMA OF THE VAGINA*

Association of Maternal Stilbestrol Therapy with Tumor Appearance in Young Women

ARTHUR L. HERBST, M.D., HOWARD ULFELDER, M.D., AND DAVID C. POSKANZER, M.D.

Abstract Adenocarcinoma of the vagina in young women had been recorded rarely before the report of several cases treated at the Vincent Memorial Hospital between 1966 and 1969. The unusual occurrence of this tumor in eight patients born in New England hospitals between 1946 and 1951 led us to conduct a retrospective investigation in search of factors that might be associated with tumor appearance. Four matched controls were established for each patient; data were obtained by personal interview. Results show maternal bleeding during the current pregnancy and previous pregnancy loss were more common in the study group. Most significantly, seven of the eight mothers of patients with carcinoma had been treated with diethylstilbestrol started during the first trimester. None in the control group were so treated (p less than 0.00001). Maternal ingestion of stilbestrol during early pregnancy appears to have enhanced the risk of vaginal adenocarcinoma developing years later in the offspring exposed.

CANCER of the vagina is rare, occurring usually as epidermoid carcinoma in women over the age of 50 years.[1] Between 1966 and 1969, however, seven girls 15 to 22 years of age with adenocarcinoma of the vagina (clear-cell or endometrial type) were seen at the Vincent Memorial Hospital.[2] Although isolated case reports of histologically similar adenocarcinomas of the vagina had previously been published,[3-8] these carcinomas, too, were usually in older patients. No such case in the younger age group had been seen at this institution before 1966.

The tumor typically caused prolonged vaginal bleeding that, occurring in young women, was mistaken for anovulatory bleeding and delayed the correct diagnosis. Routine vaginal cytology was often negative, and the tumor was not palpated on rectal examination. The correct diagnosis was arrived at only after vaginal examination had been performed.

Histologically, one of the tumors resembled endometrial carcinoma, but the remainder were characterized by tubules and glands lined by clear cells containing glycogen or "hobnail" cells. The clear cells also appeared in solid nests. There was a high prevalence of benign adenosis of the vagina in this group of patients. Although these tumors with clear cells and hobnail cells have been termed "mesonephroma," there is evidence that they are of Müllerian origin.[2]

Because of the apparent clustering of these cases, which appeared within four years, attention was focused on possible other similarities among them. However, they did not uniformly use any intravaginal irritant, douches or tampon. Only one patient had had sexual exposure. Before the onset of the present illness, none had been given birth-control pills. We then decided to conduct a case-control, retrospective study that would compare in detail these patients and their families with an appropriate control group to uncover factors that might be associated with the sudden appearance of these tumors.

METHODS

Four matched controls for each patient with vaginal carcinoma were selected by examination of the birth records of the hospital in which each patient was born. Females born within five days and on the same type of service (ward or private) as the eight propositae were identified. Women who gave birth to daughters closest in time to each patient with carcinoma were first considered. Interviewing of all mothers was done from a standard questionnaire by personal interview carried out by a trained interviewer.

In addition to the seven cases cited above, an eighth identical case of clear-cell adenocarcinoma of the vagina occurred in 1969 in a 20-year-old patient, who was treated at another Boston hospital. † Because she and her family with their matched controls were as available as our own cases, this patient has been included with the original group, and these eight cases form the basis of this study.

Comparison of the data obtained from patients and controls was carried out with the use of the paired t-test for parametric data and the matched control method suggested by Pike and Morrow[9] for nonparametric data. Unpaired t-tests and chi-square tests with Yates correction were also carried out but were not significantly different from the results obtained with the paired methodologies.

RESULTS

Table 1 summarizes chronologic details of each patient with her therapy and results. The table demonstrates the clustering of patients for time of birth and occurrence of tumor. In Table 2 the data for seven pertinent areas of inquiry for each patient

*From the Vincent Memorial Hospital (Gynecological Service of the Massachusetts General Hospital) (address reprint requests to Dr. Herbst at the Vincent Memorial Hospital, Fruit St., Boston, Mass. 02114).

Supported by a grant (1393-C-1) from the American Cancer Society (Massachusetts Division), Inc.

†We are indebted to Dr. Donald P. Goldstein, of Boston, for permission to include his case in this study.

Table 1. Summary of Cases with Carcinoma.

CASE No.	AGE AT 1ST SYMPTOMS (YR)	YR OF BIRTH	YR OF TREATMENT	THERAPY	STATUS 1971
1	20	1949	1969	Posterior exenteration & vaginectomy	Living & well
2	15	1951	1967	Radical hysterectomy & vaginectomy, with vaginal replacement	Living & well
3	14	1950	1968	Exploratory laparotomy	Died (1968)
4	15	1950	1966	Wide local excision	Living & well
5	19	1949	1969	Radical hysterectomy & vaginectomy, with vaginal replacement	Living & well
6	16	1951	1967	Radical hysterectomy & vaginectomy, with vaginal replacement	Living & well
7	18	1949	1968	Anterior exenteration, with bowel substitution of vagina	Living & well
8	22	1946	1968	Anterior exenteration, with bowel substitution of vagina	Living & well

and her matched controls are displayed, including maternal age at the birth of the child, maternal smoking (at least 10 cigarettes per day before the birth of the child), bleeding during study pregnancy, any prior pregnancy loss, maternal estrogen therapy during study pregnancy, breast feeding of infant and intrauterine x-ray exposure.

There is a highly significant association between the treatment of the mothers with estrogen diethylstilbestrol during pregnancy and the subsequent development of adenocarcinoma of the vagina in their daughters (p less than 0.00001). Other factors found to be different between propositae and controls but at lower levels of significance are maternal bleeding in the study pregnancy (p less than 0.05) and any prior pregnancy loss (p less than 0.01). No significant differences between the populations were found for maternal age at time of birth of patient, smoking in parents, intrauterine x-ray exposure and breast feeding. Other topics covered in the questionnaire that also were not statistically significant are listed in Table 3.

All the mothers who took stilbestrol began therapy in the first trimester of pregnancy. They received either a constant dose administered throughout the pregnancy, or a continually increasing dose given almost to term. Six of the seven mothers volunteered the information that stilbestrol had been prescribed for them. The seventh was uncertain, but her obstetrician identified the drug as diethystilbestrol. Bleeding during this pregnancy or previous pregnancy loss (or both) led to the administration of stilbestrol in all seven cases. The programs of management for these pregnancies occasionally included vitamins, iron or calcium.

DISCUSSION

By the choice of a control group consisting of females born within five days of the birth of the propositae in the same hospital and on the same type of service, socioeconomic differences are reduced. Of the candidates for the control group found on hospital birth lists 25 per cent could not be located. A selection bias is therefore possible because only the families

Table 2. Summary of Data Comparing Patients with Matched Controls.

CASE No.	MATERNAL AGE (YR)		MATERNAL SMOKING		BLEEDING IN THIS PREGNANCY		ANY PRIOR PREGNANCY LOSS		ESTROGEN GIVEN IN THIS PREGNANCY		BREAST FEEDING		INTRA-UTERINE X-RAY EXPOSURE	
	CASE	MEAN OF 4 CONTROLS	CASE	CONTROL	CASE	CONTROL	CASE	CONTROL	CASE	CONTROL	CASE	CONTROL	CASE	CONTROL
1	25	32	Yes	2/4	No	0/4	Yes	1/4	Yes	0/4	No	0/4	No	1/4
2	30	30	Yes	3/4	No	0/4	Yes	1/4	Yes	0/4	No	1/4	No	0/4
3	22	31	Yes	1/4	Yes	0/4	No	1/4	Yes	0/4	Yes	0/4	No	0/4
4	33	30	Yes	3/4	Yes	0/4	Yes	0/4	Yes	0/4	Yes	2/4	No	0/4
5	22	27	Yes	3/4	No	1/4	No	1/4	No	0/4	No	0/4	No	0/4
6	21	29	Yes	3/4	Yes	0/4	Yes	0/4	Yes	0/4	No	0/4	No	1/4
7	30	27	No	3/4	No	0/4	Yes	1/4	Yes	0/4	Yes	0/4	No	1/4
8	26	28	Yes	3/4	No	0/4	Yes	0/4	Yes	0/4	No	0/4	Yes	1/4
Total			7/8	21/32	3/8	1/32	6/8	5/32	7/8	0/32	3/8	3/32	1/8	4/32
Mean	26.1	29.3												
Chi square (1 df)*			0.53		4.52		7.16		23.22		2.35		0	
p value			0.50		<0.05		<0.01		<0.00001		0.20			
	(N.S.)†		(N.S.)								(N.S.)		(N.S.)	

* Matched control chi-square test used as described by Pike & Morrow.⁹   † Standard error of difference 1.7 yr (paired t-test); N.S. = not statistically significant.

218

Table 3. Additional Factors Compared in Patients and Controls Not Found to Be Significantly Different.*

Birth weight
Age at onset of menses
Complications & outcome of study pregnancy
Ingestion of other medications during pregnancy
Childhood diseases of mothers & patients
History of tonsillectomy
Childhood ingestions
Household pets
Noteworthy illnesses of patients & parents
Cosmetic use in patients & mothers
Cigarette smoking in patients
Alcohol consumption in parents
Occupation & yr of education of parents

*Events compared before date of onset of present illness for each study patient & her matched controls.

remaining in the same area could be reached for comparison. However, all eight of the families of our patients are still living in or near the community where the patients were born. Control subjects still living in the community may be a more suitably matched study population. One potential control family was excluded because the birth record indicated that the offspring had Down's syndrome. It was necessary to locate only 34 women to obtain 32 control families who would collaborate with this study.

It should be emphasized that among the eight study mothers there was a total of 10 prior pregnancy losses and only six among the 32 controls. As can be seen from Table 2, bleeding during pregnancy was also more frequent in the study group. The fact that these were truly high-risk pregnancies was the indication for stilbestrol administration. The associations observed with bleeding in the study pregnancy and with previous pregnancy loss may reflect the characteristics of the population that was selected for estrogen treatment. In one of the eight mothers whose daughter had clear-cell adenocarcinoma, there was no evidence that estrogens were administered during pregnancy, nor had she experienced prior pregnancy loss or bleeding during the study pregnancy. Furthermore, these tumors were known to occur, though rarely, in women born before the availability of oral estrogens. Thus, factors other than maternal stilbestrol ingestion appear to be operative in their development. Moreover, the stilbestrol pills prescribed for these mothers were those available between 1946 and 1951. The ingredients of these tablets, the estrogenic potency of stilbestrol and its other chemical properties must all be recognized as possible elements in the association observed. Finally, among four of the eight families there are five female siblings, ranging in age from 18 to 22 years, who are also products of pregnancies during which their mothers took diethylstilbestrol. Up to the present, a vaginal tumor has not developed in any of these girls.

To try to estimate the frequency of stilbestrol administration and the risk of development of these tumors in female offspring whose mothers took stilbestrol during pregnancy, we have examined the files of one of the hospitals in this study for the years 1946 through 1951. During this interval there was a special high-risk pregnancy clinic at the Boston Lying-in Hospital in which stilbestrol was prescribed to 675 ward patients. There were approximately 14,500 ward deliveries, indicating that at that time roughly one in 21 ward patients at the Boston Lying-in Hospital were treated during pregnancy with stilbestrol. Thus, it appears to be well within the range of statistical expectation to have a control group in which the frequency of stilbestrol use was 0 in 32. In the interval 1946 to 1951 the private service at the Boston Lying-in Hospital had more deliveries than the ward service. We have knowledge of only one case of clear-cell adenocarcinoma developing in a patient born at the Boston Lying-in Hospital, and she was delivered on the private service. Whatever the risk of tumor development in the exposed offspring, it appears to be small.

The high concurrence of benign vaginal adenosis with these adenocarcinomas suggests that an anomaly of vaginal epithelial development may be a predisposing condition. Previous reports have described an association between adenosis and this tumor in older women,[3,8] and their concurrence in younger patients was initially noted in the present cases.[2] It may be that an increase in adenosis occurs at menarche in these patients and results in greater quantities of benign tissue at risk for malignant change. It is also possible that stilbestrol alters fetal vaginal cells in utero, with changes that do not become manifest in a malignant form until years later. Animal experiments as well as further follow-up data on patients who were exposed to estrogens in utero may provide some answers. Regardless of the ultimate explanation, histologic observations of associated adenosis combined with the known estrogenic effect of stilbestrol further support a Müllerian and not a mesonephric origin for these adenocarcinomas.

The time of birth of these patients (1946 to 1951) coincides with the beginning of the widespread use of estrogens in support of high-risk pregnancy.[10] It is likely that more patients with this tumor will appear as girls who were exposed in utero come to maturity. Furthermore, although our oldest patient was discovered at the age of 22 years, it is possible that these tumors will appear in even older women as the "at-risk" population matures. Although the chance of development of these tumors appears to be very small, the results of this study suggest that it is unwise to administer stilbestrol to women early in pregnancy. Furthermore, abnormal bleeding in adolescent girls can no longer be assumed to be due to anovulation, and the possibility of vaginal tumor should be excluded by a physician's examination.

We are indebted to Miss Jean Sheridan, who carried out the interviews and helped with analyses and preparation of the manuscript, to Dr. Theodore Colton, of the Department of Preventive Medicine, Harvard Medical School, for helpful suggestions with statistical analysis, to Dr. Robert E. Scully, of the Department of Pathology, Massachusetts General Hospital and Harvard Medical School, for assistance, and to the directors and record librarians of the participating hospitals for co-operation.

REFERENCES

1. Herbst AL, Green TH Jr, Ulfelder H: Primary carcinoma of the vagina: an analysis of 68 cases. Am J Obstet Gynecol 106:210-218, 1970
2. Herbst AL, Scully RE: Adenocarcinoma of the vagina in adolescence: a report of 7 cases including 6 clear-cell carcinomas (so-called mesonephromas). Cancer 25:745-757, 1970
3. Plaut A, Dreyfuss ML: Adenosis of vagina and its relation to primary adenocarcinoma of vagina. Surg Gynecol Obstet 71:756-765, 1940
4. Novak E, Woodruff JD, Novak ER: Probable mesonephric origin of certain female genital tumors. Am J Obstet Gynecol 68:1222-1242, 1954
5. Studdiford WE: Vaginal lesions of adenomatous origin. Am J Obstet Gynecol 73:641-656, 1957
6. Nix HG, Wright HL: Mesonephric adenocarcinoma of the vagina. Am J Obstet Gynecol 99:893-899, 1967
7. Droegemueller W, Makowski EL, Taylor ES: Vaginal mesonephric adenocarcinoma in two prepubertal children. Am J Dis Child 119:168-170, 1970
8. Sandberg EC, Danielson RW, Cauwet RW, et al: Adenosis vaginae. Am J Obstet Gynecol 93:209-222, 1965
9. Pike MC, Morrow RH: Statistical analysis of patient-control studies in epidemiology: factor under investigation an all-or-none variable. Br J Prev Soc Med 24:42-44, 1970
10. Smith OW: Diethylstilbestrol in the prevention and treatment of complications of pregnancy. Am J Obstet Gynecol 56:821-834, 1948

PAPERS 33, 34 AND 35

33. Janz, D. and Fuchs, U. (1964). Are anti-epileptics harmful in pregnancy? *Dtsch. Med. Wochenschr.*, **89**, 241–243. (Extract)
34. Meadow, S. R. (1968). Anticonvulsant drugs and congenital abnormalities. *Lancet*, **ii**, 1296
35. Meadow, S. R. (1970). Congenital abnormalities and anticonvulsant drugs. *Proc. R. Soc. Med.*, **63**, 48–49

COMMENTARY

As indicated by Janz and Fuchs (Paper 33), the number of married women with epilepsy has increased because of the advances made in the treatment of this illness. Alarmed by the thalidomide tragedy, the influence of antiepileptic drugs on pregnancy and on the fetus was examined in a retrospective study of 426 pregnancies, involving 246 epileptic mothers. There were a total of 358 live births, of which 225 were exposed to antiepileptic drugs. In five cases, congenital anomalies (cleft lip, cleft palate, cardiac defect, and torticollis) were detected; these infants were all born to mothers who had received treatment. The authors, however, concluded that the association between the occurrence of malformations and the maternal use of antiepileptic drugs was not significant.

In 1968, Meadow in a letter to the *Lancet* (Paper 34) reported six infants with malformations, born to epileptic mothers treated with anticonvulsant drugs. Severe cleft lip and cleft palate were present in all cases, and four also had congenital heart defect and minor skeletal anomalies. The suggestion was made that the congenital anomalies might have been caused by folic acid deficiency induced by the anticonvulsant drugs (see also Paper 25). At a meeting of the Royal Society of Medicine, convincing evidence was presented in support of the hypothesis that anticonvulsant drugs might be teratogenic (Paper 35). Because of the considerable clinical value of these substances, Meadow cautiously implored that all his findings 'prove nothing' but are 'sufficiently provocative to demand large scale investigation'.

During the past few years, such studies have been carried out and all evidence now seems to indicate that certain anticonvulsant drugs may indeed be teratogenic in humans (Speidel and Meadow, 1974; Zellweger, 1974; Annegers *et al.*, 1974). From a more recent survey of births (2403 children) in epileptic mothers, the overall incidence of malformations was found to be 5·4%. However, when mothers receiving anticonvulsants were compared to those not treated, the incidence of malformations was 6·0 and 1·4%, respectively. Thus, the risk of birth defects occurring in mothers receiving anticonvulsant drugs is about three times that of the general population (Smithells, 1976).

There has been some speculation as to the role of epilepsy itself in the aetiology of the birth defects (Speidel and Meadow, 1974; Smithells, 1976; Shapiro *et al.*, 1976). It has been suggested that the anomalies might be caused by both the illness and the anticonvulsant, rather than the treatment alone. Findings from two large studies (Finnish Register of Congenital Malformations and Collaborative Perinatal Project, USA) of epileptic mothers revealed that the increased risk of having a child with malformations might be related to the illness, rather than to the treatment. Furthermore, the malformation rates did not differ significantly with respect to the anticonvulsants used (Shapiro *et al.*, 1976).

When maternal anticonvulsant therapy is

strongly indicated, the benefits of the treatment to the mother against possible teratogenic effects on the embryo should be seriously considered. It is the opinion of many, that the health and welfare of the mother warrants greater priority even if there is a risk that the fetus might be damaged.

Of all types of anticonvulsants administered to epileptic mothers, diphenylhydantoin, phenobarbital, or a combination of both, were used in the majority of cases (Annegers *et al.*, 1974; Speidel and Meadow, 1974). It appears that diphenylhydantoin is far more teratogenic than phenobarbitone, but when used together increases further the teratogenic risk (Smithells, 1976).

The mechanism of action of anticonvulsant drugs during pregnancy is not known. Most of the suggestions made have implicated the inhibition of folic acid metabolism. The teratogenicity of certain folic antagonists has been demonstrated repeatedly in animal studies, and several well-documented cases of human malformations associated with the

use of these substances during pregnancy have been reported (Paper 25). There is, however, no real evidence to indicate that a similar mechanism may be involved in the case of the anticonvulsants (Speidel and Meadow, 1974; Annegers *et al.*, 1974).

REFERENCES

Annegers, J. F., Elveback, L. R., Hauser, W. A. and Kurland, L. T. (1974). Do anticonvulsants have a teratogenic effect? *Arch. Neurol.*, **31**, 364–373

Shapiro, S. *et al.* (1976). Anticonvulsants and parental epilepsy in the development of birth defects. *Lancet*, **i**, 272–275

Smithells, R. W. (1976). Environmental teratogens of man. *Br. Med. Bull.*, **32**, 27–33

Speidel, B. D. and Meadow, S. R. (1974). Epilepsy, anticonvulsants and congenital malformations. *Drugs*, **8**, 354–365

Zellweger, H. (1974). Anticonvulsants during pregnancy: a danger to the developing fetus. *Clin. Pediatr.*, **13**, 338–346

From D. Janz and U. Fuchs (1964). Dtsch. Med. Wochenschr., 89, 241–243. Copyright (1964), by kind permission of the authors and Georg Thieme Verlag, Stuttgart, Germany

Sonderdruck

DEUTSCHE MEDIZINISCHE WOCHENSCHRIFT

Schriftleitung: F. GROSSE-BROCKHOFF, DUSSELDORF / H. KRAUSS, FREIBURG/BR. W. v. BRUNN, TUBINGEN H. POSTHOFEN, STUTTGART / R. H. ROSIE, STUTTGART / K. KOBCKE, MUNCHEN. GEORG THIEME VERLAG, STUTTGART

89. Jahrgang — Stuttgart, 7. Februar 1964 — Nr. 6, Seite 241—243

From the Neurological Clinic of Heidelberg University
(Head: Prof. Dr. P. Vogel)

Are Anti-Epileptics Harmful in Pregnancy?

By D. Janz and U. Fuchs

Summary

Retrospective investigations were carried out in 246 mothers with a total of 426 pregnancies that went to term during epileptic diseases. Of these cases, 262 had been treated with anti-epileptics throughout, 130 had received no treatment, while in 34 the question of treatment could not be definitely answered. The results were as follows: In the group of treated mothers, there were 12.1% miscarriages or stillbirths, among the untreated the rate was 7%. The incidence of obstetric complications such as premature births, post-maturities and abnormal presentations was not above average either, and was about the same for treated as well as untreated mothers. In the treated group 5 (2·2%) malformations were observed (cleft lip three times, heart defect once, spastic torticollis once). There were no malformations of the extremities. A relationship with medication is unlikely since, despite continuous medication, the incidence of malformations is not significantly greater than the number of malformations to be expected on average.

DECEMBER 14, 1968   THE LANCET

Letters to the Editor

ANTICONVULSANT DRUGS AND CONGENITAL ABNORMALITIES

SIR,—I should be interested to know if your readers have seen babies with hare-lip, cleft palate, and certain other specific abnormalities born to mothers who receive regular anticonvulsant therapy.

Three years ago after encountering 3 such infants I contacted 48 mothers in the Brighton area who had children with hare-lip and cleft palate. None had epilepsy, and only 1 had had an anticonvulsant (phenobarbitone) during the pregnancy. However, recently I have seen 2 more babies with the abnormalities and have been informed of another, all born to epileptic mothers.

The 6 children seen have severe hare-lip and cleft palate. 4 are known to have other abnormalities, including congenital heart lesions and minor skeletal abnormalities. All have unusual facies and skulls which are not thought to be merely the result of the hare-lip and cleft palate. The features include: short neck and low posterior hair-line, broad nose-root with wide-spaced prominent eyes, and deformities of the pinna. The skulls have been of unusual shape—for instance, pointed in the frontal area with a prominent ridged suture line—or there have been minor bone defects.

The particular point of interest is that the same abnormalities have been reported following the unsuccessful abortifacient use of folic-acid antagonists in early pregnancy.[1] Deficiency of folic acid itself has been shown to cause cleft lip and palate in rats.

Folic-acid deficiency is relatively common in pregnancy, and anticonvulsant drugs, particularly primidone, are known to act as if antagonising folic acid. The epileptic mothers of these 6 children took combinations of the following drugs: primidone (5), phenytoin (5), troxidone (1), and phenobarbitone (5). One of the mothers was proved to be severely deficient of folic acid during the pregnancy.

It is easy therefore to postulate how anticonvulsants might be added to the list of factors that may cause hare-lip and cleft palate. However, before creating anxiety about useful drugs, it would be helpful to know if other people have encountered the association.

Department of Pædiatrics,
Guy's Hospital, London S.E.1.   S. R. MEADOW.

1. Milunsky, A., Graef, J. W., Gaynor, M. F. *J. Pediat.* 1968, **72,** 790.

From S. R. Meadow (1970). Proc. R. Soc. Med., **63**, 48–49. *Copyright* (1970), *by kind permission of the author and the Royal Society of Medicine*

Congenital Abnormalities and Anticonvulsant Drugs

by S R Meadow MRCP DCH
(*Department of Pædiatrics, Guy's Hospital, London*)

By chance, some babies with congenital abnormalities will be born each year to mothers who are being treated for epilepsy. However, after encountering six babies with cleft lip and palate who had epileptic mothers, the question arose whether factors other than chance might be operating. Of these six children, two had ventricular septal defects, and all had minor skull and facial abnormalities apart from the cleft lip and palate.

Similar abnormalities have been reported following the unsuccessful abortifacient use of aminopterin and methotrexate in early pregnancy (Milunsky *et al.* 1968). These two drugs are folic acid antagonists, and it is recognized that anticonvulsant drugs seem to act as if antagonizing folic acid in many patients, for instance in producing folic acid deficiency anæmia. Whether this action of anticonvulsants might harm the human fœtus is not known.

Therefore, a letter was written to the *Lancet* (Meadow 1968) asking for the details of babies with cleft lip and palate who had been born to mothers receiving anticonvulsant therapy.

Results

From the replies a list of 32 children with cleft lip and/or palate was compiled. Thirty-one had cleft lip and/or palate, only one had isolated cleft palate.

Their mothers had epilepsy, and about a quarter were known to have had a fit during the first three months of pregnancy. All the mothers took substantial doses of anticonvulsants throughout pregnancy, and all but two took a combination of two or more drugs. The drugs taken are shown in Table 1, and are much as would be anticipated. No single drug appears in an unexpected position in that table.

Seven families had two similarly affected children; there were four pairs of siblings, two pairs of monozygotic twins, and one pair of dizygotic twins.

Table 1
Drugs received by mothers of 32 children with cleft lip and palate

	No. of cases	Mean daily dose (mg)
Phenobarbitone	29	120
Phenytoin	19	350
Primidone	16	700
Troxidone	7	1,000
Other drugs	8	

Eleven of the 32 children had other major congenital abnormalities. Eight had a congenital heart lesion, which in seven was a ventricular septal defect. Four of these children had developed infundibular stenosis which had led to reversal of the intracardiac shunt and cyanosis.

Eleven had marked facial abnormalities. It is difficult to define the additional abnormalities of a face already marred by a cleft lip. Nevertheless, the doctors concerned considered there were abnormalities in addition to those associated with the cleft. There were two or more of the following: skull bone defects and trigonocephaly, short neck with low posterior hair line, broad nose root and hypertelorism, prominent eyes and low-set ears with deformities of the pinna. Because of the facial abnormalities, some had been transferred to special units for chromosome investigation, Patau's syndrome being suspected. The chromosome studies were normal.

Six of the children were known to have minor peripheral skeletal abnormalities.

Full details of all siblings were not available, but there were five siblings reported who had a major congenital abnormality with a normal lip and palate. Four had ventricular septal defects.

Discussion

Of the 32 cases reported, 20 children with cleft lip and/or palate were born in the five-year period 1964–68. One can estimate how many of these babies would be expected to be born to epileptic mothers by chance. Each year 850,000 mothers come to term in Britain. The number with epilepsy requiring substantial doses of anticonvulsants continuously is not known, but it is most unlikely to be more than 1 in 400. On that assumption 2,100 such mothers are delivered of babies each year. As the incidence of cleft lip and/or palate in Britain is 1·2 per 1000, 2·5 babies with that defect would be expected to be born to them each year.

For the last five years my list shows an average of 4 cases every year. The actual figure is certainly more, as my list was compiled merely from replies to a letter in a medical journal. It must be incomplete and is known to be so, for other cases have been notified to the Committee on Safety of Drugs.

Therefore, unless the number of epileptic mothers on substantial doses of anticonvulsant drugs is much greater than is thought, there have been born to those mothers in the last five years more children with cleft lip and palate than expected.

Other aspects of the cases reported are also suggestive. There is an apparently high incidence of congenital heart disease (25%) compared with the 3–5% found in other series of children with cleft lip and/or palate (Drillien *et al.* 1966). There is also an apparently high incidence of both cleft lip and/or palate and other congenital abnormalities in the siblings. These facts cannot be critically examined because of the way in which the information was collected. It may be that appeals to a correspondence column result in the most severe and multiple abnormalities being preferentially reported. As it is there is certainly a suggestion that several of the children had a syndrome of abnormalities involving the lip and palate, cardiovascular and skeletal systems.

All these facts prove nothing. They are merely suggestive, but the suggestion is sufficiently provocative to demand large scale investigation. The first step is to find out if there really is an increased incidence of cleft lip and/or palate in babies born to epileptic mothers. One small survey (Janz & Fuchs 1964) of 262 epileptic mothers receiving treatment reported three children with cleft lip and/or palate. If an increased incidence is found, the next step is to try to find if it is linked with the maternal disease or the drugs.

Anticonvulsant drugs cross the placenta well. Melchior *et al.* (1967) found phenobarbitone levels in the human umbilical cord to be 95% that of the maternal serum. This work was done on 32 pregnant mothers, and it is noteworthy that they produced two babies with cleft lip and/or palate.

Genetic factors are known to play a part in the etiology of cleft lip and/or palate: there is a positive family history in just over a third of cases (Fogh Anderson 1968). Any exogenous factors must act by the eighth week of fœtal life when the lip and palate are closed. It is during these early weeks that aminopterin and other folic acid antagonists have been shown to cause cleft lip and/or palate. Animal experiments are needed to find out if anticonvulsants predispose towards clefts in animals and if so whether the addition of folic acid prevents it.

It is important not to exaggerate the hypothesis that has been put forward. There is no proof: the information is merely suggestive. Anticonvulsant drugs are of immense value to the community and even if it were shown that anticonvulsant drugs were associated with an increased incidence of certain congenital abnormalities, it is likely that for the individual epileptic mother it would still be a small chance of such abnormality.

REFERENCES
Drillien C M, Ingram T T S & Wilkinson E M
(1966) The Causes and Natural History of Cleft Lip
and Palate. Edinburgh & London
Fogh Anderson C (1968) Cranio-facial Anomalies. Philadelphia
Janx D & Fuchs U (1964) *Dtsch. med. Wschr.* 89, 241
Meadow S R (1968) *Lancet* ii, 1296
Melchior J C, Svensmark O & Trollo D
(1967) *Lancet* ii, 860
Milunsky A, Graef J W & Gaynor M F
(1968) *J. Pediat.* 72, 790

6. Yaffe, S. J. (1975). A clinical look at the problem of drugs in pregnancy and their effect on the fetus. *Can. Med. Assoc. J.*, **112**, 728–731

COMMENTARY

Many reports have been published implicating a wide spectrum of drugs as possible teratogens in man, but only few are very well documented. Drugs which are definitely teratogenic in man include thalidomide, folic acid antagonists, sex steroids, anticonvulsants, and organic mercury; the evidence available for others is less convincing. Nevertheless, caution should be exercised in the indiscriminate use of all drugs during pregnancy, because our present understanding of developmental pharmacology and the mechanisms of malformations is extremely limited.

At this stage, it seems appropriate to review briefly other clinically important drugs with teratogenic potential, but less so than those previously discussed. This is the purpose of Paper 36.

Although there has been an increased awareness of the possible harmful effects of drugs on the human conceptus because of the thalidomide tragedy, drug consumption during pregnancy has increased considerably (Nelson and Forfar, 1971; Hill, 1973; Schenkel and Vorherr, 1974). What are the risks of inducing abnormal development when drugs are used by pregnant women? It would appear that there is no real 'safe period' during prenatal development. There is ample evidence now that the conceptus is vulnerable at all stages of gestation. It is, however, fully recognized that the most susceptible period is the first trimester, the period during which organogenesis is occurring. Nonetheless, after embryogenesis other more subtle changes, including functional disturbances, may be induced in the fetus (see Paper 38). These are problems also discussed by Yaffe in his excellent overview on clinically important drugs commonly used in pregnancy.

REFERENCES

Hill, R. M. (1973). Drugs ingested by pregnant women. *Clin. Pharmacol. Ther.*, **14**, 654–659

Nelson, M. M. and Forfar, J. O. (1971). Associations between drugs administered during pregnancy and congenital abnormalities of the fetus. *Br. Med. J.*, **1**, 523–527

Schenkel, B. and Vorherr, H. (1974). Non-prescription drugs during pregnancy: potential teratogenic and toxic effects upon embryo and fetus. *J. Reprod. Med.*, **12**, 27–45

From S. J. Yaffe (1975). Can. Med. Assoc. J., **112**, 728–731. *Copyright* (1975), *by kind permission of the author and the Canadian Medical Association*

A clinical look at the problem of drugs in pregnancy and their effect on the fetus

SUMNER J. YAFFE,* MD

Summary: The first annual W. E. Upjohn Lecture concerned itself with the interrelationship between administration of drugs to the pregnant woman and fetal outcome. The epidemiology of drug intake (both prescibed and self-administered drugs) during pregnancy is reviewed, using data derived from several surveys conducted both in the United States and in Scotland. The complexities of establishing a causal relationship between drug intake during pregnancy and effects upon the fetus are considered. Special emphasis is given to the adverse effects of aspirin and cigarette smoking. The shortage of data is critical and the need for further research is stressed.

Résumé: *Considération clinique sur le problème des médicaments pris durant la grossesse et leur effet sur le fétus*

La première conférence annuelle W. E. Upjohn s'intéressait à la relation existant entre l'administration de médicaments à la femme enceinte et leur effet sur le fétus. On y a passé en revue l'épidémiologie de la question des médicaments pris pendant la grossesse (tant ceux obtenus par ordonnance que les autres), utilisant à cet effet les renseignements provenant de plusieurs enquêtes, américaines et écossaises. On a admis qu'il s'agissait d'un problème complexe, rendant difficile l'établissement d'une relation de cause à effet. On y a souligné particulièrement les effets nocifs de l'aspirine et de l'usage de la cigarette. La pénurie de données sur le sujet atteint un point critique qui exigera de nouvelles recherches.

Presented at the 107th annual meeting of The Canadian Medical Association, June 28, 1974 as the first annual W. E. Upjohn Lecture

*Professor of pediatrics, State University of New York at Buffalo and Children's Hospital of Buffalo

Reprint requests to: Dr. Sumner J. Yaffe, Children's Hospital, Division of pharmacology, 219 Bryant St., Buffalo, NY 14222, USA

Drugs are an inescapable element in the environment of 20th-century man (and woman) and are likely to remain so in the foreseeable future. Contact with drugs begins before birth for our species in most advanced countries and the degree and variety of contact appear to be increasing. Up to now drugs have been used during pregnancy mainly to treat maternal disease. Under these circumstances it is evident that the fetus will also function as a drug recipient. Consequently, it is not surprising that such endeavours often produce unexpected and occasionally tragic results in the developing fetus for whom the drug was not intended in the first place.

Before 1961 most reports of drug effects on the fetus were concerned with the perinatal period, particularly with the effect of narcotics and analgesics on the fetus at the time of delivery. Thalidomide changed that and, if any positive action was derived from that disaster, it was that attention was focused on the possibility that other drugs less teratogenic than thalidomide had not yet been recognized as such. Until the thalidomide catastrophe there was not a great deal of interest in the subject and hence there had been little clinical research into the problem. We now know that any drug or chemical substance administered to the mother is able to penetrate the placenta to some extent unless it is destroyed or altered during passage. Placental transport of maternal substances to the fetus and of fetal substances to the mother is established at about the 5th week of embryonic life. Foreign substances cross the placenta, primarily by simple passive diffusion, to establish an equilibrium between the maternal and fetal blood, with the rate of passage primarily dependent upon the concentration gradient. The "placental barrier" is a myth and the use of this term should be discontinued.

Hence, administration of a drug to a pregnant woman presents a unique problem to the physician: not only must he consider maternal pharmacologic mechanisms, but also he must be constantly aware of the fetus as a potential recipient of the drug. When malformations observed in an infant at birth are apparently the result of drug administration during the first trimester the drug is considered to be a teratogen.

Drugs in early pregnancy

Experiments with laboratory animals have yielded considerable information regarding embryopathic effects of drugs but unfortunately these experimental findings cannot be extrapolated from species to species or even from strain to strain within the same species, much less from animals to man. For example, ordinary animal tests for teratogenicity would not have incriminated thalidomide (except in the rabbit) but would have incriminated aspirin, which is not known to be a human teratogen. It is also apparent that a single teratogen can produce a variety of malformations and conversely the same malformations can be caused by a variety of teratogens. Hence, because of the lack of specificity of both cause and effect, it is difficult to establish in man a relationship between events during pregnancy and malformations manifested after birth. It has been said that the teratogenic nature of thalidomide was recognized only because the drug produced a rare and rather specific combination of defects. If it had produced a more common type of defect, such as cleft palate or harelip, it probably would not have been suspected. It may well be that drug and chemical contacts during early intrauterine life are responsible for the defects in a number of all malformed infants.

The difficulties of ascertaining the relationship between drug administration and congenital malformations are compounded also by the fact that people in the Western world are unaware of their own drug and chemical exposures. Yet this would seem to be a first requirement in studying this problem.

Studies on drug use during pregnancy

Recently several investigators have tried to assess the number of drugs ingested by women during pregnancy.[1,2] From Table I the similarity in prevalence of consumption of various drugs during pregnancy between Scotland and the United States is quite apparent but there are some differences that reflect regional practice habits. In the Texas study the mean number of drugs consumed by the 156 women followed was 10.3;[1] in Scotland 97% of 911 mothers were prescribed drugs during pregnancy.[2] A third study, reported from California shortly after the thalidomide tragedy, demonstrated that drug consumption during pregnancy had not decreased.[3]

Preliminary analysis of the prospective collaborative study of 50 000 pregnancies conducted by the National Institutes of Health in the United States reveals that 900 pharmacologic compounds were used by mothers during pregnancy.[4] Table II lists the different drugs used during different stages of pregnancy. During early pregnancy bronchodilators and antihistamines are employed to control bronchospasm, a symptom more prominent at that time than in later pregnancy. The analgesics and barbiturates used in late pregnancy are most often prescribed for headaches and functional and emotional disturbances. Dyspeptic symptoms, treated with antacids, occur predominantly later in pregnancy, as does edema.

The duration of consumption of drugs during pregnancy and the timing of drug administration are important if one is to ascertain clinical effects upon the fetus. In the Scottish study two of every three mothers took aspirin in full dosage for 6 weeks during pregnancy. Barbiturates were the next most widely used single drug in terms of doses consumed per pregnancy. In fact the Scottish study demonstrated that every mother consumed one drug in normal daily dosage throughout 60% of her pregnancy.

Teratogenic drugs

Table III lists those drugs that have been classified as possibly teratogenic; that is, those that possibly will essentially affect the embryo during the first 3 months of pregnancy. The list is very short because no drug used in therapy has shown the same teratogenic potency as thalidomide. It should be emphasized again that it was only after nearly 4 years of extensive use that the profound teratogenic effects of that drug were recognized. Recognition was also made easier because the limb deficiencies that thalidomide caused were otherwise very rare abnormalities.

The powerful folic acid antagonists aminopterin and methotrexate are also abortifacients. If they fail as such, the liveborn infant who has been subject to their influence is very likely to be severely malformed. Given early in pregnancy, synthetic progestogens and androgens can cause masculinization of the female fetus. Progestational agents

given in large doses over prolonged periods of time, usually in the treatment of threatened abortion, account for the majority of cases, but the incidence of masculinization under these circumstances is probably less than 1%. A very delayed effect of diethylstilbestrol has been the occurrence of carcinoma of the vagina in female offspring 20 years after their mothers had received this drug during pregnancy.[5]

The remaining drugs on the list have been implicated in several case reports as responsible for the production of congenital malformations. With the exception of the powerful folic acid antagonists (in prolonged use) and thalidomide, for most of the drugs listed the evidence suggests no more than a slight increase in the risk of teratogenicity; the great majority of children born to mothers taking these drugs will be normal.

Drugs affecting fetal and neonatal function

Table IV is only a partial listing of drugs that have been identified as affecting the functioning of the fetus, usually late in pregnancy or at the time of delivery. The narcotics, inhalational and local anesthetics, and barbiturates in large doses may depress the fetus's central nervous system so that respiration is not adequately established. Addiction of the mother to morphine, heroin or alcohol may result in withdrawal symptoms such as hyperirritability, vomiting and shrill cry in the baby after delivery. Diazepam administered to the mother may result in hypothermia and hypotonia in the infant. Atropine may exert a sympathomimetic effect. Succinylcholine may result in a temporary ileus. Reserpine may cause nasal congestion associated with

Table I—Prevalence of drug consumption during pregnancy

Drug type	Study area	
	Scotland (%)	Texas (%)
Analgesic	63	64
Antihistamine	7	52
Diuretic	18	57
Antibiotic	16	41
Antacid	34	35
Sedative	28	24
Antiemetic	16	36
Iron	82	41

Table II—Drugs used during pregnancy

In early pregnancy	In late pregnancy	Throughout pregnancy
Antiemetics	Antacids	Antibiotics
Antihistamines	Analgesics	Cough medicines
Appetite suppressants	Barbiturates	Iron
Bronchodilators	Diuretics	Tranquillizers
Hormones	Hypnotics	
	Sulfonamides	
	Vitamins	

Table III—Possibly teratogenic drugs

Aminopterin	Aspirin
Methotrexate	Phenytoin
Progestogens	Dexamphetamine
Estrogens	Antacids
Androgens	Nicotinamide
Barbiturates	Iron
	Thalidomide

Table IV—Drugs affecting fetal and neonatal function

Morphine	Tetracyclines
Heroin	Streptomycin
Meperidine	Thiazide diuretics
Inhalation anesthetics	Warfarin
Local anesthetics	Dicumarol
Alcohol	Diphenylhydantoin
Barbiturates	Antithyroid drugs
Diazepam	Nitrofurantoin
Atropine	Chlorpropamide
Succinylcholine	Vitamin K
Reserpine	Smoking

excessive mucus production, lethargy and bradycardia.

Local anesthetics

Local anesthetics are the most widely used anesthetic agents in obstetrics. Their popularity can be attributed in part to the widespread belief that they have few depressant effects on the fetus and newborn. Shnider and Way,[6] however, have shown that lidocaine does cross the placenta and may cause CNS depression in the newborn. They determined the concentration of lidocaine in maternal arterial and fetal umbilical vein blood at the time of delivery, after multiple paracervical and pudendal injections of the anesthetic at varying times before delivery. The concentration in maternal blood tended to be higher than that in fetal blood, but more important was the actual concentration in fetal blood; CNS depression was observed in only 4 of the 23 infants in this series, each of whom had a blood lidocaine concentration of more than 2.5 μg/ml. It is also important to realize that any route of administration (caudal or lumbar, epidural, continuous epidural or paracervical block) will allow sufficient anesthetic agent to cross the placenta.

Teramo and Rajamäki[7] in Helsinki obtained frequent measurements of the concentration of mepivacaine in maternal and fetal blood and found that an equilibrium was established. They found, from serial measurements of acid-base balance, that paracervical blockade with amide-type local anesthetics tends to produce fetal bradycardia and acidosis. Although these changes are usually transient, perhaps we should take another look at the use of these drugs as routine anesthetic agents during labour.

Obstetric analgesics

The goal in obstetric analgesia is to provide pain relief for the mother without affecting the fetus or the delivery process. Meperidine, a synthetic substitute for opiates, has been hailed by many as the safest non-narcotic strong analgesic for both mother and infant. Nevertheless, a demonstrable depression of neonatal respiration and oxygen saturation has been noted. Both the time interval before the infant sustains his own respiration and the Apgar score appear to be related to the administration of the drug and more particularly with the time of administration. The peak depressive effect appears when the drug is administered 2 to 3 hours before birth. This delayed effect can be explained by the slow rate of passage of meperidine, not only across the placenta but also across the blood-brain barrier of the fetus.

It has been assumed from clinical observation that depression of the newborn from maternal meperidine is self-limited and of several hours' duration. This conclusion is based on the misapprehension that infant functioning can be adequately evaluated by such gross indices as respiratory function, muscle tone and motor activity. The use of more sophisticated measures of infant psychophysiologic functioning indicates that effects of the analgesic may be detected up to 30 days after delivery. The ability to respond to stimuli and the learned inhibition of response were significantly decreased in treated infants. The duration of these effects and their ultimate consequence for the child are not clear at present.

Aspirin

Aspirin is generally used freely throughout pregnancy. Although the activity of the mechanisms for its metabolism (glucuronide formation and coupling with glycine) is low in the fetus and newborn, and high concentrations of unaltered salicylate are found in cord blood immediately after delivery, overt toxic effects on the fetus and newborn have rarely been noted. This is perhaps related to the difficulties of surveillance of drug ingestion during pregnancy and also to the limited scope of our observation of adverse effects — two factors of tremendous importance.

Recently, a prospective study has been reported in which accurate prenatal drug histories were obtained in 42 pregnant women during the last 2 months of gestation and compared with clinical and laboratory studies performed post partum.[8] In 14 newborn infants whose mothers had taken more than 5 grains of aspirin during the week before delivery, there was significant evidence of platelet dysfunction and diminished factor XII (Hageman factor) in the cord blood. There was a significant difference between mean factor XII activity in the drug group (46%) and that in the control group (62%). A direct correlation was also observed between factor XII activity and the interval between the last ingestion of aspirin and birth. These findings occurred after ordinary doses of aspirin had been ingested by the mother as long as 2 weeks before delivery. There was a significant lack of platelet aggregation in both newborn and mother when aspirin had been ingested and this was also related to the time of administration of aspirin; no such lack was detected when the aspirin had been ingested more than 2 weeks before delivery. Diminished factor XII activity is of uncertain clinical importance since bleeding in patients with a Hageman

trait is unusual. Aspirin-induced platelet dysfunction, however, may have clinical relevance, particularly during difficult traumatic deliveries. Hemorrhagic phenomena in this series were noted at birth in 3 of the 14 aspirin-exposed newborn. One newborn had transient gastrointestinal tract bleeding (guaiac-positive stools), another had a cephalohematoma and the third had bilateral periorbital purpura. The bleeding in each case resolved spontaneously without residual morbidity. It would appear prudent to avoid aspirin during the week before delivery until the clinical significance of these findings is further evaluated.

As far as drug surveillance during pregnancy is concerned, aspirin also affords another excellent illustrative example. In a series of 272 consecutively delivered infants at the University of Alabama Medical Center in Birmingham, Palmisano and Cassady[9] determined the concentration of salicylate in cord serum. After delivery several women were asked whether or not they had taken aspirin before labor and delivery. The answer was uniformly negative, yet 9.5% of the infants had significant concentrations of salicylate ($>$ 1 mg/dl) in cord blood. When the investigators rephrased their question and asked about the intake of specific proprietary products the truth came out. This points out the difficulties one encounters in eliciting an obstetric drug history. It has been suggested that, instead of asking about the ingestion of certain drugs by generic name, terms be employed that the pregnant woman will understand, for example "pain medication" for headache and arthritis, "heart medicine", "water pills" for diuretics, "blood pressure medicine" for antihypertensives and "blood thinner" for anticoagulants.

Smoking

It is now universally agreed that cigarette smoking during pregnancy affects fetal development. Many investigators have demonstrated that smokers produce smaller babies, have a greater incidence of premature delivery and an increased incidence of abortion, stillbirth and neonatal death. Opinions vary as to the exact meaning of these observations and doubts have been cast on their validity because of inevitable differences of social class and background. However, these factors have been taken into consideration in prospective studies and it is quite evident that the clinical findings can be justifiably attributed to the smoking. Furthermore, there are a number of animal experiments that have indicated nicotine to be the principal toxic product in tobacco.[10] Unfortunately, the doses that have to be employed are much greater than those attained during smoking in man. Nicotine's action in this instance is probably via its effect on blood supply to the fetus.

More recent studies have correlated the smoking habits of a group of pregnant women with the level of carboxyhemoglobin in the circulating blood.[11] Furthermore, when simultaneous estimates of maternal and fetal carboxyhemoglobin levels were made at delivery the fetal levels were on the average 1.8 times higher than the respective maternal level. Carboxyhemoglobin is a stable compound formed when carbon monoxide combines with a portion of hemoglobin. The total oxygen-carrying capacity of both maternal and fetal blood is thereby reduced. In addition, the oxygen dissociation of the remaining active oxyhemoglobin is impaired by the presence of carbon monoxide, so that less oxygen is available to the tissues. Fetal blood normally requires a tissue oxygen tension of about 18 mm Hg to provide an oxygen saturation of 35%, whereas blood containing carboxyhemoglobin requires a much lower tension to deliver a similar quantity of oxygen to the tissues. Also, maternal arterial oxygen tension is reduced by a direct effect of carbon monoxide on the pulmonary vasculature. These factors must certainly contribute to the low birth weight and other reported consequences of smoking during pregnancy.

The dilemma

What is the solution to the dilemma the physician faces? How can he advise his pregnant patient as to whether any particular drug is likely to be dangerous to her fetus? Certainly animal tests are not predictive and cannot protect the patient, particularly in a society that consumes medication en masse upon the insistence of the TV screen rather than upon physician prescription. Labels on medicines warning the doctor and his patient that the enclosed pills are "not to be taken during pregnancy" will do no good. The chief source of protection lies in an understanding by the obstetrician of his role as the pediatrician of the unborn. In this situation he must lead the crusade for a widespread acceptance of a sensible attitude towards drug consumption during pregnancy. This period can be rendered safe only by practising therapeutic nihilism for all women between the ages of 14 and 40. In view of the fact that most people in our contemporary society (as well as their physicians) seem to regard life as a drug-deficient disease, to be cured or even endured only with the aid of innumerable medications, this will be a slow and difficult crusade. We must also keep in mind that with the advent of intrauterine diagnosis the need for prescription of drugs to the pregnant woman for the treatment of her fetus is already at hand. We must acquire sufficient data from human studies to make fetal therapeutics as founded upon fact as is therapeutics in the adult organism. This requires more research into, and a greater understanding of, the disposition of drugs within the maternal–fetal–placental unit and the effects of drugs upon the fetus. Furthermore, this information can be gained only from studies in pregnant women and at this time the social and political climate is decidedly against fetal research.

It has been estimated[12] that 75 to 85% of all therapeutic agents are not approved for use in infants, children and pregnant women because conclusive evidence of their safety and efficacy in this population is not available, but many are administered in ignorance with potential hazard to the patient. Resolution of this vexing problem will be achieved only if fundamental and clinical investigative activities in the area of obstetric and pediatric pharmacology are expanded in many directions.

References

1. HILL RM: Drugs ingested by pregnant women. *Clin Pharmacol Ther* 14: 654, 1973
2. FORFAR JO, NELSON MM: Epidemiology of drugs taken by pregnant women: drugs that may effect the fetus adversely. Ibid, p 632
3. YERUSHALMY J, MILKOVICH L: Evaluation of the teratogenic effect of meclizine in man. *Am J Obstet Gynecol* 93: 553, 1965
4. SLONE D, HEINONEN OP, MONSON RR, et al: Maternal drug exposure and fetal abnormalities. *Clin Pharmacol Ther* 14: 648, 1973
5. HERBST AL, ULFELDER H, POSKANZER DC: Adenocarcinoma of the vagina: association of maternal stilbesterol therapy with tumor appearance in young women. *N Engl J Med* 284: 878, 1971
6. SHNIDER SM, WAY EL: Plasma levels of lidocaine (Xylocaine®) in mother and newborn following obstetrical conduction anesthesia. *Anesthesiology* 29: 951, 1968
7. TERAMO K, RAJAMAKI A: Foetal and maternal plasma levels of mepivacaine and foetal acid-base balance and heart rate after paracervical block during labour. *Br J Anaesth* 43: 300, 1971
8. BLEYER WA, BRECKENRIDGE RT: Studies on the detection of adverse reactions in the newborn. *JAMA* 213: 2049, 1970
9. PALMISANO PA, CASSADY G: Salicylate exposure in the perinate. *JAMA* 209: 556, 1969
10. BECKER RF, LITTLE CRD, KING JE: Experimental studies on nicotine absorption in rats during pregnancy. *Am J Obstet Gynecol* 100: 957, 1968
11. COLE PV, HAWKINS LH, ROBERTS D: Smoking during pregnancy and its effects on the fetus. *J Obstet Gynaecol Br Commonw* 79: 782, 1972
12. EDWARDS CC JR (Commissioner of the FDA): Address to the 1972 annual meeting of the American Academy of Pediatrics, New York, NY

PAPERS 37 AND 38

37. Amin-Zaki, L., Elhassani, S., Majeed, M. A., Clarkson, T. W., Doherty, R. A. and Greenwood, M. (1974). Intra-uterine methylmercury poisoning in Iraq. *Pediatrics*, **54**, 587–595
38. Spyker, J. M. (1975). Assessing the impact of low level chemicals on development: behavioral and latent effects. *Fed. Proc.*, **34**, 1835–1844

COMMENTARY

Methylmercury is a major environmental pollutant and its toxic effects are well documented. During the past decade, several outbreaks of mercury poisoning have occurred (Shephard, 1976). There is now ample evidence that organic mercury can also harm the fetus *in utero*. The Minamata tragedy provided the first real observations. Children with mental retardation and severe neurological deficits, not unlike cerebral palsy, were born to mothers who had eaten fish and shell-fish contaminated with high levels of methylmercury. The condition was diagnosed as congenital (fetal) Minamata disease and attributed to the transplacental passage of mercury. Forty such cases were recorded by the end of 1974 (Harada, 1975).

Other reports have now confirmed the observations made in Minamata regarding the fetal toxicity of methylmercury. The paper by Amin-Zaki and his colleagues describes 15 cases (infant–mother pairs) of fetal intoxication with organic mercury. This occurred during a severe epidemic of mercury poisoning caused by ingestion of home-made bread made from wheat treated with methylmercury fungicide. In all cases except one, the blood mercury levels were higher in the infants than in the mothers, but congenital malformations were not present. In five infants, there were signs of 'gross impairment of motor and mental development, with cerebral palsy, deafness and blindness in four'. Methylmercury also produced fetotoxic effects during the last trimester of pregnancy and was readily transferred from the mother to the infant via maternal milk.

In contrast to gross anomalies which are recognizable at birth, functional and behavioural disturbances are not readily evident. Special toxicity tests and other parameters of evaluation are often required for the detection of such latent and subtle effects in the newborn. The concept of teratogenesis has now rightly been expanded to include these functional disturbances and behavioural deficits as latent teratological responses manifesting themselves during the postnatal period. The comprehensive review by Spyker (Paper 38) deals with several important aspects of this problem.

REFERENCES

Harada, M. (1975). Minamata disease. Chronology and medical report. In W. E. Smith and A. M. Smith (eds.). *Minamata*, pp. 51–71. (New York: Holt, Rinehart and Winston, Inc.)
Shephard, D. A. E. (1976). Methylmercury poisoning in Canada. *Can. Med. Assoc. J.*, **114**, 463–472

From L. Amin-Zaki et al. (1974). Pediatrics, **54**, 587–595. *Copyright* (1974), *by kind permission of the authors and the American Academy of Pediatrics*

Intra-uterine Methylmercury Poisoning in Iraq

Laman Amin-Zaki, M.D., Sami Elhassani, M.D., Mohamed A. Majeed, M.D., Thomas W. Clarkson, Ph.D., Richard A. Doherty, M.D., *and* Michael Greenwood, B.S.

From the University of Baghdad, Baghdad, Iraq, and the University of Rochester School of Medicine, Rochester, New York

ABSTRACT. A disastrous epidemic of methylmercury poisoning occurred in rural Iraq early in 1972, due to the ingestion of home-made bread prepared from wheat treated with a methylmercury fungicide. We report the clinical and laboratory evaluation of 15 infant-mother pairs exposed to methylmercury during pregnancy, including mercury determinations in blood samples of mothers and infants, and in milk samples from mothers, during the first seven months following the epidemic.

In all cases except one, the infants' blood mercury levels were higher than their mothers' during the first four months after birth. Our results indicate that methylmercury passes readily from mother to fetus and that neonatal blood mercury levels are maintained through ingestion of mercury in mothers' milk.

Clinical manifestations of methylmercury poisoning were evident in six of 15 mothers and in at least six of 15 infants. In five severely affected infants there was gross impairment of motor and mental development. However, in only one infant-mother pair was the infant affected and the mother free of signs and symptoms—a marked contrast to the reports of Japanese mother-infant pairs from Minamata.

Careful follow-up studies of these and other Iraqi infants will determined where signs and symptoms of methylmercury poisoning will appear as these children continue to develop. Studies of these and additional infant-mother pairs may allow determination of the prenatal period of greatest fetal sensitivity to methylmercury poisoning. *Pediatrics* 54:587, 1974, METHYLMERCURY POISONING, INTRA-UTERINE MERCURY POISONING, FETAL MERCURY POISONING, PLACENTAL MERCURY TRANSFER. CEREBRAL PALSY, MILK MERCURY.

Retrospective studies of Japanese poisonings have established the occurrence of fetal poisoning and provided data which suggest that the fetus is more sensitive than the mother to toxic effects of methylmercury.[1,2] The majority of the mothers showed no toxic signs during pregnancy, yet their offspring were markedly affected when observed postnatally. It has also been shown that methylmercury is fetotoxic in nonhuman mammalian species (for a review, see Clegg[3]). Recently, behavioral abnormalities have been observed in mice exposed prenatally to doses of methylmercury which had no apparent effect on their mothers.[4]

The sources and uses of mercury have recently been reviewed by Wallace *et al.*[5] Methylmercury compounds have found their principal use as anti-fungal-seed-dressing agents. General contamination of terrestrial animals has been noted in countries where methylmercury fungicides are used. Community poisoning in Iraq,[6] Pakistan[7] and Guatemala[8] have been reported from the misuse of seed grain treated with methylmercury or ethylmercury fungicides. The outbreak in Japan from the consumption of contaminated fish has been ascribed to the release of methylmercury as a waste product from industrial plants using mercury as a catalyst for the manufacture of acetaldehyde and vinyl chloride. The finding that all the mercury in fish muscle from species caught in both fresh and oceanic waters was in the form of methylmercury indicated a more widespread source. One source is the microbial conversion of other forms of mercury to methylmercury in sediments of lakes and rivers and possibly also in the oceans. Thus, all major sources of mercury ultimately entering water in whatever form are potential precursors to methylmercury. These sources would include natural sources from the land mass itself, from geothermal processes and from man-made sources such as chlorine-alkali plants using mercury as an electrode, as well as smelting and the burning of fossil fuels. The accu-

(Received September 4, 1973; revision accepted for publication April 8, 1974.)
ADDRESS FOR REPRINTS: (T.W.C.) Department of Radiation Biology and Biophysics, University of Rochester School of Medicine, Rochester, New York 14642.

234

mulation of methylmercury in swordfish reached levels well above the guideline of 0.5 parts per million imposed by the Food and Drug Administration.

An opportunity to study the effects of prenatal exposure to methylmercury occurred during a recent large epidemic of methylmercury poisoning in Iraq, resulting from ingestion of home-made bread prepared from wheat treated with a methylmercury fungicide.[10] Body content of mercury would be expected to rise to a maximum at the end of approximately a two-month period of consumption (Fig. 1). Thereafter, it should undergo an exponential decline to preexposure values at the end of one year, assuming a biologic half-time in the adult human of 70 days.[9] Thus, possibilities existed for prenatal fetal exposure, and for postnatal exposure of suckling infants due to transmission of methylmercury in their mothers' milk. Infants born during the 12-month period immediately prior to the epidemic could have received methylmercury from maternal milk ingestion. Infants approximately 12 to 18 months of age at the time of the epidemic might have also ingested methylmercury in contaminated bread. Many categories of prenatal exposure were also possible. Without going into detail, it is clear that those infants born during and shortly after maternal consumption of contaminated bread received maximum exposure late in gestation and had a relatively large postnatal intake from milk. Infants born six to nine months after maternal consumption of

methylmercury were maximally exposed early in pregnancy and received minimal intake from milk ingestion.

Isotope studies in human volunteers have shown that the blood mercury concentration is proportional to total body mercury.[11] Samples of maternal blood collected during pregnancy and of infant blood collected at birth and subsequently should provide the most direct index for prenatal and postnatal exposure.

This report is based on clinical examinations and on mercury determinations in blood samples of mothers and infants, and in milk samples from mothers, during the first seven months following the epidemic. All infants were exposed prenatally.

METHODS
Sampling and Analysis for Mercury

Blood and milk samples were collected from hospitalized patients in Baghdad and from individuals in rural farms and in villages within a radius of 100 kilometers from Baghdad. Milk samples were expressed by hand and refrigerated or frozen until assayed. Blood samples were collected with dried heparin to prevent coagulation and were refrigerated. All mercury assays on unfrozen milk or blood samples were completed within 48 hours. Total and inorganic mercury were determined in blood and milk by selective atomic absorption.[12]

Clinical Examinations

Standard clinical neurological tests were used to evaluate mothers and babies approximately every 15 days. The milestones of development of the babies were evaluated according to Gesell's developmental screening tests. Observations made in the first examination are reported in this paper.

Fifteen infant-mother pairs are subjects of these preliminary observations. The first examination took place on March 6, 1972, and the last new infant-mother pair was examined for the first time on November 14, 1972. Thus, the observations to be reported took place within a period ranging from approximately one month after cessation of consumption of the contaminated bread to 11 months later (Fig. 1). Some of the infant-mother pairs were studied in hospitals; others were visited in their rural homes and examined there. In general, at least one blood sample was collected from the mother and the infant, and in some cases blood mercury levels were followed for a period of many months. The recording of blood levels of mercury after the end of 1972 is of little value, since blood mercury concentrations would have fallen to virtually normal background levels by this time. With the exception of one infant-mother pair, all

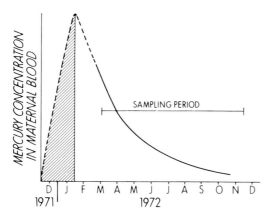

FIG. 1. A diagrammatic representation of the levels of mercury in mothers' blood during and after consumption of contaminated bread. The period over which blood and milk samples were collected from the mothers, and blood samples from the infants, was March 6, 1972, to November 14, 1972. The shaded area is the period of exposure, and the broken line is the estimated presampling blood levels.

the examinations and blood collections were carried out between March and August 1972.

RESULTS

The signs and symptoms of methylmercury poisoning in the mothers are indicated in Tables I and II. Six of 15 mothers showed one or more clinical manifestations of methylmercury toxicity. The most frequent symptoms were malaise (a feeling of general bodily discomfort without clear signs of a particular illness), vague muscle and joint pains and loss of sensation in the perioral region and in the extremities (glove and sock areas). Motor weakness and exaggerated reflexes were observed in five cases. Visual changes (constricted fields, blurred vision, dimness) were also reported with high frequency. Ataxia, auditory changes and dysarthria were not very frequent. One woman (MK46) who had a severely affected infant refused medical examination but claimed to be quite well.

The clinical manifestations observed during the first examination of the 15 infants are listed in Table IV. Five of 15 infants exhibited fairly severe clinical manifestations of methylmercury poisoning, and one had exaggerated reflexes in the lower extremities but seemed normal otherwise. An exhaustive evaluation of the infants is not possible at this time, but the main findings are listed below.

Pregnancy. All the infants were born at full term. One woman gave a history of repeated hemorrhage per vaginum during the third month, but her baby seemed to be normal.

Delivery. In five cases, all of them multiparous, there was a history of an unduly prolonged labor in women who had had easier deliveries before.

Sex and age. There were eight male and seven female infants in this series. The youngest baby was examined at the age of 6 days, and the oldest at the age of 6.5 months. Eleven of the infants were examined at an age below 2 months, and of these eight were below 1 month at the time of first examination.

Feeding. All the babies were breast-fed and the mothers insisted on breast-feeding even when they were advised against it in hospitalized cases.

Early neonatal period. There was no difficulty in sucking and swallowing in any of the infants. There was no cyanosis, jaundice, fever, or convulsions in these 15 babies. The five severely affected infants were noted to be "sick" by their families at an early age.

Congenital malformations. No congenital anomalies were seen in any of the cases.

Anthropometric measurements. WEIGHT AND LENGTH: These measurements do not seem to be very much deviated from the normal during the

TABLE I
CLINICAL MANIFESTATIONS IN MOTHERS°

Clinical Manifestation	No. of Mothers	
Early symptoms	6	
Headache		4
Malaise		6
Insomnia		2
Joint and muscle pain	6	
Sensory changes	5	
Limbs (glove and sock regions)		5
Perioral		5
Motor weakness	5	
Increased deep tendon reflexes	5	
Visual changes	4	
Blurring		4
Constricted visual fields		4
Ataxia	3	
Speech changes	1	
Hearing	2	
Tremor of extremities	1	
Mental changes	1	
Gastrointestinal tract symptoms (abdominal pain)	1	

°One mother refused to be examined and claimed to be well.

neonatal period. The weight of older infants seems to be more affected.

HEAD CIRCUMFERENCE: Three of the infants with severe clinical manifestations had a head circumference which was below the third percentile for their age, according to the standards of Harvard School of Public Health for white children in Boston.

EXCESSIVE CRYING: Fretfulness, irritability and excessive crying, especially in the evening, were present in 6 infants.

Sight. Four babies were completely blind and one had reaction to light, but seemed to have impaired vision. Nystagmus was seen in one infant and strabismus in two. The corneal and conjunctival reflexes were normal. The reaction of the pupils to light was absent in two cases.

FUNDOSCOPY: Fundi were examined by us and by an ophthalmologist in the hospitalized cases only. Of three cases, two infants seemed to have normal fundi. One infant who was severely affected and who was blind had retinae that looked paler than normal with generalized narrowing of the retinal blood vessels. His optic disks appeared normal.

Hearing. Four infants were found to have a severely impaired hearing, while the rest reacted to sudden noise.

Muscle tone. Increased muscle tone was found

TABLE II

OBSERVATIONS ON INFANT-MOTHER PAIRS IN WHICH THE INFANT HAD BEEN PRENATALLY EXPOSED TO METHYL-MERCURY (MOTHER)

Pair No.	Ser. No.	Date of First Examination (mo/day/yr)	Blood Total Hg (ppb)	Signs and Symptoms°
1	MC30	3/ 6/72	2390	1, 2, 3, 4, 5, 6, 7, 8, 9, 10, 11
2	MC101	4/11/72	1505	2, 3
3	SP38	4/11/72	1083	1, 2, 3, 4, 5, 6
4	SP82	4/18/72	40	None
5	SP59	5/ 9/72	97	None
6	SP96	6/ 1/72	253	None
7	SP73	6/ 1/72	416	1, 2, 3, 4, 5, 9
8	SP61	6/ 1/72	187	None
9	MC144	7/15/72	602	1, 2, 3, 4, 5, 6, 7, 9, 12
10	MK23	7/25/72	170	None
11	MK17	8/ 1/72	5	None
12	MK46	8/ 6/72	173	—⁺
13	MK63	8/ 7/72	300	1, 2, 4, 5, 6, 7
14	MK65	8/ 8/72	180	None
15	MK27	11/14/72	37	None

°See Table I.
⁺Refused examination but clamied to be well.

in three infants, one of them with severe opisthotonus. Two infants had decreased muscle tone.

Muscle power. Four infants had severe generalized paralysis, and one infant had reduced motor power.

Tendon reflexes. Five infants had hyperactive reflexes in the 4 limbs; one infant had brisk knee jerks only but had no other clinical manifestations.

BABINSKI'S REFLEX: When the foot was stroked from toe to heel, 12 children gave an extensor response. This is a finding frequently seen in the normal neonates as well.

ABDOMINAL AND CREMASTERIC REFLEXES: The abdominal reflexes were absent in two infants, and the cremasteric reflex was absent in three of eight male infants.

SENSATIONS: Response to pin prick was present in all the infants, but other sensations could not be evaluated.

MENTALITY: The mental power seemed to be severely affected in four infants.

The lowest concentration of mercury in an initial blood sample associated with maternal signs and symptoms of poisoning was 300 parts per billion (ppb), recorded on August 7, 1972 (Table II). The next higher level was 416 on June, 1, 1972. Allowing for differences in time of collection, maternal exposures projected from these two values would be more or less equivalent, assuming a clearance half-time of 70 days. All mothers who had measured blood levels in excess of 400 ppb exhibited signs and symptoms of poisoning. Eight mothers had recorded blood levels in the range 5 to 253 ppb without signs or symptoms of poisoning.

Those infants having blood levels in excess of 3,000 ppb, when sampled and examined in March and April of 1972, were severely affected (MC42, MC104, SP41; Tables III and IV). One infant having a blood level of 1,053 ppb when examined on

TABLE III

OBSERVATIONS ON INFANT-MOTHER PAIRS IN WHICH THE INFANT HAD BEEN PRENATALLY EXPOSED TO METHYLMERCURY (INFANT)

Pair No.	Ser. No.	Sex	Date of Birth (mo/day/yr)	Date of First Examination	Trimester of Start of Exposure	Blood Total Hg (ppb)	Signs and Symptoms
1	MC42	M	1/ 6/72	3/ 6/72	3	4220	Yes
2	MC104	F	2/11/72	4/11/72	3	3190	Yes
3	SP41	M	2/11/72	4/11/72	3	3190	Yes
4	SP85	F	2/18/72	4/18/72	3	200	No
5	SP60	M	2/ 1/72	5/ 9/72	3	162	N.A.
6	SP97	F	5/ 1/72	6/ 1/72	2	387	No
7	SP74	M	4/16/72	6/ 1/72	2	636	No
8	SP87	M	5/20/72	6/ 1/72	2	122	No
9	MC143	F	1/ 1/72	7/15/72	3	476	No
10	MK24	M	7/19/72	7/25/72	1	284	No
11	MK25	M	7/ 7/72	8/ 1/72	1	N.A.	No
12	MK47	M	1/ 7/72	8/ 6/72	3	1053	Yes
13	MK64	F	2/20/72	8/ 7/72	2	18	No
14	MK66	F	7/23/72	8/ 8/72	1	564	Yes
15	MK180	F	10/24/72	11/14/72	1	290	No

TABLE IV

CLINICAL MANIFESTATIONS IN INFANTS PRENATALLY EXPOSED TO METHYLMERCURY[*]

Ser. No.	Age at Exam (days)	Weight (lb)	Length (cm)	Head Circumference (cm)	Primitive Reflexes Moro; Grasp; Tonic Neck; Rooting	Babinski Reflex	Motor System Tone	Motor System Paralysis	Opisthotonus	Hearing	Sight	Nystagmus	Strabismus	Irritability; Excessive Crying
MC42	17	8	48	35	—	+	↑	sp.	+	↓	—	+	—	+
MC104	56	12	51	36	—	+	↑	sp.	—	↓	—	—	+	+
SP41	60	8	50	35.5	—	+	↑	sp.	+	↓	—	—	+	—
SP85	50	7.5	58	39	—	+	nor.	—	—	+	+	—	—	—
SP60	165	15	64	43	—	+	nor.	—	—	+	+	—	—	—
SP97	30	8.75	55	39	nor.	+	nor.	—	—	+	+	—	—	+
SP74	20	7.4	52	35	nor.	+	nor.	—	—	+	+	—	—	—
SP87	10	9	56	36	nor.	+	nor.	—	—	+	+	—	—	—
MC143	195	17	66	45	—	—	nor.	—	—	+	+	—	—	—
MK24	6	7	53	37	nor.	+	nor.	—	—	+	+	—	—	—
MK25	23	N.A.	N.A.	N.A.	nor.	+	nor.	—	—	+	+	—	—	+
MK47	210	10.5	60	38.5	—	+	↓	fl.	—	↓	—	—	—	+
MK64	135	15.25	67	43	—	—	nor.	—	—	+	+	—	—	—
MK66	15	8.5	56	36.5	nor.	+	↓	fl.	—	+	±	—	—	+
MK180	20	8	54	34	nor.	—	nor.	—	—	+	+	—	—	—

[*]*Abbreviations:* N.A. = not available; nor. = normal; ↑ = increased: ↓ = decreased; sp. = spastic; fl. = flaccid; + = present; — = absent.

August 6, 1972, was also severely affected (MK47). This blood level would have been approximately 3,000 ppb in March and April 1972, assuming a 70-day clearance half-time. The lowest blood level associated with signs of poisoning was 564 ppb in an infant examined in August 1972 (MK66). The signs were relatively mild. It is noteworthy that seven infants had blood levels in the range of 122 to 636 ppb, but were free of signs of poisoning when first examined.

Some mothers had signs of methylmercury poisoning and their infants did not. For example, a mother having a blood level of 416 ppb on June 1, 1972, had signs of poisoning, but her 1½-month-old infant, with a blood level of 636 ppb, had no detectable signs of poisoning (SP73, SP74; Tables II and IV). In another infant-mother pair, the mother had signs and symptoms of poisoning when examined on June 15, 1972, and had a blood level of 602 ppb, yet her 7½-month-old infant with a blood level of 476 ppb showed no signs of poisoning (MC144, MC143).

The data in Tables II and III generally indicate that blood samples from infants have higher concentrations of mercury than simultaneously collected samples from their mothers. This finding is corroborated by the data in Figures 2 and 3. The data in Figure 2 describe the changes in blood mercury concentrations in the blood of an infant and a mother and in the mother's milk over a period of several months of study (MC104, MC101).

In this particular infant-mother pair, the concentration of mercury in infant blood was consistently higher than that seen in the mother. The concentration of mercury in the mother's milk was considerably lower than seen in mother's blood, as reported previously.[9,10] The concentrations of mercury in blood of both infant and mother declined in a linear fashion when plotted on semilogarithmic paper (Fig. 2). In this infant-mother pair, the clearance half-time was approximately 50 days for both infant's and mother's blood. The concentration of mercury also declined in milk samples collected over a period from April to May. The subsequent level of mercury in milk cannot be determined, since only one further sample was collected at the end of September 1972. It is unlikely that the mercury concentration in milk actually rose. The concentration of mercury in milk is low, giving rise to possible analytical errors. Fluctuation in the recorded levels of mercury in milk may also be expected if the concentration of the sample varies from day to day.

The ratio of mercury concentrations in infant's blood to mother's blood in samples collected at the same time is plotted in Figure 3 as a function of the age of the infant. In all cases except one, the infant's blood level was substantially higher than the mother's blood during the first four months after birth. Furthermore, in the one infant-mother pair in which the infant exhibited lower blood levels than the mother, at the age of 8 months, the

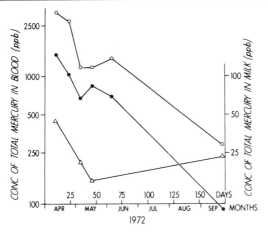

FIG. 2. The concentration of total mercury in infant blood *(open circles)* and in maternal blood *(solid circles)* and milk *(triangles)* over the period of April to September 1972. The date of birth was February 11, 1972 (approximately).

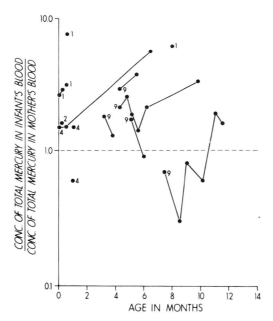

FIG. 3. The ratio of the concentration of total mercury in infant's blood to the concentration in maternal blood in infant-mother pairs according to the age of the infant. Points from the same infant-mother pair are connected by straight lines. The numbers adjacent to the points indicate the estimated month in gestation when the mother ceased consuming contaminated bread.

ratio steadily rose until eventually the infant's blood mercury level was higher than that of the mother's. During the 12-month period of study recorded in Figure 3, no definite trend in this ratio could be seen with time. If anything, in the three infant-mother pairs in which three or more consecutive samples had been collected, there was a tendency for the ratio to increase. The results indicate that infants prenatally exposed to mercury and postnatally exposed to mercury from the mothers' milk, will in general reach a higher blood total mercury concentration than those seen in their mothers.

DISCUSSION

Our results indicate that methylmercury passes readily from mother to fetus. In the 15 infant-mother pairs reported, all but one of the infant blood levels taken at birth and up to four months after birth were either equal to or higher than corresponding maternal levels. Furthermore, the blood level in the suckling infant is maintained by the transmission of methylmercury via maternal milk, as described in other publications.[9,10] One reason for the higher blood levels at birth could be that newborn infants have higher hematocrit readings than their mothers. Since most methylmercury in blood is contained in red blood cells, one would expect to see a higher concentration on this account. However, high hematocrits are not maintained for very long after birth and certainly do not explain the higher levels seen in infants at 4 months of age and older.

Clinical manifestations of methylmercury poisoning were evident in six of 15 mothers. The signs and symptoms are similar to those reported in other studies in Iraq[10] and Japan.[13] The prolonged labor experienced by five multiparous women at the time of birth of the infants in question might be due to the associated muscular weakness. On the other hand, it could be attributed to the psychological disturbance suffered by the members of poisoned families.

Tables III and IV show that at least six of the 15 infants had clinical evidence of poisoning. In the five infants severely affected, there was evidence of gross impairment of motor and mental development, with cerebral palsy, deafness and blindness in four. Blindness was not observed in any of the 22 Japanese cases of congenital Minamata disease,[1,2] but was present in the case of Pierce *et al.* in New Mexico.[14] In the Japanese cases, slight to moderate microcephaly was reported in seven of 26 cases.[2] In our series, three of the infants had microcephaly at an early age. In the prenatal case reported from New Mexico,[15] no mention is made of head size. The poor nutritional state seen in two thirds of the Japanese series was not present in hospitalized infants (Fig. 6), but infants examined in the field were under the expected weight for their age (Figs. 4 and 5). The difficulty in mastication and swallowing, reported to be present in all of Harada's cases, could not be confirmed in our series since the infants were breast-fed. There was no observed difficulty in sucking or swallowing milk. Fretfulness, excessive crying and irritability were outstanding complaints in six cases in this series, and were also reported in three of the Japanese cases and in the case reported by Snyder.

The fact that infant blood levels remain higher than those of their mothers during the first 12 months after birth suggests that these infants may face a higher risk of methylmercury poisoning than their mothers. The dose-response relationship seen in the mother, or adults in general, cannot be applied to prenatal exposure. Nevertheless, our observations to date do not point to a remarkable increase in frequency of signs and symptoms in those prenatally exposed. The lowest measured blood level in infants associated with signs of poisoning was 564 ppb. This is considerably higher than the minimum toxic levels of 200 ppb for adults, as reported by a Swedish Expert Committee.[16] Furthermore, six infants all had blood levels of 200 ppb or more at the times of examination and exhibited no signs of poisoning. In some of these cases, the reported blood levels were measured some months after birth and at an even longer period after consumption of contaminated bread by the mother. These are probably not the maximum blood levels attained by the infants. Clearly, in order to resolve the questions of sensitivity of the fetus to methylmercury, these infants and others similarly exposed must be followed for a long period of time to see if brain damage due to methylmercury poisoning may manifest itself in later years.

In the 15 infant-mother pairs reported here, only one pair was noted in which the infant had signs of poisoning and the mother claimed to be free of any symptoms or signs of methylmercury poisoning. This is in contrast to what has been reported from the outbreak of methylmercury poisoning in Minamata Bay, Japan, in the late 1950s. In the Minamata report, it was indicated that 22 infants were born with severe brain damage, whereas their mothers had only minimal signs and symptoms of poisoning or had no discernible effects of mercury at all.[1] In that series the ages of the patients with prenatal poisoning ranged from 1 to 7 years at the time of the first examination. Thus, the brain damage inflicted prenatally may

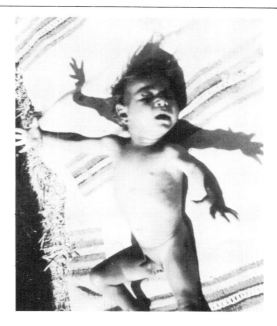

FIG. 4. Congenital methylmercury poisoning with a cerebral palsy syndrome dominated by hypertonicity, mental retardation and blindness at 20 months of age.

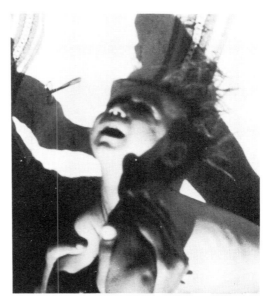

FIG. 5. The same infant (Fig. 4), illustrating hypertonicity and opisthotonus.

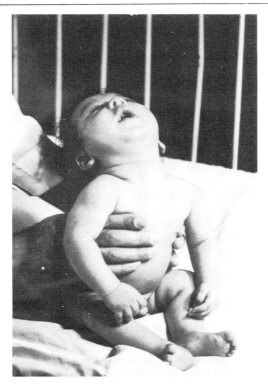

FIG. 6. Congenital methylmercury poisoning. At the age of 4 months the infant is showing clinical manifestations of cerebral palsy, with severe motor and mental handicap, blindness and deafness.

mester is one stage of pregnancy during which the fetus is sensitive to methylmercury poisoning. The other severely affected infant was exposed throughout gestation with maximal exposure during the first trimester. Studies in progress of more infant-mother pairs should aid in resolving the prenatal period of greatest fetal sensitivity to methylmercury poisoning.

Some conversion of methylmercury to inorganic mercury has been reported in patients in Iraq.[10] For example, it was reported that inorganic mercury accounted for 22% and 39%, respectively, of the total mercury in samples of plasma and milk. The question arises as to why acrodynia or pink disease was not seen in the infants reported in this paper. This disease, seen only in infants, is associated with a plethora of signs and symptoms making diagnosis difficult.[17] Peripheral spasms in the extremities causing cold hands and feet, pink color of the extremities and cheeks, edema and blistering and desquamation of skin are frequently reported. Other effects include salivation, profuse sweating, photophobia and anorexia, extreme irritability, insomnia, apathy, and hypotonia. The classic papers of Warkany and Hubbard identified mercury as one important causative agent and the subsequent withdrawal of calomel-containing teething powders has led to the virtual disappearance of this disease.[17-19] Only a small fraction of children exposed to mercury ever developed acrodynia and it would be statistically highly improbable to expect a single case in the 15 infants reported in this paper.[19]

have had time to manifest itself in the Japanese infants. In this study, the infants were examined at a much earlier time (six to seven months after birth). Careful follow-up studies of these and other Iraqi infants are in progress to determine whether signs and symptoms will appear at later ages as these children continue to develop.

The data in Tables II and III indicate that consumption of contaminated bread took place at various times during pregnancy. Presumably maximum blood levels in the pregnant woman were reached at the end of consumption of contaminated bread. In four infant-mother pairs, maximum maternal levels occurred in the first trimester of pregnancy, in four pairs in the second trimester, and in seven pairs in the third trimester. The numbers of pairs are too small to show which trimester of pregnancy is most hazardous to the fetus in terms of methylmercury exposure. Three severely affected infants were exposed only in the last three months of gestation, indicating that the third tri-

REFERENCES

1. Harada, Y.: Study group on Minamata disease. *In* Katsuma, M. (ed.): Minamata Disease. Japan: Kumamoto University, 1966, pp. 93-117.
2. Murakami, U.: The effect of organic mercury on intrauterine life. Advances Exp. Med. Biol., 27:301, 1972.
3. Clegg, D. J.: Mercury in Man's Environment. Ottawa: Royal Society of Canada, 1971, pp. 141-148.
4. Spyker, J. M., Sparber, S. B., and Goldberg, A. M.: Subtle consequences of methylmercury exposure: Behavioral deviations in offspring from treated mothers. Science, 177:621, 1972.
5. Wallace, R. A., Fulkerson, W., Shuits, W. D., and Lyon, W. S.: Mercury in the environment. Oak Ridge National Laboratory, ORNL NSF-EP-1, 1971.
6. Jalili, M. A., and Abbasi, A. H.: Poisoning by ethyl mercury ptoluene sulphonanilide. Brit. J. Industr. Med., 18:303, 1961.
7. Haq, I. U.: Agrosan poisoning in man. Brit. Med. J., 5335:1579, 1963.
8. Ordonez, J. V., Cavvillo, J. A., Miranda, M., and Gale, J. L.: Epidemiological study of a disease in the Guatemalan highlands believed to be encephalitis. Bol. Ofic. Sanit. Panamer., 60(6):510, 1966.
9. Amin-Zaki, L., Elhassani, S., Majeed, M. A., Clarkson, T. W., Doherty, R. A., and Greenwood, M. R.

Studies of infants postnatally exposed to methyl-mercury. J. Pediat., 85:81, 1974.

10. Bakir, F., Damluji, S. F., Amin-Zaki, L., Murtadha, M., Khalidi, A., Al-Rawi, N. Y., Tikriti, S., Dhahir, H. I., Clarkson, T. W., Smith, J. C., and Doherty, R. A.: Methylmercury poisoning in Iraq, an inter-university report. Science, 181:230, 1973.

11. Miettinen, J. K.: Absorption and elimination of dietary mercury (Hg^{2+}) and methylmercury in man. *In* Miller, M. W., and Clarkson, T. W. (eds.): Mercury, Mercurials and Mercaptans. Springfield, Ill.: Charles C Thomas, Publisher, 1973, pp. 233-243.

12. Magos, L., and Clarkson, T. W.: A method for determining total, inorganic and organic mercury in normal and exposed populations. J. Assoc. Anal. Chem., 55:966, 1972.

13. Tokuomi, H.: Minamata disease in human adults. Study Group of Minamata Disease, Kumamoto University, Japan, 1968.

14. Pierce, P. E., Thompson, J. F., Likosky, W. H., Nickey, L. N., Barthal, W. F., and Hinman, A. R.: Alkyl mercury poisoning in humans: Report of an outbreak. JAMA, 220:1439, 1972.

15. Snyder, R. D.: Congenital mercury poisoning. New Eng. J. Med., 284:1014, 1971.

16. Berglund, F., Berlin, M., Birke, G., Cederlof, R., von Euler, U., Fviberg, L., Holmstedt, B., Johsson, B., Luning, K. G., Ramel, C., Skerfving, S., Swensson, A., and Jejning, S.: Methylmercury in fish. Nord. Hyg. T., Suppl. 4, 1971.

17. Warkany, J., and Hubbard, D. M.: Mercury in the urine of children with acrodynia. Lancet, I:829, 1949.

18. Warkany, J., and Hubbard, D. M.: Acrodynia and mercury. J. Pediat., 42:365, 1953.

19. Warkany, J., and Hubbard, D. M.: Adverse mercurial reactions in the form of acrodynia and related cardilions. Amer. J. Dis. Child., 81:335, 1951.

ACKNOWLEDGMENTS

The analytical data on mercury were supplied by the Mercury Research Laboratory under the direction of Dr. Hashim I. Dhahir. We wish to acknowledge Mrs. Patricia Dhahir for supervising the analytical team and for data processing. The analytical determinations were made by Mrs. Ilham M. Al-Jubouri, Mr. Amir Khayat, Miss Salwa M. Matook and Mr. Mansour Al-Muntasir. This laboratory is a collaborative project sponsored by the Universities of Baghdad, Iraq, and Rochester, New York.

We wish to thank Dr. A. Harith for assisting in the study of patients at Salman Pak, and Dr. D. Hardan, director-general for administrative support for our studies in Mussayeb al-Kabeer Irrigation Project.

We wish to thank Dean Muallah of the Medical School, University of Baghdad, and Dean Orbison of the University of Rochester School of Medicine for helping to arrange the interuniversity collaboration. Grateful thanks are due to Dr. Mardan Ali, Director of the Medical City Hospital Center, for facilities at the hospital. We are grateful for helpful advice and useful discussions with Dr. A. W. Mufti of the Ministry of Health, Iraq, and the invaluable assistance given by the Ministry.

The University of Rochester acknowledges support from NSF (RANN) GI-300978, the FDA, the NIGMS, Pharmacology-Toxicology Program (GM 15190).

From J. M. Spyker (1975). Fed. Proc., **34**, 1835–1844. *Copyright* (1975), *by kind permission of the authors and the Federation of American Societies for Experimental Biology*

Assessing the impact of low level chemicals on development: behavioral and latent effects[1,2]

JOAN M. SPYKER

University of Virginia Medical School, Department of Anatomy, Charlottesville, Virginia 22901

Industrial wastes, pesticides, food and fuel additives, drugs, herbicides, fungicides, and numerous environmental pollutants represent chemicals to which humans are routinely exposed. Methylmercury and lead are familiar examples of contaminants that have accumulated slowly through time, reached critical levels, and unexpectedly caused permanent, deleterious effects in humans and other organisms. There is a pressing need to find out what effects the substances accumulating in our environment may be having on us.

Detection of the insidious onset of toxically induced pathological processes presents a major challenge. Modern toxicology has the capability of predicting, attenuating and even preventing deleterious effects that may result from the ubiquitous chemicals found in man's environment. Behavioral teratology and toxicology play key roles here.

BEHAVIORAL TOXICOLOGY

Behavioral changes may serve as the earliest indicators that some, as yet covert, toxic action is occurring—perhaps at a time when the process can still be reversed. There is growing evidence that nervous tissue, especially the brain, is more sensitive to many foreign chemical substances than has previously been suspected, and that toxic effects may be manifested as subtle disturbances of behavior long before any classical symptoms of poisoning become apparent (4, 24, 25, 33).

The detection of an insidious toxic process and its cumulative effects

ABSTRACT

There is growing evidence that nervous tissue, especially the brain, is more sensitive to many foreign chemical substances than has previously been suspected, and that toxic effects may be manifested as subtle disturbances of behavior long before any classical symptoms of poisoning become apparent. Early detection of an insidious toxic process (behavioral toxicology) may enable the prevention or attenuation of harm to humans and other organisms. Adding to both the sensitivity and complexity of behavioral toxicologic testing is the increasing evidence that individuals are more vulnerable to adverse factors during the period of development (conception → puberty) than at any other time in life. Subtle functional disturbances in organisms exposed while immature (behavioral teratology) may be one of the most sensitive indicators of chemical toxicity. Furthermore, defects in a developmental process may have only delayed effects. A morphological or biochemical lesion can be dormant and not manifest itself until later in life as a behavioral disorder, mental deficiency, or overt functional impairment. Longitudinal evaluation is required to detect long-term or delayed effects of a particular developmental influence on biological and behavioral functions. Examples from research on the subtle and latent consequences of prenatal and early postnatal exposure to methylmercury that illustrate the above principles are presented. It is concluded that behavioral and long-term evaluation of organisms exposed during development are essential for a thorough assessment of the impact of certain low level chemicals on human health.— SPYKER. J. M. Assessing the impact of low level chemicals on development: behavioral and latent effects. *Federation Proc.* 34: 1835–1844, 1975.

through time may be greatly facilitated by sensitive and reliable behavioral evaluation procedures. Repeated behavioral samples can measure the extent of reversibility of toxic effects and reveal delayed and progressive impairments. Thus, changes in either isolated or functionally related behaviors can serve as early warning indicators of potential damage to organisms and their environment.

Behavioral processes are also important in themselves. Deficits in intellectual processes, sensory function, motor control (especially coordination and skilled performance), emotional responses and so forth, may be exceedingly disadvantageous to an organism even though morbidity and mortality may remain unaffected.

VULNERABILITY OF DEVELOPING ORGANISMS

Adding to both the sensitivity and complexity of behavioral toxicologic testing is increasing evidence that exposure to chemicals while immature is more likely to produce toxic effects than exposure as an adult. It

[1] From the Symposium on *Current Status of Behavioral Pharmacology*, sponsored by the American Society for Pharmacology and Experimental Therapeutics and the Division of Psychopharmacology of the American Psychological Association, presented at the 58th Annual Meeting of the Federation of American Societies for Experimental Biology, Atlantic City, N.J., April 9–10, 1974.

[2] Supported in part by a grant from The National Foundation/March of Dimes and Public Health Service Grant FR05431.

is now fairly well accepted that an individual is more vulnerable to certain adverse factors during the period of development than at any other time in life. Distinguishing features that contribute to the developing organism being more vulnerable to chemical insult than the mature organism include differences in metabolizing enzymes (12), excretory capacity (2), degree of development of protective systems like the blood–brain barrier (20), binding capacities of the serum and tissue proteins (14), proportion and distribution of various tissues (3), and differences in tissue concentrations of the chemical (20).

An organism continues to develop both prenatally (embryo → fetus) and postnatally (neonate → infant → child → adolescent) until puberty is reached. Thus, reference will be made to developing organisms as encompassing all immature stages. Although prepubertal individuals (because they are incompletely developed) are still at more risk than adults, most of our evidence for the vulnerability of developing organisms comes from humans and experimental animals exposed during the prenatal period.

It was previously believed that a placental barrier protected the fetus. Although the maternal organism may alter a chemical or at least reduce its concentration, the function of the placenta as a barrier is limited and molecules of most substances can cross the "barrier" either by simple diffusion or by some type of active transport system. Consequently, many chemicals entering the pregnant woman ultimately will be found in the fetus. Furthermore, the immature organism does not have the same capacities as the adult to metabolize and detoxify noxious substances. It has been shown that the fetus and newborn have not yet developed the mechanisms to detoxify and excrete a variety of drugs and environmental chemicals (8, 17). Perhaps nowhere is the vulnerability of the unborn more dramatically evident than in the thousands of congenital malformations and severe functional deficits resulting from prenatal exposure to certain drugs, radiation, industrial wastes, and other chemicals in our environment (9, 15, 18, 21). Almost without exception, the mothers were unaffected.

Testing of new drugs in pregnant experimental animals has been required in the United States ever since the thalidomide tragedy of the 1960's —which revealed for the first time that a drug, given with the best intentions for the benefit of the mother, could have disastrous consequences for the human fetus. These teratological testing procedures are primarily designed to uncover the potential of a substance, when given to the mother, to cause death, structural abnormalities, growth retardation, or overt functional impairment in the young. However, it is unlikely that prenatal exposure to chemicals at levels routinely encountered in our environment will result in clinically evident birth defects. The problem is that, in the absence of obvious impairment, subclinical damage may still exist and may be overtly expressed with age.

BEHAVIORAL TERATOLOGY

Assessment of the subtle functional consequences of an insult (e.g., exposure to a toxic substance) during development has been termed "Behavioral Teratology." The underlying theme is that teratogens may have special affinities for particular developing fetal brain centers, that the developing brain is very vulnerable to insult, and that alterations in neurodevelopment become manifest as alterations in behavior. The developmental deviation is thought to be of a neuroanatomical (perhaps seen only at the ultrastructural level) or neurochemical nature. However, since behavior represents an integrated response of the organism, an impairment in the functioning of systems other than the nervous system may also be reflected as a behavioral change.

Teratology can be defined as the study of the adverse effects of the environment (i.e., everything outside the organism) on developing systems. A more comprehensive definition is that teratology is the science dealing with the causes, mechanisms, and manifestations of developmental deviations of either structural or functional nature (37). Behavior is at least as susceptible to teratogenic influence as other developing systems. However, unlike structural birth defects, subtle behavioral abnormal-

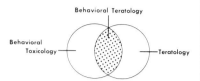

Figure 1. Schematic representation of the areas of responsibility and overlap in behavioral teratology; the principles of teratology as well as of behavioral toxicology must be considered.

ities are not readily evident and may be revealed only by special tests during postnatal life. Particularly at low levels, teratogens may cause behavioral changes in the absence of gross functional or structural defects (1, 7, 11, 30, 31, 34, 35, 38).

In behavioral evaluation of subjects exposed to a toxin during development, the factors affecting both teratology and behavioral toxicology testing should be taken into account. Figure 1 schematically illustrates the areas of responsibility and overlap in the emerging science of behavioral teratology. Basic considerations in teratology and behavioral toxicology, respectively, are briefly summarized in the following two paragraphs; these factors are discussed in detail in the references cited.

Although many questions remain to be answered regarding the behavioral consequences of teratogens, it appears that those factors that determine the type and extent of structural abnormality also influence the type and extent of behavioral abnormality. These five, basic factors can be outlined as follows: a given inherited *genetic predisposition*, linked together with a *particular teratogen*, administered at a certain *dosage level*[3], during a specific *stage of development*[3] results in the observed abnormality. Finally, since the maternal organism provides the environment for the developing organism, *maternal/fetal-offspring interaction* is also a factor that must be considered (13, 36).

Results of behavioral tests are likewise influenced by a number of factors. The most important influences

[3] In many behavioral teratologic tests to stimulate the real-life situation, the dosage level employed is well below the "teratogenic range," per se, (i.e., dosage sufficient to interfere with specific developmental events without destroying the whole embryo) and the organism is exposed during all stages of development (i.e., the mother is treated throughout pregnancy).

include the housing and testing environments that constrain and shape the organism's behavior (16), the consequences of various responses that organisms perform during the tests (22), past experience in laboratory and natural settings (10), and the adaptive significance and evolutionary history of the behaviors chosen for observation (6). All of these factors must be considered when evaluating the significance of behavioral test results.

LATENT EFFECTS

Defects in a developmental process may not become evident for years. A morphological or biochemical lesion can be dormant and not manifest itself until later in life as a behavioral disorder, mental deficiency, or overt functional impairment (19, 26, 32). Perhaps there are compensatory mechanisms that initially mask the defect, but are not adequate as aging, repeated exposure to stress, and cell death occur. Delayed effects can be uncovered by long-term evaluation.

Long-term evaluation of animals chronically exposed as adults to a particular drug or substance is part of standard toxicologic testing procedure. Long-term assessment of subjects exposed while immature is seldom done, yet may be a more revealing indicator of the potential toxicity of the substance in question. This approach is especially warranted if children, adolescents and women of child-bearing age are anticipated to be in the "exposed population."

Determination of long-term or delayed effects of a particular developmental influence on biological or behavioral functions requires the use of a "longitudinal"[4] research design (Fig. 2). This involves following specific individuals from birth through maturity, satisfactorily controlling or monitoring genetic background and environmental experiences, and periodically assaying biological and behavioral functions.

Since changes may be seen at one period in life and not at another, it is important to assay functions at each major stage of the subject's life-span. Tests in animal subjects with a short life-span permit the complete study of developmental effects from conception to death in a relatively brief

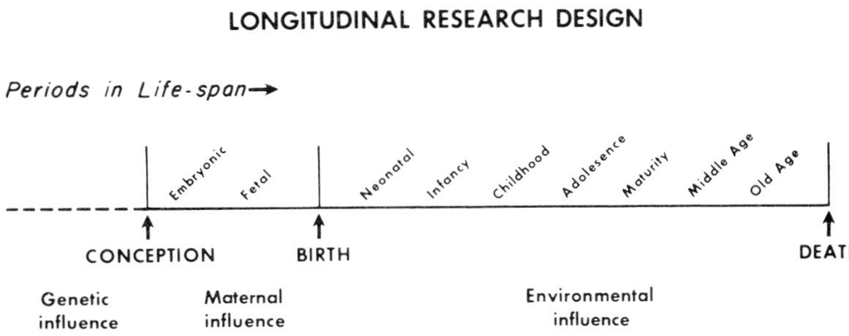

LONGITUDINAL RESEARCH DESIGN

Figure 2. A longitudinal research design must be employed to detect delayed and long-term consequences of an insult during development. This involves following specific individuals, controlling or monitoring genetic background, controlling or monitoring prenatal and postnatal influences, and periodically assaying biological and behavioral functions during the subject's life-span.

period (e.g., the life-span in mice is approximately 2 years).

MATURATIONAL AND BEHAVIORAL EVALUATION

One form of behavior may be affected and not another following interference with a particular developmental process. Since it is extremely difficult to predict what types of subtle or delayed effects will be seen, or when, it is best to utilize a variety of maturational and behavioral measures at various periods of the life-span.

The discriminative power of any behavioral analysis increases as a function of the range of behavioral end points examined. The following categories are frequently included in postnatal functional evaluation:

1) Morphological and physical characteristics: e.g., congenital defects; sex; general appearance, such as posture, fur condition; objective signs, such as cyanosis, ptosis.

2) Maturational landmarks: e.g., age of ear opening, eye opening, piliation, rearing, mating; delay in these parameters often implies that other processes will be retarded or otherwise affected.

3) Growth: e.g., weight gain at normal rates; growth is frequently used as the best index of general health.

4) Specific reflexes, responses and sensory-motor capacities: e.g., righting reflex, corneal reflex, grasping, orienting, response to nose and tail pinch; test especially during the first few weeks of life to assess maturation.

5) Activity levels: e.g., measures of hyper- or hypoactivity at various ages, such as spontaneous activity in home cage, activity wheel, open-field; distinguish type of activity change, such as tremor or locomotion.

6) Neuromuscular ability: e.g., tests of coordination, strength, speed, endurance, agility; gait evaluation.

7) Sensory functions: e.g., tests of the "intactness" of various sensory processes, such as vision, audition, olfaction, somesthesia.

8) Learning ability: e.g., measures of learning, reasoning and retention; vary difficulty from simple classical conditioning to complex operant behavior.

9) Emotionality: e.g., measures to assess role of autonomic nervous system, such as response to a foreign environment; techniques may be parallel to evaluating role of personality variables in man.

10) Sexual parameters: e.g., sexual development, sex role, reproductive efficiency, mating behavior, maternal behavior, fertility rate.

The categories listed above are relatively exhaustive. Even if money, time and expertise were no object, it is impractical—as well as impossible—to test every biological and behavioral function. The results of cost:risk:benefit analysis of the chemical in question, knowledge of its distribution and mechanism of action in the

---

[4] Most developmental research uses the "cross-sectional" (versus longitudinal) method, which involves studying several age periods concurrently, with the assumption that antecedent events would have been held constant. This method cannot address those questions concerned with long-term changes.

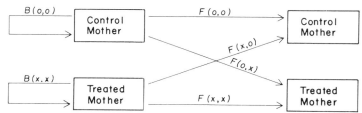

Figure 3. Schema of experimental groups generated according to maternal treatment and rearing-mother type, where: B = litters remained with their *biological* mother, F = litters were transferred to a *foster* mother. The figures in parentheses represent dosage (e.g., x = 2 mg methylmercury/kg mouse): first figure = dosage to biological mother, second figure = dosage to rearing mother. These procedures are employed at birth (before progeny nurse) in order to discriminate prenatal from postnatal influences in subsequent maturation and development.

pregnant organism, as well as results from an initial dose-response evaluation will help guide the investigator in choice and number of test procedures to be employed. In addition, careful, periodic observation of an experimental colony in a well-controlled environment can often provide good clues as to where to look. In fact, one of the most useful applications of this type of research design is to *predict* — that is, to give clues of what to look for and monitor in exposed human populations in order to pick up deficits early — hopefully at a time when they are still reversible.

The evaluation should be done during the early stages of the animals' life-span, i.e., in the mouse, birth through puberty (3–4 wks) and into young adulthood (2–6 months). If no deviations are detected during the maturational screen, some offspring should be maintained for longitudinal testing and biological and behavioral functions periodically assayed to determine if delayed effects can arise from prenatal or early postnatal exposure to the chemical in question. Initially, a dose-response function for readily observable central nervous system effects should be obtained.

CROSS-FOSTERING PROCEDURES

Longitudinal research in behavioral teratology is fraught with potentially confounding variables that may obscure or contribute to real effects. One of the most subtle such influences is that of postnatal effects induced by the mother. In mammals, any experimental maternal treatment producing prenatal effects (i.e., chemical effects on the fetus directly via placental transfer or indirectly by interfering with placental function) must also be considered capable of affecting offspring postnatally. Maternal residual (postnatal) chemical effects may be mediated directly via the milk of the nursing mother, or indirectly through maternal neglect of offspring and other early experience factors (e.g., aberrant maternal retrieving, grooming and activity).

In order to separate prenatal from postnatal influences on subsequent maturation and development, fostering (exchanging offspring with similarly treated mothers) and cross-

fostering (exchanging treated progeny with control mothers and vice versa) procedures should be employed prior to nursing. In addition, a proportion of both control and experimental offspring should be raised by the biological mother to control for the fostering variable itself (Fig. 3). (Described in Spyker (25)).

EXAMPLES FROM RESEARCH

Generally speaking, the objective of research in our laboratory is to investigate the effects of environmental pollutants on immature organisms. Of special interest is the evaluation of subtle and long-term effects resulting from low-level exposure. In addition to detecting and describing effects at all stages of the life-span, attempts are being made to identify sites and mechanisms of action.

Longitudinal research design

Figure 4 schematically represents our experimental design and procedures for long-term evaluation of mice exposed to a chemical during development. The broken line represents the possible period of exposure either prenatally (via placental transfer) or postnatally (via mother's milk or treatment) or both.

At birth, the neonates are physically examined (P) and suitable proportions are fostered and cross-fostered (x-f). Various maturational parameters are evaluated between birth and puberty, at which time the offspring are weaned (21 days). At four major stages in the animals' life-span, i.e., adolescence (1 mo), maturity (6 mo → 1 yr), middle age (1 → 1.5 yr), and old age (1.5 → 2 yr), mice are examined for physical signs and

symptoms (P) and then functionally evaluated (F).

When maturational or behavioral deficits are detected, neurochemical, neuroanatomical, or other indicated procedures (e.g., immunological; see below) are done to complement functional findings.

The longitudinal research design illustrated in Fig. 4 is now being used in our laboratory to assess the subtle and delayed consequences of exposure to methylmercury[5] during development. This protocol for long-term evaluation was arrived at after my co-workers and I carried out developmental, behavioral, biochemical and morphological studies over the lifetime of mice from mothers exposed to methylmercury (MeHg) at different stages of gestation (5, 23–30).

In these studies, the pregnant female was treated on specific days during gestation in order to determine the vulnerability of the embryo or fetus at different ages. In addition, some offspring were exposed to the chemical postnatally via mother's milk; others were cross-fostered to a control dam and thus were only exposed prenatally. (An alternate treatment approach is to chronically expose the mother to low doses prior to conception and throughout gestation. This method probably simulates the real-life situation better; however, it cannot answer the question of when in development the or-

---

[5] Methylmercury is a cumulative environmental contaminant, is currently affecting a large number of people, crosses blood–brain and placental barriers, concentrates in the fetus, and has primarily neurotoxic effects that may be reversible to some extent if detected early enough.

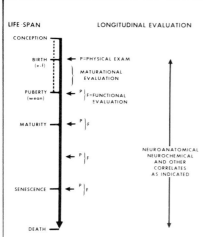

LIFE-SPAN   LONGITUDINAL EVALUATION

Figure 4. Schematic representation of the experimental design and procedures for long-term evaluation of mice exposed to a chemical during development. The broken line represents the possible period of exposure either prenatally (via placental transfer) or postnatally (via mother's milk or treatment) or both. (x-f) = cross-fostering procedures employed at birth.

ganism is most susceptible to adverse effects or what type of functional deficit is associated with the stage of development when exposed).

Methods

On one of days 7, 9, 12 or 13 of pregnancy, nulliparous mice (strain 129/SvSl) received a single intraperitoneal (i.p.) injection of 0, 0.5, 1, 2, 4, or 8 mg/kg MeHg dicyandiamide (Panogen)[6] freshly dissolved in 0.5 ml of 0.9% NaCl/100 g body weight.[7] Females receiving only saline served as controls. One day prior to term (day 18), the females were put in separate cages and allowed to deliver. Sixty-two treated females produced 372 neonates that were apparently normal at birth. Subsequent developmental, behavioral, biochemical and morphological evaluation of these "normal" offspring during their life-spans produced some interesting and unexpected results. A summary of some of these findings are presented below. The detailed methodology and results are described separately (25).

Abnormal development

Although, on close inspection, treated and control neonates were indistinguishable at birth, MeHg retarded general growth and development in a significant number of offspring by 1 mo of age. Many of these animals never attained normal size. Not only did a larger number of prenatally exposed offspring, overtly normal at birth, grow less rapidly than controls, but a significant number died before weaning. As one might expect, both survival time and weight-gain data were dose-dependent. Functionally, neither control nor MeHg young exhibited any discernible neuromuscular deficits (such as retarded righting response, tremor, ataxic gait, leg dragging, hind-leg crossing) during maturation.

Behavioral deviations

The majority of offspring in the experimental colony appeared unaffected at the time of weaning, even though a significant number either were under-developed or did not survive. In an attempt to further elucidate how maternal MeHg exposure may affect postnatal development of apparently normal offspring, behavior was assessed. Our objective was to determine if behavioral deviations were detectable in prenatally and postnatally exposed animals that were grossly indistinguishable from controls. Treated and control mothers were also observed for possible differences in behavioral tests; no differences were found. Summaries of two behavioral tests are included here.

Open-field test: The open-field is an effective, widely used instrument for observing and quantifying basic behavior. This testing device is frequently used to measure the response of an organism to an unfamiliar environment. When 30-day-old, overtly normal offspring were tested in the open-field on 2 consecutive days, there was a significant difference between MeHg and control animals with respect to four of eight parameters evaluated (Table 1). When control animals were placed in the center of the field they proceeded forward and began exploratory activity. In addition to differences in the two indexes used most frequently to assess emotionality (defecation and urination), offspring from MeHg-treated mothers took a significantly longer time to begin exploration and when they did, a significant number took three or more backward steps initially or during the test period (30).

Swimming evaluation: Following the last period in the open-field, mice were placed in a glass tank filled with water at room temperature and their swimming behavior was observed for a period of 10 min. Video tape recordings were made for subsequent evaluation and confirmation of findings. In spite of the fact that all treated animals were grossly indistinguishable from controls at time of testing, behavioral differences were observed

TABLE 1. The effect of prenatal exposure to methylmercury dicyandiamide on open-field performance

Parameter	Treatment[a]		Sex[a]	
	Saline[b]	MeHg[c]	Female	Male
Center latency, sec	5.5	7.1[e]	6.1	6.5
Center squares entered[d]	4.1	2.9	3.7	3.3
Peripheral squares entered	34.9	34.1	35.4	33.6
Defecation	2.9	1.7[e]	2.9	1.7[f]
Urination	0.89	0.52[f]	0.92	0.50[f]
Rearing	3.6	3.3	3.4	3.6
Grooming	1.3	0.65	0.58	1.3
Backing	0.03	0.37[e]	0.18	0.22

[a] Mean number of responses from 2-min trials on 2 consecutive days beginning at 30 days of age. [b] No. = 19 (8 female, 11 male). [c] No. = 20 (11 female, 9 male). Mother of test animal injected with 0.16 mg MeHg dicyandiamide/20 g body weight. [d] Entering is defined as placing all four legs into any square. [e] $P < 0.05$, [f] $P < 0.01$, 2-way least squares analysis of variance, no interactions significant.

[6] Donated by NOR-AM Agricultural Products, Inc., Woodstock, Ill. The highest dose used (8 mg/kg) corresponds to approximately one-fourth the LD_{50} (median lethal dose) for the nonpregnant adult mouse.

[7] This experimental design (i.e., days of injection, doses of MeHg, strain of mouse) was employed because in a previous study to determine the effects of MeHg on prenatal development, using this design, 490 of 498 viable fetuses appeared normal when recovered at term (28). This surprising result prompted the postnatal study to see if deviations were detectable after birth in apparently unaffected offspring.

in a simple swimming apparatus. Figure 5 illustrates some of the deviant swimming behavior characteristic of the treated group (30).

Neuromuscular deficits

As the offspring reached adulthood (6 mo–1 yr), those exposed to the highest dose began showing signs of overt neurological impairment (e.g., tremor, incoordination, ataxia, difficulty righting). However, the majority of the colony was unremarkable upon routine observation. This observation prompted a behavioral study to assess motor ability in the apparently unaffected group.

From the colony of 12 to 15 month-old mice that appeared normal when observed in home cages, 10 animals were randomly selected from the following three treatment groups: *1*) controls (born and reared by a saline mother), *2*) prenatally exposed (born of a MeHg mother; reared by a saline mother), and *3*) postnatally exposed (born of a saline mother; reared by a

TABLE 2. Results of neuromuscular evaluation of mature mice exposed to methylmercury during prenatal or postnatal development

Treatment	Number tested	Number abnormal in test situation		
		Inclined plane	Horizontal surface	Vertical grid
Control	10	0	0	0 ⎤[a]
Prenatally exposed	10	3	4	5 ⎬
Postnatally exposed	10	1	2	2 ⎦

[a] $P < 0.05$.

MeHg-mother). In each case the MeHg-mother had received the 4 mg/kg dose. These 30 offspring were evaluated in each of the following test situations: *1*) horizontal surface, *2*) inclined plane, and *3*) vertical grid (described in Spyker (25)). Table 2 shows the number of animals, according to treatment, exhibiting neuromuscular deficits when evaluated in the three test situations listed above. Evaluation of these older animals on the vertical grid was the most discriminating of the tests whereas assessment of motor ability on the in-

clined plane was the least sensitive. As indicated in Table 2, for each test situation more offspring were found abnormal in the group exposed to MeHg in utero than in the group that was exposed postnatally via the treated, rearing mother.

Immuno-deficiencies

Among the unexpected findings during long-term postnatal evaluation was an increased incidence of infection (usually eye infections) in older treated animals. Infections were seldom found in controls or younger treated animals. On laboratory evaluation, the afflicted animals proved culture positive for pneumococci and streptococci. This higher incidence of infection in the treated group was suggestive of a deficiency in the immune system. Preliminary evaluation of immunological competence revealed a significant difference in immune response between MeHg and control animals (See under *Immunological evaluation*, next section).

Generalized debilitation

Without the use of special tests, most of the treated mice were indistinguishable from controls—while they were young. However, as the animals approached middle age (1–1.5 yr), a variety of differences between the treated and control groups began to emerge. The relative incidence of neurological damage, postural defects, muscular atrophy, eye lesions, weight change, and general debilitation rose markedly in offspring exposed to methylmercury prenatally, via mothers' milk, or both. Some of these obvious differences are illustrated in Fig. 6. Subtle behavioral tests were no longer needed to significantly discriminate the treated group; CNS involvement had generally become obvious.

Figure 5. A significant number of apparently normal offspring from MeHg-treated mothers exhibited deviant behavior during swimming. Controls swam with *a*) front legs tucked, hind legs alternately kicking to turn or propel, and tail under water for balance and propulsion (note general posture with respect to waterline). Characteristic of the treated group were frequent episodes of incoordination and impaired swimming ability such as *b*) "freezing" in the water with all legs extended for periods up to 2 min (compare posture to that of control in Fig. 5*a*); *c*) floating suspended in a vertical position with only head above water; and *d*) swimming with legs askew and inability to maintain normal orientation in water. (From (30). Copyright 1972 by the American Association for the Advancement of Science.)

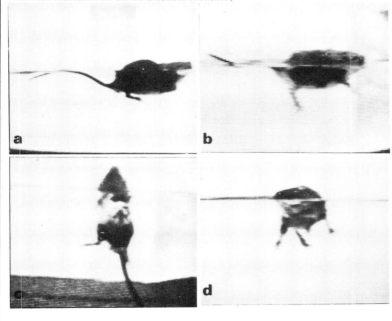

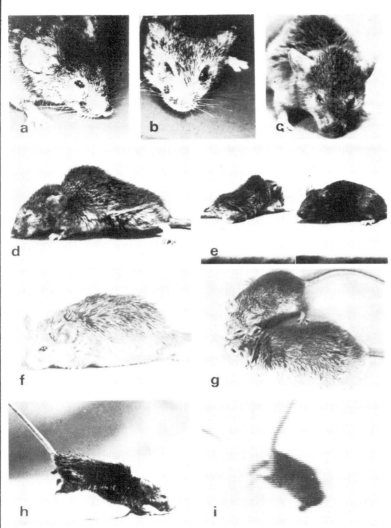

Figure 6. Figure illustrates representative abnormalities found during long-term evaluation of mice prenatally exposed to methylmercury. *a)* Purulent exudate apparent in right eye of offspring at 14 months of age. *b)* Same animal as in Fig. 6a three months later. Cornea of right eye is now dense, dull and opaque. Left eye appears unaffected. *c)* Same animal as in Fig. 6a and *b* when 2 yr old. Right eye has completely atrophied leaving only a sunken orbit filled with connective tissue. Left eye is now also undergoing atrophy, although no exudate was present. *d)* Kyphosis, an abnormally increased convexity of the thoracic spine, occurred frequently in the treated group after 1 yr of age. *e)* After kyphosis had developed, most of the deformed animals displayed muscular atrophy in the hind legs (left). Control (right) *f)* Treated offspring (1.5 yr old) which became obese within a 2-week period. *g)* Control (above) compared to obese animal from treated group (below). *h)* Generally debilitated female with prolapsed uterus photographed just before dying at 15 mo of age. *i)* Many offspring that behaved abnormally when young had severe neuromuscular deficits when older. Animal shown here is unable to right itself when placed on its side.

biochemical, histopathological and other studies as indicated to permit correlation of these parameters with data from functional evaluation (see next section).

Summary of lifetime findings

The progression of major findings from this long-term research is schematically illustrated in Fig. 7 in the order in which they were detected. In summary, offspring from treated mothers, although apparently normal at birth, responded differently from controls when tested for maturational and behavioral deviations at various stages throughout postnatal development. These early behavioral indications of trouble were indeed forewarnings of later, more severe developments such as obvious motor impairment, neuropathology, postural problems, immuno-deficiencies, generalized debilitation, and early aging. The severity of the deficit and the length of time before it was detected were generally dose-dependent. The mothers were not affected.

MORPHOLOGICAL AND BIOCHEMICAL CORRELATES OF BEHAVIORAL DEFICITS

Neuroanatomical assessment

Brains of behaviorally abnormal offspring were studied in an attempt to correlate subtle deficits with neuropathology. Initially, no morphological changes were observed at the light microscope level. However, a variety of ultrastructural changes were observed when tissue samples from cerebellums were examined with the electron microscope (5, 26).

Increased lysosomal number, size and activity were observed in many Purkinje neurons and granule cells; discharge of lysosomal material was also noted (Fig. 8a). Formation of giant sized lysosomes or autophagosomes, and disintegration of the rough endoplasmic reticulum were additional features seen in these cells. All of these changes in fine structure probably denote early signs of cellular degeneration of neurons. Indeed, brains from *older*, more severely involved animals in the treated group weighed significantly less than controls, and dead or dying cells were apparent when brains were studied under the light microscope.

Premature death

As might be expected, many offspring that deviated from normal in the ways described above died sooner than controls. However, survival time could not be calculated for a large number of test subjects found to be functionally abnormal. These animals were sacrificed for morphological,

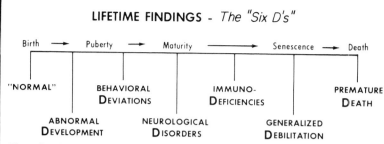

LIFETIME FINDINGS - *The "Six D's"*

Birth ⟶ Puberty ⟶ Maturity ⟶ Senescence ⟶ Death

"NORMAL" BEHAVIORAL **D**EVIATIONS IMMUNO- **D**EFICIENCIES PREMATURE **D**EATH

ABNORMAL **D**EVELOPMENT NEUROLOGICAL **D**ISORDERS GENERALIZED **D**EBILITATION

Figure 7. Schematic summary of six major ways animals prenatally exposed to methylmercury were found to be significantly different from controls as they grew older. All 372 offspring evaluated postnatally were apparently normal at birth. None of these deviations from normal would have been detected without long-term evaluation.

Perhaps the most significant findings were the incomplete myelination of some nerve fibers (Fig. 8b) and absent or diminutive post-synaptic densities in many synaptic junctions (Fig. 8c and d). The size of the post-synaptic membrane is thought to be an indicator of synaptic activity. Such malformations of the nerve fibers and synaptic complexes, together with the pathological changes in the nerve cells described above, may have contributed to the behavioral deficiencies observed in these animals.

Neurochemical analysis

In an attempt to correlate the observed behavioral differences with neurotransmitter enzymes, choline acetyltransferase and cholinesterase determinations were done on the brains of 24 randomly chosen mice (equally distributed between treated and controls, males and females). A

Figure 8. Electron micrographs showing alterations in ultrastructure of cerebellar cells from mice prenatally exposed to low levels of methylmercury. a) Purkinje neuron, treated. Note increased lysosomal activity. Release of lysosomal enzymes into the cytoplasmic matrix (→) is also apparent. ×17,000 b) Longitudinal section through a large nerve fiber at the node of Ranvier, treated. Reduction in myelination in one segment of the nerve fiber (S_2) as compared to the neighboring segment (S_1) of the same fiber is shown. Degenerative changes are also evident at the node of Ranvier. ×18,000. c) Mossy fiber terminal, control. Note the regularly arranged densities (→) and normal synaptic pattern. ×48,000. d) Mossy fiber terminal, treated. Note the reduction and absence of synaptic densities (→) in contrast to control in Fig. 8c.

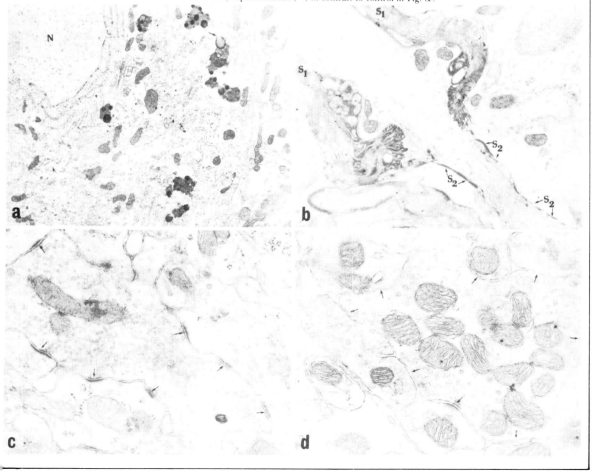

two-way (MeHg by sex) analysis of variance was done for each of the following parameters: diencephalic-telencephalic weight (everything above the superior colliculus); cerebellar weight; total milligrams protein in whole brain; and activity of choline acetyltransferase and cholinesterase (in μmoles/gram protein per hour or μmoles/brain per hour. The only significant ($P < 0.05$) effect was a sex difference in cerebellar weight (males > females). No significant alteration was found in any parameter between MeHg and saline offspring when evaluated at 1 mo of age (30). Perhaps neurochemical differences would have been detected if we had made determinations by brain region rather than by whole brain, or if we had assessed the animals later in their life-span.

Immunological evaluation

Awareness of an increased incidence of bacterial infection in older animals that had been exposed to MeHg in utero prompted a preliminary evaluation of the dual-natured immune system. Sheep red blood cells were used to selectively challenge the T-cell immune system (responsible for the expression of cellular immunity) and *Brucella abortus* antigen was used to challenge the B-cell system (responsible for the expression of humoral immunity). Ten young (4 mo) and 10

Figure 9. Impaired immune function may be a delayed effect of prenatal exposure to methylmercury. Sheep red blood cells (SRBC) and *Brucella abortus* antigen were used to selectively challenge the T-cell and B-cell immune systems, respectively. A highly significant low antibody response was detected in *older* treated animals injected with *Brucella* antigen.

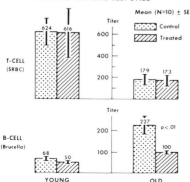

mature (14 mo) randomly chosen female offspring from both treated and control groups were immunized with the two antigens and antisera were collected to measure hemagglutinin titers (primary antibody producing capacity).

A highly significant low antibody response was detected in the older group injected with *Brucella* antigen (Fig. 9). No other significant differences were found (27). These preliminary results indicate that the thymus-dependent (T cell) immune function was left intact, whereas thymus-independent (B cell) immune function, which resists infections caused by bacteria, was impaired in mature offspring from MeHg-treated mothers. The results may, in part, explain the increased incidence of bacterial infections in the older animals. This humoral deficiency may in turn relate to a plasma cell dysfunction as suggested by a high percentage of abnormal plasma cells found in the spleens of these animals (Chang and Spyker, unpublished observations).

Although this is a preliminary study, impaired immune function may indeed be a delayed effect of prenatal exposure to MeHg. Like other systems, the immune system is differentiating during fetal development. Furthermore, the two-compartment immune system can be distinguished quite early. Therefore, it is possible that insult during embryogenesis could affect one immune system and not the other.

I would like to emphasize here that this delayed effect, as well as many others, could not have been detected without the use of a longitudinal research design. This apparent dysfunction of the immune system may also be an example of how impairment of a system other than the nervous system can affect behavior. On the other hand, decreased immunological competence may be altering nervous system function and thus indirectly affecting behavior.

SUMMARY AND CONCLUSIONS

Behavioral toxicology

Behavioral assessment is an important component in the evaluation of adverse effects for two main reasons: *1*) Subtle, behavioral changes may

serve as early indicators or predictors of later, more severe, consequences. Early detection of toxic effects may enable the prevention or attenuation of harm to humans and other organisms; *2*) Behavioral deficits may be extremely disadvantageous to an organism and, therefore, are important in their own right.

Developing organisms

Individuals are more vulnerable to adverse factors during the period of development (conception → puberty) than at any other time in life. Thus, the fetus and child are at greater risk from toxic effects than the adult. Subtle functional disturbances in offspring from exposed mothers (behavioral teratology) may be one of the most sensitive indicators of chemical toxicity.

Latent effects

Defects in a developmental process may be dormant and not manifest themselves until later in life as a behavioral disorder, mental deficiency, or overt functional impairment. Longitudinal evaluation is required to detect long-term or delayed effects of a particular developmental influence on biological and behavioral functions.

Safety standards

Exposure to certain substances during development can have subtle and/or delayed consequences that almost certainly would remain undetected by the test procedures currently required. There is need for continual review of the tests required for safety evaluations—and of the protocols for carrying out these tests—both from the point of view of protecting the public health and of assuring efficient utilization of scientific resources.

Due to the nature of behavioral changes, the vulnerability of developing organisms, the fact that we normally are exposed to low concentrations of chemicals, and finally, to the implications of the research already done in Behavioral Teratology, I believe that behavioral and long-term evaluation of organisms exposed during development are essential for a thorough assessment of the impact of low level chemicals on human health.

REFERENCES

1. ARMITAGE, S. G. Effects of barbiturates on behavior of rat offspring as measured in learning and reasoning situations. *J. Comp. Physiol. Psychol.* 45: 146, 1952.

2. BERNSTEIN, J. Postnatal development of the kidney. *Am. J. Pathol.* 66: 16a, 1972.

3. BOYD, E., AND C. KRIJNEN. Tolerated doses of phenacetin in relation to body weight and organ weights. *Jpn. J. Pharmacol.* 19: 386, 1969.

4. BRYCE-SMITH, D. Behavioral effects of lead and other heavy metal pollutants. *Chem. Br.* 8: 240, 1972.

5. CHANG, L. W., AND J. M. SPYKER. Ultrastructural changes in the nervous system after in utero exposure to low doses of methylmercury. *Acta Neuropath.* In press.

6. EIBL-EIBESFELDT, I. *Ethology, the Biology of Behavior.* New York: Holt, Rinehart & Winston, 1970.

7. FURCHTGOTT, E. Behavioral effects of ionizing radiations: 1955–1961. *Psychol. Bull.* 60: 157, 1963.

8. HAGERMAN, D., AND C. A. VILLEE. Transport functions of the placenta. *Physiol. Rev.* 40: 313, 1960.

9. HICKS, S. P., C. J. D'AMATO AND M. J. LOWE. The development of the mammalian nervous system. *J. Comp. Neurol.* 113: 435, 1959.

10. HINDE, R. A. *Animal Behavior: A Synthesis of Ethology and Comparative Psychology.* 2nd ed. New York: McGraw-Hill, 1970.

11. HOFFIELD, D. R., AND R. L. WEBSTER. Effect of injections of tranquilizing drugs during pregnancy on offspring. *Nature* 205: 1070, 1965.

12. JONDORF, W., R. MAICKEL AND B. BRODIE. Inability of newborn mice and guinea pigs to metabolize drugs. *Biochem. Pharmacol.* 1: 352, 1959.

13. KALTER, H. *Teratology of the Central Nervous System.* Chicago: University of Chicago Press, 1968.

14. KOBYLETZKI, D. Basis of prenatal medications: maternal-fetal distribution, peripartal elimination. In: *Prenatal Infections,* edited by O. Thalhammer. Stuttgart: Georg Thieme-Verlag, 1971.

15. LENZ, W. Thalidomide and congenital abnormalities. *Lancet* 1: 45, 1962.

16. MARLER, P., AND W. J. HAMILTON III. *Mechanisms of Animal Behavior.* New York: Wiley, 1966.

17. MOYA, F., AND B. E. SMITH. Distribution and placental transport of drugs and anesthetics. *Anesthesiology* 26: 45, 1965.

18. MURAKAMI, U. Embryo-fetoxic effect of some organic mercury compounds. *Annu. Rep. Res. Inst. Environ. Med., Nagoya Univ.* 18: 33, 1971.

19. NAIR, V., AND K. P. DUBOIS. Prenatal and early postnatal exposure to environmental contaminants. *Chicago Med. Sch. Q.* 27: 75, 1968.

20. NYHAN, W. Toxicity of drugs in the neonatal period. *J. Pediatr.* 59: 1, 1961.

21. RUGH, R., AND M. WOHLFROMM. Previous reproductive history and the susceptibility to X-ray induced congenital anomalies. *Nature* 210: 969, 1966.

22. SKINNER, B. F. *Contingencies of Reinforcement: A Theoretical Analysis.* New York: Appleton-Century-Crofts, 1969.

23. SPYKER, J. M. Methylmercury, mice and men. (Ph.D. Thesis), Minneapolis: Univ. of Minnesota, 1971 (summarized in *Diss. Abstr. Int.* 32: 8, 1972).

24. SPYKER, J. M. Subtle consequences of methylmercury exposure. *Teratology* 5: 267, 1972.

25. SPYKER, J. M. Behavioral teratology and toxicology. In: *Behavioral Toxicology,* edited by B. Weiss and V. G. Laties. New York: Plenum, 1975, p. 311–344.

26. SPYKER, J. M., AND L. W. CHANG. Delayed effects of prenatal exposure to methylmercury: brain ultrastructure and behavior. *Teratology* 9: A37, 1974.

27. SPYKER, J. M., AND G. FERNANDES. Impaired immune function in offspring from methylmercury-treated mice. *Teratology* 7: 28, 1973.

28. SPYKER, J. M., AND M. SMITHBERG. Effects of methylmercury on prenatal development in mice. *Teratology* 5: 181, 1972.

29. SPYKER, J. M., AND S. B. SPARBER. Behavioral teratology of methylmercury in the mouse. *Pharmacologist* 13: 275, 1971.

30. SPYKER, J. M., S. B. SPARBER AND A. M. GOLDBERG. Subtle consequences of methylmercury exposure: Behavioral deviations in offspring from treated mothers. *Science* 177: 621, 1972.

31. VAN GELDER, G. A., T. L. CARSON AND W. B. BUCK. Slowed learning in lambs prenatally exposed to lead. *Toxicol. Appl. Pharmacol.* 25: 466, 1973.

32. VORSTER, D. W. Psychiatric drugs and treatment in pregnancy. *Br. J. Psychol.* 3: 431, 1965.

33. WEISS, B., J. BROZEK, H. HANSON, R. C. LEAF, N. K. MELLO AND J. M. SPYKER. Effects on behavior, Chap. X. In: *The Evaluation of Chemicals for Societal Use,* edited by N. Nelson. Washington, D.C.: National Academy of Sciences, 1974.

34. WEISS, B., AND J. M. SPYKER. Behavioral implications of prenatal and early postnatal exposure to chemical pollutants. *Pediatrics* 53: 851, 1974.

35. WERBOFF, J. Developmental psychopharmacology. In: *Principles of Psychopharmacology,* edited by W. G. Clark and J. del Guidice. New York: Academic, 1970.

36. WILSON, J. G. Embryological considerations in teratology. In: *Teratology: Principles and Techniques,* edited by J. G. Wilson and J. Warkany. Chicago: University of Chicago Press, 1965.

37. WILSON, J. G. *Environment and Birth Defects.* New York: Academic, 1973.

38. YOUNG, R. G. Developmental psychopharmacology: a beginning. *Psychol. Bull.* 67: 73, 1967.

39. Simpson, W. J. (1957). A preliminary report on cigarette smoking and the incidence of prematurity. *Am. J. Obstet. Gynecol.*, **73**, 808–815. (Extract)
40. Lowe, C. R. (1959). Effect of mothers' smoking habits on birth weight of their children. *Br. Med. J.*, **2**, 673–676

COMMENTARY

Simpson (1957) first reported that the weight of infants born to mothers who smoked during pregnancy was less than that of non-smokers. The incidence of premature births (2500 g or less) in mothers who smoked was twice that of non-smokers and this increased with the number of cigarettes (Paper 39). Lowe (1959) confirmed that the birth weight was reduced in mothers who smoked; he attributed this effect to fetal growth retardation and not to a shortening of the gestational period (Paper 40). Other reports showed that maternal smoking was associated not only with fetal growth retardation, but also with an increase in abortion, premature deliveries, and perinatal deaths.

Numerous studies have been carried out to determine the fetal effects of maternal smoking. The results are conflicting and emphasize the complexity of the problem. It has been rightly argued that the many 'associations' reported between maternal smoking and fetal well-being are not necessarily 'cause–effect' relationships.

Blood level of carboxyhaemoglobin (CoHb) in mothers who smoke during pregnancy is significantly more than that of non-smokers. The fetal concentration of CoHb was found to be 1·8 times greater than maternal in mothers who smoked during pregnancy. In these pregnancies less oxygen is carried by maternal and fetal blood. In addition, oxygen release to fetal tissues is decreased because of an impairment in the oxygen dissociation curve. It was assumed that the resulting fetal hypoxia may

account for the intrauterine growth retardation (Cole *et al.*, 1972). However, in view of the finding that placental weight in smokers was not affected Targett and his colleagues (1973) considered hypoxia unlikely to be of importance in the aetiology of this growth retardation.

Andrews (1973) suggested that the fetal growth retardation seen in smokers might be due to the increased levels of thiocyanate present in maternal and cord blood. Other studies, however, have incriminated nicotine as producing this effect.

Because birth weight is strongly related to maternal weight gain during pregnancy, it was thought that the low birth weight of infants born to mothers who smoke might be mediated by a low caloric intake or reduced weight gain. This hypothesis was investigated in 162 mothers from a poor black, urban community. It was concluded that a decrease in maternal weight gain or caloric intake was likely the most important factor for the fetal growth retardation (Rush, 1974). Recently, Davies *et al.* (1976) in a study of 1159 mother–infant pairs confirmed this observation. In addition, the offspring of heavy smokers were found to be shorter and had smaller heads, thus lending further support to Lowe's suggestion that smoking during pregnancy impaired intrauterine growth.

In mothers who smoke during pregnancy, fetal breathing movements were markedly reduced (Manning *et al.*, 1975; Gennser *et al.*, 1975). This response was attributed to an impairment of placental blood flow, possibly mediated by nicotine

Fedrick *et al.* (1971) found that the incidence of congenital heart diseases was significantly increased in those mothers who smoked in pregnancy. This association was not related to maternal age, parity, and social class. Little is known concerning the long-term effects of cigarette smoking on fetal health. In children studied at ages 7 and 11 years, both physical and mental development was seriously affected as a result of the mothers smoking during pregnancy (Butler and Goldstein, 1973). Of considerable interest is a report by Mau and Netter (1974) that the incidence of perinatal deaths and congenital malformations was also significantly increased in the offspring of fathers who smoked. These fetal effects of paternal smoking were independent of maternal and paternal age, number of births, socio-economic conditions, and previous obstetrical history.

There is no satisfactory explanation to account for the reported adverse influence of maternal and paternal smoking on the fetus. The results of many studies have been inconclusive, but because of the widespread use of tobacco further investigations are clearly warranted.

REFERENCES

Andrews, J. (1973). Thiocyanate and smoking in pregnancy. *J. Obstet. Gynaecol. Br. Commonw.*, **80**, 810–814

Butler, N. R. and Goldstein, H. (1973). Smoking in pregnancy and subsequent child development. *Br. Med. J.*, **4**, 573–575

Cole, P. V., Hawkins, L. H. and Roberts, D. (1972). Effects on the fetus of smoking during pregnancy. *J. Obstet. Gynaecol. Br. Commonw.*, **79**, 782–787

Davies, D. P., Gray, O. P., Ellwood, P. C. and Abernethy, M. (1976). Cigarette smoking in pregnancy: associations with maternal weight gain and fetal growth. *Lancet*, **i**, 385–387

Fedrick, J., Alberman, E. D. and Goldstein, H. (1971). Possible teratogenic effect of cigarette smoking. *Nature (London)*, **231**, 529–530

Gennser, G., Marsal, K. and Brantmark, B. (1975). Maternal smoking and fetal breathing movements. *Am. J. Obstet. Gynecol.*, **123**, 861–867

Manning, F., Pugh, E. W. and Boddy, K. (1975). Effect of cigarette smoking on fetal breathing movements in normal pregnancies. *Br. Med. J.*, **1**, 552–553

Mau, G. and Netter, P. (1974). Die Auswirkungen des väterlichen Zigarettenkonsums auf die perinatale sterblichkeit und die Mißbildungshäufigkeit. *Dtsch. Med. Wochenschr.*, **99**, 1113–1118

Rush, D. (1974). Examination of the relationship between birthweight, cigarette smoking during pregnancy and maternal weight gain. *J. Obstet. Gynaecol. Br. Commonw.*, **81**, 746–752

Targett, C. S., Gunesee, H., McBride, F. and Beischer, N. A. (1973). An evaluation of the effects of smoking on maternal oestriol excretion during pregnancy and on fetal outcome. *J. Obstet. Gynaecol. Br. Commonw.*, **80**, 815–821

From W. J. Simpson (1957). Am. J. Obstet. Gynecol., **73,** 808–815. *Copyright* (1957), *by kind permission of the author and the C. V. Mosby Company, St Louis,* Mich., USA

A PRELIMINARY REPORT ON CIGARETTE SMOKING AND THE INCIDENCE OF PREMATURITY

WINEA J. SIMPSON, M.D., LOMA LINDA, CALIF.

(From the San Bernardino County Health Department and the Department of Preventive Medicine and Public Health, School of Medicine, College of Medical Evangelists)

Summary

This report, which is based upon data gathered from 7,499 patients, shows an incidence of premature births at private hospitals which is approximately twice as great for smoking mothers as it is for nonsmoking mothers. The prematurity rate increases with the number of cigarettes smoked per day. The highest prematurity rates are for heavy smokers and the lowest rates for nonsmokers.

The County Hospital represents a different population in which socio-economic factors may affect the picture. The prematurity rate for nonsmokers is relatively higher at the County Hospital than at the private hospitals and there is less difference between the prematurity rate for smokers and nonsmokers. Mexicans delivered at the County Hospital report less smoking than any other ethnic group and show the lowest prematurity rate.

The writer is grateful to Dr. William B. Michael for his expert guidance in tabulating and interpreting the data presented. To the following doctors who critically previewed this report goes a vote of thanks: M. E. Cosand, L. Corsa, Jr., C. H. Thienes, L. H. Lonergan, H. N. Mozar, B. W. Halstead, F. R. Lemon, and W. F. Norwood.

Much credit is due to the following supervisors and their assistants who were responsible for gathering the information for the questionnaires: Mary Hyatt, County Hospital Obstetrical Supervisor; Sister Mary Elaine, St. Bernardine's Hospital Records Librarian; Ruth Wipperman, Loma Linda Sanitarium and Hospital Obstetrical Supervisor.

From C. R. Lowe (1959). Br. Med. J., **2**, 673–676. *Copyright* (1959),
by kind permission of the author and the British Medical Association

EFFECT OF MOTHERS' SMOKING HABITS ON BIRTH WEIGHT OF THEIR CHILDREN

BY

C. R. LOWE, M.D., Ph.D., D.P.H.

Lecturer in Social Medicine, University of Birmingham

It has been reported that when pregnant rats and rabbits are exposed to tobacco smoke their offspring weigh less than those of control animals (Essenberg, Schwind, and Patras, 1940 ; Schoeneck, 1941). A similar observation has been made in respect of pregnant women. Simpson (1957) collected data over a three-year period from American maternity hospitals and found that the incidence of premature births (those weighing 5½ lb.—2.5 kg.—or less) among women who smoked was double that among non-smokers and increased fairly regularly with the amount smoked. No explanation was offered for this observation, but it is clear from the data that age, parity, and social circumstances had little to do with it.

The subject seemed to be of sufficient importance to require further investigation, particularly since Simpson's report left a number of important questions unanswered. For example, it did not indicate whether the low birth weight was attributable to retardation of foetal growth or to early onset of labour.

The present paper gives the results of an inquiry into the effect of smoking upon the pregnancies of 2,042 women delivered in six Birmingham maternity hospitals during the summer of 1958.

Material

In order to obtain accurate information about smoking during pregnancy, it was thought desirable to limit the inquiry to recent deliveries. Two social workers visited six maternity hospitals in Birmingham at frequent intervals over a period of five months. At each visit they completed a questionary for every woman

TABLE I.—*Percentage Distribution of Birth Weights of Infants Related to Maternal Smoking Habits during Pregnancy*

Smoking Habits During Pregnancy	Birth Weight (lb.)							Total	Mean±S.E.
	<4	4–	5–	6–	7–	8–	9+		
Never smoked*	1·7 (19)	1·9 (22)	6·5 (74)	23·8 (273)	39·8 (456)	21·5 (241)	5·4 (61)	100 (1,146)	7·33±0·03
Gave up early in pregnancy	0·6 (1)	2·2 (4)	6·7 (12)	26·7 (48)	38·3 (69)	18·3 (33)	7·2 (13)	100 (180)	7·36±0·29
Gave up but later began again	2·6 (1)	2·6 (1)	10·5 (4)	28·9 (11)	34·2 (13)	15·8 (6)	5·3 (2)	100 (38)	7·11±0·59
Smoked regularly	2·7 (18)	2·4 (16)	13·9 (92)	32·3 (214)	30·8 (204)	14·8 (98)	3·1 (20)	100 (662)	6·93±0·05

* Women who never smoked during pregnancy are referred to as " non-smokers " in the figures and in subsequent tables.

TABLE III.—*Percentage Distribution of Non-smokers and Regular Smokers According to Duration of Gestation**

Gestation (Days)	<250	250–	260–	270–	280–	290–	300+	Total	Mean±S.E.
Non-smokers	3·7 (33)	2·7 (24)	9·2 (81)	26·9 (237)	39·1 (345)	14·9 (131)	3·5 (31)	100 (882)	279·9±1·5
Regular smokers	5·5 (30)	5·1 (28)	10·5 (57)	24·6 (134)	35·8 (195)	14·3 (78)	4·2 (23)	100 (545)	278·5±1·7

* Pregnancies terminated by surgical induction or elective caesarean section are excluded.

delivered in the hospital since the previous visit. An obstetrical history was recorded in the ward day-room from the hospital record card and a smoking history at the bedside from the mother. In addition each woman was asked what her weight was immediately before she became pregnant. Non-Europeans and women who had had twin births were excluded.

Results

The sample of 2,042 women contained 1,155 who did not smoke at any time during their pregnancy (women who had never smoked or had given up smoking before they conceived), 181 who smoked during the early months of pregnancy but gave up later (all but 7 of them before the end of the fifth month), 38 who stopped early in pregnancy but later began to smoke again, and 668 who smoked regularly throughout pregnancy. Since the data were not complete in every detail for every woman, it will be found that the numbers in these four categories vary a little from table to table.

Birth Weight

The basic data of the investigation are presented in Table I and Fig. 1. Infants of mothers who smoked regularly throughout pregnancy were on the average more than 6 oz. (170 g.) lighter than infants of those who never smoked during pregnancy, referred to

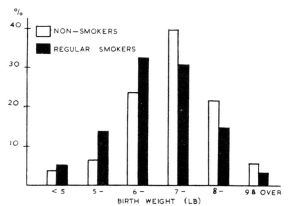

Fig. 1.—Birth weight of infants related to their mothers' smoking habits.

subsequently as non-smokers (6.93 lb. and 7.33 lb. respectively—a difference of 0.40 ± 0.06 lb.). There were only 38 women who gave up smoking early in pregnancy but later began to smoke again, so no significance can be attached to the mean weight of their infants. There was no difference between weights of infants of non-smokers and of women who gave up early in pregnancy and did not begin to smoke again. This suggests that the influence of smoking upon birth weight may possibly be greater during the second than during the first half of pregnancy ; but again the numbers are rather small. The analysis which follows is concerned only with the non-smokers (1,155) and the regular smokers (668), women in the two small intermediate categories being excluded.

Table II shows that the mean weight of infants of heavy smokers (10 or more cigarettes a day) was less than that of infants of light smokers (fewer than 10

TABLE II.—*Mean Birth Weight (lb.) of Infants Related to Maternal Smoking Habits During Pregnancy*

Sex of Infant	Non-smokers	Regular Smokers		Total
		< 10 Cigs. a Day	10 or More Cigs. a Day	
Male ..	7·43 (607)	7·18 (187)	7·05 (165)	7·32 (959)
Female ..	7·23 (539)	6·74 (163)	6·67 (147)	7·04 (849)
Total ..	7·33 (1,146)	6·98 (350)	6·87 (312)	7·18 (1,808)

cigarettes a day). This was true of both male and female infants. The influence of smoking on birth weight was so pronounced that male infants of regular smokers were appreciably lighter than female infants of non-smokers—a reversal of the usual sex difference in weight.

Duration of Gestation

The possibility that the low birth weight of infants of women who smoked during pregnancy was attributable to shortening of the duration of gestation was examined. Intravenous nicotine is known to release antidiuretic hormone, which can be found in human urine after smoking (Burn, 1951), so it is not impossible that smoking might have an oxytocic effect.

To explore this possibility the duration of gestation was examined in smokers and non-smokers. Since the question considered was whether tobacco smoking induces early onset of labour, it was of course necessary to exclude from the comparison pregnancies which had been terminated by surgical induction and elective caesarean section. There was no substantial difference between duration of gestation of smokers and of non-smokers (Table III). That tobacco does not have an oxytocic effect was confirmed by the observation that, with one interesting exception, whatever the duration of gestation the mean birth weight of children born to smokers was always less than that of children born to non-smokers (Fig. 2). The fact that gestations of less than 260 days did not conform to this general pattern lends some support to the suggestion made in the preceding section, that the influence of smoking upon birth weight may lie mainly in the later months of pregnancy. Further confirmation of the finding that smoking has little or no effect upon duration of gestation is provided in Table IV, in which it is shown that for a given birth weight the percentage of mothers who were smokers bore little relation to duration of gestation. On the other hand, at each duration of gestation there was a striking inverse relation between birth weight and percentage of smokers. For gestations of 290 days and over, 57% of the mothers of infants weighing 6 lb. (2.7 kg.) or less were smokers, compared with 17% of those of infants weighing 9 lb. (4 kg.) or more. Again the shorter durations of gestation (less than 260 days) were exceptional.

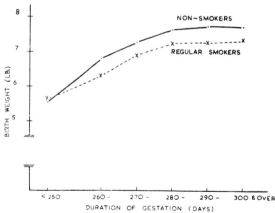

FIG. 2.—Birth weight related to duration of gestation and maternal smoking habits.

Maternal Weight

Although the matter does not appear to have been scientifically investigated, it is common knowledge that tobacco has an adverse effect upon appetite and that smokers who give up the habit tend to put on weight. Since the birth weight of an infant is directly related to the weight of its mother (McKeown and Record, 1957) the possibility has to be considered that the observed relationship between smoking and birth weight may be due to the effect of smoking upon maternal nutrition. It was indeed found (Table V) that smokers weighed significantly less than non-smokers. (Maternal weights were based on mothers' statements about their weights immediately before pregnancy, but there seems to be no reason why they should be biased in relation to smoking habits.) However, the difference—less than 4 lb. (1.8 kg.)—hardly seems sufficient to account for the difference in birth weight, since dietary deficiencies have little influence upon birth weight unless they are severe (Thomson, 1951). This view is supported by the observation that when the mothers were grouped according to their weights the infants or non-smokers were heavier than the infants of smokers for each maternal weight group (Table VI). At the same time, of course, for both smokers and non-smokers birth weight increased regularly with maternal weight.

TABLE VI.—Mean Birth Weight (lb.) of Infants Related to Mother's Weight (st.)

Mother's Weight (st.)	Non-smokers (a)	Regular Smokers (b)	Difference (a–b)
<7 ..	6·50 (19)	6·05 (20)	+0·45
7– ..	6·87 (156)	6·46 (121)	+0·41
8– ..	7·24 (328)	6·80 (201)	+0·44
9– ..	7·24 (313)	7·23 (153)	+0·01
10– ..	7·50 (149)	7·14 (84)	+0·36
11+ ..	7·82 (117)	7·59 (46)	+0·23
Total ..	7·33 (1,082)	6·92 (625)	+0·41

Maternal Age and Parity

It is necessary now to inquire whether the relation between birth weight and maternal smoking habits is influenced by maternal age or parity. It is known that birth weight increases with parity fairly consistently to the third birth rank (McKeown and Gibson, 1951), and it is not unlikely that smoking habits may be related either to parity or to age (with which parity is closely

TABLE IV.—*Percentage of Mothers who Were Smokers Related to Birth Weight and Duration of Gestation (all Deliveries)*

Gestation (Days)	Birth Weight (lb.)						Total
	<6	6-	7-	8-	9+	Total	
<260	45·8 (83)	41·0 (39)	42·1 (19)	(6)	(1)		43·2 (148)
260-	46·9 (49)	42·6 (61)	22·4 (58)	16·7 (12)	—		35·6 (180)
270-	50·9 (53)	34·8 (158)	28·2 (174)	27·1 (70)	21·4 (14)		32·6 (469)
280-	57·1 (35)	40·1 (167)	27·6 (286)	26·2 (164)	17·9 (39)		31·3 (691)
290+	57·1 (21)	48·3 (87)	28·8 (170)	27·3 (110)	16·7 (36)		32·8 (424)
Total	51·5 (241)	40·2 (512)	28·0 (707)	26·2 (362)	18·9 (90)		33·3 (1,912)

TABLE V.—*Percentage Distribution of Mothers According to Their Weight Before Pregnancy*

Mother's Weight (st.)*	<7	7-	8-	9-	10-	11-	12+	Total	Mean ± S.E.
Non-smokers	1·7 (19)	14·5 (158)	30·2 (330)	28·8 (314)	13·8 (151)	6·8 (74)	4·1 (45)	100 (1,091)	9·29 ± 0·04
Regular smokers	3·2 (20)	19·2 (121)	32·2 (203)	24·6 (155)	13·5 (85)	5·1 (32)	2·4 (15)	100 (631)	9·02 ± 0·05

*14 lb.

TABLE IX.—*Percentage Incidence of Complications of Pregnancy*

	Toxaemia	Threatened Abortion	Ante-partum Haemorrhage	Post-partum Haemorrhage	Other*	None	Total
Non-smokers	5·8 (67)	1·8 (21)	1·9 (22)	2·3 (27)	7·7 (89)	80·4 (929)	100 (1,155)
Regular smokers	3·3 (22)	1·9 (13)	2·8 (19)	2·1 (14)	6·6 (44)	83·2 (556)	100 (668)

* Albuminuria from causes other than toxaemia, severe oedema, pyelitis, etc.

correlated). The data showed no consistent change in smoking habits with age, but there was a marked and rather unexpected relationship with parity (Table VII).

TABLE VII.—*Percentage of Mothers who were Smokers Related to Age and Parity (All Deliveries)*

Age	Parity*				Total
	1	2	3	4+	
<25	27·8 (724)	42·5 (181)	41·9 (43)	50·0 (10)	32·0 (958)
25–	31·2 (285)	31·8 (132)	34·7 (49)	40·5 (42)	31·3 (508)
30–	40·4 (99)	32·6 (92)	38·5 (39)	50·0 (64)	32·5 (294)
35+	31·8 (44)	23·3 (60)	35·3 (34)	42·2 (102)	34·6 (240)
Total	29·9 (1,152)	35·1 (465)	37·6 (165)	44·5 (218)	33·3 (2,000)

* In assessing parity, stillbirths were included.

Although the change was greatest for young mothers, the proportion of women who smoked regularly throughout pregnancy increased fairly regularly with parity for each age group. Under 25 years of age 43.4% of the women in their third or later pregnancy were regular smokers, compared with only 27.8% of the primiparae. Clearly this can have played no part in determining the relationship between smoking and birth weight. Indeed, since both the proportion of smokers and birth weight increased with parity, it will, if anything, have decreased the overt effect of the one upon the other. This point is underlined in Table VIII.

TABLE VIII.—*Mean Birth Weight (lb.) Related to Maternal Parity*

Parity	Non-smokers	Regular Smokers	Total
1	7·27 (684)	6·83 (342)	7·12 (1,026)
2+	7·43 (462)	7·03 (319)	7·27 (781)
Total ..	7·33 (1,146)	6·93 (661)	7·19 (1,807)

For both primiparae and multiparae the infants of smokers weighed less than the infants of non-smokers. The effect of smoking is so marked that it can apparently override the usual pattern of parity and birth weight, for the infants of primiparous non-smokers were heavier than the infants of multiparae who smoked.

Complications of Pregnancy and Labour

Apart from reports by Mgalobeli (1931) and Athayde (1948) that women who work in the tobacco industry are more subject to abortion and stillbirth than women in the general population, there does not appear to be

any reference in the literature to the effect of tobacco upon the frequency of complications of pregnancy and labour in the human female. So far as the present inquiry is concerned there was nothing to suggest that cigarette smoking was related to complications of pregnancy. The incidence of toxaemia and of ante-partum and post-partum haemorrhage was much the same for smokers and for non-smokers (Table IX), and there was no great difference in the frequency with which delivery was effected by caesarean section or with obstetrical forceps (Table X).

TABLE X.—*Type of Delivery*

	Caesarean Section	Forceps	Other	Total
Non-smokers ..	5·5 (63)	6·8 (79)	87·7 (1,013)	100% (1,155)
Regular smokers	5·5 (37)	5·1 (34)	89·4 (597)	100% (668)

However, smoking had one noticeable effect upon the course of pregnancy. It was shown in Table III that the tobacco habit had little effect upon the length of gestation when it was naturally determined—that is, when labour began spontaneously. But the proportion of pregnancies in which labour was surgically induced was substantially lower among the women who smoked throughout pregnancy than among those who did not smoke (Table XI). The difference, although small, was

TABLE XI.—*Percentage of Pregnancies in Which Labour was Surgically Induced**

Sex of Infant	Percentage of Surgical Inductions		Difference±S.E. (a–b)
	Non-smokers (a)	Regular Smokers (b)	
Male ..	20·0 (610)	16·4 (353)	3·6±2·6
Female ..	20·7 (545)	13·3 (315)	7·4±2·6
Total ..	20·3 (1,155)	15·0 (668)	5·3±1·8

* Includes elective caesarean section.

highly significant. Smoking apparently provides a measure of insurance against surgical interference with the normal course of pregnancy. This is not altogether unexpected. Suspected disproportion is a common reason for surgical induction, and, as we have shown, the size of the foetus is influenced by maternal smoking habits.

Foetal Complications

The question whether maternal smoking habits have any effect upon the foetus other than upon its birth weight is clearly of considerable importance. There is no answer to this question in the literature, and the evidence in the present inquiry is inconclusive. Minor foetal abnormalities are irregularly and incompletely recorded in hospital records (from which the data were obtained), and major abnormalities are relatively uncommon. A much larger sample would therefore be required to uncover any but the grossest effects.

When stillbirths and deaths within the first 24 hours were grouped together, mortality among the infants of smokers was a little higher than among those of non-smokers (30 and 23 per 1,000 total births respectively). Since the total number of deaths was only 47, this could easily be a chance effect. In the same way, although the incidence of major malformations was rather higher among smokers than among non-smokers (15 and 11 per 1,000 respectively), the numbers were too small to permit any conclusion to be drawn (Table XII).

TABLE XII.—*Major Malformations*

Malformation	Non-smokers	Regular Smokers
Anencephalus (with or without spina bifida)	6	2
Hydrocephalus (with or without spina bifida)	4	3
Spina bifida alone	—	1
Renal conditions	2	—
Imperforate anus	—	2
Exomphalos	1	1
Congenital heart	—	1
Total	13	10
Number of pregnancies	1,155	668
Incidence per 1,000 births	11	15

Smoking appeared to have no influence upon the incidence of foetal asphyxia, which was 70 per 1,000 for smokers and 81 per 1,000 for non-smokers.

Discussion

In this investigation it is shown that smoking during pregnancy reduces the birth weight of the infant. The reduction in weight is by no means trivial. Infants of mothers who smoked throughout pregnancy weighed on the average 6 oz. (170 g.) less than infants of mothers who did not smoke. This was much more than the difference between male and female infants and between first and later births. It appeared to be great enough to lower significantly the incidence of surgical induction among smokers.

Since the effect of smoking upon birth weight is not due to a shortening of gestation, it must be attributed to a direct retardation of foetal growth. It is not difficult to suggest possible explanations for this. It is conceivable, for example, that tobacco might have a direct pharmacological action on the foetus, since the foetal heart rate increases when a pregnant woman smokes a cigarette (Sontag and Wallace, 1935; Doerfel, 1952). An even more credible explanation is that smoking during pregnancy may restrict the placental circulation, retarding the growth of the foetus by limiting its blood supply. In most normal adults smoking causes a peripheral vasoconstriction which may last for half an hour or longer, and is associated with a rise in both systolic and diastolic blood pressures and a measurable decrease in the temperature of fingers and toes (Simon, Iglauer, and Braunstein, 1954; Eckstein, Wood, and Wilkins, 1957; Roth and Shick, 1958). Moreover, there is some evidence that women are more sensitive than men to these effects (Friedell, 1953). It is therefore quite possible that vasoconstriction, repeated ten or more times a day, might have an appreciable effect upon the nutrition of the foetus, particularly during the later months of pregnancy.

If the effect of smoking on birth weight is as considerable as this inquiry indicates, it is evident that it must make a substantial contribution to the frequency of " premature births," defined according to weight. Moreover, it suggests a possible explanation for the observation that there has been no significant decline in the incidence of premature births in a period when obstetric services have improved considerably. In the same period the proportion of women who smoke has risen steadily, and this must have contributed in some degree to the relative constancy of the proportion of infants born at low weights.

Summary

Obstetrical and smoking histories were recorded for 2,042 pregnant women delivered in six Birmingham maternity hospitals during the summer of 1958.

The mean weight of infants of mothers who smoked regularly throughout pregnancy was 6 oz. (170 g.) less than that of infants of mothers who never smoked during pregnancy (6.93 lb. and 7.33 lb. respectively). This was more than the difference in weight between male and female infants and between first and later births. It was sufficient to lower significantly the incidence of surgical induction among smokers.

The effect of smoking upon birth weight was unrelated to maternal weight, age, and parity, or to the complications of pregnancy. It was not due to shortening gestation (brought about by early onset of labour). It is concluded, therefore, that smoking during pregnancy substantially retards foetal growth.

It is with pleasure that I acknowledge my indebtedness to the obstetricians at Dudley Road, the Queen Elizabeth and St. Chad's Hospitals, and at Heathfield Road, Lordswood, and Marston Green Maternity Hospitals. I also thank Miss Ida Giles and Mrs. Eileen Armstrong, who interviewed the patients and helped to sort the data.

REFERENCES

Athayde, E. (1948). *Brasil-méd.*, **62**, 237.
Burn, J. H. (1951). *Brit. med. J.*, **2**, 199.
Doerfel, G. (1952). *Z. ges. inn. Med.*, **7**, 227.
Eckstein, J. W., Wood, J. E., and Wilkins, R. W. (1957). *Amer. Heart J.*, **53**, 455.
Essenberg, J. M., Schwind, J. V., and Patras, A. R. (1940). *J. Lab. clin. Med.*, **25**, 708.
Friedell, M. T. (1953). *J. Amer. med. Ass.*, **152**, 897.
McKeown, T., and Gibson, J. R. (1951). *Brit. J. soc. Med.*, **5**, 98.
—— and Record, R. G. (1957). *J. Endocr.*, **15**, 410.
Mgalobeli, M. (1931). *Mschr. Geburtsh. Gynäk.*, **88**, 237.
Roth, G. M., and Shick, R. M. (1958). *Circulation*, **17**, 443.
Schoeneck, F. J. (1941). *N.Y. med. J.*, **41**, 1945.
Simon, D. L., Iglauer, A., and Braunstein, J. (1954). *Amer. Heart J.*, **48**, 185.
Simpson, W. J. (1957). *Amer. J. Obstet. Gynec.*, **73**, 808.
Sontag, L. W., and Wallace, R. F. (1935). Ibid., **29**, 77.
Thomson, A. M. (1951). *Brit. J. Nutr.*, **5**, 158.

PAPER 41

41. Jones, K. L. and Smith, D. W. (1975). The fetal alcohol syndrome. *Teratology*, **12**, 1–10

COMMENTARY

The process of fermentation for the production of alcoholic beverages represents one of primitive man's earliest achievements. It has been suggested that 'the development of man's ingenuity and intellect can almost be measured with the variety and complexity of his alcoholic beverages and the uses to which they have been extended both medically and socially' (Forney and Hughes, 1968). The problem of alcohol abuse in present-day society has reached alarming proportions. Despite the increasing number of reports concerned with the medical, social, and economical aspects of alcoholism, the production of alcoholic spirits continues to increase by about 10% annually (WHO, 1975a, b).

Since antiquity, suspicion had existed that alcohol consumption before and during pregnancy could adversely influence the development of the offspring. A special committee of the British House of Commons reported in the early part of the 19th century that the children of alcoholic mothers presented a 'starved, shrivelled, and imperfect' appearance. In other studies, a high incidence of early fetal and perinatal death, prematurity, and low birth weight were found in association with maternal alcoholism.

More recently, Lemoine *et al.* (1967) and Jones *et al.* (1973) described a pattern of specific malformations (Fetal Alcohol Syndrome) in children born to chronically alcoholic women. Prenatal and postnatal growth retardation, developmental delay, microcephaly, an unusual dysmorphic facies, and short palpebral fissures were detected in most cases; maxillary hypoplasia, joint anomalies, abnormal palmar creases, cardiovascular malformations, abnormal external genitalia, micrognathia, and cleft palate were also found in some of the children. Sufficient evidence has accumulated to indicate a high risk of fetal damage to pregnant women who are chronic alcoholics. In Paper 41, Jones and Smith discuss the clinical aspects of this syndrome and its possible aetiology.

As yet we know very little about the way alcohol acts during pregnancy and alters fetal growth and morphogenesis. Ethanol is readily transmitted across the placenta and accumulates in fetal tissues and in amniotic fluid. Both ethanol and its degradation product, acetaldehyde, are embryotoxic and teratogenic in laboratory animals. Whether the adverse effects are produced by direct toxic action on the fetus or mediated via alterations in placental circulation remains to be determined. The possible involvement of the nutritional status and socioeconomic conditions of the mothers in the etiology of Fetal Alcohol Syndrome is strongly suspected and needs to be fully evaluated. Clearly, further studies are warranted.

An unusual facies, fetal growth retardation, and microcephaly are found in Trisomy 19, Cornelia de Lange, Noonan, and Smith–Lemil–Opitz syndromes, and in rubella embryopathy. This should be taken into consideration in the differential diagnosis of the Fetal Alcohol Syndrome. Apparently, this condition is not fully manifested in all offspring of alcoholic mothers. Christoffel and Salafsky (1975) reported an interesting case of a pair of fraternal twins born to an alcoholic mother. Only one infant was severely affected; the changes in the other were minimal and recognized only because of the affected sibling. It was therefore suggested that all infants born to alcoholic mothers should be routinely screened with long-term follow-up for the more subtle lesions of maternal intoxication so that early remedial measures may be implemented to compensate for possible developmental delay.

REFERENCES

Christoffel, K. K. and Salafsky, I. (1975). Fetal alcohol syndrome in dizygotic twins. *J. Pediatr.*, **87**, 963–967

Forney, R. B. and Hughes, F. W. (1968). *Combined Effects and Other Drugs*. (Springfield, Illinois: Charles C. Thomas)

Jones, K. L., Smith, D. W., Ulleland, C. W. and Streissguth, A. P. (1973). Pattern of malformation in offspring of chronic alcoholic women. *Lancet*, **i**, 1267–1271

Lemoine, P. H., Harousseau, H., Borteyru, J. P. and Menuet, J. C. (1967). Les enfants de parents alcooliques: anomalies observées à propos de 127 cas. *Arch. Fr. Pediatr.*, **25**, 830–832

WHO (1975a). Alcohol: a growing danger. *WHO Chronicle*, **29**, 102–105

WHO (1975b). Problems of non-medical drug use. *WHO Chronicle*, **29**, 87–102

From K. L. Jones and D. W. Smith (1975). Teratology, **12**, 1–10. *Copyright* (1975), *by kind permission of the authors and the Wistar Institute Press*

The Fetal Alcohol Syndrome [1,2,3]

KENNETH L. JONES AND DAVID W. SMITH
Dysmorphology Unit, Department of Pediatrics, University of Washington School of Medicine, Seattle, Washington 98195, and Department of Pediatrics, University of California, San Diego School of Medicine, San Diego, California 92103

ABSTRACT A specific pattern of malformation involving prenatal-onset growth deficiency, developmental delay, craniofacial anomalies, and limb defects is now recognized in offspring of chronic alcoholic women. Historical evidence suggests that this is not a new observation. A recent French study of 127 offspring of alcoholic mothers indicates that this specific syndrome has been recognized in other parts of the world. Many of the features of this disorder could be related to the kind of malorientation of brain structure seen at the autopsy of one patient described herein. The frequency (43%) of adverse outcome of pregnancy for chronic alcoholic women suggests that serious consideration be given to early termination of pregnancy in severely chronic alcoholic women.

A pattern of altered growth and morphogenesis, referred to as the fetal alcohol syndrome, has now been reported in 16 children, all of whom were born to severely and chronically alcoholic women who continued heavy alcohol consumption throughout pregnancy (Jones et al., '73; Jones and Smith, '73; Ferrier et al., '73; Hall and Orenstein, '74; Palmer et al., '74).

HISTORICAL PERSPECTIVE

Since the initial discrimination of the fetal alcohol syndrome historical evidence has been brought to our attention indicating that an association between maternal alcoholism and serious problems in the offspring is not a new observation. Evidence is even available from classical Greek and Roman mythology suggesting that maternal alcoholism at the time of conception can lead to serious problems in fetal development. This led to an ancient Carthaginian ritual forbidding the drinking of wine by the bridal couple on their wedding night so that defective children might not be conceived (Haggaro and Jellinek, '42). In 1834 a select committee of the British House of Commons was established to investigate "drunkenness" prior to the establishment in that same year of an Alcoholic Licensure Act. Evidence presented to that committee indicated that infants born to alcoholic mothers sometimes had a "starved, shriveled and imperfect look." In 1900 Sullivan investigated female alcoholics at the Liverpool Prison. He documented an increased frequency of early fetal death and early infant mortality in their offspring. Other investigators have found increased frequency of prematurity and decreased weight of surviving children born to chronic alcoholic mothers (Ladraque, '01; Roe, '44; Lecomte, '50; Christiaens et al., '60).

A study reported in 1967 of 127 children born to alcoholic parents was recently brought to our attention by Dr. W. Lenz of Germany (Lemoine et al., '67). Abnormalities frequently noted in the children were growth deficiency of prenatal onset, an unusual facies, and a 25% incidence of malformations (in particular cleft palate and cardiac malformations). Psychomotor retardation (IQ 70) associated with "agitation" and "character disturbances" occurred often.

Animal experiments on the effects of ethanol on early morphogenesis have led

Received Feb. 18, '75. Accepted April 14, '75.
[1] Supported by the Maternal and Child Health Services, Health Services and Mental Administration, Department of Health, Education and Welfare Project 913, NIH grants HD05961 and GM15253, and the National Foundation — March of Dimes.
[2] Reprint address: Dr. David W. Smith, Department of Pediatrics, RR234 Health Sciences, RD-20, University of Washington School of Medicine, Seattle, Washington 98195.
[3] Presented as a Special Lecture at the 14th Annual Meeting of the Teratology Society, July 7–10, 1974, University of British Columbia, Vancouver, B. C., Canada.

to variable results (Sandor, '68). However, recent experiments demonstrated ethanol-induced dysmorphogenesis in chick as well as rat embryos (Sandor, '68a,b; Sandor and Amels, '71). This consisted in chicks of deformed brain vesicles and spinal cord, abnormal development of somites, and retardation of general growth.

PATTERN OF MALFORMATION

Features shared by the 11 children who were initially evaluated with this syndrome are summarized in figure 1. One child from each of the ethnic groups in which the fetal alcohol syndrome has been recognized are depicted in figure 2.

Prenatal growth deficiency has been more severe with regard to length than weight at birth. This is in direct contrast with most studies of generalized maternal undernutrition in which the newborn infants are underweight for their length.

Severe postnatal growth deficiency occurred in each of the 9 patients followed for longer than 1 year. The linear growth rate averaged 65% of normal whereas the average rate of weight gain was only 30% of normal despite the fact that 6 of the children were hospitalized on numerous occasions for failure to thrive, during which time adequate caloric intake was well documented, and despite the fact that 3 of them were receiving excellent foster-care. The most striking example of postnatal growth deficiency in this syndrome occurred in an American Indian girl who, at the age of 7 months had a length and weight that were in the 50th percentile for 35 weeks' gestation.

Intelligence quotients ranged from below 50 to 83 with a mean of 63.

Relative to the microcephaly, head circumference was less than the 3rd percentile for chronological age at birth in 10 out of 11 patients; and in all but 1 evaluated at 1 year of age it was below the 3rd percentile for height-age as well.

The short palpebral fissures were initially interpreted as being secondary to decreased growth of the eyes. Frank mi-

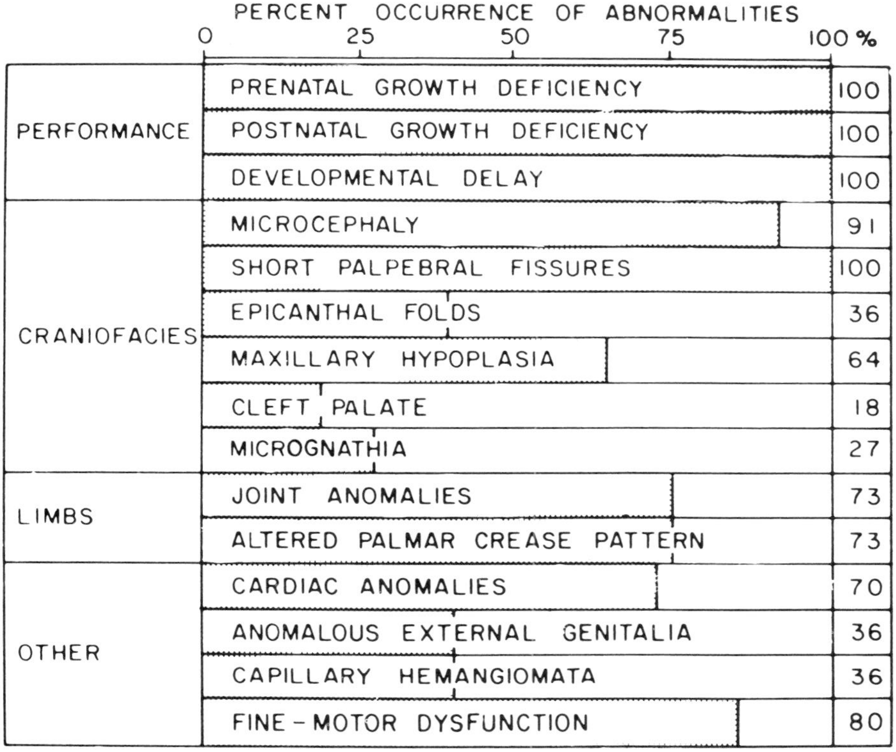

PERCENT OCCURRENCE OF ABNORMALITIES

		%
PERFORMANCE	PRENATAL GROWTH DEFICIENCY	100
	POSTNATAL GROWTH DEFICIENCY	100
	DEVELOPMENTAL DELAY	100
CRANIOFACIES	MICROCEPHALY	91
	SHORT PALPEBRAL FISSURES	100
	EPICANTHAL FOLDS	36
	MAXILLARY HYPOPLASIA	64
	CLEFT PALATE	18
	MICROGNATHIA	27
LIMBS	JOINT ANOMALIES	73
	ALTERED PALMAR CREASE PATTERN	73
OTHER	CARDIAC ANOMALIES	70
	ANOMALOUS EXTERNAL GENITALIA	36
	CAPILLARY HEMANGIOMATA	36
	FINE-MOTOR DYSFUNCTION	80

Fig. 1 Pattern of malformation.

THE FETAL ALCOHOL SYNDROME

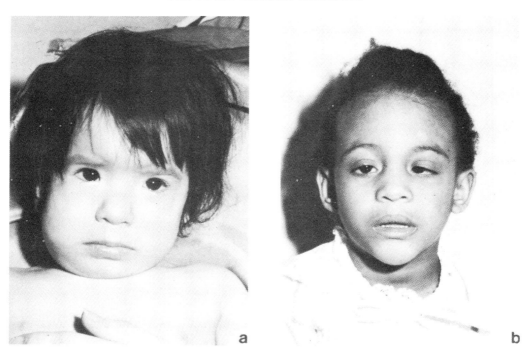

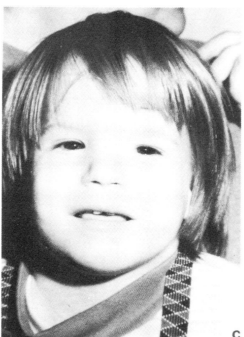

Fig. 2 Three children with the fetal alcohol syndrome, (a) a 1-year-old American Indian girl, (b) a 3 9/12-year-old black girl, and (c) a 2 6/12-year-old white boy. Note the short palpebral fissures in all children and the strabismis and asymmetric ptosis in the black girl.

KENNETH L. JONES AND DAVID W. SMITH

crophthalmia, noted in 2 newborn infants with the syndrome, tends to support this interpretation.

The joint anomalies were variable and consisted of congenital hip dislocation in 3, inability to extend the elbows completely in 3, camptodactyly of toes in 2, and inability to flex the metacarpal-phalangeal joints completely in 2 patients.

The following alterations of palmar-crease patterns were present: rudimentary palmar creases, and aberrant alignment of the palmar creases and a single upper palmar crease, or both.

Cardiac anomalies consisted of atrial septal defect in 1 patient, patent ductus arteriosus in 1 patient, and grade III/VI systolic murmurs interpreted as representing ventricular septal defect in 6 patients.

Anomalies of the external genitalia consisted of hypoplastic labia majora in 3 patients and a septate vagina in 1.

Fine-motor dysfunction was manifest by a weak grasp, poor eye-hand coordination, and tremulousness in the newborn period.

RECOGNITION OF THE FETAL ALCOHOL SYNDROME IN EARLY INFANCY

Two babies with the fetal alcohol syndrome, initially evaluated in the newborn period, are depicted in figures 3 and 4. Pertinent data relative to the maternal history of alcoholism, early neonatal course, and subsequent performance are presented in the following case reports.

Case reports

Patient 1. A 2-day-old American Indian male was ascertained because his mother was a severe chronic alcoholic. Her 7 other living children, all born prior to her becoming an alcoholic, are allegedly of normal stature and intelligence. Six years before the birth of patient 1 she began drinking 2 quarts of red wine daily. She developed cirrhosis and nutritional anemia and experienced delirium tremens. During that time she also had 3 1st-trimester spontaneous abortions. Throughout her pregnancy with the patient she continued to drink wine heavily. Her nutritional sta-

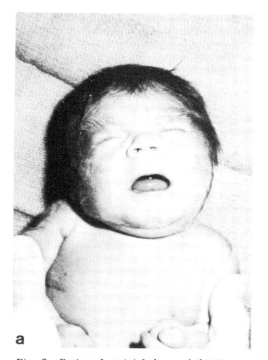 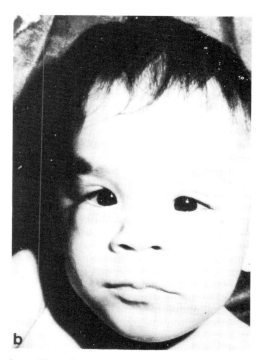

Fig. 3   Patient 1 at (a) 1 day and (b) 10 months of age. Note short palpebral fissures and hirsutism. Similarity in the newborn period to the deLange syndrome was not present at 10 months of age.

THE FETAL ALCOHOL SYNDROME

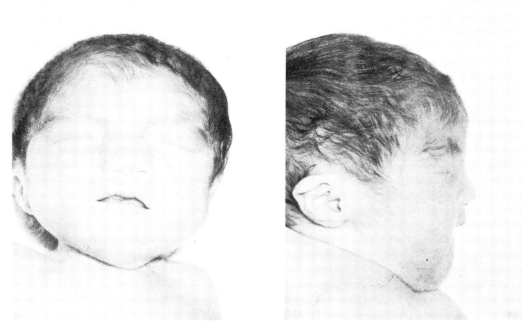

Fig. 4   Necropsy picture of patient 2 at 5 days of age. Note the short palpebral fissures, hirsutism, and the flat facies with maxillary hypoplasia.

tus, evaluated shortly after delivery, was normal except for iron deficiency. Serum vitamin A, vitamin C, folic acid, and total protein were normal. Maternal weight gain during pregnancy totaled 6.75 kg. Delivery was from a breech presentation after a 38-week gestation, during which time there was decreased fetal activity. One- and 5-min Apgar scores were 1 and 6, respectively. The attending physician noted "alcohol on his breath." Birth weight was 2020 g (50th percentile for 34 weeks' gestation), birth length was 43 cm (50th percentile for 32.5 weeks' gestation), and head circumference was 29 cm (below the 3rd percentile). There was a striking degree of hirsutism especially over the forehead. The palpebral fissures were short, measuring 1.1 cm on the right and 1.2 cm on the left. A grade II/VI systolic murmur was thought to represent a ventricular septal defect. There was left congenital hip dislocation and bilateral simian creases. A deep pilonidal sinus over a prominent coccyx was present. The immediate neonatal period was complicated by mild respiratory distress lasting 5 days and requiring 40% ambient oxygen concentration, transient hypoglycemia lasting 24 h, and hyperbilirubinemia. Tremulousness, noted soon after birth, was thought to represent "alcoholic withdrawal" but did not respond to phenobarbital sedation and was still present at 10 months of age. Since being discharged from the newborn nursery he has had excellent foster care, but despite optimum stimulation and caloric intake his growth rate and development have been markedly retarded. At the time of writing he was 13 months old and was 65.5 cm long (50th percentile for 5 months), weighed 5.7 kg (50th percentile for 3 months), and had a head circumference of 41 cm (below the 3rd percentile). His developmental age was estimated at 7 months. Seizures precipitated by hyperventilation and followed by postictal lethargy were first noted at 8 months of age. Minor nonspecific electroencephalographic signs have improved, and the seizures, despite the absence of therapy, have decreased in frequency.

KENNETH L. JONES AND DAVID W. SMITH

Patient 2. A newborn American Indian girl was ascertained because her 40-year-old mother was a severe chronic alcoholic of unknown duration. Although no complications of alcoholism were known a blood-alcohol level determined 1 week after the child's birth, at a time when the mother did not seem intoxicated, was 157 mg/100 ml. Maternal weight gain during pregnancy was 4.95 kg. Delivery, at 32 weeks' gestation, was from a vertex presentation. Apgar scores at 1 and 5 min were 5 and 8, respectively. Birth weight was 1300 g (50th percentile for 30 weeks' gestation), birth length was 38.5 cm (50th percentile for 29 weeks' gestation), and head circumference was 27 cm. She had marked hirsutism, especially over the forehead, microphthalmia, and a cleft of the soft palate. The following joint anomalies were present: overlapping of the 3rd over the 2nd fingers; clinodactyly of the left 5th finger; and camptodactyly of the right 3rd finger with absence of the distal interphalangeal crease. There was a systolic murmur along the left sternal border. The vagina was septated. There were only 2 vessels in the umbilical cord. Because of the phenotypic similarity to the 18-trisomy syndrome a chromosome study was done which was interpreted as normal. Cyanosis developed at 5 h of age and multiple apneic episodes culminated in death at 5 days of age.

The autopsy of that child is, to our knowledge, the first performed on a patient as having the fetal alcohol syndrome. The brain findings were of special pertinence. There were extensive developmental anomalies which resulted primarily from aberration of neuronal migration and thereby in multiple heterotopias throughout the leptomeninges and cerebral mantle as well as the subependymal regions. The strikingly abnormal external appearance of the brain (fig. 5) was due to sheets of neuronal and glial cells that had abnormally migrated out over the surface of the cerebral hemispheres. These changes, plus cellular disorganization of the cere-

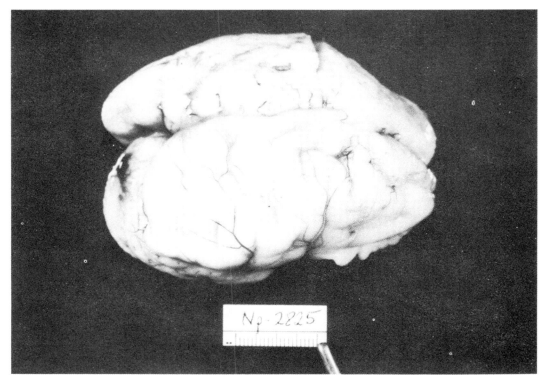

Fig. 5 External appearance of brain from patient 2. Note the smooth surface of the cerebral cortex bilaterally.

THE FETAL ALCOHOL SYNDROME

Fig. 6 Section through cerebral cortex of brain of patient 2. Note the apparently normal cells which have extended through small defects in the pia and have infiltrated the meninges. Disorganization of cellular elements is present throughout the cerebral mantle.

bral mantle, are demonstrated microscopically in figure 6. Incomplete development of the cerebral cortex was evidenced by enlarged lateral ventricles, the inner surface of which were studded with numerous nodules of heterotopic neurons (fig. 7). In addition there was agenesis of the corpus callosum.

Some of the structural and functional abnormalities in this syndrome, such as microcephaly, developmental delay, and motor dysfunction, may all be secondarily related to the type of malorientation of the brain observed in the patient. Even the joint anomalies could well be related to neurological impairment of the fetus, including diminished movement in utero resulting from this type of malorientation of brain structure.

Recognition of the fetal alcohol syndrome can be particularly difficult in the newborn. Patient 1 was initially diagnosed as having DeLange syndrome and patient 2, 18 trisomy syndrome. Incorrect diagnosis could lead to inappropriate counseling regarding the risk of malformations in future offspring. The risk of the fetal alcohol syndrome in future children is potentially high, as indicated by reports of multiple affected children. The 7 normal children born to the mother of patient 1 before she became a chronic alcoholic suggest that the recurrence risk might be related to control of maternal alcoholism.

OUTCOME OF PREGNANCY IN CHRONIC ALCOHOLIC WOMEN

The incidence and nature of problems of morphogenesis and function in the offspring of a group of women ascertained purely by the history of chronic alcoholism have recently been set forth (Jones et al., '74).

The sample of 23 was drawn from the Collaborative Perinatal Study of the National Institute of Neurological Disease and Stroke. This was a prospective study of 55,000 pregnant women and their off-

KENNETH L. JONES AND DAVID W. SMITH

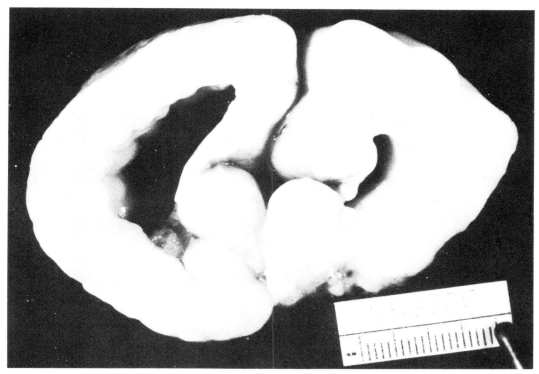

Fig. 7   Section through the cerebral cortex. Note the markedly enlarged ventricle, the inner surface of which is studded with numerous nodules representing heterotopic neurons.

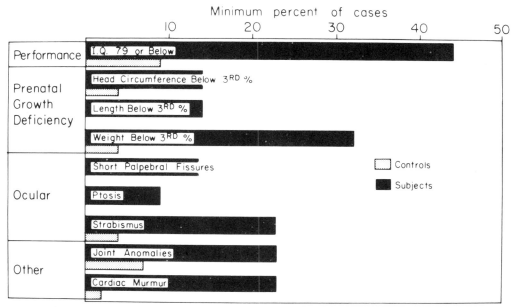

Fig. 8   The minimum frequency of abnormalities noted in children born to chronically alcoholic mothers compared with matched controls.

spring who were followed up to 7 years postnatally in 12 medical centers. Two nonalcoholic control women were matched for each of the 23 study cases. These were matched for socioeconomic status, maternal education, race, maternal age, parity, marital status, and institution where the mother and child were followed.

The results of that study suggest the overwhelming magnitude of the handicapping problems that maternal alcoholism can impose on the developing fetus.

Four of the 23 offspring of women who drank before and during pregnancy died before 1 week of age, a perinatal mortality of 17% as opposed to 2% for the control group.

The relative frequencies of problems in the 19 surviving offspring are set forth in figure 8. The structural anomalies listed are all common features in the fetal alcohol syndrome. It is important to realize that only the minimum frequency of individuals with each anomaly is depicted because all children were not systematically evaluated for such features as short palpebral fissures, ptosis, and strabismus as well as joint anomalies and cardiac murmurs.

Regarding the incidence of the fetal alcohol syndrome 6 of the 19 (32%) surviving children born to chronically alcoholic women had enough abnormal features to suggest the possibility of the syndrome from the physical findings alone, whereas not one of the matched controls was so affected.

The frequency of adverse outcome of pregnancy for chronically alcoholic women from this study was 43% (4 who died in the perinatal period and 6 with the fetal alcohol syndrome) as opposed to 2% of their controls. Because of the magnitude of this risk it is recommended that serious consideration be given to early termination of pregnancy in severely chronically alcoholic women.

DISCUSSION

The similarity in the overall pattern of anomalies in these children suggests a single etiology, most likely environmentally determined, by some as yet unknown effect of maternal metabolism. Regarding direct toxicity to the developing fetus the most obvious possibility is ethanol itself.

There is good evidence in human beings and other animals that ethanol freely crosses the placenta (Waltman and Iniquez, '72). Animal studies have shown it to be distributed in the amniotic fluid and throughout multiple fetal tissues, at least during late gestation (Ho et al., '72). Other possibilities involving direct toxicity include one of the breakdown products of ethanol such as acetaldehyde or an unknown toxic agent in the alcoholic beverages the mothers were consuming.

The adverse affect on growth and morphogenesis could also be the indirect consequence of generalized maternal undernutrition or deficiency of a specific nutrient or vitamin. However, neither this degree nor this pattern (birth length more severely affected than birth weight) of growth deficiency nor the pattern of malformation herein described have been reported in offspring of severely undernourished nonalcoholic women (Smith, '47).

Further studies are now clearly needed to examine the amount and duration of maternal alcoholism necessary to result in offspring with the fetal alcohol syndrome. All affected children recognized to date have been the offspring of severely chronically alcoholic women who drank heavily throughout pregnancy.

In addition the total spectrum of the disorder needs to be more fully delineated. Experience with other environmental teratogens would lead one to expect variable severity of this pattern of malformation and function in offspring of chronic alcoholic women.

Finally, basic studies must be performed with respect to the specific cause and possible prevention of this tragic disorder.

ACKNOWLEDGMENTS

The authors wish to thank Dr. Richard Leech for interpretation of the neuropathological specimens, Mrs. Lyle Harrah and Mrs. Mary Ann Harvey for the library research studies, Mr. Bradley Gong for photography, and Mrs. Beverly Gonsowski and Mrs. Christine Hansen for secretarial assistance.

LITERATURE CITED

Christiaens, L., J. P. Mizon and G. Delmarle 1960 Sur la descendance des alcooliques. Ann. Pédiat., 36: 37–42.

KENNETH L. JONES AND DAVID W. SMITH

Ferrier, P. E., I. Nicod and S. Ferrier 1973 Fetal alcohol syndrome. Lancet, 2: 1496.

Haggard, H. W., and E. M. Jellinek 1942 Alcohol Explored. Doubleday, Doran, New York.

Hall, B. D., and W. A. Orenstein 1974 Noonan's phenotype in an offspring of an alcoholic mother. Lancet, 1: 680.

Ho, B. T., G. E. Fritchie, J. E. Idänpään-Heikkilä and W. M. Moissac 1972 Q. J. Stud. Alcohol, 33: 485–494.

Jones, K. L., and D. W. Smith 1973 Recognition of the fetal alcohol syndrome in early infancy. Lancet, 2: 999–1001.

Jones, K. L., D. W. Smith, A. P. Streissguth and N. C. Myrianthopoulous 1974 Outcome in offspring of chronic alcoholic women. Lancet, 1: 1076–1078.

Jones, K. L., D. W. Smith, C. W. Ulleland and A. P. Streissguth 1973 Pattern of malformation in offspring of chronic alcoholic women. Lancet, 1: 1267–1271.

Ladraque, P. 1901 Alcoholism et Enfants. Steinheil, Paris.

Lecomte, M. 1950 Elements d'hérédopathologie. Scalpel, 103: 1133–1145.

Lemoine, P., H. Harousseau, J. P. Borteyru, J. C. Menuet 1967 Les enfants de parents alcohol-

iques: anomalies observées à propos de 127 cas. Arch. Fr. Pédiat., 25: 830–832.

Palmer, R. H., E. M. Ouellette, L. Warner and S. R. Leichtman 1974 Congenital malformations in offspring of a chronic alcoholic mother. Pediatrics, 53: 490–494.

Roe, A. 1944 The adult adjustment of children of alcoholic parents raised in foster homes. Q. J. Stud. Alcohol., 5: 378–393.

Sandor, S. 1968a The influence of aethyl-alcohol on the development of the chick embryo. Rev. Roum. Embryol. Cytol., Ser. Embryol., 5: 51–76.

——— 1968b The influence of aethyl-alcohol on the developing chick embryo. Rev. Roum. Embryol. Cytol., Ser. Embryol., 5: 167–171.

Sandor, S., and D. Amels 1971 The action of aethanol on the praenatal development of albino rats. Rev. Roum. Embryol. Cytol., Ser. Embryol., 8: 105–118.

Smith, C. J. 1947 Effects of maternal undernutrition upon the newborn infants in Holland (1944–1945). Pediatrics, 30: 229–243.

Sullivan, W. C. 1900 The children of the female drunkard. Med. Temp. Rev., 1: 72–79.

Waltman, R., and E. S. Iniquez 1972 Placental transfer of ethanol and its elimination at term. Obst. Gyn., 40: 180–185.

PAPER 42

42. Renwick, J. H., Possamai, A. M. and Munday, M. R. (1974). Potatoes and spina bifida. *Proc. R. Soc. Med.*, **67**, 360–364

COMMENTARY

On the basis of epidemiological data, Renwick (1972) proposed that anencephaly and spina bifida are due to mothers eating or coming into contact with blighted potatoes, i.e. potatoes infected with the fungus *Phytophthora infestans*. An antifungal product in the potato tubers was suspected as the aetiological factor.

Teratological testing of freeze-dried blighted potatoes in marmosets initially provided some evidence in support of the hypothesis (Poswillo *et al.*, 1972), but subsequent epidemiological (Elwood and MacKenzie, 1973; Emanuel and Sever, 1973; Kinlen and Hewitt, 1973; Clarke *et al.*, 1973; Spiers *et al.*, 1974) and experimental studies (Poswillo *et al.*, 1973; Swinyard and Chaube, 1973; Ruddick *et al.*, 1974) have failed to confirm it. There is, however, no substantial evidence to refute the hypothesis.

Perhaps the most important comment one could make regarding the involvement of blighted potatoes in the aetiology of neural tube defects is that too little information is available as yet. However, because of the importance of neural tube defects and the novelty of the suggestion regarding their origin, Paper 42 is included. Renwick reviews and discusses further aspects of his interesting hypothesis. In this context, reference should also be made to the proceedings of a symposium on *Potatoes and Birth Defects*, which was sponsored by the Teratology Society (see *Teratology*, **8**, 317–361, 1973).

REFERENCES

Clarke, C. A., McKendrick, O. M. and Sheppard, P. M. (1973). Spina bifida and potatoes. *Br. Med. J.*, **3**, 251–254

Elwood, J. H. and MacKenzie, G. (1973). Associations between the incidence of neurological malformations and potato blight outbreaks over 50 years in Ireland. *Nature (London)*, **243**, 476–477

Emanuel, I. and Sever, L. E. (1973). Questions concerning the possible association of potatoes and neural-tube defects, an alternative hypothesis relating to maternal growth and development. *Teratology*, **8**, 325–331

Kinlen, L. and Hewitt, A. (1973). Potato blight and anencephalus in Scotland. *Br. J. Prev. Soc. Med.*, **27**, 208–213

Poswillo, D. E. *et al.* (1973). Investigations into the teratogenic potential of imperfect potatoes. *Teratology*, **8**, 339–348

Poswillo, D. E., Sopher, D. and Mitchell, S. (1972). Experimental induction of foetal malformation with 'blighted' potato: a preliminary report. *Nature (London)*, **239**, 462–464

Ruddick, J. A., Harwig, J. and Scott, P. M. (1974). Non-teratogenicity in rats of blighted potatoes and compounds contained in them. *Teratology*, **9**, 165–168

Spiers, P. S., Pietrzyk, J. J., Piper, J. M. and Glebatis, D. M. (1974). Human potato consumption and neural-tube malformation. *Teratology*, **10**, 125–128

Swinyard, C. A. and Chaube, S. (1973). Are potatoes teratogenic for experimental animals? *Teratology*, **8**, 349–358

From J. H. Renwick et al. (1974). Proc. R. Soc. Med., **67**, 360–364. *Copyright* (1974), *by kind permission of the authors and the Royal Society of Medicine*

Dr James H Renwick,
Mrs Anne M Possamai
and Mrs Madeleine R Munday
(*London School of Hygiene & Tropical Medicine, London WC1E 7HT*)

Potatoes and Spina Bifida

Anencephaly and spina bifida (ASB) are important human malformations: four in every 1000 births, including stillbirths, have one or other of these major birth defects in the UK as a whole (0.4%). In the Western world, spina bifida, though usually more frequent than anencephaly, behaves more or less the same as anencephaly in its epidemiology. *Where* one is common, the other is common, e.g. in Ireland. *Where* one is rare, the other is rare, e.g. in London, where it is about five times rarer than in Belfast. *When* one is common, the other is common, e.g. in winter, and a bad year for one tends to be a bad year for the other. Both afflict the poor more than the wealthy by a factor of about four. Both occur at higher rates in older mothers and among those mothers with more children. The previous birth of an anencephalic leads the mother to have a 5% risk of anencephaly or spina bifida in a later pregnancy; the previous birth of a spina bifida child also leads to a comparable risk of either malformation.

For these reasons of similarity, particularly this mutual relationship within sibships, and because both are defects of one or other end of the neural tube, probably in the fourth week of embryonic life, we can treat the two as one condition (ASB), in this country at least.

Preventability
Most of these variables – time, place, class, mother's age and parity – are in principle controllable. An extremely favoured child has a risk over a thousand times smaller than a disfavoured child has, so there is certainly preventability in principle.

Two years ago, and until 8.11.73, our hypothesis was that short-term potato avoidance would prevent 95% of ASB in this country. Apparently, ASB is not so simple and the present position is as follows.

The seasonal peak of ASB incidence rates suggests damage particularly in May, as noted by Leck & Record (1966). They later recognized (unpublished) that this is the time of year when the overwintered potatoes are at their worst quality.

Then there is the rough regional concordance within countries between the birth incidence rates of ASB and the prevalence of potato blight, a fungal disease of potato. The wet west of the British Isles has a high incidence of both blight and ASB; the dry east has less of each. In the USA, the humid east has some blight and some ASB; the dry west has little of either, and the same is true of Canada. It has been doubted whether France and Sweden fit the geographical relationship, but there is no cause for this doubting. Given the unreliability of inferences across international boundaries when there are so many uncontrolled variables (potato varieties, cooking habits, &c.), the low ASB rates are quite reconcilable with a large consumption of potatoes. It is quality that matters rather than quantity. Tuber blight in most of France or Sweden is of low frequency by British standards despite the blighting of the haulms. Culinary pride is perhaps more prevalent there than here and may lead to the more frequent discarding of partly blemished potatoes. The ASB rate is accordingly rather low.

From the seasonal and geographical relationships, we predicted that an epidemic of late blight, caused by *Phytophthora infestans*, would be followed by an ASB epidemic. The eating of an

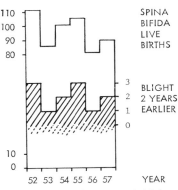

WEST OF SCOTLAND

Fig 1 Histogram showing yearly blight scores for West Scotland (Cox & Large 1960), two calendar years previous to the live spina bifida births for West Scotland (Findlay 1969). The yearly number of such births is adjusted to constant birth population size (55 000 live births per annum). P = 2! 2! 2!/6! = 0.011. (After Renwick 1972a)

overwintered potato in, say, May 1901 that was blighted in the autumn of 1900 would perhaps damage an embryo later to be born in the following February, 1902. So, when the data are available only for calendar years, as are those in Fig 1 from West Scotland, we expect a phase lapse of two calendar years between the blight and the spina bifida births. There is a clear relationship as predicted between these variables.

Fig 2 gives another confirmation of the prediction of year-to-year correlation. This is much more impressive, particularly in numbers – seven million births are involved; this time in England and Wales in the 1960s. The correlation coefficient is +0.85 and statistically highly significant. This one study embodies nearly twice as many births as all previous and subsequent studies put together. The anencephaly data were given in quarter years by Knox (1972) and, by averaging, the interval between blight and birth was fixed, as it should be, at $1\frac{1}{8}$ years from the end of the blight year, reflecting in part the storage of potatoes over the winter and in part the storage of the embryo in the uterus. The latter period is shortened by about 7 weeks by anencephaly (modal estimate), by comparison with normal or spina bifida gestations.

So we have three relationships, seasonal, regional, and year-to-year, one of which was predicted from the other two and then found. The jump from these to preventability by potato avoidance involves certain untested assumptions.

One of these assumptions, not explicitly recognized at the time, is that the effect of the teratogen, whatever substance that may be, can be avoided by short-term exclusion from the current diet. But maternal blood levels of any teratogen may reflect in part a background of slow release from body stores as well as current intake. The precise proportion of ASB that may be preventable by avoiding current intake then depends on the relative magnitudes of the two contributions. The blight correlations demand merely that the contribution from current intake is not rendered negligible by the blood level from storage sites.

If we make the perhaps rash supposition that fresh intake ceases altogether at one season of the year, then the relative contribution of the fresh intake to the total teratogenic effect can be estimated (but unfortunately overestimated) by the proportional excess from seasonal fluctuations over the minimal monthly rate. From Kinlen & Hewitt (1973), the estimate for Scotland is 11.6% (273/2348) for 1959–1963 and slightly larger, 14.7%, for 1939–1958. Rather less than 11% of anencephaly in Scotland might, on this model, be preventable by short-term avoidance of fresh intake of the teratogen – a small effect too

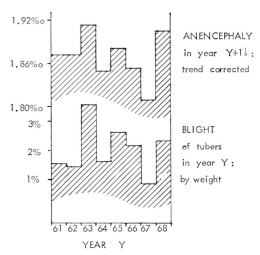

ENGLAND & WALES

Live and still births

> 0.7 million per annum

Fig 2 Anencephaly incidence rates (Knox 1972), for year Y+1⅛, based on live and still births in excess of 700 000 per annum and corrected for annual time trend of −0.05%. The lower histogram represents the percentage of potato tubers (by weight) blighted in year Y (Cox & Large 1960). r = +0.85, P = 0.005 (one-tailed test). (After Renwick (1973) incorporating various corrections)

Proc. roy. Soc. Med. Volume 67 May 1974

difficult to detect by a preventive trial. For most of the remaining 89%, body stores would have to be depleted. Further, the special population of mothers who have already borne one ASB child would tend, on this model, to have above-average body stores of the teratogen, so the degree of preventability by short-term avoidance of teratogen by these mothers would be even smaller.

For Birmingham, England, the size of the contribution from fresh intake is also falling, relatively and in absolute terms; but it is estimated to be greater than in Scotland: 41.2% for 1940–1958 and 20.7% for 1958–1963 (Leck & Record 1966). The diminishing influence of season in both Scotland and Birmingham is consistent with a decline in fresh intake which in turn would accord with the overall downward trend in anencephaly incidence, a 25% fall in the past decade in England and Wales (Knox 1972). Here, about 6.2% of the current incidence may be related to fresh intake, if this intake is entirely seasonal, and if the rest is attributable to body stores.

What is the chance that this sort of retention of the unknown teratogen occurs? No answer can yet be given but there are many toxins that are known to be retained for periods of months or years, among them DDT, some steroids, iophenoxic acid – which has a plasma halflife of $2\frac{1}{2}$ years in dogs (Wade *et al.* 1971) – methyl mercury and chloramphenicol. Some are stored in the fat or in various organs; others are excreted in the bile then reabsorbed in a perpetual recycling process, the enterohepatic recirculation. Since we do not know what the potato-related or blight-related teratogen is, we cannot test its storage behaviour; but solanine, a known potentially lethal toxin in potatoes, particularly green ones, is one of the possible candidates. It is itself a steroid derivative and it is stored for a time in rats (Nishie *et al.* 1971). Solanine is antifungal, so there is likely to be more in those potatoes that survive a winter after a bad blight year.

The work of Goldman (1972) hints at another type of storage mechanism. One interpretation of his work on rats is that teratogenic quantities of one specific enzyme inhibitor are bound by the ovum. The relevant ASB teratogen, if stored at all, may be stored in the body in any of these ways – in storage depots, in the enterohepatic circulation or in the ovum itself. If it is stored, removal of risk would require a period of potato avoidance preceding conception and the corresponding abative hypothesis would be extremely difficult to test.

This possibility of storage in the body becomes of potential importance now that a Belfast study has shown that short-term avoidance of potato does not prevent ASB. On 8.11.73, Dr Norman Nevin in Belfast told me of 2 ASB and 15 normal infants born to mothers who chose to exclude potatoes from the house during and shortly before conception; these mothers had at least one ASB child, the mean number of such previous ASB children being 1.22. The standard recurrence risk in each of these pregnancies would be about 6%. It was clearly not reduced to the 95% degree demanded by the potato hypothesis that 95% of ASB could be prevented in the UK by short-term potato avoidance. The hypothesis must therefore be abandoned and a new one sought that accommodates the new facts. So far, we have not framed a new, testable hypothesis. The Belfast exceptions, and four similar but anecdotal failures of potato avoidance elsewhere, have caused us to reconsider the assumptions, particularly the non-storage assumption. As mentioned above, storage of a natural toxin in the body, with slow release into the blood over several months or even years, might not be a rare phenomenon and could conceivably account for the failures of short-term potato avoidance.

Experimental Teratology

Can any guidance be obtained from experiments on animals? Such experiments are being undertaken in several centres following the demonstration of teratogenesis for marmosets of a potato preparation (Poswillo *et al.* 1972, 1973). The 4 out of 11 young that were affected with an osseous cranial defect were the dizygotic twin offspring of the two marmoset mothers that had been on the potato-containing diet for the longest time before conception. This is consistent with a cumulative effect and with a storage effect. Of the various classes of chemical agents that might conceivably be responsible for the marmoset defect, two are noteworthy – the cytochalasins and the solanines.

Cytochalasin B produces spina bifida in chick embryos (Linville & Shepard 1972), and another member of the cytochalasin family was found in the teratogenic potato preparation of Poswillo *et al.* Solanine increases the spina bifida rate in chick embryos from 20% in controls to 80% (Hughes 1973), and produces a different spinal and and rib anomaly in rats (Swinyard & Chaube 1973). Cytochalasins and solanines have not yet been adequately studied from the storage angle, and nor have their teratogenic potentialities been explored in the marmoset or other primate. Inference from animals to man may be dangerous and, even from primates, it must be treated cautiously.

Non-potato Interpretations

Some alternative interpretations of the blight correlations involve neither consumption nor body storage of a potato-related teratogen. The spores liberated from the fungus growing on the

278

Section of Epidemiology & Preventive Medicine

potato tops, and from other fungi that flourish in bad blight years, alight on other food crops and might initiate synthesis of antifungal substances (phytoalexins). It is known that most if not all higher plants respond to fungi by such syntheses and that pathogenicity of the fungus is, in general, not required for this. Other vegetables must therefore be considered and the requirement of a time lag before the effect on births is visible suggests that root vegetables and some of the Brassicæ might repay study.

Discussion
A solution to this important problem of ASB prevention seems to be coming closer, though we are not yet ready to put forward a testable new hypothesis. In the meantime, we do have the blight correlations as pointers and, to consolidate these, criticisms that have been raised concerning them are discussed.

The year-to-year correlation discovered on the massive data from England and Wales was attacked by Carter (1973). First, he objected to the lack of a zero on the histogram. Its insertion would, of course, not alter the correlation coefficient of +0.85 (P=0.005 by a one-tailed test). Secondly, he found no significant deviation from a linear time trend. But the point under test was not the linearity of the trend but rather the resemblance or otherwise between the patterns of ASB incidence and of blight severity over the years. He neglected to state that even the incomplete data he chose to analyse, livebirths excluded, gave a correlation coefficient of +0.34. He would have obtained a higher and more nearly correct coefficient if he had allowed for the fact that an embryo damaged by a dietary teratogen in, for instance, May may be born as late as mid-February of the following year. (This allowance could not be made on births for 1970 so he, like us, would have had to ignore that year.)

What was described inaccurately as 'a similar set of data' by Smith *et al.* (1973) comprised malformations among births in a single hospital in Edinburgh – a matter of 4300 births annually compared with 700 000 annually in the data from England and Wales. No effect was seen.

Kinlen & Hewitt (1973) did not find a year-to-year relationship with tuber blight rates at harvest even in the whole of Scotland. This failure is unexpected but may indicate that, in Scotland, where burning of the potato tops (haulms) is still not extensively practised, at least on the ware crop, blight infection of the tubers by contact with infected haulms at lifting still occurs. The rate of visible blighting among tubers at lifting would then be a poor guide to what is consumed months later. Under such conditions, the haulm

score may be a better guide to final tuber rate, and it was indeed the haulm score for West Scotland that was shown to be positively correlated with spina bifida incidence in West Scotland (P=0.011, Renwick 1972a) and with initiation rates for anencephaly in the whole of Scotland (P=0.0012, Renwick 1972b). The correlation coefficient with initiation rates should be even higher in the West itself, but the attempt by Kinlen & Hewitt to demonstrate this by subdividing the 1950s data by region was spoilt by their having to accept the wrong blight-birth interval. A large part of the seasonal excess of anencephalic stillbirths, and therefore a large part of the annual variation, falls after 1 January, and this part is assigned to the wrong blight year in Kinlen & Hewitt's analysis.

MacMahon *et al.* (1973) tested the year-to-year prediction using hospital births in Boston, Massachussetts, which are about four times as numerous as in Edinburgh. The sixteen years of slight or no blight are followed by an ASB rate that is 20% lower than the rate following the 14 years of severe blight. The moderate blight years show an intermediate rate. The effect in this small sample is not significant but the prediction is upheld. The stagewise analysis of the authors obscures this and would indeed be expected to do so.

In Canada, the Provinces of Nova Scotia and New Brunswick have small populations. Each yields only about twenty anencephalic births annually, even when the latter Province is augmented by Prince Edward Island. The lack of correlation observed by Elwood (1973) is therefore not necessarily of great moment. The lack extends to Quebec and Ontario. These are more populous, each producing about 150 anencephalics annually but, as the author says, the potatoes imported from Prince Edward Island and New Brunswick 'might mask a local effect'. It would be interesting to look for a correlation with blight (or other disease) in these imported tubers.

In North America there is less storage of potatoes than in the UK and when practised is indoors in partially controlled conditions of temperature and humidity. Hence the effects of blight on secondary invasion by other organisms and on the protective synthesis of antifungal agents (phytoalexins) are likely to be smaller than in the UK. Correlations between blight and ASB incidence would be loose, so a failure to demonstrate them in North America, even in the long term, need not influence the interpretation of those found in the UK. The lack of cyclic fluctuation of ASB rates with season in most USA data is also perhaps related to the shorter and better storage of potatoes.

Proc. roy. Soc. Med. Volume 67 May 1974

Elwood & McKenzie (1973) note that in Ireland the year-to-year correlation coefficient is small between the number of blight outbreaks on haulms by the end of June and the ASB rate in Dublin hospital births during the following year. There is, however, a weakness in the analysis. As already mentioned, when data are available only by year, there ought to be two calendar years between the blight and the spina bifida birth. The analysis given allowed only one. For anencephaly, with a modal gestation of 33 weeks, the situation is less simple, since the cyclical peak falls near the end of the year. The effect of blight is therefore spread over two calendar years and the analysis should have taken account of this. Further, the authors themselves mention serious limitations of the data: the June count of blight outbreaks is an inadequate measure of tuber blight at harvest in the autumn, because the weather varies so much in the intervening months, and it is an even worse measure of tuber quality at consumption after storage.

Summary

The year-to-year blight/ASB correlation is open to definitive testing. So far, no other workers have been able to confirm it, but we have found it to be upheld on three large sets of published data totalling over 8 000 000 births. The simplest possible interpretation of it seems, from the recent data of Nevin (1973, personal communication), not to be the correct one. We are not decided at present which of the alternative interpretations has the most to commend it, but it is reasonable to hope than an effective preventative measure will be discovered within the next ten years.

REFERENCES

Carter C O (1973) *British Medical Journal* i, 290
Cox A E & Large E C (1960) Agricultural Handbook,
Agricultural Research Service, Washington; no. 174
Elwood J H & MacKenzie G (1973) *Nature* 243, 476
Elwood J M (1973) *Lancet* i, 769
Findlay F A
(1969) *Developmental Medicine & Child Neurology* 20, Suppl. p 86
Goldman A S (1972) *Gynecological Investigation* 2, 213
Hughes A (1973) Personal Communication
Kinlen L & Hewitt A
(1973) *British Journal of Preventive & Social Medicine* 24, 208
Knox E G
(1972) *British Journal of Preventive and Social Medicine* 26, 219
Leck I & Record R G
(1966) *British Journal of Preventive and Social Medicine* 20, 67
Linville G P & Shepard T H
(1972) *Nature New Biology* 236, 246
MacMahon B, Yen S & Rothman K J (1973) *Lancet* i, 598
Nishie K, Gumbmann M R & Keyl A C
(1971) *Toxicology & Applied Pharmacology* 19, 81
Poswillo D E, Sopher D & Mitchell S J
(1972) *Nature (London)* 239, 462
Poswillo D E, Sopher D, Mitchell S J, Coxon D T,
Curtis R F & Price K R (1973) *Nature (London)* 244, 367
Renwick J H
(1972a) *New Scientist* 56, 277
(1972b) *British Journal of Preventive &
Social Medicine* 26, 67–89, 269 errata
(1973) *British Medical Journal* i, 172
Smith C, Watt M, Boyd A E W & Holmes J C
(1973) *Lancet* i, 269
Swinyard C A & Chaube S (1973) *Teratology* 8, 349
Wade D N, Desbiens N, Strewler G J jr, Brendt W O
& Mudge G H (1971) *Journal of Pharmacology
& Experimental Therapeutics* 178, 173

PAPERS 43 AND 44

43. Murphy, D. P. (1929). The outcome of 625 pregnancies in women subjected to pelvic radium or roentgen irradiation. *Am. J. Obstet. Gynecol.*, **18**, 179–187. (Extract)

44. Sternberg, J. (1973). Radiation and pregnancy. *Can. Med. Assoc. J.*, **109**, 51–57

COMMENTARY

In 1920, Aschenheim reported a case of an infant born with microcephaly and mental retardation following maternal exposure to x-rays during pregnancy. This observation was confirmed by Murphy (1929) in a survey of 625 pregnancies of women who received radiation treatment, either before or after conception. He recommended that irradiation of the lower abdomen should be avoided in pregnant women, and that pregnancy should be terminated in cases of accidental exposure to radiation (Paper 43).

Subsequent studies, both epidemiological and experimental, have shown that congenital defects may be caused by exposing the conceptus to high levels of radiation. The extent of fetal damage was related not only to the dose of radiation, but also to the stage of gestation when the exposure occurred. In addition to microcephaly and mental retardation, spina bifida, cleft palate, and skeletal and visceral malformations were detected in offspring whose mothers had abdominal and pelvic irradiation early in pregnancy. The infants irradiated *in utero* by the atomic bomb explosion in Hiroshima, before the 18th week of pregnancy, also showed a high incidence of microcephaly and mental retardation (Hicks and D'Amato, 1966; Sternberg, 1973). Of considerable importance is the reported increased risks of leukaemia and Down's syndrome in association with irradiation before conception, and of leukaemia, other cancers, an increased death rate, and changes in the sex ratio resulting from irradiation after conception.

Maternal exposure to radiation occurs either on a selective basis, because of a medical indication, or on a non-selective basis during routine pelvimetry or atomic bomb radiation, as in Hiroshima. Comparing several selective and non-selective epidemiological studies, Oppenheim and his colleagues (1975) found that the results conflicted and in each instance a significant discrepancy was evident. It was suggested that the 'selection of subjects on the basis of medical indication might have introduced biases into the various studies'; this possibility cannot be ruled out. It would be difficult to resolve whether the effects on the fetus of maternal exposure to diagnostic radiation are due to maternal factors or to the radiation itself.

A recent survey in the United Kingdom (Carmichael and Berry, 1976) indicated that fetal radiography was undertaken in 22·7% of all pregnancies (21 105 deliveries). This is a surprisingly high figure and emphasizes the need for establishing diagnostic criteria and also a re-evaluation of the situation. Because of the potential risks to the fetus of radiation during pregnancy (see Paper 44), the recommendation of the Royal College of Radiologists should be followed. It is suggested that radiological examination of the lower abdomen should be carried out within 10 days from the beginning of the last menstrual cycle. There are, however, obvious difficulties in the implementation of this '10-day rule'. Fochem (1975) recommended that x-ray examinations in pregnant women should be undertaken as a final step in diagnosis and only after the fifth month of pregnancy when the risk to the fetus is minimal.

REFERENCES

Aschenheim, E. (1920). Schädigung einer menschlichen Frucht durch Röntgenstrahlen. *Arch. Kinderheilkd.*, **68**, 131–140

Carmichael, J. H. E. and Berry, R. J. (1976). Diagnostic x-rays in late pregnancy and in the neonate. *Lancet*, **i**, 351–352

Fochem, K. (1975). Zur Röntgendiagnostik während der Schwangerschaft. *Wien. Klin. Wochenschr.*, **87**, 699–701

Hicks, S. P. and D'Amato, C. J. (1966). Effects of ionizing radiations on mammalian development. In D. H. M. Woollam (ed.). *Advances in Teratology*, Vol. 1, pp. 195–259. (New York: Academic Press)

Oppenheim, B. E., Griem, M. L. and Meier, P. (1975). The effects of diagnostic x-ray exposure on the human fetus: an examination of the evidence. *Radiology*, **114**, 529–534

Sternberg, J. (1973). Radiation and pregnancy. *Can. Med. Assoc. J.*, **109**, 51–57

From D. P. Murphy (1929). Am. J. Obstet. Gynecol., **18**, 179–187. *Copyright* (1929), *by kind permission of the author and the C. V. Mosby Company, St Louis, Mich., USA*

THE OUTCOME OF 625 PREGNANCIES IN WOMEN SUBJECTED TO PELVIC RADIUM OR ROENTGEN IRRADIATION*

By Douglas P. Murphy, M.D., Philadelphia, Pennsylvania

(*From the Gynecean Hospital Institute of Gynecologic Research, University of Pennsylvania*)

SUMMARY AND CONCLUSIONS

1. Six hundred and twenty-five pregnancies in women subjected to pelvic irradiation treatment have been studied to ascertain the influence of the irradiation upon the length of pregnancy and upon the health and development of the subsequent children.

2. Irradiation *before conception* may be followed by the birth of unhealthy or defective children. It cannot definitely be stated that such maternal treatment has a detrimental influence on the health of subsequent children.

3. *Irradiation of the pregnant woman is extremely likely to be followed by the birth of seriously defective offspring.* The frequency of these defects and their conformity to a type, of which microcephaly is the most common, strongly suggest that they are the result of the irradiation received by the embryos in utero.

4. It is believed that diagnostic curettage should always precede pelvic radiotherapy, in order to avoid possible irradiation of a growing embryo.

5. The conclusion is reached that the pregnant uterus should never be subjected to radiotherapeutic exposures.

6. It is further deemed advisable that should a growing embryo unwittingly be irradiated and its existence later be discovered, such a pregnancy should be terminated at the earliest possible moment.

---

*Read, by invitation, at a meeting of the New York Obstetrical Society, December 11, 1928.

*From J. Sternberg (1973). Can. Med. Assoc. J., **109**, 51–57. Copyright (1973), by kind permission of the author and the Canadian Medical Association*

Radiation and pregnancy

Joseph Sternberg, M.D., *Montreal*

Summary: Irradiation during pregnancy may occur either as the result of radioactive pollution of the environment, or during a medical procedure using x-rays or radionuclides. While the former is usually unforeseeable, the latter is known and accepted by both physician and patient.

Recent statistics estimate that about one quarter of pregnant women have had a radiographic experience during the pregnancy, either for obstetrical reasons or in the course of medical and dental examinations. The amount of radiation delivered to the fetus is in the range of one rad or less. Radionuclidic procedures may result in fetal radiocontamination, chiefly after placental transfer and fetal uptake. Radioiodine, radioactive calcium and selenomethionine are dangerous for the fetus, since they cross the placenta freely and are taken up by fetal tissues. The labelled proteins, radiocolloids and some mercury compounds remain in the maternal compartment and therefore can affect the fetus only through their gamma radiation at some distance from the fetus.

The teratogenic effect, the leukemogenic threshold and the lowered resistance to neonatal infections have been demonstrated after irradiation with doses far higher than those encountered during diagnostic applications of ionizing radiation. Statistical data suggest an increase of susceptibility to leukemia in infancy after intra-uterine irradiation at a diagnostic level. Cytogenic analysis may offer valuable data for the establishment of the extent of radiation damage.

Résumé: L'irradiation au cours de la vie intra-utérine peut se produire soit durant la radiocontamination du milieu, soit après un acte médical fait à l'aide des rayons x ou des molécules marquées. Dans le premier cas, l'irradiation se fait sans le consentement du sujet, tandis que dans le second cas, le patient est au courant et accepte le procédé.

Des statistiques récentes indiquent qu'environ un quart des femmes enceintes au Etats-Unis ont eu un examen radiologique au cours de la gestation, soit pour des raisons obstétricales, soit pour autres examens médicaux ou dentaires. En général il faut compter la quantité de radiation absorbée par le foetus entre quelques fractions de rad et 1-2 rads. La radiocontamination foetale exige un transfert placentaire et une distribution tissulaire foetale de la molécule marquée. L'utilisation de l'iode radioactif, du calcium ou du strontium marqués, ainsi que la sélénométhionine radioactive, comporte un danger considérable pour le foetus, car ces composés traversent le placenta et sont concentrés dans les tissus foetaux. Par contre, les protéines marquées et les radiocolloides restent exclusivement dans le compartiment maternel et peuvent irradier le foetus seulement par leur radiation gamma agissant à travers la paroi utérine.

L'effet tératogénique et leucémogénique, ainsi que la susceptibilité aux infections en bas âge, ont été obtenus avec des doses considérablement plus élevées que celles notées durant les applications diagnostiques de la radiation. Des données statistiques suggèrent une augmentation de la susceptibilité à la leucémie infantile après irradiation *in utero* pour des radiographies diagnostiques. Les examens cytogénétiques peuvent offrir des informations précieuses pour l'appréciation des radiolésions.

Fashion in medicine is as changing and illogical as in other areas of human endeavour. The recent emphasis placed by mass media upon chemical and biological pollution of the environment seems to have rendered obsolete the concern about radioactive contamination. Yet the problem is far from being obsolete. Nor did it diminish with the temporary lull in the atmospheric testing of nuclear weapons; industrial uses of nuclear energy are steadily growing and diversifying, while biomedical applications of radionuclides develop at an unprecedented pace.

Observations on the effects of radiation during pregnancy are almost as old as medical applications of x-rays. In 1902 Boullé and Bar reported a severe burn of the abdominal skin after local exposure to x-rays in a pregnant woman. Surprisingly, the report mentions that the woman delivered a set of apparently healthy twins.[1] About the time of World War I, irradiation over the abdominal region was considered a relatively innocuous and convenient procedure for therapeutic abortion; with a dose around 350 R., abortion occurred after three to four weeks. In some cases the fetus survived this assault and was delivered at term with severe developmental defects — stunted growth, microcephaly and mental retardation.[2] This procedure continued to be applied until the late thirties, for we find a report in 1936 presenting statistics of 200 cases performed in a New York hospital.[3]

The advent of World War II and the tragic events in Hiroshima sensitized public opinion against radiation, be it x-rays or fall-out. The children born of women exposed during pregnancy to the nuclear radiation in Hiroshima and Nagasaki exhibited var-

Reprint requests to: Professor J. Sternberg, Head, Laboratory of Radiobiology and Nuclear Medicine, University of Montreal, P.O. Box 6128, Montreal 101, P.Q.

ious degrees of microcephaly and mental retardation similar to those noted after unsuccessful attempts at radiotherapeutic abortion.[4]

In the early fifties the pendulum of public concern swayed to a limit of extreme caution and almost unreasonable fear of radiation. This was understandable at the time, since the menace of world-wide nuclear war loomed in the background of every human activity. Simultaneously, industrial uses of nuclear energy began to acquire importance and medical applications of radionuclides started their spectacular development, to continue with the same momentum until now.

What is the present situation and to what extent must we fear fetal radiation damage when applying a radiation procedure during pregnancy?

The details of the problem have been analysed extensively in recent reviews and symposia.[5,6] This article stresses only the salient points and offers some guidelines to the clinician.

Parameters of study

A semantic clarification is necessary for better understanding of the terms employed in this review. One distinguishes irradiation from radiocontamination in the sense that the former implies the effects of electromagnetic rays (x-rays or γ-rays) delivered from a source external to the body and acting simultaneously on the mother and the fetus. Radiocontamination is a more intimate process, since the radiation carrier is first distributed systemically into maternal tissues, reaches and crosses the placenta and is taken up finally by fetal tissues. In this case, not only the γ-rays are effective, but also the particulate α- and β-rays, with a shorter range but a markedly higher ionizing power.

The mechanism of radiation damage has by no means been entirely elucidated, but a simplified version distinguishes the "direct hit" which provokes breakage in intracellular bonds, such as in the DNA molecule. Concurrently, the production of free radicals in the irradiated cell inhibits the repair process in the damaged molecule. If radiobiology could find an effective method of repairing the damaged DNA molecule, then a large measure of radioprotection could be offered. Nature shows us that this is possible, since recently a microorganism was found in effluents of high radiation sources. The microorganism, appropriately baptized *Micrococcus radiodurans*, is capable of repairing rapidly and effectively the damaged DNA molecule (Fig. 1).

Both irradiation and radiocontamination occur as environmental factors, be they natural or man-made. Man receives about 150 to 300 mrads/year

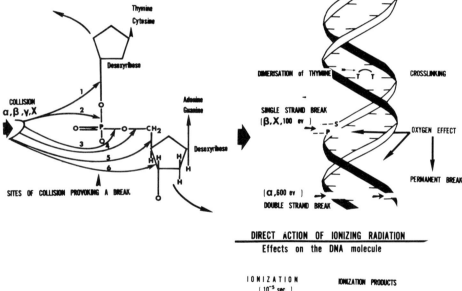

DIRECT ACTION OF IONIZING RADIATION
Effects on the DNA molecule

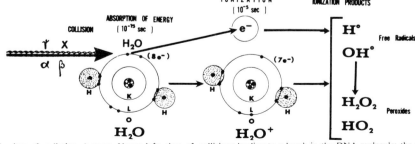

FIG. 1—Mechanism of radiation damage. Upper left: sites of collisions leading to a break in the DNA molecule; the most frequent site is in the proximity of the PO₄ residue. Upper right: radiation damage of the DNA molecule: break of a single strand provoked by about 100 electron-volts (β- or x-rays); break of a double strand provoked by an α-ray (600 electron-volts). Lower: production of free radicals and peroxides after interaction of ionizing radiation with water: the peroxides will hamper the repair process in the broken DNA molecule and will render the damage permanent.

from natural sources, about 30% of which originates from cosmic rays, a similar proportion from the ground and buildings and less from food. There are areas in the world with a higher component of one or other factor, but thus far no clear-cut results have been obtained which point to a harmful effect of an increased level of natural radioactivity. A doubling or even tripling of cosmic irradiation does not appear to have deleterious effects on the inhabitants of the high plateaus of Peru, Bolivia or Tibet. Also, the population in the thorium-containing regions of Brazil and Kerala, India, live in areas with a tenfold increase of irradiation from the ground and dwellings without exhibiting notable effects attributable to excess irradiation. Finally, the so-called radioactive waters in the European spas of Pistyan, Bad Gastein, etc. seem to have contributed amply to the benefit of both patients and physicians during the epoch when radium was considered a cure for many ailments (Fig. 2).

The man-made sources of environmental radiocontamination are produced by the industrial uses of nuclear energy, if one omits nuclear weapons. There are at present about 275 nuclear power

plants throughout the world, functioning or under construction; also, there are a considerable number of nuclear-powered ships. This represents an enormous amount of fissionable material and radioactive wastes. Even with the most stringent safeguards, accidents have happened in the past and are bound to occur in the future.

Environmental irradiation or radio-contamination occurs without the knowledge and approval of the persons subjected to its action. In contrast, the patient submitted to iatrogenic irradiation or radiocontamination is well aware of the reasons and accepts the possible risks of a procedure intended for his benefit. Iatrogenic irradiation comprises the diagnostic and therapeutic applications of x-rays, while medical uses of radiopharmaceuticals enter the category of radiocontamination.

The diagnostic use of x-rays during pregnancy constitutes the most common source of intra-uterine irradiation. A study carried out in 1966 in the United States revealed that of the total of 4,071,000 pregnant women in the country 1,086,000 (26%) underwent a radiographic examination and 478,-000 (11%) had a dental x-ray. Half of

the examinations (54%) were made during the third trimester, 25% during the second and 21% during the first trimester. Almost all obstetrical radiography was carried out during the last trimester, and included pelvimetry, placentography and scout films for the determination of fetal position. The nonobstetrical radiography — about 10% of the total amount during the last trimester — included gastrointestinal series, barium enema, cholecystography, etc. (Fig. 3). The large majority of the radiographic procedures carried out during the first and second trimesters were routine chest radiographs, with a small percentage of fluorograms, heart films, etc. Similar statistics were published in Great Britain, where pelvimetry and placentography dominated the list of requests. To our knowledge, there are no similar statistics from Canada. The application of the National Health Insurance Plan does not appear to have changed the proportion of radiographic procedures during pregnancy if one compares the data in Britain with those in the United States. On the other hand, the development of sonar procedures for placentography and estimate of fetal maturity may have

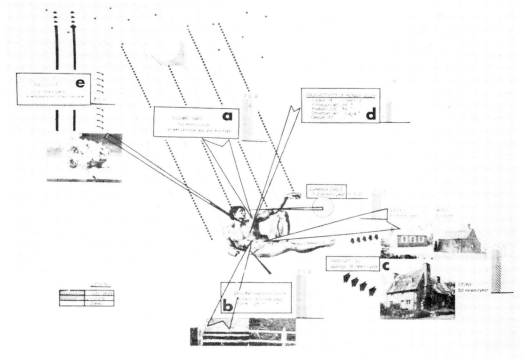

FIG. 2—Environmental sources of irradiation and radiocontamination. Total average: 200-300 mrads/yr. (rad: unit of energy absorption in matter, 1 rad corresponding to the absorption of energy produced by ionizing radiation, equivalent to 100 ergs/g. matter): (a) cosmic rays, 50 mrads/yr., at sea level; (b) ground radioactivity, 25-90 mrads/yr.; (c) habitations radioactivity, 30-50 mrads/yr.; body radioactivity (K, Ra, ¹⁴C), 60 mrads/yr.; (e) fall-out from nuclear testing, 1-2 mrads/yr.

brought about a drastic change in the number of requests for x-rays during pregnancy.

The amount of radiation received by the fetus during a radiological procedure in the mother ranges from a fraction of a rad to a maximum of 2 to 2.5 rads; this excludes fluoroscopic examinations, in which the exposure can be considerably higher.

The last statistical analysis concerning nuclear medical procedures dates from 1968, but the rapid developments in this field have rendered the data obsolete. At an educated guess there were about 2,000,000 radionuclidic *in vivo* procedures in 1972 in the United States and about 180,000 in Canada. The major areas of application are thyroid studies, brain and liver scanning, followed by imaging of kidneys, lungs and bones, hematologic studies, etc.

The dosimetry of internally administered radionuclides is more complex than that of x-ray procedures. It must take into account the physical nature of the radiation, the metabolic pathway of the radiopharmaceutical in the maternal compartment, its rate of placental transfer as well as the distribution pattern in fetal tissues. The critical factor is the degree of placental permeability for a given radiation carrier. The placenta can be entirely permeable to mineral metabolites, small molecules of sugars, amino acids, etc.; it becomes impermeable to large protein molecules, colloidal suspensions, or small molecules which attach themselves to protein carriers along their metabolic pathway.

A classification of nuclear medical procedures according to their potential danger to the fetus places in the first rank the thyroid imaging and function studies carried out with radioactive iodine or pertechnetate. Not only does iodine cross the placenta freely, but the fetal thyroid is about six to seven times more avid for iodine than maternal thyroid. Inadvertent administration of radioiodine constitutes a danger of radiation damage to the fetus — considerably greater if the dose is in the therapeutic range. In the past, there have been many reports of complete destruction of the fetal gland with severe exophthalmos and marked diminution of the brain; all dealt with millicurie-range applications of radioiodine in unknown pregnancies. Today the physician is well aware of this possibility and accidents are very rare. The simplest way to avoid them is to perform diagnostic and especially therapeutic procedures during the two weeks following the menstrual period.

Another procedure with potential danger to the fetus is pancreas scanning with ^{75}Se selenomethionine. The labelled amino acid crosses the placenta freely and remains in fetal tissues for a considerably long period of time. Whenever the possibility of an early pregnancy exists the test must be proscribed, and after its administration to a woman of child-bearing age a course of an ovulation-suppressing agent is indicated for a few months.

Bone scanning with radioactive calcium ([47]Ca) or strontium ([85]Sr) is also dangerous to the fetus, since the mineral crosses the placenta freely then is avidly taken up by the fetal skeleton if radiocontamination occurs after the onset of ossification.

Brain scanning constitutes a more complex problem: while imaging of tumour vascularization can be carried out with labelled albumin, the extracellular distribution pattern can be achieved with pertechnetate and the intracellular uptake of tumour cells appears better with labelled mercury. Both labelled albumin and mercury compounds remain in the maternal compartment, while pertechnetate has the same distribution pattern as iodine. Therefore, if a brain scan becomes mandatory during pregnancy, ^{99m}Tc-labelled albumin appears safer than the other compounds.

Radioactive gases (^{133}Xe and [85]Kr) became popular for lung function and organ irrigation studies; they have even been used for the determination of uteroplacental irrigation in normal and pathologic pregnancies. However, they must be proscribed, for the inert gases are rapidly transferred across the placenta, probably at an early stage of pregnancy when radiosensitivity of the embryo is considerably higher.

On the other hand, lung scanning with macroaggregates of labelled albumin should be less dangerous since the labelled compound remains restricted to the maternal system.

Liver scanning with radiocolloids ([198]Au or ^{99}Tc-sulfide) appears to be relatively safe since the radiopharmaceutical remains exclusively confined to the maternal compartment. A similar situation occurs in the case of kidney scanning with [197m]Hg compounds which bind rapidly to plasma proteins after intravenous administration. However, the amount of radiation delivered to the kidney is high enough (close to 10 rads) to suggest a transuterine irradiation by the γ-ray of the isotope. Labelled iodohippuran is also retained in the maternal compartment and is less hazardous, being rapidly excreted in the urine.

In essence, organ visualization with radiopharmaceuticals appears to be less dangerous to the fetus than one would think, with the exception of thyroid, pancreas and bone scanning. The advent of scintillation cameras as well as the availability of short-lived isotopes contributed to the reduction of radiation exposure. For the radiopharmaceuticals confined to the maternal space, fetal irradiation by γ-rays from the maternal side should be roughly equal to or less than the amount of irradiation received as a result of the usual x-ray diagnostic procedures.

Therapeutic applications of radiopharmaceuticals represent about 2% of the total radionuclidic procedures and include radioiodine therapy, ^{32}P therapy

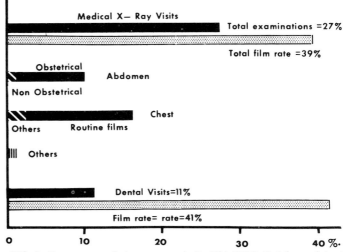

FIG. 3—X-ray exposure during pregnancy in the USA (1966). Statistics carried out on 4,071,000 pregnancies. Total amount = 27% of the pregnant women, but total film rate = 39%, about 1.44 films/patient. The ratio of dental films is markedly higher — 3.7 films per patient.

of polycythemia and some regional applications of colloidal ^{198}Au, especially intra-articular injections for arthritic disease. Both radioiodine and radiophosphorus must be prohibited, while radiogold can be safely used during pregnancy since it remains localized at the site of injection.

Effects of intra-uterine irradiation

The effects of prenatal irradiation vary considerably with the age of the progeny. Little is known about the effect of irradiation during the very early stages between conception and implantation of the egg (the first 9 to 10 days in man). Irradiation during the phase of primordial organs (up to the 18th to 20th day postconception) is likely to provoke death and expulsion of the ovum. The effects are best known for the phase of organogenesis (between the 20th and the 50th days postconception). Irradiation with about 100 to 200 rads will provoke major developmental anomalies in the central nervous system, eyes, skeleton, etc. Larger doses induce neonatal death. Radiocontamination with millicurie doses of ^{32}P is followed by severe damage to the central nervous system, usually lethal. On the other hand, administration of radioiodine before the onset of thyroid function can be less damaging than later, when the thyroid gland becomes functional.

In humans, the organogenetic phase ends on the 50th day and is followed by the fetal phase, which lasts about three quarters of the intra-uterine life. Irradiation during this phase does not induce teratogenesis, but slows down or even arrests the fetal growth, either of the entire body or only of the skull and the brain (Figs. 4A and 4B).

The critical factor in determining the degree of severity of radiation damage is the correlation between the threshold of irradiation and a given pathological manifestation. There are thresholds for different types of damage, such as the 100 rads level, established as the lowest amount known to produce leukemia in adults. In children irradiated in utero in Hiroshima with doses between 50 and 100 rads, there was a significant degree of microcephaly and mental retardation but no increase in childhood leukemia.

Clinical reports in this matter are scarce and incomplete; one report of granulocytic leukemia in a 10-month-old infant attempts to correlate this disease to prenatal irradiation with about 25 rads in a series of obstetrical radiographies. The report is incomplete and subject to dispute; the correlation may have been coincidental, for the entire dose of 25 rads was protracted over five radiographies, ranging from 1.4 to 8.4 rads.[7]

Another case, far better studied, presents a complete cytogenetic analysis of both mother and infant.[8] The mother underwent radiation treatment for breast cancer during the sixth month of pregnancy. The total amount of radiation delivered to the breast and axilla was estimated at 19,000 rads in protracted doses; there is no indication of the dose to the abdomen, which was adequately shielded. The newborn showed growth impairment as well as severe generalized infection. A detailed karyotype analysis showed a considerable amount of chromosomal damage to an average of 63% of the examined cells. In a single cell, the author reported no fewer than 17 chromosome breaks (Figs. 5A and 5B).

The gap between 50 rads and the usual 1 to 2 rads level encountered during diagnostic uses of x-rays or radiopharmaceuticals is very great indeed. The chief question is whether this small amount is capable of provoking damage when applied during preg-

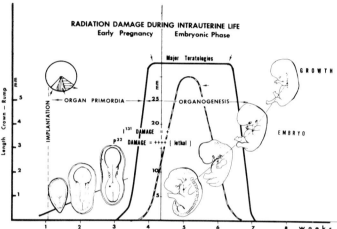

FIG. 4A—Radiation damage during early pregnancy. The phases of embryonic development are schematized as size in function of age in days. The circle gives the relative proportion of each developmental phase as a fraction of the duration of term. The three phases, i.e. implantation, organ primordia, and organogenesis, constitute about 23% of intra-uterine life (in man, far more in mouse). The major teratisms occur after irradiation with about 100-200 R. during organogenesis. Large amounts of radiophosphorus provoke major teratisms, but radioactive iodine is relatively less damaging than after onset of thyroid function

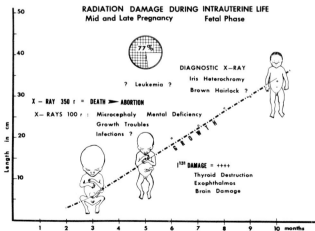

FIG. 4B—Radiation damage during fetal life. Circle illustrates the proportion of fetal life (77% of total term) in humans. Radioactive iodine provokes severe damage, while teratisms are far less frequent than during organogenetic phase.

nancy. The answer is far from being unequivocal and extrapolation from animal experimentation cannot be accepted without strong reservations. Results of statistical investigations in humans were interpreted by some authors as an argument for an increase of susceptibility to leukemia after intrauterine irradiation at the diagnostic level.[9] This has been criticized by other investigators and the argument is not yet settled. Another statistical study suggests an increase of iridian heterochromy (eyes of different colours) in children irradiated *in utero* at the 0.5-3 rads level.[10] Thus far, no comprehensive study has been carried out on other parameters, especially the effects of intra-uterine irradiation on the susceptibility to childhood infections. Experimental data suggest that this area deserves to be explored.

Medico-legal problems

In view of the increasing number of malpractice suits, the practitioner must be well aware of his legal responsibility when performing a radiation procedure. In some cases a genetically transmitted birth defect could be claimed by the plaintiff to have been caused by prenatal irradiation, carried out without expert advice. Brent[11] establishes four categories of causative agents in teratogenesis: definite (e.g. thalidomide), probable relationship, improbable and no relationship. Radiation teratogeny enters the category of "probable rela-

tionship" when a single dose of 50 rads is given during the time of organogenesis. A dose of 25 rads is considered to have an "improbable relationship", comparable to physical or psychological trauma during pregnancy.

This classification should be supplemented with more evidence, as a framework for future reference. Legal-

ly, the report mentioned above of acute leukemia occurring in an infant who had received 25 rads *in utero* could be taken as an instance of "probable relationship", even if the scientific value of such an assertion is far from being established. The legal value of cytogenetic examination has not been fully exploited; even if we ignore the rela-

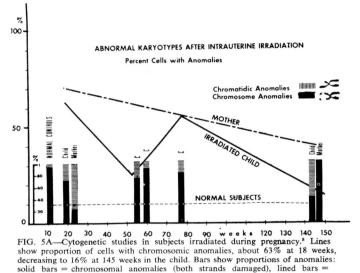

FIG. 5A—Cytogenetic studies in subjects irradiated during pregnancy.[8] Lines show proportion of cells with chromosomic anomalies, about 63% at 18 weeks, decreasing to 16% at 145 weeks in the child. Bars show proportions of anomalies: solid bars = chromosomal anomalies (both strands damaged), lined bars = chromatidic anomalies (one strand damaged).

CHROMOSOME DAMAGES AFTER INTRAUTERINE IRRADIATION

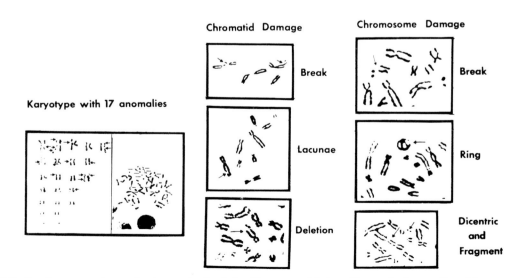

FIG. 5B—Chromosome damage after intra-uterine irradiation. Karyotype at left shows 17 anomalies in one cell; at right, most common anomalies encountered after irradiation.

tionship between a given chromosomal damage and a pathological manifestation, excluding well known genetic entities, a karyotype could constitute a weighty argument in court for or against radiation damage as the causative agent of disease in childhood.

Another aspect concerns the legality of prenatal irradiation as a valid reason for interruption of pregnancy. According to the presented data, only amounts of approximately 350 rads applied to the abdomen can cause intra-uterine death and abortion. Except for radiation therapy to the abdomen during an unknown pregnancy, such a high dose would be very unlikely. If such a situation were to arise, interruption of pregnancy ought to be considered. Also, administration of therapeutic doses of radioiodine and radiophosphorus may be invoked as a reason for interruption of pregnancy, but it is not automatically accepted as a valid argument. Tests employing diagnostic levels of irradiation are not admissible as reasons for therapeutic abortion.

The clinician has also the responsibility to inform the woman of childbearing age receiving a therapeutic dose of ^{131}I or ^{32}P that she should follow a course of ovulation-suppressing agents for about four to five months after treatment, in order to avoid a pregnancy while the isotope is still present in her organism in relatively large amounts.

Conclusions

What conclusions should one draw from this exposé of the complex problem of radiation fetopathology?

The first point to be stressed is that, regardless of the nature of radiation, be it iatrogenic or environmental, provoked by x-rays or radionuclides, the crucial problem is the dose-effect relationship. The extent of radiation damage at the low diagnostic level has not yet been determined; statistical arguments suggesting an increase in childhood leukemia must be supported with more convincing data to justify total abstention from radiological examination during pregnancy. The thalidomide tragedy has started a type of "backlash" against hyperdiagnosis and hypermedication during pregnancy. However, there are instances where failure to apply a proved procedure could have very serious consequences; a rapid and accurate localization of the placenta by x-rays or radiopharmaceuticals could be life saving and should not await sonar techniques for fear of fetal irradiation. Medical practice entails continuous risks taken in good faith for the benefit of the patient. If, with equally satisfactory results, the risk of radiation damage could be avoided by choosing a non-radiation procedure, then by all means the latter should be used.

In view of the risks to the embryo, it may be concluded that radiological investigations in women exposed to the possibility of pregnancy should be confined to the first two weeks of the menstrual cycle. If they are thought to be indicated after this time limit has passed, it has been stated that a pregnancy test should first be performed. While immunological tests of pregnancy can yield positive results from the 21st to the 23rd days post-conception coinciding with the onset of the organogenetic period of the embryo, the possibility of false results must not be disregarded. The responsibility for eliciting the menstrual and coital history and interpreting the results of the pregnancy test should be assumed by the referring physician and not delegated to the radiologist.

There is no clear-cut position for or against radiation procedures during pregnancy. The reason for this attitude is that each case must be considered individually and the decision has to be taken as in any other medical act. To establish a rule of thumb is dangerous and unscientific.

To borrow the expression of the classic hero of Racine, one may say with regard to radiation procedures during pregnancy: *"Cela ne mérite ni cet excès d'honneur, ni cette indignité."*

References

1. BAR PJ, BOULLÉ T: Ulcérations profondes et troubles trophiques graves de la paroi abdominale produits par les rayons X chez une femme enceinte; heureuse influence des rayons rouges. *Bull Soc Obstet Gynecol (Paris)* 4: 251, 1902
2. GANZONI M, WIDMER H: Erfahrungen uber des Rontgenabort. *Strahlentherapie* 19: 485, 1925
3. MAYER MD, HARRIS W, WIMPELMEYER S: Therapeutic abortion by means of X-rays. *Am J Obstet Gynecol* 32: 945, 1936
4. WOOD JW, JOHNSON KG, OMORI Y: *In utero* exposure to the Hiroshima atomic bomb. An evaluation of the head size and mental retardation twenty years later. *Pediatrics* 39: 385, 1967
5. STERNBERG J: Radiation risk in pregnancy. *Clin Obstet Gynecol* 16: 235, 1973
6. ARTHURE H: Proceedings of the symposium on the effects of low radiation doses on the maturation of the developing ovum and fetus. *Br J Radiol* 30: 714, 1968
7. GUNZ FW, BORTHWICK RA, ROLLESTON GL: Acute leukemia in an infant following excessive irradiation. *Lancet* II: 190, 1958
8. JALBERT P, PATET J, BACHELOT C, et al: Evolution cytogénétique et hématologique d'un nourrisson irradié *in utero*. *Arch Fr Pediatr* 26: 185, 1969
9. STEWART A, WEBB J, GILES D, et al: Malignant disease in childhood and diagnostic irradiation. *Lancet* II: 190, 1958
10. TUBIANA M, MAYER M, LEJEUNE J, et al: Données actuelles sur les risques pour l'embryon, le foetus et l'enfant de la radiologie médicale. *Rev Hyg Méd Soc* 11: 751, 1963
11. BRENT RL: Medico-legal aspects of teratology. *J Pediatr* 71: 288, 1967

PART VI

DETECTION OF ENVIRONMENTAL TERATOGENS

45. Persaud, T. V. N. (1974). Environmental factors in the etiology of human malformations: perspectives and problems of evaluation. In F. Coulston and F. Korte (eds.). *Environmental Quality and Safety*, Vol. 3, pp. 164–172. (Stuttgart: Georg Thieme Verlag)

46. Doll, R. (1973). Hazards of the first nine months: an epidemiologist's nightmare. *J. Irish Med. Assoc.*, **66**, 117–126

COMMENTARY

These review articles deal with the difficult problem of identifying potential human teratogens in the environment. The first paper is concerned with laboratory studies, in particular the design of teratological experiments and the relevance of the information obtained to the human situation (Paper 45); in the other, the epidemiological and clinical perspectives are presented (Paper 46).

The teratological screening of drugs, chemicals, and environmental pollutants represents a complex type of toxicological problem. Multiple factors, including the mother, embryo and placenta, are involved. Because studies of this nature are neither ethical nor justifiable in humans, the results of carefully planned animal studies should continue to provide essential data for predicting possible harmful effects in the pregnant woman. It is recognized, however, that teratological studies in animals are unlikely to provide conclusive evidence which would incriminate any given substance as being teratogenic in humans. This evidence can only be obtained from detailed clinical observations; all proven human teratogens have been first identified in this manner.

In many countries at the present time, a system of reporting birth defects to a regional centre is proving useful for monitoring the incidence, pattern, and variation of congenital malformations occurring in the population at large. Such an approach may also direct our attention to causal environmental influences.

From T. V. N. Persaud (1974). Environmental Quality and Safety, Vol. 3, 164–172. *Copyright* (1974), *by kind permission of the author and Georg Thieme Verlag, Stuttgart, Germany*

Environmental Factors in the Etiology of Human Malformations: Perspectives and Problems of Evaluation

T.V.N. Persaud
The University of Manitoba, Winnipeg, Manitoba, Canada

Summary Teratogenic compounds are discussed, i.e. active products which probably have teratogenic effects in man. For environmental chemicals, the general principles for the causation of deformities are enumerated and evaluated. The difficulties of predicting possible teratogenic effects of any chemical from animal experiments are pointed out, especially as there are no standardized methods.

Zusammenfassung Zunächst werden Wirkstoffe vorgestellt, die mit Sicherheit teratogen sind bzw. die mit einer gewissen Wahrscheinlichkeit im Menschen teratogene Effekte haben. Für Umweltchemikalien werden die allgemeinen Prinzipien zur Entwicklung von Mißbildungen aufgezählt und bewertet. Es wird auf die Schwierigkeit der Voraussage möglicher teratogener Effekte irgendeiner Chemikalie aus Tierexperimenten hingewiesen, besonders da keine standardisierten Methoden vorhanden sind.

Congenital malformations have assumed great importance in recent years, due not only to the thalidomide tragedy, but also to improved antenatal care and better management of traditional infectious and nutritional diseases. The mortality rate from birth defects has risen proportionally as the mortality rate from infection and malnutrition has decreased. The severe damage done to unborn children by the use of thalidomide during pregnancy has helped to focus attention on the potential hazards of adverse environmental agents to the pregnant woman and her offspring. It is now established that most birth defects have an environmental component in their multifactorial etiology.[10, 11, 15, 34, 75] Some measure of control will only become possible with the identification of potential environmental hazards and an understanding of their envolvement in the production of developmental defects. The increasing contamination of the human environment with harmful substances[3, 12, 20, 21, 25, 29, 42, 67] makes this an urgent problem.

Human Teratogens

In 1942 the first environmental factor recognized as causing human malformations was described. Cataract, microcephaly, deaf-mutism and heart lesions were observed in infants of mothers who had contracted German measles during early pregnancy.[26] Since then numerous reports have been published implicating other viruses and infectious agents in the etiology of human malformations. Apart from rubella, cytomegalic inclusion virus,[33] syphilis [5] and toxoplasmosis,[30, 55] the evidence is not conclusive that other *maternal infections* can lead to fetal damage and fetal abnormalities.[4, 18, 19, 45, 60, 61] Particular attention should be directed to the increasing contamination of the human environment with various ionizing and non-ionizing *radiations* and their potential harmful effect on the human conceptus. The teratogenic hazards of ionizing radiations during early pregnancy are well established.[28, 29, 53] Microcephaly, spina bifida, cleft palate, visceral malformations and limb defects have been observed following irradiation of the abdomen and pelvis in early pregnancy. There is some relationship between the dose level and time of irradiation and the adverse effects produced.

Aminopterin, an antagonist of folic acid, produced malformed fetuses when administered during early pregnancy to tuberculous women for the purpose of inducing therapeutic abortion [70] and in cases of illegal abortion.[43, 63, 76] Intrauterine growth retardation, anencephaly, hydrocephaly, meningocele, cleft palate, and skull anomalies were observed on the fetuses recovered.

Progestational compounds are used clinically for the prevention of threatened **abortion, but maternal** treatment with synthetic progestins in early pregnancy has caused masculinization of female infants.[57, 59, 74, 79]

Thalidomide provided an almost perfect example of a causal relationship between a specific teratogen and human congenital malformations. The teratogenicity of this substance in man was demonstrated during its use as a sedative which resulted in the birth of thousands of severely malformed infants.[14, 35, 40, 77] A wide spectrum of congenital malformations, including limb defects (Figure 1), absence of the

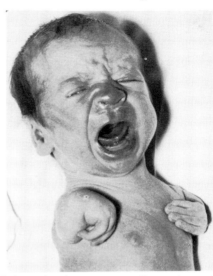

Fig. 1 *Infant showing severe malformations of the upper limbs and ears induced by thalidomide. (Courtesy of Professor W. Lenz)*

internal and external ears, deafness, haemangioma on the forehead, and malformations of the cardiovascular, digestive and urogenital systems were detected in the offspring of mothers who ingested thalidomide during early pregnancy.

The use of *psychotropic substances,* in particular marihuana and LSD (lysergic acid diethylamide), has increased considerably in the past few years.[7, 8, 39, 73] It is not surprising that there is wide-spread concern that these substances may prove to be harmful to the pregnant woman and her offspring,[46] particularly since two cases of multiple malformations in infants of mothers, who used cannabis in combination with other psychotropic drugs, have been reported.[9, 27] The results of animal experimental studies lend support to these observations.[22, 23, 50, 51]

Of 161 infants born to parents who took LSD before or during pregnancy, 5 showed gross malformations. The incidence rate of abortion is apparently increased following the use of LSD during pregnan-

Environmental Teratology

cy. However, the results of animal studies with LSD have been conflicting and do not support the view that LSD is teratogenic in man.[36]

There have been isolated reports relating other environmental agents to the occurrence of congenital abnormalities in pregnant women.[2, 24, 38, 62, 64, 65, 66, 75] Many of these observations must be interpreted with caution, since they are invariably based on fragmentary and inconclusive evidence.[17, 38, 47, 71]

Experimental Studies

Numerous reports have appeared on the teratogenic effects of a wide spectrum of environmental agents in laboratory animals [12, 20, 47, 58, 69, 71, 81, 82] and it has been suggested that almost any environmental agent is capable of inducing developmental defects under appropriate conditions. Investigations of this nature are neither ethical nor justifiable in man. On this account, the data derived from experimental studies in animals will remain an important source, not only for predicting possible harmful effects of environmental agents on the human fetus, but also in determining the underlying mechanisms operating at various phases of intrauterine existence.

Although the exact *mechanisms* by which the majority of environmental teratogens may interfere with embryonic development and so produce abnormalities remain obscure, certain general principles and guidelines relating to the occurrence of abnormalities have emerged. These are presented in summary as follows:

1. The site of primary action of teratogens may be either the embryo itself, the mother, the placenta or hormonal and other regulatory mechanisms involved in pregnancy.

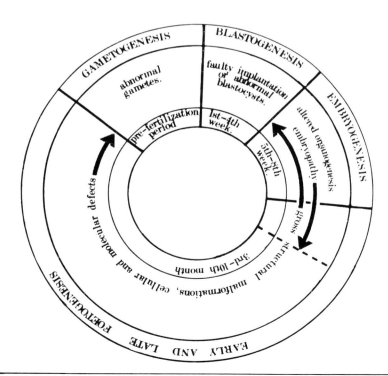

Fig. 2 Gestational periods and the timing of teratogenicity

Experimental Studies

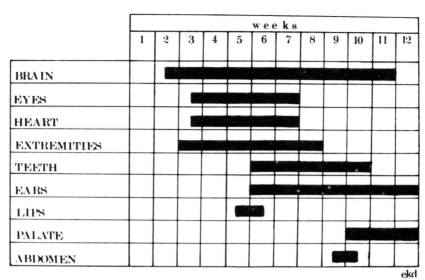

Fig. 3 Critical periods during organogenesis

2. The period of gestation during which the teratogen is administered influences the teratogenic responses (Figure 2). These "critical phases" during embryonic and fetal development are related to the degree of differentiation of specific organs; as differentiation proceeds susceptibility to teratogenesis decreases (Figure 3). For this reason gross structural defects hardly ever occur after organogenesis is completed.

The concept that congenital abnormalities cannot be induced during the pre-implantation period of the blastocyst is invalid. The early conceptus is highly susceptible to teratogenesis, particularly during implantation and placentation.

3. Teratogenic activity of the noxious agent is often dependent on the species and strain of animals involved. Our studies on the teratogenicity of hypoglycin and diethyl barbituric acid demonstrate the significance of species differences in *susceptibility to teratogenesis.*[48, 52]

4. Congenital malformations are generally induced by a dosage of the teratogenic agent which is slightly higher than that which has no effect on the embryo, but much smaller than that which will kill the mother. If small doses of the teratogen are administered, the embryos will not be affected and will appear quite normal at birth. Large doses of the teratogen will invariably kill the conceptus. The *teratogenic zone* is a relatively small range of dosage. Within this range the mortality and malformation rates tend to follow a parallel course and vary with both the dosage and period of treatment.

5. *Hereditary influences* are of considerable importance in determining the occurrence of congenital abnormalities. In particular the following genetic conditions should be taken into consideration in the evaluation of teratological data:

(a) Mutant genes which are the source of a wide variety of malformations probably influence the structure or rate of synthesis of polypeptides during embryonic development. The resulting biochemical errors may induce abnormal morphological changes.

(b) Chromosomal aberrations invariably produce major congenital abnormalities;

chromosomal breaks and rearrangements and abnormal metaphase figures have been observed following maternal exposure to various teratogens.

(c) The most frequent of the genetically influenced malformations are multifactorial in nature. These are the results of interactions between multiple genetic and environmental factors. It is now recognized that all developmental processes, normal and abnormal, are due to the complex interplay between maternal genes, the genotype of the embryo and environmental influences.

Teratological Evaluation

Animal studies, designed to uncover teratogenic side-effects of environmental agents, have a poor predictive value for the human fetus. The validity and some of the limitations of these tests have been discussed in previous reports.[1, 6, 13, 16, 32, 37, 41, 49, 54, 58, 72, 78]

There is some agreement that mammals, in particular rodents and primates,[69, 72, 81, 82] are best suited for teratological evaluation studies. However, the high cost of maintenance, the lengthy period of gestation and the small numer of offspring produced by primates would limit their extensive use in teratological investigations.

Any recommended *experimental procedure* in these species involves production and verification of pregnancy in the selected animals under controlled laboratory conditions. The test animal is exposed to a suitable and measured dose of the suspected environmental factor, on one or more days during pregnancy, which should include the period of organogenesis. Fetuses are recovered by Caesarean-section immediately before or at term in order to prevent the mothers from devouring damaged fetuses. Fetuses of both the control and treated groups of animals are weighed, measured and subjected to the same detailed and systematic examination for abnormalities.

A small number of fetuses are usually fixed in Bouin's solution and sectioned by the Wilson's technique[80] for the identification of gross visceral malformations. Other fetuses are subjected to histological examination of selected tissues, and selected fetuses are fixed in 95% ethyl alcohol in order to examine the skeletal system after clearing and staining by the Alizarin S technique. It is desirable also that the fetuses be studied further for cellular and metabolic changes.

The occurrence of congenital abnormalities in the offspring of treated animals can only suggest *possible* teratogenicity for the human conceptus, and with this a substantial risk that if the child was born it may suffer from such physical or mental abnormalities as to be seriously handicapped. On the contrary, negative results give no positive clearance for safety in man.

In the design and interpretation of these laboratory evaluation, consideration must be given to factors such as age, nutritional requirements, general health and maintenance of the animals, and the number and size of the litters. During gestation, the pregnant animals should regularly be weighed and subjected to frequent physical examinations for the presence of obvious signs of harm.

The teratological evaluation of chemicals, drugs and natural products represents a complex type of toxicological problem, where multiple factors involving the mother, fetus, placenta and the suspected noxious agent itself influence the response of the developing conceptus. Because of species and strain variation in susceptibility to teratogenesis, these environmental agents must be tested in several species and possibly of different strains. As a rule, screening should be carried out in two or more species for a preliminary evaluation of possible teratogenic activity.

Surprisingly, very few teratological studies, involving a specific environmental agent in several animal species, have been reported from the same laboratory. This would facilitate the evaluation of data obtained since individual investigators have worked out their own screening procedures. Invariably these are carried out under different methodological, laboratory and environmental conditions.

Because of the varying conditions under which teratological testing of suspected environmental agents is carried out, every effort should be made to standardize methods and define clearly the objective of these investigations. Taking this into consideration, teratological evaluation in laboratory animals would continue to provide useful information on the ability of exogenous agents to induce developmental deviations and also in determining the underlying mechanisms operating at various stages of prenatal development.

It is unlikely that laboratory evaluation of any environmental factor can provide conclusive evidence of possible harmful effects for the human conceptus. This data can only be derived from detailed clinical observations of pregnant women and their abnormal offsprings. The application of *epidemiological techniques* is contributing significantly to the recognition of environmental teratogens and in increasing our understanding of the nature of birth defects.[31, 38, 44, 56, 62, 68, 75] For this reason, the systematic collection and analysis of reports of adverse effects produced on the human conceptus should also be considered important for the early recognition of deleterious environmental teratogens.

References

1 Baker, S. B., and Davey, D. G. (1970): The predictive value for man of toxicological tests of drugs in laboratory animals. Br. med. Bull. 26, 208–211

2 Batstone, G. F., Blair, A. W., and Slater, J. M. (1972): A handbook of prenatal paediatrics for obstetricians and paediatricians. J. B. Lippincott Company, Philadelphia and Toronto

3 Brent, R. L. (1972): Protecting the public from teratogenic and mutagenic hazards. J. Clin. Pharmacol. 12, 61–70

4 Brown, G. C. (1970): Maternal virus infection and congenital anomalies. Arch. Environ. Health 21, 362–365

5 Bulova, S., Schwartz, E., and Harrer, W. V. (1972): Hydrops fetalis and congenital syphilis. Pediatrics 49, 285–287

6 Cahen, R. L. (1964): Evaluation of the teratogenicity of drugs. Clin. Pharmacol. Ther. 5, 480–514

7 Cannabis – Report by the Advisory Committee on Drug Dependence. Her Majesty's Stationery Office, Lond., 1968

8 Cannabis – A report of the commission of inquiry into the non-medical use of drugs. Ottawa, 1972

9 Carakushansky, G., Neu, R. L., and Gardner, L. I. (1969). Lysergide and cannabis as possible teratogens in man. Lancet 1, 150–151

10 Carter, C. O. (1967): Congenital malformations. WHO Chronicle 21, 287–292

11 Carter, C. (1970): The genetics of congenital malformations. In Scientific Foundations of Obstetrics and Gynaecology (Eds. E. E. Philipp, J. Barnes, and M. Newton), William Heinemann Medical Books Ltd., London. pp. 655–660

12 Clegg, D. J. (1971): Embryotoxicity of chemical contaminants of foods. Fd. Cosmet. Toxicol. 9, 195–205

13 Cook, M. J., Fairweather, F. A., and Hardwick, M. (1969): Further thoughts on teratogenic testing. In Teratology (Eds. A. Bertelli and L. Donati), Excerpta Medica Foundation, Amsterdam. pp. 34–42

14 Curran, W. J. (1971): The thalidomide tragedy in Germany. The end of a historic medicolegal trial. N. Eng. J. Med. 284, 481–482

15 de la Cruz, M. V., mu Noz-Castellanos, L., and Nadal-Ginard, B. (1971): Extrinsic factors in the genesis of congenital heart disease. Brit. Heart J. 33, 203–213

16 Delahunt, C. S. (1970): Detection of teratogenic action. In Methods in Toxicology (Ed.

Environmental Teratology

G. E. Paget), Blackwell Scientific Publ. pp. 132–157

17 Döring, G. K., and Hossfeld, C. (1964): Über die Gefahren einer übertriebenen Medikamentenfurcht in der Schwangerschaft. Dtsch. med. Wschr. 89, 1069–1072

18 Dudgeon, J. A. (1968): Fetal infections. J. Obstet. Gynaec. Br. Commonw. 75, 1229–1233

19 Dudgeon, J. A. (1968): Breakdown in maternal protection: infections. Proc. roy. Soc. Med. 61, 1236–1243

20 Durham, W. F., and Williams, C. H. (1972): Mutagenic, teratogenic, and carcinogenic properties of pesticides. Annual Rev. Entomol. 17, 123–148

21 Epstein, S. (1972): Environmental Pathology. Am. J. Pathol. 66, 252–374

22 Geber, W. F., and Schramm, L. C. (1969a): Effects of marihuana extract on fetal hamsters and rabbits. Toxicol. Appl. Pharmacol. 14, 276–282

23 Geber, W. F., and Schramm, L. C. (1969b): Teratogenicity of marihuana extract as influenced by plant origin and seasonal variation. Arch. Int. Pharmacodyn. Ther. 177, 224–230

24 Gerfeldt, E. (1964): Frequenz, Aetiologie und Prophylaxe von angeborenen Entwicklungsstörungen. Med. Klin. 59, 1287–1292

25 Goldberg, L. (1971): Trace chemical contaminants in food: Potential for harm. Fd. Cosmet. Toxicol. 9, 65–80

26 Gregg, N. M. (1942): Congenital cataract following German measles in the mother. Trans. Ophthal. Soc. Aust. 3, 35–46

27 Hecht, F., Beals, R. K., Lees, M. H., Jolly, H., and Roberts, P. (1968): Lysergic-acid-diethylamide and cannabis as possible teratogens in man. Lancet 2, 1087

28 Hicks, S. P., and D'Amato, C. J. (1966): Effects of ionizing radiations on mammalian development. In Advances in Teratology (Ed. D. H. M. Woollam) Logos and Academic Press, New York. Vol. 1, pp. 195–259

29 Hueper, W. C. (1971): Public health hazards from environmental chemical carcinogens, mutagens and teratogens. Health Phys. 21, 689–707

30 Hume, O. S. (1972): Toxoplasmosis and pregnancy. Am. J. Obstet. Gynecol. 114, 703–715

31 Kennedy, W. P. (1967): Epidemiologic aspects of the problem of congenital malformations. Birth Defects Original Article Series 3, 1–18

32 Keplinger, M. L. (1971): Assessment of toxicity of substances. J. Occup. Med. 13, 2–7

33 Krech, U., Jung, M., and Jung, F. (1971): Cytomegalovirus infections of man. S. Karger A. G., Basel

34 Leck, I. (1972): The etiology of human malformations: Insights from epidemiology. Teratology 5, 303–314

35 Lenz, W., and Knapp, K. (1962): Die Thalidomid-Embryopathie. Dtsch. med. Wschr. 87, 1232–1242

36 Long, S. Y. (1972): Does LSD induce chromosomal damage and malformations? A review of the literature. Teratology 6, 75–90

37 Lorke, O. (1963): Zur Methodik der Untersuchungen embryotoxischer und teratogener Wirkungen an der Ratte. Arch. exp. Path. Pharmak. 246, 147–151

38 Lowe, R. (1972): Congenital malformations and the problem of their control. Brit. med. J. 3, 515–520

39 Marihuana and health – A report to Congress from the Secretary, U. S. Department of Health, Education and Welfare. Washington, 1971

40 McBride, A. (1961): Thalidomide and congenital abnormalities. Lancet 2, 1358

41 McKenzie, J. (1969): The chick embryo grown in vitro. In Teratology (Eds. A. Bertelli and L. Donati). Excerpta Medica Foundation. Amsterdam. pp. 43–54

42 McLeod, H. A., Grant, D. L., and Phillips, W. E. (1971): Pesticide residues and metabolites in placentas. Can. J. Publ. Hlth. 62, 341–433.

43 Meltzer, H. J. (1955): Congenital anomalies due to attempted abortion with 4-aminopteroglutamic acid. J. Am. med. Ass. 161, 1253

44 Miller, J. R. (1964): The use of registries and vital statistics in the study of congenital malformations. In: Second International Conference on Congenital Malformations (Ed. M. Fishbein) International Medical Congress, New York. pp. 334–340

45 Monif, G. R. G. (1969). Viral infections of the human fetus. The Collier-MacMillan Company, Toronto, Canada

46 Neuberg, R. (1972): Drug addiction in pregnancy: Review of the problem. Proc. roy. Soc. Med. 65, 867

47 Persaud, T. V. N. (1968): Aspects of teratology. W. I. Med. J. 17, 74–82

48 Persaud, T. V. N. (1972a): Teratogenic activity of hypoglycin-A. In Advances in Teratology (Ed. D. H. M. Woollam), Logos and Academic Press. Vol. 5, pp. 77–95

49 Persaud, T. V. N. (1972b): Effect of intra-amniotic administration of hypoglycin B on foetal development in the rat. Exp. Pathol. 6, 55–58

[50] Persaud, T. V. N., and Ellington, A. C. (1968a): Teratogenic activity of cannabis resin. Lancet 2, 406–407

[51] **Persaud, T. V. N.**, and Ellington, A. C. (1968b): The effects of cannabis sativa L. (Ganja) on developing rat embryos-preliminary observations. W. I. Med. J. 17, 232–234

[52] Persaud, T. V. N., and Henderson, W. M. (1969): The teratogenicity of barbital sodium in mice. Arzneim.-Forsch. (Drug. Res.) 19, 1309–1310

[53] Plummer, G. (1952): Anomalies occurring in children exposed *in utero* to the atomic bomb in Hiroshima. Pediatrics 10, 687–693

[54] Poswillo, D. E., Hamilton, W. J., and Sopher, D. (1972): The marmoset as an animal model for teratological research. Nature (Lond.) 239, 460–462

[55] Remington, J. S. (1968): Toxoplasmosis and congenital infection. Birth Defects Original Article Series 4, 47–56

[56] Renwick, J. H. (1972): Anencephaly and spina bifida are usually preventable by evidence of a specific but unidentified substance present in certain potato tubers. Brit. J. prev. soc. Med. 26, 67–88

[57] Rice-Wray, E., Cervantes, A., Gutierrez, J., and Marquez-Monter, H. (1971). Pregnancy and progeny after hormonal contraceptive studies. J. Reprod. Med. 6, 101–104

[58] Robson, J. M. (1970): Testing drugs for teratogenicity and their effects on fertility. The present position. Br. Med. Bull. 26, 212–216

[59] Schreiner, W. E. (1971): Nebenwirkungen der medikamentösen Antikonzeption. Schweiz. Med. Wochenschr. 100, 778–784

[60] Sever, J. L. (1970): Viruses and embryos. In Congenital Malformations (Ed. F. C. Fraser and V. A. McJusick), pp. 180–186. Excerpta Medica Foundation, Amsterdam

[61] Sever, J. L. (1971): Virus infections and malformations. Fed. Proc. 30, 114–117

[62] Shapiro, S., Ross, L. J., and Levine, H. S. (1965): Relationship of selected prenatal factors to pregnancy outcome and congenital anomalies. Am. J. Publ. Hlth. 55, 268–282

[63] Shaw, E. B., and Steinbach, H. L. (1968): Aminopterin-induced fetal malformation, survival of infant after attempted abortion. Am. J. Dis. Child. 115, 477–482

[64] Skoupý, M., Skoupá, M., and Saxl, O. (1967): Angeborene Mißbildungen und Arzneimittel. Dtsch. Ges. Wesen. 22, 1267–1273

[65] Smithells, R. W. (1966): Drugs and human malformations. In Advances in Teratology (Ed. D. H. M. Woollam), Logos Press Ltd., London. Vol. 1, pp. 251–278

[66] Sutherland, J. M., and Light, I. J. (1965): The effect of drugs upon the developing fetus. Pediat Clin. North America 12, 781–806

[67] Sutton, H. E. (1971): Workshop on monitoring of human mutagenesis, Teratology 4, 103–107

[68] Stevenson, A. C., Johnston, H. A., Stewart, M. I. P., and Golding, D. R. (1966): Congenital malformations. A report of a series of consecutive births in 24 centres. Bull. Wld. Hlth. Org. 34, Suppl. 1–127

[69] Tanimura, T. (1972): Effects on macaque embryos of drugs reported or suspected to be teratogenic to humans. Acta endocrin. (suppl. Number) 166, 293–308

[70] Thiersch, J. B. (1952): Therapeutic abortions with folic acid antagonist, 4-aminopteroyl-glutamic acid (4-amino-P. G. A.) administered by oral route. Am. J. Obstet. Gynec. 63, 1298–1325

[71] Tuchmann-Duplessis, H. (1970): The effects of teratogenic drugs. In Scientific Foundations of Obstetrics and Gynaecology (Eds. E. E. Phillip, J. Barnes, and M. Newton), William Heinemann Medical Books Ltd., London. pp. 636–648

[72] Tuchmann-Duplessis, H. (1972): Teratogenic drug screening. Present procedures and requirements. Teratology 5, 271–286

[73] United Nations Commission on Narcotic Drugs. Document E/3648, E/CN 7/432. W. H. O., Geneva, 1962

[74] Venning, G. R. (1965): The problem of human foetal abnormalities with special reference to sex hormones. In Embryopathic Activity of Drugs (Eds. J. M. Robson, F. M. Sullivan, and R. L. Smith), Little, Brown and Company, Boston

[75] Villumsen, A. L. (1970): Environmental factors in congenital malformations. A prospective study of 9006 human pregnancies. F. A. D. L. S. Forlag, Copenhagen, Aarhus, Odense

[76] Warkany, J., Beaudry, P. H., and Hornstein, S. (1959): Attempted abortion with aminopterin, malformations of the child. Am. J. Dis. Child. 97, 274–281

[77] Weicker, H., and Hungerland, H. (1962): Thalidomid-Embryopathie. I. Vorkommen inner- und ausserhalb Deutschlands. Dtsch. med. Wschr. 87, 992–994

[78] WHO (1967): Principles for the testing of drugs for teratogenicity. WHO Tech. Rep. Ser. No. 364, Geneva

Environmental Teratology

[79] Wilkins, L. (1960): Masculinization of female fetus due to use of orally given progestins. J. Am. med. Ass. 172, 1028–1033

[80] Wilson, J. G. (1965): Methods for administering agents and detecting malformations in experimental animals. In Teratology, Principles and Techniques (Eds. J. G. Wilson and J. Warkany). University of Chicago Press, pp. 262–277

[81] Wilson, J. G. (1969): Teratological and reproductive studies in non-human primates. In methods for teratological studies in experimental animals and man (Eds. H. Nishimura and J. R. Miller) Igaku Shoin, Tokyo, pp. 16–31

[82] Wilson, J. G. (1972): Abnormalities of intrauternie development in non-human primates. Acta endocrin. (Suppl. Number) 166, 261–272

[83] Herbst, A. L., Ulfelder, H., and Poskanzer, D. C. (1971) Adenocarcinoma of the vagina. Association of maternal stilbestrol therapy with tumor appearance in young women. New Engl. J. Med. 284, 878–881

[84] Moore, K. L. (1973) The developing human. W. B. Saunders Co., Philadelphia. pp. 108–124

Addendum

Recently, Herbst et al.[83] made the important observation that vaginal adenocarcinoma developed in some young women many years after administration of stilboestrol to their mothers during pregnancy. This is the first report drawing attention to the possible carcinogenic action of drugs on the human fetus and to the prenatal origins of certain cancers. For a discussion on the embryological basis of congenital malformations and a comprehensive survey of known and suspected human teratogens, see Moore.[84]

From R. Doll (1973). J. Irish Med. Assoc., **66**, 117–126. Copyright (1973), by kind permission of the author and the Irish Medical Association

Hazards of the First Nine Months: an Epidemiologist's Nightmare*

RICHARD DOLL
Regius Professor of Medicine
University of Oxford

FEW fields of medicine have seen such dramatic success as has been achieved by the combined efforts of obstetricians, paediatricians, medical officers of health, and laboratory workers to reduce the mortality of children. Vital records in England and Wales, which are typical of those of industrialized countries, show that, over the last 40 years, the stillbirth rate has been reduced by 68 per cent, infant mortality by 71 per cent, and the mortality of children at 1 to 9 years of age by 87 per cent. As a result, the odds on a foetus completing a decade of extra-uterine life, once it comes officially under starter's orders 28 weeks from its mother's last menstrual period, have shortened from 13 to 2 to 27 to 1.

But even these odds are not the best that can be achieved. Examination of the figures for intervening years shows that the decline continues—rapidly in the case of the stillbirth rate, but more slowly in the case of infant mortality and more slowly still at older ages (Fig. 1). Past trends, however, are poor predictors in the field of vital statistics, as anyone knows who has tried to predict the rate of growth of the population, and it is more encouraging to know that lower rates have already been obtained in other countries—notably in Scandinavia (Table I). Moreover, examination of the figures for individual causes of death, which are given in broad categories for the years 1961 and 1970 in Fig. 2, shows that a large proportion of the early deaths are still attributed to the complications of pregnancy and labour. These it would be neither proper nor possible for me to comment on in detail; but it is not controversial to say that they could be reduced substantially by better education and the full and equal application of current knowledge and skills. They will, I suspect, be reduced still more by the advances that are now being made in our knowledge of foetal physiology.

*Bartholemew Mosse Lecture, Rotunda Hospital, 1972.

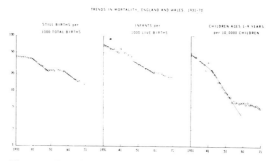

Figure 1. Trends in stillbirth rate, infant mortality, and childhood mortality at 1-9 years of age in England and Wales, 1931 to 1970.

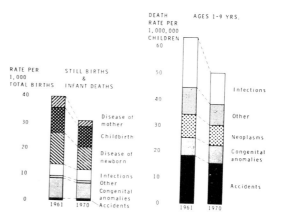

Figure 2. Causes of (i) stillbirths and infant deaths and (ii) childhood deaths at 1-9 years of age in England and Wales in 1961 and 1970.

But if we can be optimistic about the stillbirth and infant mortality rates, the position with regard to childhood mortality is different. Violence, con-

Table I
Countries with low stillbirth and infant mortality
rates, 1969

| Country† | Rate per 1000 live births | |
	Stillbirths*	Infants under one year
England & Wales	13.3	18.0
Australia	—	17.8
New Zealand	10.0	16.9
Switzerland	9.4	15.4
Denmark	8.6	14.8
Finland	—	14.4
Norway	11.2	13.8
Netherlands	11.1	13.2
Iceland	11.2	11.7
Sweden	—	11.7

*Stillbirths recorded per 1000 *live* births (Demographic Yearbook, U.N.)
†Ireland, infant mortality rate, 20.6.

genital malformations, and cancer already account for 60 per cent of all deaths at 1 to 9 years of age, and the prospect for the early prevention of any of these categories of disease is small. To some extent the two latter groups of conditions are genetic in origin but few can be attributed to genetic factors alone. More often the expression of the genes is dependent on the environment in which the child develops; and it is now becoming plain that environmental agents, which operate during the mother's pregnancy and are potentially capable of control, may be determining causes. Such agents can sometimes be detected more easily by epidemiological methods than by experiment, and it is to these agents and the methods by which their effects can be investigated, that I should like to draw attention this evening. I shall not attempt to review them all, but will pick out for consideration a few that are of particular interest.

Ionizing Radiations
Cancer. Consider first the carcinogenic effect of X-rays. That children who are irradiated *in utero* are more likely to develop cancer than other children has now been demonstrated so often and so consistently that it cannot be seriously challenged. With minor exceptions all studies have pointed to the conclusion that the increase in risk associated with exposure to x-rays *in utero* is approximately 50 to 100 per cent. When Stewart and her colleagues (Stewart, Webb, Giles and Hewitt, 1956; Stewart, Webb and Hewitt, 1958) first described the effect they relied on a comparison of the histories given by mothers whose children had died of cancer with those given by mothers of living children of the same sex, who were born in the same area and at the same period as the children who had died. It was, therefore, possible to argue that the results were an artefact due to differential recall of past events by mothers whose children had died of a mysterious disease, particularly if those events related to the pregnancy in question. That this was not so, however, was finally demonstrated by a detailed examination of the medical records of the mothers who gave a positive history of irradiation, and of a sample of the mothers who did not (Hewitt, Sanders and Stewart, 1966).

If any element of doubt remained, it was excluded by MacMahon's (1962) study of children born in selected hospitals in the United States in which records of x-ray examinations during pregnancy had been maintained. In this study, x-ray exposures were determined solely by reference to hospital records compiled before the children were born, so that opportunities for bias were effectively excluded.

The fact of the association is, to my mind, proved; but it does not necessarily follow that the radiation caused the disease. Some women who were x-rayed in pregnancy were x-rayed routinely; but others were x-rayed for medical reasons. It may be, therefore, that the carcinogenic factor was associated in some way with these reasons rather than with the x-ray examination. So far every effort to identify such an association has failed. MacMahon (1962), in particular, showed that the results could not be explained by the separate association of x-rays and carcinogenesis with the economic status, age, or religion of the mother, with the birth order of the child, or with Caesarean section, head or forceps delivery, placenta praevia, or toxaemia of pregnancy.

Belief in a causal relationship has been strengthened by the demonstration of a linear relationship between risk and dose received down to approximately 200 mrads (Stewart and Kneale, 1970; Newcombe and McGregor, 1971). Conversely it has been weakened by the lack of any increased mortality from cancer among the children who were irradiated *in utero* by the atomic bomb explosions in Japan (Jablon and Kato, 1970). The Japanese data, however, are few and relate principally to children whose mothers had been heavily irradiated at all periods in pregnancy. Whether the effect of this type of irradiation would be comparable, dose for dose, with that produced by small doses in the third trimester is doubtful. It may be that the damage to the marrow cells in those Japanese children in whom leukaemia would have been produced was too great to allow them to survive.

The crucial test is, of course, the test of practical prevention. Unfortunately, this is not easy to apply. According to Stewart's estimates, diagnostic radiology might have accounted for about 6 or 7 per cent of all cancer deaths in children under 10 years of age, so that even if exposure was greatly reduced a corresponding reduction in mortality would be difficult to detect. In fact, the trend in mortality in Britain does show a decrease since the publication of Stewart's first article in 1956 (Fig. 3). Some of the decrease in leukaemia may plausibly be related to prolonged survival from improved treatment; but it is difficult to believe that all can be accounted for in this way, as there is no compensating increase at older ages. Moreover, the mortality from other cancers has also decreased without any corresponding improvement in survival. It may be, therefore, that there has been a genuine decrease in incidence. Certainly medical practice has altered and the pregnant uterus now receives much less irradiation—a trend which, in the days of improving stillbirth and infant mortality rates, one would hesitate to reverse.

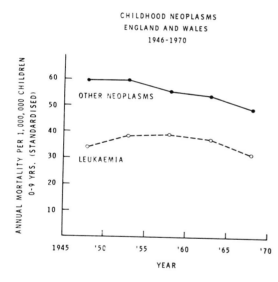

CHILDHOOD NEOPLASMS
ENGLAND AND WALES
1946-1970

Figure 3. Trends in mortality from (i) leukaemia and (ii) other cancers under 10 years of age in England and Wales, 1946 to 1970.

Congenital malformations. That ionizing radiations can also produce congenital malformations was shown by the high incidence of microcephaly among infants irradiated *in utero* by the atomic bomb explosions in Japan. Detailed observations, recently reported by Miller and Blot (1972), allow the incidence of this abnormality to be related to the dose of radiation for the first time. Among 1010 control children, approximately 4 per cent had a head circumference that was smaller than the average for their age and sex by at least two standard deviations and none showed gross mental retardation. Among children who were exposed to the bombs when their gestational age was less than 18 weeks, the proportion rose from 8 per cent, when the radiation dose was less than 20 rads, to 59 per cent when the dose was 150 rads or more; while the proportion who showed gross mental retardation rose from 2 per cent to 36 per cent (Table II). That any effect was observed with doses of less than 50 rads is surprising, but may perhaps be explained by the fact that the irradiation at Hiroshima was partly by neutrons. The small size of the head is presumably a secondary effect due to the reduction in the number of cells in the developing brain and hence in the stimulus to skull growth.

A similar lesion has also been observed on a number of occasions in which pregnant women have been exposed therapeutically or by mistake to X-ray doses of the order of 200 rads.

Other abnormalities of the central nervous system, eye, and skeleton have been attributed to irradiation but the evidence is inconclusive. Despite the ease with which multiple deformities can be produced in rats, mice and guinea pigs, there is no firm evidence of a teratogenic effect from a large dose of x-rays other than the production of microcephaly, possibly because doses that are large enough to cause malformations during the period of major organogenesis are lethal.

Whether any abnormalities can be produced by doses of the order of those given in the course of diagnostic radiography is uncertain. The only con-

Table II

Children irradiated in utero and surviving to 10 years of age (after Miller & Blot, 1972)

| Radiation dose (rads) | Gestational age at irradiation | | | | | |
| | Less than 18 weeks | | | 18 weeks or more | | |
	No. of children	Percent with small head	Percent with gross mental retardation	No. of children	Percent with small head	Percent with gross mental retardation
less than 20	125	8	2	124	3	0
20-49	58	26	0	46	7	0
50-149	35	31	6	50	6	0
150 or over	22	59	36	17	18	12

crete evidence that bears examination relates to the production of heterochromic wedges in the iris as a result of irradiation during the seventh month (Lejeune et al, 1960, 1962; Cheeseman and Walby, 1963). The various reports that have purported to relate the incidence of congenital malformations to the amount of background radiation are open to too many criticisms to justify consideration.

Drugs

Cancer. That drugs can also produce both cancer and congenital malformation is now well established; but it is only recently that we have had examples of the production of cancer by exposure to a drug *in utero*. The recognition by Herbst, Ulfelder and Poskanzer (1971) that adenocarcinoma of the vagina in women was due to the mothers' use of stilboestrol during pregnancy was an astute clinical observation, comparable to Gregg's (1941) observation of the relationship between congenital cataract and rubella and MacBride's (1961) observation of the relationship between phocomelia and thalidomide — an observation which, you will remember, was rejected by the medical press until after the first reports of Lenz's (1962) study, on the grounds that it would give rise to unnecessary anxiety.

Adenocarcinoma of the vagina in young women is normally so rare that Herbst and his colleagues could be confident that a new situation had arisen when they learnt of eight cases within the space of four years, six of which had been treated at one Boston Hospital. No similar cases could be traced in the records of the hospital before 1966. Enquiry showed that at least 7 of the mothers had taken stilboestrol during the relevant pregnancy to stop a threatened abortion. None of the mothers of 32 healthy girls of the same ages, who had been selected as controls, had taken stilboestrol and common experience confirmed that the use of stilboestrol during pregnancy, even at the height of its popularity, was unusual. It was, therefore, impossible to believe that the association was due to chance. The belief that the relationship was causal was greatly strengthened when it was shown that an 'epidemic' had also occurred in New York State, 9 cases having been reported to the Cancer Registry in girls aged 15 to 19 years in the period 1966-72. Once again no such case had been reported previously, and enquiries showed that 8 and possibly all 9 mothers had taken stilboestrol or a similar oestrogen (Greenwald et al, 1971). In these two series the dose of stilboestrol appears to have been of the order of 25 to 125 mg. a day spread out over several weeks. Smaller doses, however, may also have been carcinogenic, and Herbst (1972) refers to one girl in a total of over 80 with the disease who have now been reported from all over the United States, whose mother is believed to have taken no more than 1.5 mg. a day.

These findings provide no indication of the size of the risk and it could be that it was relatively small. Certainly stilboestrol was used fairly widely in some parts of the United States in the treatment of threatened abortion during the late forties and early fifties, probably in 1 per cent of all pregnancies or more. A few obstetricians used it in Britain, but so far we appear to have escaped the epidemic. Cancer registry data, which cover perhaps 80 per cent of all cases in the country, reveal records of 7 cases in women aged 15 to 24 years spread out evenly over an 11 year period; none appears to have been associated with the use of stilboestrol (Inman, personal communication).

Whether any other drugs that are taken in pregnancy can produce cancer in the child is an open question. Only very few drugs have been shown to be carcinogenic in adults and then nearly always because of some peculiar circumstances. Either the risk has been very great, as in the case of cancer of the bladder following the use of chlornaphazine, or the development of the disease has been accompanied by some pathognomonic feature which directed attention to the use of the drug, as in the case of squamous carcinoma of the palm of the hands in arrenicism. A relatively small risk of a common cancer is easily overlooked unless special and exhaustive enquiries are made. In this field, as in the field of teratogenesis, animal experiments are a poor guide to human experience—irrespective of whether the results are positive or negative—and we must keep our minds open to the possibility that other childhood cancers may also be iatrogenic in origin.

Congenital Malformations. The few drugs that are known to produce congenital malformations are listed in Table III. I have included anticonvulsants as a group as all that are commonly used may be responsible. The idea that they might have a teratogenic effect arose when it was discovered that phenytoin could produce megaloblastic anaemia by reducing the serum folic acid. It was already known that folic acid antagonists produced congenital malformations when used as abortifacients and it seemed reasonable to suggest that phenytoin could exert a similar mechanism. The results of seven epidemiological enquiries are summarized in Table IV. All agree in showing an excess of congenital malformations, particularly hare lip with or without cleft palate, in children whose mothers had been taking anticonvulsants during the first trimester. The extent of the excess varies greatly, however, from about 10 to 90 per 1,000 children. Examination of the case histories shows that the excess is not confined to the children of women who took phenytoin, but is found also (if not predominantly) with the use

Table III

Teratogenic Drugs

Drug	Main Anomaly
Thalidomide	Phocomelia
Aminopterin, methotrexate	Deformities of skull and bones, cleft palate
Androgens, progestogens	Virilization of female genitalia
Tetracyclines	Discolouration and deformity of teeth
Iodides	Goitre
Anticonvulsants	Hare lip ± cleft palate

Table IV

Malformations in children associated with the use of anticonvulsants

Country	Epileptic	Mothers not on anticonvulsants				Mothers on anticonvulsants			
		Children		Children with hare lip ± cleft palate		Children		Children with hare lip ± cleft palate	
		No.	Percent malformed	Percent of total	Percent malformed	No.	Percent malformed	Percent of total	Percent malformed
Germany	yes	130	0.0	0.00(0)+	0.0	225	2.2	1.3(3)+	60
Netherlands I	no	325,776*	1.4	0.13(427)	9.7	—	—	—(10)	56
Netherlands II	no	11,986	1.8	0.23(27)	12.2	65	15.4	7.7(5)	50
Denmark						32	6.3	6.3(2)	100
Wales	no	23,345*	2.7	0.18(43)	6.9	93	5.4	1.1(1)	20
London	no	7,865	2.4	0.12(10)	5.3	22	9.1	9.1(2)	100
	yes	9	0.0	0.00(0)	0.0				
Leeds	no	448	1.6	0.22(1)	14.3	315	5.4	1.0(3)	18
	yes	56	0.0	0.00(0)	0.0				

*A total population including an unknown but small proportion on anticonvulsants.
+Numbers of cases in parentheses.

For references, see Janz and Fuchs (1964), Germany; Elshove and Eck (1971), Netherlands; Melchior, Svensmark, and Trolle (1967), Denmark; Lowe (personal communication), Wales; South (personal communication), London; and Speidel and Meadow (1972), Leeds.

of barbiturates and possibly also of primidone. Laboratory experiments show that cleft palate can be produced by the administration of phenytoin to pregnant mice of a strain in which clefts are normally rare, and similar defects have been produced by very large doses of phenobarbitone and primidone (Sullivan, 1972). According to Elshove (1970) the phenytoin effects in mice can be reduced by the addition of folic acid to the diet, but it remains to be seen whether this also applies to man.

Another drug which may have to be regarded as teratogenic is ergometrine. That this may be so is suggested by the report of 24 cases of the Poland anomaly at a hospital centre in Bristol. The anomaly, which is characterized by unilateral absence of the the sternocostal head of the pectoralis major and ipsilateral syndactyly and may be complicated by short or absent fingers, rib and costal cartilage defects, absence or hypoplasia of the nipple or breast, and possibly genito-urinary anomalies, is normally rare. In the epidemic, which has recently been described by David (1972) and personal communica-

tion), five of the 24 patients were adopted and five others were illegitimate. There was a strong suspicion that the mothers of seven of the children who were not adopted had tried to secure an abortion, two had taken ergometrine tablets, one crude ergot infusion, one 'tablets', while the method used by the other three was not known—rudimentary evidence indeed, but enough, I think, to justify a more extensive enquiry.

Viral Infections

Congenital Malformations. But enough of iatrogenic hazards. Real though they are, they are not the only ones that the embryo has to face and I have given them priority only because of my increasing realization of the difficulty of avoiding Sir Thomas More's admonition 450 years ago that 'It is a pretty poor doctor who cannot cure one disease without giving you another'. Indeed, the diseases that the pregnant woman is likely to develop may present greater dangers. One, that has come under suspicion on a number of occasions, is influenza. Most often the suspicion has been that it might cause congenital malformations. When Coffey and Jessop (1959, 1963) described their observations of 1,343 infants who were born in Dublin following the epidemic of Asian influenza in 1957 the case seemed strong. Eight out of 108 infants whose mothers said they had influenza in the first trimester had malformations compared with 16 out of 554 whose mothers said they had influenza in the second or third trimester (2.9 per cent), and 10 out of 663 whose mothers said they did not have influenza at all (1.5 per cent) —moreover all 8 infants in the first group had anencephaly, spina bifida, or meningocele, compared with 5 out of 16 and 4 out of 10 in the other two groups.

A similar observation was made in Finland (Hakosalo and Saxen, 1971) but not, in general, by other investgators and an examination of vital records shows that there has been no regular increase in the prevalence of anencephaly, or of any other malformation, following influenza epidemics (Leck, 1963; Rogers, 1972). On present evidence the case for a specific teratogenic effect of the influenza virus must be regarded as not proven.

Prematurity. Now two other effects have been suggested. In his annual report for 1970, the chief medical officer (1971) of the English Department of Health and Social Security noted that infant mortality had increased in comparison with the previous year—a change in direction that had occurred only once before in the last 25 years, and then in 1951 when there was also an influenza epidemic. Following this report, Wynne Griffith, Adelstein, Lambert and Weatherall (1972) examined the vital statistics relating to stillbirths and infant mortality. These showed that the stillbirth rate and the late neonatal and postnatal death rates were all lower in 1970 than they had been in 1969. Only the early neonatal death rate (that is, the death rate in the first week of life) was raised. Furthermore, this increase occurred predominantly in the second quarter of the year following the period when the influenza epidemic was at its height. Examination of the mortality from influenza shows that there were five major epidemics in which more than 5,500 deaths from influenza were recorded in the first quarter of the year and six non-epidemic years when less than 500 deaths were recorded. Comparison of the trends in these two groups of years shows that the trend line for the epidemic years was consistently above that for the non-epidemic years for early neonatal deaths but only for the first six months; for stillbirths and late neonatal deaths and for all three rates in the last half of the year, the trend lines were indistinguishable. Similar results were also observed

in the United States for the shorter period 1950-67 for which data are available. Examination of the causes of death shows that the excess in the June quarter of 1970 compared with 1969, was due not to congenital malformations, but to anoxic and hypoxic conditions and to immaturity unqualified, which together rose from 4.7 to 5.8 per 1,000. Wynne Griffith and his colleagues, therefore, suggested that the effect might be due to an increase in the proportion of infants born prematurely some months after the peak of the epidemic was passed— a suggestion for which they were able to obtain a good deal of support from published data.

Leukaemia. The second effect was suggested by Fedrick and Alberman (1972) from examination of the results of the British Perinatal Mortality Survey (Butler and Bonham, 1963) and its continuation the National Childhood Development Study (Davie, Butler and Goldstein, 1972). In this survey, questionaires were completed by midwives for 98 per cent of the babies notified as having been born in Great Britain during the first week of March 1958. Of the 17,418 babies, all but 348 (2 per cent) were followed successfully to 11 years of age. Of those who survived for 4 weeks (16,750) nearly 2,000 were born to mothers who gave a history of influenza during pregnancy. Among them the incidence of cancer was 4.1 per 1,000 compared to an incidence of only 0.8 per 1,000 in the remainder. Classification of the cancers by type showed that the excess in the influenza group was limited to leukaemia and other reticuloses. Cancer, other than reticuloses, occurred with the expected frequency in both groups, as did the reticuloses in the children without a history of maternal influenza.

The number of reticuloses is small (7 in one group and 6 in the other), but even so the probability of finding so large a difference by chance is less than 1 in 1,000. It must, of course, be remembered that the observations were made as a result of searching the records to see which factors distinguished the children who developed cancer. Many factors were examined but only one was found to discriminate. In these circumstances, the result of a statistical test is less impressive than it would have been had the observation been made to test a pre-existing hypothesis. It is, therefore, important to see whether the results can be confirmed independently. Fedrick and Alberman (1972) tried to do this by comparing the proportion of children born each year between 1955 and 1969 who were destined to die of leukaemia under 5 years of age with the rate of incapacity from influenza among employed women during the 12 month period from the beginning of June in the preceding year. The results showed a positive correlation between the two rates which seemed to provide a good check on the hypothesis. Unfortunately, however, the authors had to confine themselves to data for children who died under 5 years of age, as it is possible to deduce from published data the year of birth of children who develop leukaemia only for these ages. It now appears that the more extensive data that have been collected by Dr Stewart and her colleagues in the course of the Oxford Childhood Cancer Survey do not support the hypothesis when more years of birth are studied and the age limit is extended (Draper, personal communication)—something that was certainly desirable as the majority of the cases in the influenza series did not appear until after 6 years of age or older. If, therefore, there is an association between a maternal history of 'influenza' and childhood leukaemia, it would seem likely that the agent is not the influenza virus but another respiratory virus that produces symptoms which are mistaken for influenza during an epidemic.

The only other data that bear on this question were obtained retrospectively by Stewart and her colleagues in the course of the Oxford Childhood Cancer survey (Draper, personal communication). Enquiries of the mothers of a large proportion of all the children who died of cancer under 10 years of age in Britain between 1953 and 1967 showed that rather more of them said they had had chicken pox, rubella, or influenza during pregnancy than of the mothers of the control children, whereas no difference was noted in respect of other virus infections. The extent of the difference in the history of influenza was less than would be expected from Fedrick and Alberman's data, but this could be attributed to incomplete recall after so many years. What is more disturbing, however, is that there was no difference between the approximately equal numbers of mothers of children with leukaemia and other cancers. On the whole I am now inclined to think that Fedrick and Alberman's results are a statistical fluke.

Smoking

Other agents over which the mother has, or should have, more control include smoking and diet. That smoking during pregnancy might have an effect on the foetus was first suggested by Simpson (1957), who found that the birth weight of infants whose mothers smoked during pregnancy was less, on average, than that of infants whose mothers did not. These results were rapidly confirmed by others, when it appeared that the reduction in birth weight was of the order of 150 to 250 g. The largest of these studies, the British Perinatal Mortality Survey, which has been referred to previously in relation to influenza, showed also that the reduction in birth weight was accompanied by an increase in both

foetal and neonatal mortality of 28 per cent, the excess of deaths being accounted for by causes that are normally associated with a low birth weight (Butler and Alberman, 1969). Smoking habits are not impossible to change and there must be many mothers who would willingly stop smoking in pregnancy if assured that it would have an appreciable effect on the chances of survival of their child, so it is of some importance to decide whether smoking causes the effect, or whether, as Yerushalmy (1964, 1971) suggests, the low birth weight and the high mortality are associated with a particular type of mother, who also happens to be prone to smoke—an explanation that was made plausible by the discovery that mothers who smoked in pregnancy tended to come from a poorer social background, were older, and had had more children than the mothers who did not (Butler and Alberman, 1969). In a situation like this, the ideal solution is to carry out an experiment of intervention in which women are divided into groups at random, half of whom are advised not to smoke during pregnancy. Ethical considerations, of course, require that the obstetricians in charge should have serious doubts about the meaning of the present evidence. For my part, I could not do the experiment as I am reasonably satisfied that smoking in pregnancy does in fact exert an effect on the chances of the child's survival. In reaching this conclusion, I have been impressed by Butler, Goldstein and Ross's (1972) analysis of the data obtained in the British Perinatal Mortality Survey. They showed (1) that the association between birth weight and smoking held only for the amount smoked after the fourth month of pregnancy and, when habits had been changed, was independent of the amount smoked before pregnancy had begun, and (2) that the results were practically unaltered after taking account of the sex, gestation, and survival of the infant, and of the age, parity, height, and social class of the mother (Table V).

A reduction in birth weight does not necessarily increase the risk of death, so long as the reduction is relatively small, the initial weight is adequate, and the obstetric and paediatric services are good. These conditions are, I believe, sufficient to account for the fact that the increase in mortality among children of smokers was negligibly small in three large scale studies of white Americans and Finns. In all their studies the overall death rate was substantially lower than in other studies in which the increase of mortality with smoking was large (for references, see Butler, Goldstein and Ross, 1972). This differential effect of smoking, depending on the basic mortality rate, was neatly demonstrated in the British Mortality Survey. In social classes 1 and 2, the excess mortality among the children of

310

Table V

Birth weight in relation to mother's smoking habits before pregnancy and after fourth month: 16,994 singleton births.

Mother's smoking habits after 4th month (cigarettes/day)	Birth weight (g) Mother's smoking habits before pregnancy (cigarettes/day)		
	0	1-9	10 or more
0	3387	3388	3387
1-9	3243	3244	3243
10 or more	3207	3208	3207

After Butler, Goldstein and Ross, 1972.

smokers was only 10 per cent; for the study as a whole it was 28 per cent.

Diet

Iodine Deficiency. That diet can be responsible for the development of congenital malformation has been recognized ever since it was realized that goitres could be produced by a deficiency of iodine. Where goitre is common, there is also 'endemic cretinism', a poorly defined condition characterized by a variety of factors varying from deaf-mutism, spastic paraplegia, and severe mental deficiency without signs of hypothyroidism, to a condition distinguishable from the sporadic cretinism due to thyroid aplasia. One or other variety of this condition has been found to be common in the Himalayas, the Andes, the Congo and East and West New Guinea. Now Pharaoh, Butterfield and Hetzel (1971) have shown by a beautiful experiment of intervention that the neurological type can be almost, if not completely, eliminated by giving the mother-to-be an injection of iodized poppyseed oil before conception takes place. A controlled trial of this method, with random allocation of treatment, was begun in the Jimi area of New Guinea in 1966. Infants born to the women in both treated and control groups were then examined at intervals over the next four years. Twenty-six cretins were diagnosed among 534 children born to the control women compared with 7 among the 498 children born to the treated women. Moreover, in 6 of the 7 affected cases in the treated group the mother was already pregnant when the oil was administered, and the seventh mother may have been also, but there was uncertainty about the child's date of birth. It would seem, therefore, that iodine is required for some process unrelated to thyroid function, but concerned with the development of the central nervous system at a stage in pregnancy before the foetal thyroid develops, and that a deficiency of iodine can lead to serious damage of the nervous system.

Water. The effect of variations in other elements of the diet is unknown. Penrose speculated that the geographical variations in the prevalence of anencephaly might be due to agents 'such as the presence or absence of trace elements in the water supply' as long ago as 1957; but the suggestion was not taken up until 1970, when Fedrick reported that the prevalence of anencephaly was closely related to the nature of the water supply in 10 large towns throughout the U.K. In her series it was notable that correlation with the calcium content of the water (correlation co-efficient —0.845) was stronger than with total water hardness (—0.801) or any other of the seven features of the water supply that were examined. In the United States, Fedrick found that areas with a high incidence of spina bifida had a mean water hardness that was little more than half that of areas with a low incidence (89 p.p.m. against 157 p.p.m.)

More detailed examination of the data for 48 local authority areas in South Wales and for 58 county boroughs in England and Wales confirms that correlation between malformations of the central nervous system and water hardness exists (Lowe, Roberts and Lloyd, 1971), but it is relatively weak and is indeed weaker than that between water hardness and infant mortality as a whole (Crawford, Gardner and Sedgwick, 1972). It may be, therefore, as Lowe and his colleagues suggest, that the softness of water supplies 'is no more than an uncertain pointer to some, as yet undetermined, specific teratogen in the non-specific poverty complex'. What we need is more detailed comparison between countries, an examination of what happened in towns that altered their water supply, and a comparison of the waters actually drunk by the mothers of affected and unaffected children. Perhaps it will eventually be shown that water supplies enter into the equation by facilitating the effect of some other agents.

Other dietary factors. That environment as well as heredity plays some part in the development of anencephaly is certain. Not only is the concordance rate as low as 11 per cent in monozygous twins (Renwick, 1972), but the incidence varies with year, season, and place, as well as with the social class and parity of the mother. For example, a major epidemic of both anencephaly and spina bifida occurred in Boston between 1920 and 1949 with a peak in 1929-32, at which time the prevalence of the two conditions was more than treble what it is now (MacMahon and Yen, 1971). The increase during the period of prohibition, 1920 to 1933, is striking and it may be that some abnormal constituent of alcohol was responsible—an idea that is at least consistant with the observation that the disparity between the rates in Boston Irish and

Boston Jews was much greater during the early thirties than it is now (Naggan and MacMahon, 1967; Naggan, 1969).

In the last few months three new hypotheses have been put forward. First Fedrick (1972) compared the prevalence of anencephaly with the consumption of eleven different foodstuffs in 5 socio-economic classes, and in 19 countries. Only one foodstuff showed a large and significant correlation in both series—namely tea. Fedrick, therefore, sent a questionnaire to some 500 mothers who had given birth to a stillborn child with anencephaly or spina bifida and 2,000 control mothers matched for date of delivery, region, and mother's age parity. The results showed an increase in risk of about 65 per cent in women who drank tea regularly compared with that in women who drank none. In soft water areas the difference increased to threefold; in hard water areas it practically disappeared.

Secondly, Renwick (1972) suggested that anencephaly and spina bifida are largely the result of exposure of the embryo to glycosides of solanine in the mother's diet. These substances which develop in and under the skin of the potato tuber on storage or exposure to ultraviolet light, are fungicidal; and it is suggested that their concentration in potatoes is increased in response to attack by the fungus of potato blight, *phytopthora infestans*. Renwick finds correlations between the geographical and temporal incidence of anencephaly and spina bifida and potato blight and produces ingenious explanations for such apparently awkward facts as the reduction in the prevalence of anencephalic stillbirths during the war, which was accompanied by an *increase* in potato consumption. It is impossible to do justice to his argument in a brief précis but perhaps it is not necessary to try and do so now that Posswillo, Sopher, and Mitchell (1972) have observed defects in the occipital region of the skull with distortion of the underlying brain in 4 out of 11 offspring born to marmosets on a diet containing large amounts of concentrate from blighted potatoes. Such defects have not been reported previously in these animals which, it appears, may be particularly suitable for testing human teratogens. At least they are sensitive to the teratogenic effects of both ionizing radiations and thalidomide (Poswillo, Hamilton and Sopher, 1972). I would not find Renwick's argument compelling in the absence of the experimental results, but it cannot now be ignored. It is difficult to see how the hypothesis can be tested effectively other than by an experiment in which young women are persuaded to cease eating potatoes whenever they are at risk of conceiving.

Thirdly Knox (1972) has suggested that the geographic and temporal variations may be largely attributed to variations in the consumption of mag-nesium salts in canned peas or of nitrates and nitrites in cured meats. Knox's suggestion is based on a detailed and objective analysis of data for England and Wales over the nine year period 1961 to 1969 and is statistically irreproachable. It is notable that Knox's analysis found a positive correlation with the consumption of new potatoes and a negative correlation with the consumption of old potatoes, in both cases with a lag interval of five months. Knox regarded these correlations as being complementary to an independent seasonal pattern; when season was eliminated other components contributed virtually nothing to the variation in the prevalence of the disease.

Conclusion

In this survey, I have described only a few of the hazards to which the embryo or foetus may be exposed *in utero*, considering particularly those that produce delay in development, congenital malformations, and malignant disease later in life. The circumstances which cause these hazards cannot always be reproduced in animal experiments, nor, if they can, can we always assume that the human animal responds in the same way as the guinea-pig, rat or marmoset. Experiment to produce disease in children is unthinkable, so that we often have to reach conclusions on the basis of observations that are, in principle, open to several different interpretations.

The variety of agents that have been implicated as a cause of these hazards, the intricate way in which some of them are interwoven with the events of daily life, and the delay before their effects are manifest, make detection particularly difficult. It is, therefore, not surprising if the epidemiologist has a haunting fear that his conclusions may not always be correct. Doctors, like other men, have their prejudices, not least when the evidence points to a deleterious effect of their favourite method of treatment, and it was bitter experience that led Sir Derrick Dunlop, until recently Chairman of our Committee on Safety of Drugs, to comment that 'the majority of our opinions are mere wish-fulfilments, like dreams in Freudian theory, and the mind of the most rational can be compared to a stormy ocean of passionate conviction based upon desire, upon which floats perilously a few tiny boats carrying their cargo of scientifically vested beliefs'. This is indeed a salutary warning, but it is possible, even for epidemiologists, to bring their boats safely into harbour, if they pay attention to the lighthouses and charts that experience and modern technology have provided.

Doubt about the interpretation of epidemiological observations should not be allowed to delay action interminably. The best sort of experiment is an experiment in prevention, and it is not a bad last resort, even if we are unable to carry it out in a properly controlled way. Proof in the strict logical sense may not have been obtained, but does this matter if the disease has disappeared?

References

Butler, N.R. and Alberman, E.D. (1969) *Perinatal problems.* Livingstone, Edinburgh.

Butler, N.R. and Bonham, D.G. (1963) *Perinatal mortality.* Livingstone, Edinburgh.

Butler, N.R., Goldstein, H. and Ross, E.M. (1972) *Brit. med. J.,* **2,** 127-130.

Cheeseman, E.A. and Walby, A.L. (1963) *Ann. hum. Genet., Lond.,* **27,** 23-29.

Chief Medical Officer (1971) On the state of the public health. *Annual report of the Chief Medical Officer for the year 1970* H.M.S.O., London.

Coffey, V.P. and Jessop, W.J.E. (1959) *Lancet,* **2,** 935-938.

Coffey, V.P. and Jessop, W.J.E. (1963) *Lancet,* **1,** 748-751.

Crawford, M.D., Gardener, M.J. and Sedgwick, P.A. (1972) *Lancet,* **1,** 988-992.

David, T.J. (1972) *New. Engl. J. Med.,* **287,** 487-489.

Davie, R., Butler, N.R. and Goldstein, H. (1972) *From birth to seven.* Longmans, London.

Elshove, J. (1970) *Teratogene werking von fenytoine* Proefschrift, Groningen.

Elshove J. and Van Eck, J.H.M. (1971) *Ned. T., Geneesk.,* **115,** 1371-1375.

Fedrick, J. (1970) *Nature,* **227,** 176-177.

Fedrick, J. (1972) to be published.

Fedrick, J. and Alberman, E.D. (1972) *Brit. med. J.,* **2,** 485-488.

Greenwald, P., Barlow, J.J., Nasca, P.C. and Burnett, W.S. (1971) *New Engl. J. Med.,* **285,** 390-392.

Gregg, N.M. (1941) *Trans. ophthal. Soc. Aust.,* **3,** 35.

Hakosalo, J. and Saxen, L. (1971) *Lancet,* **2,** 1346-1347.

Herbst, A.L. (1972) Statement presented before the United States Senate Committee on Labor and Public Welfare, Sub-committee on Health Diethylstilboestrol (DES) Hearings, July 10, 1972.

Herbst, A.L., Ulfelder, H. and Poskanzer, D.C. (1971) *New Engl. J. Med.,* **284,** 878-881.

Hewitt, D., Sanders, B. and Stewart, A. (1966) Oxford Survey of Childhood Cancers: progress report IV Reliability of data reported by case and control mothers. *Mon. Bull. Minist. Hlth.,* **25,** 80-85.

Jablon, S. and Kato, H. (1970) *Lancet,* **2,** 1000-1003.

Janz, D. and Fuchs, U. (1964) *Dtsch. med. Wcschr,* **89,** 241.

Knox, E. C. (1972) *Brit. J. prev. soc. Med.,* **26,** 219-223.

Leck, I. (1963) *Brit. J. prev. soc. Med.,* **17,** 70-80.

Lejeune, J., Turpin, R., Rethore, M-Q. and Mayer, M. (1960) *Rev. franç. Étud. clin. biol.,* **5,** 982.

Lenz, W. (1962) *Lancet,* **1,** 45.

Lowe, C.R., Roberts, C.J. and Lloyd, S. (1971) *Brit. med. J.,* **2,** 357-361.

McBride, W.G. (1961) *Lancet,* **2,** 1358.

MacMahon, B. (1962) *J. nat. Cancer Inst.,* **28,** 1173-91.

MacMahon, B. and Yen, S. (1971) *Lancet,* **1,** 31-33.

Melchior, J.C., Svensmark, O. and Trolle, D. (1967) *Lancet,* **2,** 860-861.

Miller, R.W. and Blot, W.J. (1972) *Lancet,* **2,** 784-787.

Naggan, L. (1969) *Amer. J. Epidem.,* **89,** 154-160.

Naggan, L. and MacMahon, B. (1967) *New. Engl. J. Med.,* **277,** 1119-1123.

Newcombe, H.B. and McGregor, H.B. (1971) *Lancet,* **2,** 1151-1152.

Penrose, L.S. (1957) *J. ment. Defic. Res.,* **1,** 4-15.

Pharaoh, P.O.D., Buttfield, I.H. and Hetzel, B.S. (1971) *Lancet,* **1.** 308-310.

Poswillo, D.E., Hamilton, W.J. and Sopher, D. (1972) *Nature*

Poswillo, D.E., Sopher, D. and Mitchell, S. (1972) *Nature.*

Renwick, J.H. (1972) *Brit. J. prev. soc. Med.,* **26,** 67-88.

Rogers, S.C. (1972) *Lancet,* **1,** 261.

Simpson, W.J. (1957) *Amer. J. Obstet. Gynaec.,* **73,** 808-815.

Speidel, B.D. and Meadow, S.R. (1972) *Lancet,* **2,** 839-843.

Stewart, A.M. and Kneale, G.W. (1970) *Lancet,* **1,** 1185-1188.

Stewart, A., Webb, J., Giles, D. and Hewitt, D. (1956) *Lancet,* **2,** 477.

Stewart, A., Webb, J. and Hewitt, D. (1958) *Brit. med. J.,* **1,** 1495-1508.

Sullivan, F.M. (1972) Mechanisms of teratogenesis in *Adverse Drug Reactions.* Ed. D.J. Richards and R.J. Rondel. Churchill Livingstone, Edinburgh.

Yerushalmy, J. (1964) *Amer. J. Obstet. Gynec.,* **88,** 505-518.

Yerusalmy, J. (1971) *Amer. J. Epidem.,* **93,** 443-456.

PART VII

PRENATAL DIAGNOSIS AND MANAGEMENT OF CONGENITAL ABNORMALITIES

PAPER 47

47. Milunsky, A. and Atkins, L. (1974). Prenatal diagnosis of genetic disorders. An analysis of experience with 600 cases. *J. Am. Med. Assoc.*, **230**, 232–235

COMMENTARY

Amniocentesis is now widely used for the prenatal detection of chromosomal abnormalities, sex-linked diseases, inherited biochemical disorders, and neural tube defects. The technique involves the removal of a small sample (10–20 ml) of amniotic fluid transabdominally. Between the 14th and 16th week of gestation the volume of amniotic fluid is 100–285 ml, and this is the optimal time for performing diagnostic amniocentesis.

Amniotic fluid cells, which are mainly fetal in origin, can be cultured and examined for chromosomal abnormalities or for inborn errors of metabolism. Estimation of specific metabolites in amniotic fluid itself may also give some guidance in the diagnosis of certain fetal abnormalities, such as the high α-fetoprotein levels which are found in cases of anencephaly, spina bifida, and myelocele (see Persaud, 1976).

Prior to amniocentesis, it is important to determine the exact position of the placenta in order to avoid placental damage and haemorrhage, fetal risks (abortion, puncture, congenital malformations), and maternal blood groups isoimmunization. Ultrasonography is the method of choice for the localization of the placenta; it is simple, rapid, and accurate.

Paper 47 reviews on the basis of 600 consecutive cases current perspectives in diagnostic amniocentesis. In agreement with other studies, the commonest indication for the procedure was advanced maternal age. Nineteen 'affected' fetuses were predicted. These included four male fetuses (in the group of mothers suspected for X-linked diseases), chromosomal (unbalanced D/G translocation, Klinefelter syndrome, trisomy 18 and mosaicism) and metabolic disorders (Tay–Sachs disease and

Cumulative USA and Canadian experience with amniocentesis for prenatal genetic studies*

Indications	Cases studied	'Affected' fetuses	Therapeutic abortion	Prenatal diagnosis confirmed
Chromosomal disorders				
Translocation carriers	93	17	17	17
Maternal age >40 years	347	9	7	7
Maternal age 35–39	255	4	3	3
Previous trisomy 21 (Mongolism)	485	5	4	3
Miscellaneous	188	1	1	1
X-linked disorders	115	54	40	34
Metabolic disorders	180	37	30	26
Total	1663	127	102	91

* From Milunsky, A., *The Prenatal Diagnosis of Hereditary Disorders*, 1973. Courtesy of Charles C. Thomas, Publisher, Springfield, Illinois.

Hunter's syndrome). In 13 cases, the pregnancy was terminated and the antenatal diagnosis subsequently confirmed.

Perhaps more representative of the indications and results of diagnostic amniocentesis are those observed in an exhaustive survey of 1633 cases, reported from the United States and Canada (Milunsky, 1973). The major indications were as follows: chromosomal disorders (1368), sex determination for X-linked diseases (115), and for metabolic disorders (180). The results of this study, summarized in the Table on preceding page, are self-explanatory.

REFERENCES

Milunsky, A. (1973). *The Prenatal Diagnosis of Hereditary Disorders.* (Springfield, Ill.: Charles C. Thomas, Publisher)

Persaud, T. V. N. (1976). Prenatal diagnosis and its pathologic confirmation. In H. S. Rosenberg and R. P Bolande (eds.). *Perspectives in Pediatric Pathology*, Vol. 3. (Chicago: Year Book Medical Publishers Inc.)

From A. Milunsky and L. Atkins (1974). J. Am. Med. Assoc. **230**, 232–235. *Copyright* (1974), *by kind permission of the authors and the American Medical Association*

Prenatal Diagnosis of Genetic Disorders

An Analysis of Experience With 600 Cases

Aubrey Milunsky, MB BCh, MRCP, DCH, Leonard Atkins, MD

● Prenatal diagnosis of hereditary disorders is now an established part of routine antenatal care. This report of our experience with 600 cases indicates that advanced maternal age is by far the commonest indication for amniocentesis. Chromosomal or metabolic abnormalities were diagnosed in 15 fetuses. In addition, four fetuses were determined to be male in the sex-linked group. The parents elected termination of the pregnancies in 13 cases. Reassurance was provided to more than 95% of mothers studied. Every physician is urged to offer these prenatal genetic studies when indicated or to seek consultation when in doubt.
   (*JAMA* 230:232-235, 1974)

EACH year in the United States alone, there are more than 20,000 live births with chromosomal abnormalities.[1] We estimate that in 1973, chromosomal abnormalities were diagnosed in fewer than 75 fetuses in utero. There would appear to be three major reasons to explain this remarkably small number of intrauterine genetic diagnoses made in one year: (1) obstetricians' hesitation to use amniocentesis during the second trimester because of the lack of precise information regarding the magnitude of risk for this procedure, (2) lack of awareness of the indications for prenatal genetic studies, and (3) inadequate, unproven, or no facilities for

From the Eunice Kennedy Shriver Center, Walter E. Fernald State School, Waltham, Mass (Dr. Milunsky), the Genetics Unit, Children's Service (Dr. Milunsky), and Department of Pathology (Dr. Atkins), Massachusetts General Hospital, and the departments of pediatrics (Dr. Milunsky) and pathology (Dr. Atkins), Harvard Medical School, Boston.
   Reprint requests to Eunice Kennedy Shriver Center, 200 Trapelo Rd, Waltham, MA 02154 (Dr. Milunsky).

amniotic fluid cell culture and specific studies.

While the risk of amniocentesis should be satisfactorily answered by the collaborative National Institute of Child Health and Human Development (NICHHD) study now in its closing phase, this study will provide some guidance. The indications, problems and pitfalls, and reservations for prenatal genetic studies have been fully discussed,[2] and only new points or additional useful experience will be referred to in this paper. A lack of local facilities is not sufficient reason to withhold needed studies on high-risk patients, since transport of amniotic fluid for culture is eminently feasible if done properly.

The lessons learned in this report of our carefully studied experience with 600 cases should prove useful to those not thinking daily about offering prenatal genetic studies to their higher-risk patients.

MATERIAL AND METHODS

Our Genetics Laboratory is the center for prenatal diagnosis in Massachusetts. Amniotic fluid samples aspirated during the second trimester of pregnancy are brought (usually by hand) to us for study. The vast majority of amniocenteses are performed in the offices of private obstetricians. Usually 10 to 20 ml of amniotic fluid is obtained, and delivery of the sample made usually on the same day as the amniocentesis.

Almost all samples were centrifuged and the cells resuspended in Eagle minimum essential medium with 15% fetal calf serum, and grown in 5% carbon dioxide in air at 37 C. The cells were harvested and processed according to previously described methods.[3] Efforts were made to count chromosomes in at least 30 metaphases in each case. In some instances, this was not possible because of poor quality or inadequate number of divisions. In more difficult cases, 30 to 100 cells were counted. As a general rule, at least five metaphases per case were photographed and analyzed in detail. Trypsin banding has been performed only in known or suspected cases of translocation, or those with enigmatic karyotypes.

Uusually around the 15th day, decisions are made about the need for a second amniocentesis. This cautious approach was employed to avoid the difficult situations that could (and do) arise when laboratories inform the obstetrician of failure to obtain a result four to five weeks after the first amniocentesis. As a consequence of this policy, diagnoses were provided in all cases where prenatal diagnosis was attempted in time for repeat studies where necessary.

RESULTS

Diagnoses were reported on the first amniotic fluid sample received in 89.8% of cases (Table 1). A second amniocentesis was necessary in 6.7% of cases. In a further 2.2% of cases studied, a second tap was recommended, but as it ultimately turned out, not needed (see "Comment"). In six cases, the first amniocentesis was performed too late in gestation for a repeat aspiration. Seven patients simply refused a recommended repeat tap. A second tap was not repeated in a further eight cases—two had spontaneous abortions; the obstetrician decided against a second tap in two cases, resulting in the birth of an infant with Down syndrome in one case; in four cases, half the sample was received—three sent by air from new service laboratories failed to grow, and one was contaminated. "Dry" taps (no fluid obtained) were experienced in 32 (10%) cases of 328 where data were available. In two cases, a dry tap occurred after two amniocenteses (one to two weeks apart), and in one case, failure to obtain fluid occurred after three separate amniocenteses.

Amniotic Fluid Studies

Grossly bloody samples were received in 6.6% of cases. All bloody amniotic fluid samples were cleared using the ammonium chloride lysis technique.[4] The rapidity with which results were obtained from bloody and nonbloody amniotic fluid samples differed widely. The average time for determining the karyotype was 17 days. By the 17th day, 58% of clear amniotic fluids were completed in contrast to the 39% of bloody samples. Admixture of maternal and fetal cells has as yet not been encountered. Total loss of the amniotic fluid sample by contamination occurred in only three (0.5%) instances, two samples of which were initially split elsewhere. Thus far, no errors in prenatal diagnosis, including sex determination, have been made. Transported (by air or mail) samples (27) fared poorly,

with no results being provided from ten such samples. Results were obtained from one sample in transit for seven days.

Poor cell growth (35 cases) was by far the commonest reason for failure to obtain a result on the first amniocentesis. Because of the need for a large number of cells for the prenatal diagnosis of certain biochemical disorders, second amniocenteses were called for in two cases, while in a third, we received only half the split sample, which proved insufficient. In six instances, the amniotic fluid obtained by the obstetrician was carelessly mailed and subsequently ruined by postal delay, temperature extremes, or breakage. Other reasons for a second amniocentesis were grossly bloody fluid or little or no fluid (six cases), failure of cells to har-

vest (two cases), and verification of diagnosis (one case).

A third amniocentesis was required in two cases (0.3%) because of grossly bloody fluid, little or no amniotic fluid, and poor cell growth, and was requested by one patient. In the latter instance, rubella exposure had occurred, and live virus was isolated from the amniotic fluid and the subsequently aborted fetus.[5]

Detailed Results

A detailed summary of our experience with 600 consecutive cases (Table 2) indicates that advanced maternal age is by far the commonest reason for prenatal genetic studies. Chromosomal or metabolic abnormalities were observed in 15 cases. In addition, four fetuses were determined to be male in the X-linked group.

Table 1.—Amniocentesis Data in 600 Consecutive Cases

	No. (%) of Cases
Report on first fluid sample	539 (89.8)
Second amniocentesis necessary	40 (6.7)
Second amniocentesis unnecessary	13 (2.2)
Third amniocentesis	3 (0.5)
Amniocentesis not repeated	21 (3.5)
Too late	6
Patient refused	7
Other	8*
Errors in diagnosis	0 ...
Sample loss by contamination	3 (0.5)

*See text.

Table 2.—Experience With 600 Consecutive Cases for Prenatal Diagnosis

Indications	Cases Studied	"Affected" Fetuses	Therapeutic Abortion	Prenatal Diagnosis Confirmed	Live Births
Chromosomal disorders					
Translocation carrier	10	3	3*†	3*†	5
Maternal age, 35-39 yr	157	1‡	...	1‡	117
Maternal age, ≥40 yr	146	4§‖	2‖	3‖	116
Previous Down syndrome	99	...	...	...	74¶
Family history of Down syndrome	38	1*	1*	1*	30
Miscellaneous	107	1#	...	...	79
X-linked disorders	12	4 (males)	2	4	9
Metabolic disorders	31	5**	5**	5**	21
Total	**600**	**19**	**13**	**17**	**451**††‡‡§§

*Unbalanced D/G translocation (2).
†Rubella (1).
‡Klinefelter syndrome (1).
§Mosaic (46 XY/47 X(p)X(q)Y) (1).
‖Trisomy 18 (3).
¶Down syndrome (1).
#Possible radiation/viral damage (1).
**Tay-Sachs disease (4), Hunter syndrome (1).
††Twins (8 pairs).
‡‡Partial phocomelia (1), cranio-synostosis (1), cleft lip (1).
§§Births pending (123).

Table 3.—Untoward Outcome of Pregnancies After Amniocentesis in 600 Cases*

Indications for Amniocentesis	Case No.	Outcome
Maternal age, 35-39 yr	A_1	Spontaneous abortion three weeks after tap
	A_2	Spontaneous abortion two weeks after tap
	A_3	Spontaneous abortion three days after tap
	A_4	Spontaneous abortion 20 days after tap
	A_5	Missed abortion five weeks after tap
	A_6	No fetal heart by doptone at amniocentesis (15 weeks); spontaneous abortion ten days after tap; very tight true umbilical cord knot around one leg; fetus and placenta grossly normal
Maternal age, ≥40 yr	B_1	Spontaneous abortion seven weeks after amniocentesis, yielding a normal-appearing fetus and small placenta
	B_2	Pregnancy complicated by hypertension, prediabetes, and excessive weight gain, ending with normal-appearing stillborn
	B_3	Fetal death two days after amniocentesis with the abortus affected by erythroblastosis (as were two previous intrauterine deaths)
	B_4	Dark brown amniotic fluid at the time of amniocentesis signifying probable fetal death, which was confirmed shortly thereafter
	B_5	Stillbirth in a pregnancy complicated by hypertension and placental insufficiency at seven months' gestation
Previous Down syndrome	C_1	Spontaneous abortion after amniocentesis and between 16 to 21 weeks' gestation; amniocentesis conceivably related to fetal loss
	C_2	Fetal death due to erythroblastosis fetalis at 20 weeks' gestation
Family history of Down syndrome	D_1	Vaginal bleeding from the fourth week of gestation until spontaneous abortion the 18th week, 16 days after amniocentesis; abortus appeared normal and placenta circumvallate
Miscellaneous	E_1	Spontaneous abortion; grossly malformed fetus at 32 weeks' gestation
	E_2	Premature twins at 27 weeks after a pregnancy complicated by hydramnios; one twin a macerated stillborn; other twin lived less than two hours
	E_3	Fetal death between 18 to 19 weeks' gestation; amniocentesis conceivably a cause

*Pregnancies completed in 465 cases.

The parents elected to terminate the pregnancy in 13 cases, the diagnosis being confirmed in the abortus in all cases.

In the maternal age group of 35 to 39 years, one mother aged 38 was found to be carrying a fetus with an XXY karyotype. The parents elected to continue that pregnancy and in due course, the affected child was delivered as predicted—together with a normal, unsuspected twin.

Four affected fetuses were found in the group of mothers aged 40 years and more. One fetus had trisomy 18, which was diagnosed from an amniotic fluid received at 28 weeks' gestation—too late to terminate the pregnancy. Another two cases of trisomy 18 were diagnosed in time for the parents to elect pregnancy termination. One mother had previously given birth to another child with trisomy 18. The karyotypes of the parents were normal, and this represents the first recorded instance, to our knowledge, of recurrent trisomy 18. Trypsin banding of the chromosomes confirmed the diagnosis, and the phenotypic features of the fetus after abortion were consistent with trisomy 18. The fourth affected fetus diagnosed in this category was in a 47-year-old mother who had the amniocentesis performed at 34 weeks' gestation! The prenatal diagnosis of mosaicism was made approximately one month prior to delivery, the karyotype showing a normal cell line and an abnormal line with two abnormal X chromosomes (to be reported in detail elsewhere). The prenatal diagnosis of a Klinefelter syndrome mosaic was made approximately one month prior to delivery. Blood and skin studies on this child revealed a normal karyotype after birth!

Diagnostic Dilemmas

The indications for amniocentesis in the miscellaneous category were as previously documented.[2] In one case, the mother had been subjected to diagnostic irradiation (gastrointestinal and gallbladder series) and had thereafter been subjected to amniocentesis because of the inadvertent irradiation at three weeks' gestation. At the first amniocentesis, 10% of the cells studied showed chromosomal fragmentation, a dicentric chromosome, and a ring chromosome. A second amniocentesis one month later yielded cells that showed chromosomal breakage in 13% to 14% of the cells. The parents elected to continue this pregnancy, which resulted in a karyotypically (blood and skin) normal child.

In each of two cases, a single amniotic cell with a ring chromosome was found in 90 and 60 metaphases, respectively. The parents elected to continue these pregnancies, recognizing that no accurate prenatal diagnosis was possible. A healthy infant with a normal karyotype was born in the first case. The other patient is yet to give birth.

Thus far, there have been 451 live births, including eight sets of twins. Three infants were born with disorders not diagnosable in utero, and incidental to the primary reason for prenatal studies (Table 2).

Maternal and Fetal Complications

Major complications were confined to spontaneous abortion, stillbirth, fetal death, or marked prematurity in 477 cases studied after amniocentesis and where pregnancy had been completed. There were 17 such major complications (Table 3). In seven cases (1.5%) (A_1 through A_5, C_1, and E_3), amniocentesis was considered as a probable cause of fetal loss. Information on minor complications following amniocentesis was available in only 328 cases. In four cases, there was minor vaginal bleeding with all pregnancies going to term with normal delivery and child. Vaginal amniotic fluid leakage occurred in two cases. In both instances, the pregnancy and birth continued uneventfully with normal resulting offspring.

COMMENT

We have previously discussed lessons learned from our early experience with 298 cases for prenatal diagnosis.[2,6] Comments here will be confined to new lessons or additional perspectives gained subsequently.

Mosaicism in cultured amniotic fluid cells provides serious diagnostic dilemmas. Indeed, Kajii[7] has suggested that aneuploidy may *arise* in amniotic cell cultures, and therefore may not necessarily or accurately reflect the fetal karyotype. Kardon et al[8] reported an apparent 45X/46XY mosaic in which 45X cells were found in the first amniotic fluid culture studied, and 46XY cells in the second sample. We have studied an amniotic

fluid culture that showed sex chromosome mosaicism ($46XY/47X_{1p}X_{1q}Y$). The child subsequently delivered had a normal karyotype in blood and skin.

A second amniocentesis was done in 8.9% of our cases (6.7% were necessary, and an additional 2.2% requested). Gerbie et al[9] found that second amniocenteses were done in 7% of 238 cases, and Doran[10] 8.3% of 73 cases—not really different from our experience. Grossly bloody samples were received in 6.6% of cases, compared to the 4% elsewhere.[9]

The risks to the mother and fetus from amniocentesis are still under study in the collaborative NICHHD Amniocentesis Registry Project. Nevertheless, certain useful observations can be made from our experience. No maternal mortality was noted, and maternal morbidity was minor. Fetal loss probably related to amniocentesis occurred in 1.5% of cases, which is in contrast to reported second-trimester spontaneous abortion only of 1.2% of cases.[11] However, no significant

difference is apparent between these two figures. The final assessment of risk however, must await the carefully *matched control* studies of the NICHHD. In our experience, spontaneous abortion has occurred between 14 to 16 weeks' gestation *prior* to amniocentesis in three cases where the procedure had been scheduled. Should these fetal losses have occurred after amniocentesis, they could have been viewed as complications of the tap.

Prenatal genetic studies are now an integral part of routine antenatal care. Every obstetrician is urged to offer these studies when indicated or to seek consultation when in doubt. It is no longer reasonable to withhold these studies from mothers at risk for having babies with genetic disease that could be prevented.

This investigation was supported in part by Public Health Service research grant 1-P01-HD05515-01 (NICHHD), the NICHHD contract No. 71-2451, and the Maternal and Child Health Project 906.

References

1. Lubs HA, Ruddle FH: Chromosomal abnormalities in the human population: Estimation of rates based on New Haven newborn study. *Science* 169:495-497, 1970.
2. Milunsky A: *The Prenatal Diagnosis of Hereditary Disorders.* Springfield, Ill, Charles C Thomas, Publishers, 1973.
3. Milunsky A, Atkins L, Littlefield JM: Polyploidy in prenatal genetic diagnosis. *J Pediatr* 79:303-305, 1971.
4. Dioguardi N, Agostani A, Fiorelli G, et al: Characterization of lactic dehydrogenase of normal human granulocytes. *J Lab Clin Med* 61:713-723, 1963.
5. Levin MJ, Oxman MN, Moore MG, et al: Diagnosis of congenital rubella. *New Engl J Med*, to be published.
6. Milunsky A, Atkins L, Littlefield JW: Amniocentesis for prenatal genetic studies. *Obstet Gynecol* 40:104-108, 1972.
7. Kajii T: Pseudomosaicism in cultured amniotic-fluid cells. *Lancet* 2:1037, 1971.
8. Kardon NB, Chernay PR, Hsu LY, et al: Pitfalls in prenatal diagnosis resulting from chromosomal mosaicism. *J Pediatr* 80:297-299, 1972.
9. Gerbie AB, Nadler HL, Gerbie MV: Amniocentesis in genetic counseling. *Am J Obstet Gynecol* 109:765-768, 1971.
10. Doran TA: The antenatal diagnosis of genetic disease. *Am J Obstet Gynecol* 118:314-321, 1974.
11. Javert CT: *Spontaneous and Habitual Abortion.* New York, McGraw-Hill Book Co, Inc, 1957.

75, Not 75%.—An error occurred in the ORIGINAL CONTRIBUTION, "Prenatal Diagnosis of Genetic Disorders: An Analysis of Experience With 600 Cases," published in the Oct 14 issue (230:232-235, 1974). On page 232, the second sentence of the text should read "We estimate that in 1973, chromosomal abnormalities were diagnosed in utero in fewer than 75 fetuses."

PAPERS 48 AND 49

COMMENTARY

As indicated by Santos-Ramos and Duenhoelter (Paper 49), radiography is indispensable for the rapid prenatal detection of anencephaly and hydrocephaly, but ultrasonography is useful 'to modify, specify, and expand the radiologic and clinical diagnosis'. The first paper clearly demonstrates the value of ultrasound methods in prenatal diagnosis of certain fetal anomalies, including anencephaly, hydrocephaly, iniencephaly, achondroplasia, sacrococcygeal teratoma, hydronephrosis, and polycystic kidney. Of the 13 cases presented, the initial diagnosis was made by radiography.

Compared to radiological techniques, ultrasonography does not involve radiation and is apparently safe for both the mother and fetus. Soft tissue abnormalities are best diagnosed by ultrasound. In addition to the early detection of major malformations, ultrasonography is of considerable value in assessing the growth of the chorionic sac, early fetal life, pregnancy failure, and fetal maturity. Furthermore, it is the most important single method for the localization of the placenta in cases of placental abnormalities and also before diagnostic amniocentesis (Robinson, 1975; Jouppila and Piiroinen, 1975).

The paper by Birnbaum (Paper 48) is of considerable interest. It is the first report of the prenatal diagnosis of Down's syndrome by x-ray techniques. From a review of abdominal roentgenograms, it was suggested that extreme hyperextension of the head and dorsiflexion of the cervicodorsal spine may be indicative of this relatively common genetic anomaly.

REFERENCES

Jouppila, P. and Piiroinen, O. (1975). Ultrasonic diagnosis of fetal life in early pregnancy. *Obstet. Gynecol.*, **46**, 616–620

Robinson, H. P. (1975). The diagnosis of early pregnancy failure by sonar. *Br. J. Obstet. Gynaecol.*, **82**, 849–857

From S. J. Birnbaum (1971). Obstet. Gynecol., **37**, 394–395. *Copyright* (1971),
by kind permission of the author and the American College of Obstetricians and Gynecologists

Prenatal Diagnosis of Mongolism by X-Ray

STANLEY J. BIRNBAUM, MD, FACOG

Finding extreme hyperextension of the fetal head with dorsiflexion of the cervicodorsal vertebrae in abdominal roentgenogram during the third trimester of pregnancy is highly suggestive of a fetus with Langdon-Down syndrome. Although lateral angulation may accompany this finding, it is not specific when occurring alone.

AN X-RAY FINDING WHICH SEEMS TO BE USEFUL IN PREDICTING MONGOLISM (Langdon-Down syndrome) during the third trimester of pregnancy was recently called to my attention.[1] In a retrospective study of abdominal X-rays taken near term of five patients who subsequently delivered mongoloid infants, an abnormal fetal attitude, consisting of hyperextension of the fetal head with marked dorsiflexion of the cervicodorsal vertebrae, was revealed in every case. In two of these fetuses lateral flexion of the head was also observed. Using this information, we were able to predict the birth of an infant with Langdon-Down syndrome in the following case:

CASE REPORT

RB, a 35-year-old para 4, gravida 5, was admitted to our Hospital Center at term because of mild toxemia. An abdominal X-ray, which had been taken at 35 weeks because of hy-

From the Department of Obstetrics and Gynecology, The Brookdale Hospital Center, Brooklyn, NY.

Appreciation is expressed to the staffs of the New York Lying-In Hospital and The Brookdale Hospital Center X-Ray Departments for their cooperation.

Submitted for publication Aug 7, 1970.

dramnios, had shown a cephalic presentation with marked lateral flexion of the head. The patient started labor soon after admission. A repeat abdominal film taken at this time revealed a breech presentation with marked hyperextension of the head at the cervicodorsal junction (Fig 1). The delivery of a mongoloid infant was then predicted. The patient subsequently delivered a 7 lb 10 oz male infant, after five hours of labor, which proved to have typical Langdon-Down syndrome.

To ascertain the predictive specificity of this sign, more than 100 abdominal X-rays of third-trimester pregnancies from the files of the New York Lying-In Hospital and Brookdale Hospital Center were reviewed. Another fetus was found to have had marked dorsiflexion of the cervicodorsal spine in a breech presentation. This fetus also proved to be a mongoloid baby. Three other fetuses (two breech, one vertex) were found to have had lateral flexion, but not hyperextension. Two of these were later described as being normal babies. The third, an infant of a diabetic mother with hydramnios, was not mongoloid but was moderately retarded at six months of age.

DISCUSSION

The obstetric and radiologic literature of the past ten years was reviewed, but no mention was found relating a specific X-ray finding to Langdon-Down syndrome. Hyperextension of the fetal head with normal fetal skeletal features has been described with fetal thyroid enlargement (congenital goiter), cystic hygroma (hygroma colli), and he-

DIAGNOSIS OF MONGOLISM

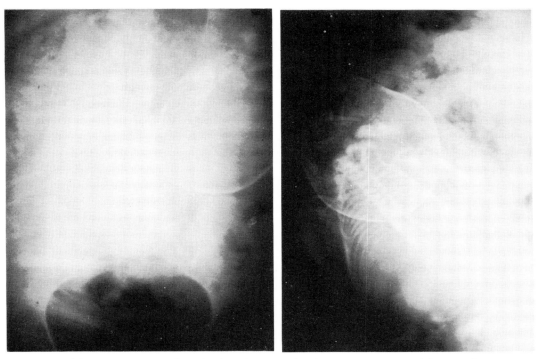

Fig 1. (left). Hyperextension of the head at the cervicodorsal junction, A-P view. **Right.** Lateral view.

mangioma.[2] These conditions must, therefore, be included in the differential diagnosis in the presence of this X-ray finding.

It is not surprising that fetuses with Langdon-Down syndrome assume bizarre attitudes while floating in amniotic fluid. One of the striking features of mongolism is extreme hypotonicity and joint laxity,[3] which apparently prevent normal muscle tonus from keeping the head in its usual habitus of flexion. Interestingly, these unusual attitudes of the head were found in both cephalic and breech presentations, and the point of maximal angulation seemed to be at the cervicodorsal junction. This is in contrast to the deflexion of the head which is seen in face and, occasionally, in breech presentations.

In these situations, the angulation is of the cervical spine only and is not as extreme.

Our review of a large number of antepartum roentgenograms, indicates that extreme hyperextension of the head and dorsiflexion of the cervicodorsal spine may be the key findings in mongoloid fetuses. Lateral angulation of the head, if it occurs alone, is apparently not specific.

The Brookdale Hospital Center
Linden Blvd at Brookdale Plaza
Brooklyn, NY 11212

REFERENCES

1. Birnberg CH: Oral Communication
2. Shaffer AJ: Diseases of the newborn. Philadelphia, WB Saunders Co, 1960, p 477
3. Nelson WE: Textbook of Pediatrics. Philadelphia, WB Saunders Co, 1959, p 1134

From R. Santos-Ramos and J. H. Duenhoelter (1975). Obstet. Gynecol., **45**, 279–283.
Copyright (1975), *by kind permission of the authors and the American College of Obstetricians and Gynecologists*

Diagnosis of Congenital Fetal Abnormalities by Sonography

RIGOBERTO SANTOS-RAMOS, MD and JOHANN H. DUENHOELTER, MD

Sonographic examinations were performed on 13 patients whose fetuses had the following congenital malformations: anencephaly (4 cases), hydrocephaly (4), obstruction of the renal excretory system (3), iniencephaly (1), and sacrococcygeal teratoma (1). In 7 cases the initial diagnosis was made by sonography, in 6 cases by radiography. Sonography was valuable *a)* in the detection of discrepant growth between fetal chest and head and *b)* in the recognition of fetal soft tissue abnormalities. It is concluded that sonography is a valuable aid in the diagnosis of congenital fetal anomalies.

OBSTETRICIANS have used sonography to localize the placenta, to measure the biparietal diameter of the fetal head, and to diagnose multiple and molar pregnancy. Hellman et al[1] described six different types of embryonic malformations based on sonographic studies of patients in early pregnancy. In some instances ultrasound has been used to diagnose fetal malformations such as anencephaly[2-9] and hydrocephaly.[10,11] During the past 2½ years, 13 pregnant women whose fetuses had major congenital malformations were examined in the sonography laboratory at Parkland Memorial Hospital. These cases are presented here because they demonstrate the usefulness

of sonography in the diagnosis of fetal abnormalities.

MATERIALS AND METHODS

Between December 1971 and March 1974, 2465 obstetric patients were examined with sonography. During the same time, 15,425 patients delivered at Parkland Memorial Hospital. In 13 fetuses congenital malformations were diagnosed before onset of labor: group I consisted of 4 fetuses with anencephaly; group II of 4 fetuses with hydrocephaly; group III of 5 fetuses with other malformations: 1 had iniencephaly, 1 a sacrococcygeal teratoma, and 3 obstruction of the renal excretory system.

With an ultrasonic laminograph (Picker Echo-view 9, Model 104), the abdomen of each patient was scanned in the longitudinal direction beginning in the midline and parallel to it in distances of 2 cm or less if indicated. Scans of the transverse planes were obtained beginning at the umbilicus, then at 2-cm intervals below and above. Studies were frequently complemented by scans of oblique planes. Between 25 and 35 Polaroid™ photographs were taken in every case.

Group I: Anencephaly

This group consisted of 4 patients with anencephalic fetuses. Clinical and laboratory data are summarized in Table 1. In all cases the diagnosis was made first by radiography and then confirmed by sonography. A consistent finding with both technics was absence of

From the Division of Maternal–Fetal Medicine, Department of Obstetrics and Gynecology, The University of Texas Southwestern Medical School, Dallas, Texas.
Submitted for publication June 1, 1974.

TABLE 1. GROUP I: ANENCEPHALY

Case No.	Age	Gravidity/Parity	Race	Anomaly suspected from:	Diagnosis made by:	Amniotic fluid volume (ml)	Fetal weight (g)
1	14	1/0	Negro	Rapid increase in uterine size	X-ray	4250	1420
2	17	1/0	Latin	Rapid increase in uterine size	X-ray	5800	1120
3	21	2/1	Latin	Prolonged pregnancy	X-ray	2850	2850
4	17	2/0	Negro	Prolonged pregnancy	X-ray	Unremarkable	2245

SANTOS AND DUENHOELTER

TABLE 2. GROUP II: HYDROCEPHALY

Case No.	Age	Gravidity/Parity	Race	Anomaly suspected from:	Diagnosis made by:	BPD* (cm)	Fetal weight (g)
5	17	2/1	Latin	Increase in uterine contents	Sonogram	11.6	2810
6	43	15/12	Negro	Increase in uterine contents	Sonogram	11.3	2530
7	24	3/2	Latin	Large mass	X-ray	13.2	3600
8	24	3/1	White	Increase in uterine contents	X-ray	10.8	2750

* BPD = biparietal diameter of the head

TABLE 3. MEASUREMENTS OF BPD* AND APD* BETWEEN 37 AND 40 WEEKS' GESTATION IN CASE 5

Week of gestation	BPD (cm)	APD (cm)
37	10.5	9.0
39	11.1	9.0
40	11.6	9.3

* BPD = biparietal diameter of head; APD = anteroposterior diameter of chest

the typical skull structure. In 2 of the patients the rapid increase in uterine size caused by polyhydramnios led the physicians to suspect an anomaly. In the other 2 cases, the diagnosis was made only after the pregnancy had progressed to 42 weeks.

Group II: Hydrocephaly

In Table 2 the data of 4 patients with hydrocephalic infants are summarized. Patient 5 had sonographic examinations at 37, 39, and 40 weeks' gestation (Table 3). The hastened growth of the head was in marked contrast to the normal growth of the chest. In case 6 (Figure 1) the difference between the biparietal diameter of the head and the anteroposterior diameter of the chest was 4.1 cm. In all 4 cases the physicians

decompressed the fetal head by removing cerebrospinal fluid to achieve delivery. Three of the infants died soon after birth, the fourth at the age of 4 weeks. In case 7 a second congenital abnormality, achondroplasia, was identified from the radiogram and confirmed at delivery.

Group III: Other Malformations

A short summary of the 5 cases in this group follows:

Case 9. A 27-year-old Latin American, gravida 5, para 4, attended the clinic first at the 25th week of gestation. Two weeks later, her physician suspected twins and obtained a roentgenogram in which the outline of a single fetus in breech presentation could be barely seen. At sonography the fetus was clearly outlined and surrounded by polyhydramnios. A fetal malformation was present which was thought to be a meningomyelocele in the region of the neck (Figure 2).

At cesarean section, the amniotic sac was decompressed and 6000 ml of amniotic fluid were drained. An Apgar 1 male infant was delivered and succumbed shortly thereafter. The malformation was typical of iniencephaly.

Case 10. A 16-year-old Latin American, gravida 1, was seen initially in the Obstetric Clinic 3 months before her delivery at an unknown duration of gestation. One month

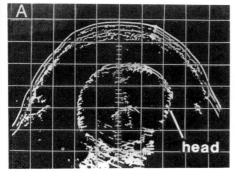
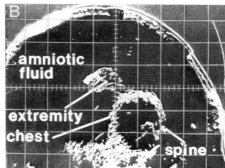

Fig 1. Case 6. A. Cross-section of fetal head; biparietal diameter, 12 cm. B. Polyhydramnios. Fetal body with anteroposterior diameter of 7.5 cm.

FETAL ABNORMALITIES

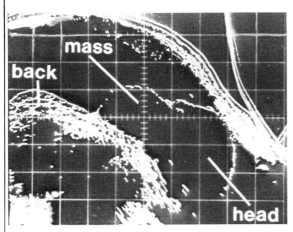

Fig 2. Case 9. Fetal head with mass attached to posterior aspect of fetal neck. Polyhydramnios.

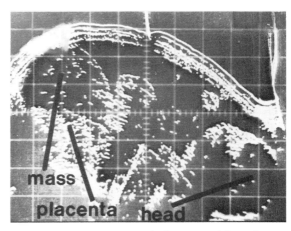

Fig 3. Case 10. Mass in uterine fundus separated from placenta, attached to caudal area of fetus.

after the initial visit, the attending physician thought that the fetus had grown more rapidly than normal. He obtained a sonogram which showed an abnormality in the lumbosacral area (Figure 3). Four weeks later, the patient developed hypertension (160/100 mmHg). She was treated with magnesium sulfate and went into spontaneous labor. A 2050-g infant was delivered which had a large sacrococcygeal tumor. The tumor ruptured at delivery and the infant succumbed shortly thereafter.

At autopsy the tumor was identified as a sacrococcygeal teratoma.

Case 11. A 26-year-old Negro, gravida 4, para 3, with chronic hypertension attended the Obstetric Clinic first at 15 weeks' gestation. To follow fetal growth, sonography was obtained first at 24 weeks' gestation. The biparietal diameter of the head was 6.5 cm. During a second sonography 9 weeks later, the head could not be measured accurately, but the fetal abdomen was distended (Figure 4).

After 36 weeks' gestation, a 3920-g male, Apgar 10, was delivered precipitously in the Emergency Room. The baby had a typical Potter facies and a distended abdomen from which the musculature was missing. On an intravenous pyelogram the calices were absent on the right; they were abnormal on the left. The urachus was markedly distended. A cystostomy had to be performed. The infant died of renal failure 2½ months after birth.

Case 12. A 16-year-old Negro primigravida was seen first in the Obstetric Clinic at 30 weeks' gestation. Seven weeks later she developed hydramnios, hypertension (160/120 mmHg), and proteinura. Therapy was begun with magnesium sulfate.

The sonograms were interpreted to show the following: excessive amount of amniotic fluid, biparietal diameter of the head 8.4 cm, distention of the fetal abdomen by

ascites, and a huge bladder or a polycystic kidney.

A 2300-g, Apgar 1 male with massive ascites was delivered by cesarean section and died 2 hours postpartum.

At autopsy, massive ascites, severe bilateral hydronephrosis, and hydroureter due to obstruction at the ureterovesical junction were found.

Case 13. A 24-year-old Negro, gravida 2, para 1, was admitted at 36 weeks' gestation with hypertension. Her physicians ordered sonography to rule out fetal growth retardation. The biparietal diameter of the head measured 99 mm and the anteroposterior diameter of the chest 100 mm. Incidentally several masses were identified in the

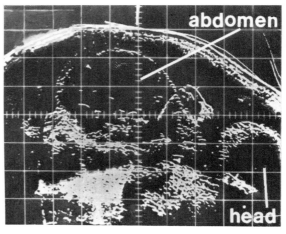

Fig 4. Case 11. Discrepancy between the size of fetal head and abdomen which is distended with fluid.

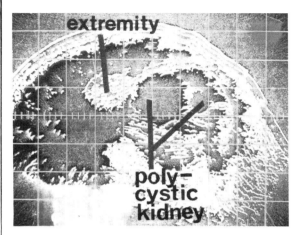

Fig 5. Case 13. Fetal abdomen with multiple cysts.

fetal abdomen to the right of the midline (Figure 5). The biggest of these cystic structures measured 62 × 59 × 59 mm. With increased gains no echoes were recorded from the inside of the masses. No change in their appearance could be detected 48 and 50 hours later. The differential diagnosis included unilateral right hydronephrosis, urachal cyst, right multicystic kidney, and hepatic cyst. After induction of labor, the patient delivered spontaneously a 3570-g female, Apgar 9/10. A mass which had similar dimensions as the large cyst seen by ultrasound could be palpated on the right at the level of the umbilicus. Two days after birth a multicystic right kidney was removed. The infant did well postoperatively.

DISCUSSION

The early diagnosis of fetal malformations is important. Radiography has been used successfully to diagnose anencephaly, gross hydrocephaly, and some forms of dwarfism. In order to diagnose soft tissue abnormalities, amniography has been employed. This involves amniocentesis, injection of radiopaque material into the amniotic sac, and several roentgenograms. Although the amount of radiation for a single x-ray of the abdomen is only 150–300 mR, the ultimate individual risk is not necessarily dose-dependent. In sonography, on the other hand, no radiation is involved. In addition, soft tissue outlines are visualized during routine scanning. Since most physicians are familiar with x-ray technics and with interpretation of radiograms, it is not surprising that the diagnosis in the 8 cases with bony abnormalities was made in 6 instances first by x-ray. In these, sonography served to confirm the diagnosis. The achondroplasia in case 7 was also initially diagnosed by radiography. On the

other hand, case 5 (Table 3) demonstrates that the diagnosis of hydrocephaly may be made with sonography before the head reaches its enormous proportions.

Both hydrocephaly and anencephaly have been studied with sonography by several authors.[2-10] While in hydrocephaly the dimensions of the head are greatly increased, in anencephaly the typical cephalic structure is missing.

In iniencephaly the brain and much of the spinal cord form a single cavity. In the case reported here, the small fetus could barely be seen on the x-ray because the uterus was extremely distended by polyhydramnios. The site of malformation could be recognized only on the sonogram (Figure 2). The lesion was interpreted to be a meningocele although it actually was a typical iniencephalus.

In case 10, a large solid mass was found from the sonograms to be attached to the lumbosacral area. The most likely diagnosis was therefore a neoplastic process rather than a meningocele.

Marked enlargement of the fetal abdomen as was demonstrated in cases 11 (Figure 4) and 12 most often is associated with high degrees of distal urinary tract obstruction. This may lead to striking dilatation of the proximal portions and is frequently associated with defective musculature formation of the abdominal wall. In both fetuses with massive ascites diagnosed prior to delivery, the urinary tract obstruction could be demonstrated later.

Garrett et al[12] reported the first case of a fetal polycystic kidney diagnosed antepartum with ultrasound. They found the abdomen distended by ascites and by a soft tissue tumor in the right flank of the fetus. The fetus died intrapartum and the autopsy findings were consistent with a polycystic kidney. The fetus of patient 13 in this report had neither marked abdominal enlargement nor ascites.

Polyhydramnios is frequently associated with fetal congenital abnormalities. In the 13 cases reported here, it was present in 8 and led to radiologic and sonographic examinations. In 3 cases, the indication for sonography was rapid or discordant fetal growth; in 2, lesions were found coincidentally.

At the present time, radiography is indispensable if one has to diagnose anencephaly or marked hydrocephaly rapidly. Sonography is helpful to modify, specify, and expand the radiologic and clinical diagnosis. In a fetus with a soft tissue tumor, sonography may be the simplest method to evaluate the outline and contents of the mass.

FETAL ABNORMALITIES

REFERENCES

1. Hellman LM, Kobayashi M, Cromb E: Ultrasonic diagnosis of embryonic malformations. Am J Obstet Gynecol 115:615–623, 1973
2. Sunden B: On the diagnostic value of ultrasound in obstetrics and gynecology. Acta Obstet Gynecol Scand 43: Suppl 6:118–123, 1964
3. Thieme VR, Johannigmann J, Zahn V: Ultraschallbilddiagnose eines Anenzephalus. Zentralbl Gynaekol 93: 1468–1470, 1971
4. Kratochwil A, Schaller A: Geburtshilfliche Ultrachalldiagnostik des Anenzephalus. Geburtshilfe Frauenheilkd 31: 564–567, 1971
5. Lüder VR: Möglichkeiten der Erkennung fetaler MiBbildungen durch Ultraschall. Zentralbl Gynaekol 94:1173–1178, 1972
6. Campbell S, Holt EM, Johnstone FD, et al: Anencephaly: Early ultrasonic diagnosis and active management. Lancet II:1226–1227, 1972
7. Thiery M, Kets HV, Yo Le Sian A, et al: Early diagnosis of anencephaly. Lancet I:599–600, 1973
8. Schlensker K-H: Pränatale Diagnostik der Anenzephalie mit der Ultraschallschnittbilduntersuchung. Geburtshilfe Frauenheilkd 33:133–136, 1973
9. Kobayashi M, Hellman LM, Cromb E: Atlas of Ultrasonography in Obstetrics and Gynecology. Edited by Butterworths. New York, Appleton-Century-Crofts. 1972, pp 233–249
10. Reed MF: Ultrasound in diagnosing hydrocephalus. Br Med J 3:762, 1972
11. Kratochwil A, Stoger H, Schaller A: Geburtshilfliche Ultraschalldiagnostik des Hydrozephalus. Geburtshilfe Frauenheilkd 33:322–325, 1973
12. Garrett WJ, Grunwald G, Robinson DE: Prenatal diagnosis of fetal polycystic kidney by ultrasound. Aust NZ J Obstet Gynaecol 10:7–9, 1970

Address reprint requests to
Rigoberto Santos-Ramos, MD
Department of Obstetrics & Gynecology
University of Texas Health Science Center
5323 Harry Hines Blvd
Dallas, TX 75235

Accepted for publication July 16, 1974.

PAPERS 50 AND 51

50. Queenan, J. T. and Gadow, E. C. (1970). Amniography for detection of congenital malformations. *Obstet. Gynecol.*, **35**, 648–657
51. Suzumori, K. and Yagami, Y. (1975). Diagnosis of human fetal abnormalities by fetography. *Teratology*, **12**, 303–310

COMMENTARY

Amniography was first described by Menees and his colleagues in 1930. In principle, a water-soluble radiopaque substance is injected into the amniotic cavity in order to outline the amniotic sac, the position of the placenta, and the external features of the fetus when examined radiologically. A modification of this technique, known as fetography, involves injection of an oil-soluble contrast medium. Because of the absorption of the fat-soluble contrast medium to the vernix caseosa of the fetus, considerably more details of fetal features are demonstrated. Papers 50 and 51 deal with the clinical importance and application of both these techniques for the intrauterine detection of congenital anomalies that are associated with polyhydramnios.

As indicated by Queenan and Gadow (Paper 50), soft-tissue abnormalities and malformations of the gastrointestinal tract are best visualized by amniography. The predictive value of amniography in the antenatal diagnosis of meningocele or myelomeningocele (soft-tissue abnormalities) is considered good, providing one takes into account the possible occurrence of false negatives in cases of a flat or unwrinkled myelomeningocele (Frigoletto Jr., 1974). Recently, Rubino (1975) reported the unusual case of an intact hydatidiform mole with associated living fetus diagnosed *in utero* by amniography.

The specific areas of clinical application of fetography include localization of the fetus prior to amniocentesis and for intrauterine transfusion;

assessment of fetal maturity; diagnosis of polyhydramnios, abnormalities of fetal soft-tissues, atresia of the foregut, fetal distress and fetal death; and the detection of multiple pregnancy and cases of conjoined twins. This technique, however, is associated with a high incidence of spontaneous labour, apparently due to placental damage by the radiopaque substances, amnionitis, and fetal damage.

Fetoscopy, the direct visualization of the fetus *in utero*, is the most recent and promising development in fetal diagnosis. A fiberoptic instrument is carefully introduced into the amniotic cavity through which the fetus can be seen, examined, and photographed. At the same time, fetal biopsy can be carried out. Until now, fetoscopy has been exploratory in nature and experience with this technique is limited. Almost invariably, fetoscopy was followed by termination of the pregnancy because the effects of the procedure on the continuing development of the fetus and its safety have not yet been evaluated.

REFERENCES

Frigoletto Jr., F. D. (1974). Amniography for the detection of fetal myelomeningocele. *Obstet. Gynecol.*, **44**, 286–290

Menees, T. O., Miller, J. D. and Holly, L. E. (1930). Amniography. Preliminary report. *Am. J. Roentgenol. and Radium Ther.*, **24**, 363–366

Rubino, S. M. (1975). Diagnosis of an intact hydatidiform mole with coexistent fetus by amniography. *Obstet. Gynecol.*, **46**, 364–367

From J. T. Queenan and E. C. Gadow (1970). Obstet. Gynecol., **35**, 648–657. *Copyright (1970), by kind permission of the authors and the American College of Obstetricians and Gynecologists*

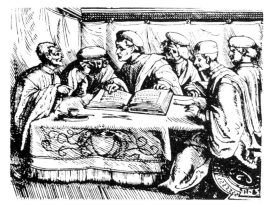

IDEAS AND ACTIONS

AMNIOGRAPHY FOR DETECTION OF CONGENITAL MALFORMATIONS

JOHN T. QUEENAN, MD, FACOG
and ENRIQUE C. GADOW, MD

The association of hydramnios with congenital malformations is helpful because it alerts the clinician to the problem. Diabetes, erythroblastosis fetalis, and multiple gestation are conditions that initially should be ruled out. In a 20-year review of 86,301 consecutive deliveries, one-third of all patients with unexplained hydramnios had fetuses with congenital malformations. Although the roentgenogram

From the Department of Obstetrics and Gynecology, The New York Hospital-Cornell Medical Center, New York, NY.

Presented at the Third International Conference on Congenital Malformations, The Hague, Netherlands, Sept 7–13, 1969.

Supported in part by the Greenwich Health Association, Greenwich, Conn.

Submitted for publication Aug 18, 1969.

The illustration at the top of the page is from a 16th-century German woodcut. (The Bettmann Archive.)

detects skeletal abnormalities, amniography is necessary to diagnose such soft-tissue malformations as encephalocele, meningomyelocele, or exstrophy of the bladder. In addition malformations involving the gastrointestinal tract can be detected. Prenatal diagnosis of congenital malformations is important in order to avoid intrapartum maternal and fetal trauma as well as to provide surgical correction immediately postpartum.

CONGENITAL MALFORMATIONS are too often unsuspected and are psychologically traumatic occurrences in the delivery room. The association of congenital malformations with hydramnios is helpful because it alerts the clinician to look for the problem. Prenatal diagnosis of congenital malformations requires additional work-up. Early detection will be reflected in a decreased perinatal mortality.

In a 20-year review (1948–1967) of 86,301 consecutive deliveries at our medical center, there were 358 cases of hydramnios, an incidence of 0.41%[5] (Table 1). Hydram-

TABLE 1. OCCURRENCE AND CLASSIFICATION OF HYDRAMNIOS IN A 20-YEAR STUDY (1948–67)

	Incidence	
	No.	%
Total deliveries	86,301	100.00
Hydramnios	358	0.41
Associated conditions		
Diabetes	88	24.6
Erythroblastosis fetalis	41	11.5
Multiple gestation	33	9.2
Congenital malformations	72	20.1
Idiopathic	124	34.6
TOTAL	358	100.0

nios was associated with diabetes in 88 instances (24.6%), erythroblastosis fetalis in 41 (11.5%), and multiple gestation in 33 (9.2%). Of the remaining 196 cases of hydramnios, congenital malformations were present in 72 instances (20.1%). From these data it is apparent that if hydramnios complicates a pregnancy and if multiple gestation, erythroblastosis fetalis, and diabetes are ruled out, more than one-third of the

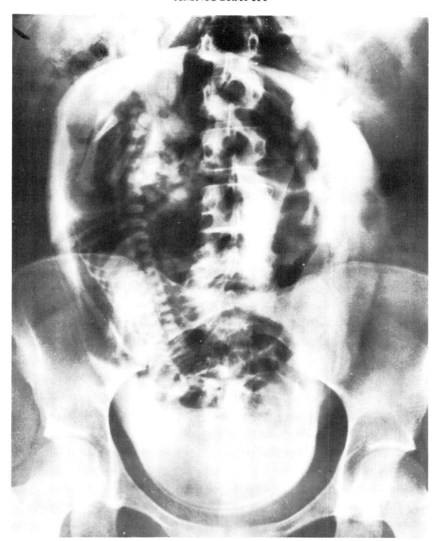

Fig 1. Amniogram of fetus at 32 weeks' gestation. Opacified amniotic fluid outlines fetal soft tissue and gastrointestinal tract. (From Queenan et al.[4])

remaining patients will deliver infants with congenital malformations.

The perinatal mortality rate in the presence of congenital malformations was 86.0%. Of the 72 patients with congenital malformations, there were 14 intrauterine, 15 intrapartum, and 33 neonatal deaths. The high incidence of intrapartum deaths was due in some instances to destructive opera-

tions for noncorrective malformations. Retrospectively, some infants proved to have correctable anomalies.

Prenatal diagnosis of congenital malformations requires radiographic procedures.[5] Although the roentgenogram detects skeletal abnormalities, amniography is necessary to diagnose soft-tissue or gastrointestinal malformations.[1-4]

MATERIALS AND METHODS

Since this review, an amniogram was done on all patients with hydramnios in whom multiple gestation, erythroblastosis fetalis, or diabetes was ruled out. The amniocentesis was performed with a 22-gauge spinal needle and 15–20 ml of diatrizoic acid (Hypaque-M, 75%)* was injected as the contrast medium.

The Amniogram

"Injected into the amniotic cavity, the radiopaque medium disperses uniformly throughout the amniotic fluid, which becomes sufficiently opacified to render the fetal soft tissue readily visible on roentgenogram."[4] Since fetal soft-tissue abnormalities displace the opacified amniotic fluid, malformations such as meningocele or exstrophy of the bladder can be identified readily. The swallowed opacified amniotic fluid outlines the fetal gastrointestinal tract and facilitates the diagnosis of such abnormalities as esophageal atresia with tracheoesophageal fistula, atresia of the gastrointestinal tract and diaphragmatic hernia.

Figure 1 is an amniogram of a normal fetus at 32 weeks' gestation. The opacified amniotic fluid outlines the fetal soft tissue. The fetal neck and back reveal no soft-tissue masses. There is no scalp edema. Radiopaque medium has been liberally swallowed, demonstrated by opacification of the fetal small intestine. On the right side of the figure there is less opacification; this represents the location of the placenta.

Figure 2 is a diagram of this amniogram. Figure 3 is an amniogram of a patient with hydramnios. Note the arrows defining the markedly distended amniotic cavity. Figure 4 is a lateral view of the same fetus 1 week later. Note the opacified gastrointestinal tract suggesting no malformation. Good definition of fetal soft tissue indicates no abnormalities as a meningocele.

---

* Winthrop Laboratories, New York, NY 10016.

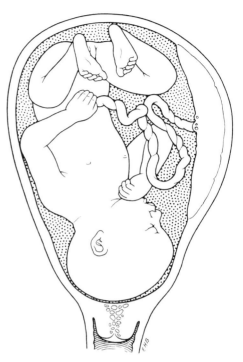

Fig 2. Diagram of amniogram in Fig 1. Note location of placenta, cord, and outlines of fetal soft tissue. (From Queenan et al.[4])

RESULTS

Prenatal diagnosis of most congenital malformations can be made by amniography. Figure 5 is an amniogram of a fetus at 38 weeks' gestation. The uterus is enlarged, out of proportion to fetal size. The upper and lower extremities, although flexed, are lying away from the abdomen. The spine is straight. The back is well outlined with no abnormalities. There is no intestinal opacification indicating a possible gastrointestinal malformation. Normal scalp thickness ruled out hydrops fetalis. Roentgenogram on the same patient indicated no fetal abnormalities. The distended abdomen caused difficulty during the delivery. An exploratory laparotomy revealed atresia of the terminal ileum with meconium ileus.

Figure 6 is an amniogram at 30 weeks' gestation with hydramnios. The patient received no antepartum care. A roentgenogram

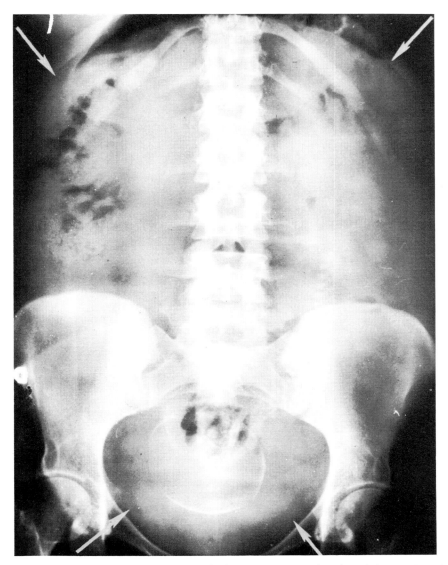

Fig 3. Amniogram of patient at 26 weeks' with hydramnios. **Arrows** outline distended amniotic cavity.

revealed no fetal abnormalities. On the amniogram the fetal extremities are extended over a markedly distended abdomen. There is no opacification of the intestinal tract. The well outlined back and spine are straight. The scalp thickness is normal.

The spontaneous delivery of the infant at 32 weeks' gestation was difficult due to an extremely distended abdomen. He expired at 1 hr of life. Postmortem examination revealed congenital infection.

Figure 7 is an amniogram at 32 weeks' gestation with hydramnios associated with anencephaly. The fetal attitude is poor with the lower extremities extended and the spine straight. The skull is absent and the

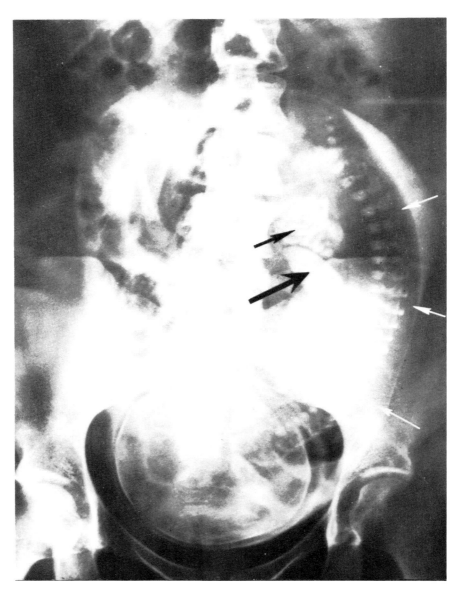

Fig 4. Lateral view of fetus in Fig 3 at 27 weeks'. **Black arrow** indicates opacified gastrointestinal tract. **White arrows** outline normal soft tissue of back.

AMNIOGRAPHY

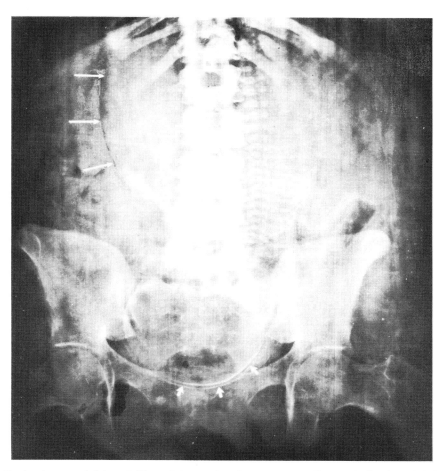

Fig 5. Amniogram of fetus at 38 weeks' gestation. **Long arrows** outline markedly distended fetal abdomen. Note lack of intestinal opacification. **Short arrows** show normal scalp thickness ruling out hydrops fetalis.

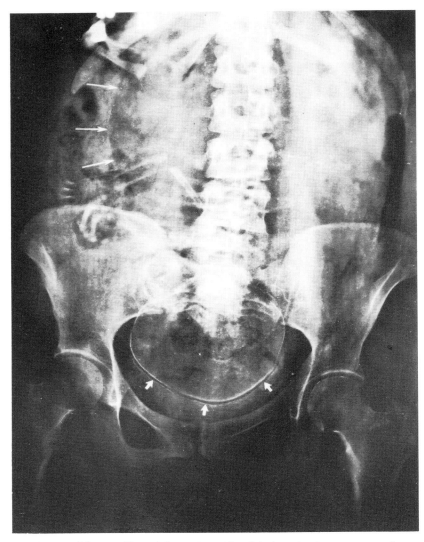

Fig 6. Amniogram of fetus at 30 weeks' gestation with polyhydramnios. **Long arrows** outline markedly distended abdomen. Note lack of opacification of gastrointestinal tract. **Short arrows** show normal scalp thickness.

AMNIOGRAPHY

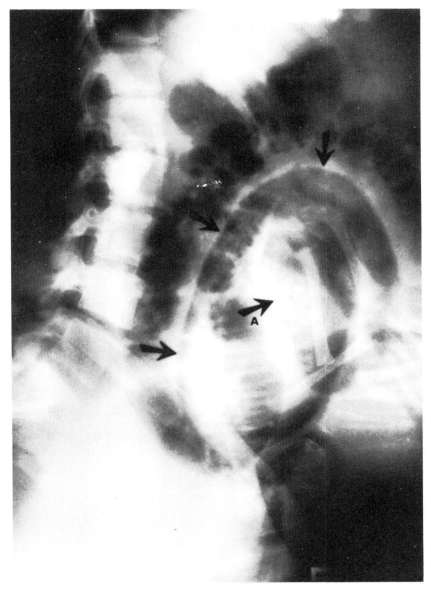

Fig 7. Amniogram of anencephalic at 32 weeks' gestation. **Arrows** outline normal soft tissue of back and buttocks. **Arrow A** indicates opacified gastrointestinal tract.

338

QUEENAN & GADOW

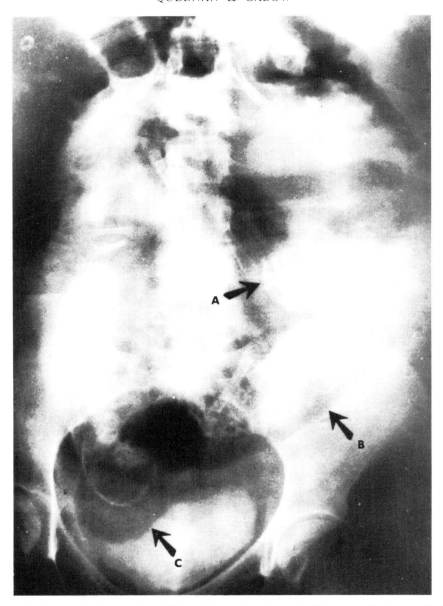

Fig 8. Amniogram of microcephalic at 32 weeks' gestation. **Arrow A** indicates opacified gastrointestinal tract; **arrow B**, the normal back and spine; and **arrow C**, a soft-tissue cephalic mass.

facial bones flat. The back and spine are well outlined with no soft tissue malformations. This anencephalic infant was delivered at 38 weeks' gestation.

Figure 8 is an amniogram at 32 weeks'

gestation of a microcephalic fetus with associated polyhydramnios. The fetal spine is curved and the extremities flexed. The skull is disproportionally small. There is no evidence of meningomylocele. At delivery this

AMNIOGRAPHY

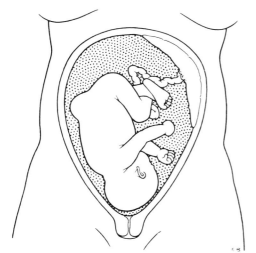

Fig 9. Diagram of amniographic findings of fetus with meningomylocele.

microcephalic infant was found to have an encephalocele. The infant expired shortly after birth.

Figure 9 is a diagram of a fetus with a meningomylocele. The opacified amniotic fluid is displaced by the soft-tissue malformation.

DISCUSSION

When the clinician is confronted with hydramnios he must determine the cause. After multiple gestation, erythroblastosis fetalis, and diabetes are ruled out, a congenital malformation must be suspected and the type and extent determined by amniography.

If a correctable congenital malfomation is found, premature labor should be prevented to enable the fetus to reach optimum maturity for better neonatal care. Knowledge of the type of malformation is crucial to select the route of delivery. Prevention of intrapartum morbidity will facilitate optimum neonatal care.

When congenital malformations are not correctable, termination of the pregnancy is indicated as soon as it is safe for the mother. The route of delivery should be that which allows the least maternal danger.

525 E 68th St
New York, NY 10021

REFERENCES

1. BISHOP PA: Roentgenologic diagnosis in soft tissue dystocia. *Radiol Clin N Amer* 5:8, 1961
2. CASH MB, KORNMESSER JG: Diagnosis of a fetal neck mass by amniography. *Radiology* 91:476, 1968
3. McLAIN CR, JR: Amniography, a versatile diagnostic procedure in obstetrics. *Obstet Gynec* 23:45, 1964
4. QUEENAN JT, VON GAL HV, KUBARYCH SF: Amniography for clinical evaluation of erythroblastosis fetalis. *Amer J Obstet Gynec* 102:264, 1968
5. QUEENAN JJ, GADOW EC: Hydramnios: Chronic versus acute. *Amer J Obstet Gynec* (in press)
6. RUSSELL JGB: Radiology in the diagnosis of fetal abnormalities. *J Obstet Gynaec Brit Comm* 76:345, 1969

340

From K. Suzumori and Y. Yagami (1975). Teratology, **12**, 303–310. *Copyright* (1975), *by kind permission of the authors and the Wistar Institute Press*

Diagnosis of Human Fetal Abnormalities by Fetography [1]

KAORU SUZUMORI [2] AND YOSHIAKI YAGAMI
*Department of Obstetrics and Gynecology, Nagoya City University,
Medical School, Nagoya, 467 Japan*

ABSTRACT   Being able to detect fetal abnormalities that may be associated with hydramnios would be extremely useful, especially when diabetes mellitus, Rh isoimmunization, and multiple pregnancy are ruled out. For this purpose the new technique of fetography, consisting of injecting a small amount of 2 radioque media (liposoluble and hydrosoluble), was used. Four out of 6 fetuses were correctly predicted to be abnormal. They were 1 case of esophageal atresia, 1 of suspicious chromosomal abnormality (after birth it was confirmed as having the Smith-Lemli-Opitz syndrome), and 2 of trisomy 18. It is felt that this simple technique should be used as an aid to the obstetrician faced with the problem of determining the basis of unexplained hydramnios.

Recently Wiesenhaan ('72) reported a new technique of fetography consisting of injecting a small amount of liposoluble and hydrosoluble contrast media. This technique mades it possible to visualize the outline of the fetus as well as the gastrointestinal tract. We predicted the nature of the condition in 4 out of 6 fetuses with hydramnios using this technique.

MATERIALS AND METHODS

The methods we used were as follows. With the patient supine the position of the fetus was determined by abdominal palpation, and diagnostic ultrasound (compound-contact B-Mode scanner) was used to observe the placental localization prior to transabdominal amniocentesis. Following this the site for the puncture was found, and usually we elected to use the area of the nape of the fetus. After the patient's bladder was emptied a 12-cm needle (19 gauge) was carefully inserted into the amniotic cavity, so as not to harm the fetus or penetrate the placenta. Twenty milliliters of amniotic fluid were withdrawn and 12 ml of 60% Urografin (an X-ray contrast medium consisting of a mixture of Na diatrizoate and methylglucamine diatrizoate, Schering, Berlin, West Germany) and 8 ml of 40% Moljodol (iodinated poppy seed oil, Daiichi, Tokyo, Japan) were injected.

X-ray films of the posteroanterior, lateral, and oblique positions were taken after 24 h and again at 72 h. The hydrosoluble Urografin made the intestine of the fetus visible and the liposoluble Moljodol outlined the skin of the fetus.

RESULTS

Since 1973, 10 patients have been referred to our University Hospital because of hydramnios, but 1 case of hydrops fetalis, 2 of diabetes mellitus, and 1 of multiple gestation were ruled out from this investigation. Therefore fetography was performed in 6 cases with unexplained hydramnios.

Diagnosis of most fetal abnormalities could be made by this technique. Figure 1 is a fetogram of a fetus at 39 weeks of gestation. This film revealed no external fetal abnormality, but there was no swallowed opacified amniotic fluid whatsoever in the intestine, indicating a possible foregut atresia. Shortly after birth the male infant (2,400 g) brought forth considerable quantities of thick tenacious mucus. The cry was hoarse, and much thick mucus was visible in the mouth and pharynx. The suspicion of esophageal atresia was confirmed by nasal catherization, the catheter meeting a solid obstruction about 7 cm from the nares. Lipiodol (another X-ray constant medium) defined the blind pouch clearly (fig. 2). An operation was performed immediately.

[1] Reported at the 14th Annual Meeting of the Congenital Anomalies Research Association of Japan, Sendai.
[2] Present address: Tokai Teishin Hospital, Matsubara, Naka-ku, Nagoya, 460 Japan.

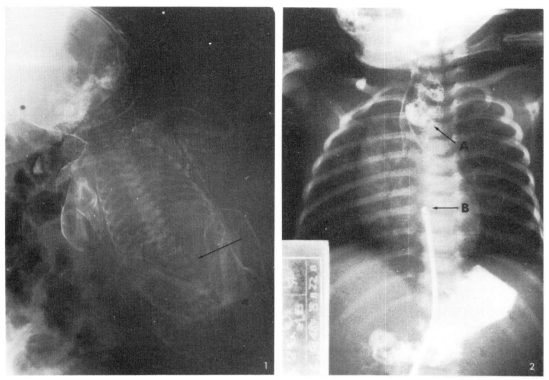

Fig. 1   Fetogram of fetus with esophageal atresia taken at 39 weeks' gestation. Note absence of opacification of the intestinal tract.
Fig. 2   Roentgenogram of the newborn in figure 1; arrow A shows the blind pouch defined by Lipiodol and arrow B the catheter inserted from his stomach.

Figure 3 is a fetogram at 39 weeks of gestation. Though opacification of the intestinal tract was observed the fetal outline showed the malformed auricles, which were seen to be slanting away from the eyelids, and micrognathia. The newborn infant was a male (3,300 g) that was distinctly hypotonic. The following physical abnormalities were noted: micrognathia, bilateral ptosis, small phallus and cryptorchidism, broad nasal tip with anteverted nostril, high-arched palate, low-set auricles slanting away from eyes, and transverse palmar crease. Chromosomal analysis by peripheral blood culture revealed a normal 46,XY karyotype. The clinical diagnosis considered was the Smith-Lemli-Opitz syndrome (Smith et al., '64; Ruvalcaba et al., '68). After 7 days the infant died of pneumonia (figs. 4a,b).

Figures 5a and b are fetograms at 32 weeks of gestation of a mother 43 years

of age. They gave a very impressive outline of the soft tissue of the fetus which showed a prominent occiput, low-set malformed ears, micrognathia, abnormal bending of the wrist joints, flexion deformities of fingers, and rocker-bottom feet. Opacification of the intestinal tract was observed. Trisomy 18 was strongly suspected. Amniotic-fluid cells obtained by amniocentesis were cultured for the detection of fetal chromosomes because of the advanced maternal age, and after 20 days of cultivation the karyotype showed a modal chromosome number of 47 with E, probably 18, trisomy and XX chromosome complement (fig. 6). The diagnosis of trisomy 18 syndrome was confirmed and the pregnancy was interrupted. The fetus was a female (980 g, 38 cm) and had phenotypic abnormalities compatible with trisomy 18 (figs. 7a,b).

Figure 8 is a roentgenogram of a fetus

at 36 weeks of gestation and indicated external abnormalities which consisted of low-set malformed ears, micrognathia, and abnormal bending of wrist joints, as also seen in the previous fetus. In this one there was no opacification of the intestinal tract. We diagnosed this as trisomy 18 with atresia of the foregut. Soon after delivery the infant died. Phenotypic findings such as cleft lip, malformed low-set ears, widespread nipples, hypertelorism, micrognathia, short sternum, small pelvis, hypoplasia of external genitalia, clubhand, flexion deformities of fingers, and rocker-bottom feet, and autopsy findings indicating esophageal atresia and horseshoe kidneys, were compatible with our antenatal diagnosis (fig. 9).

COMMENTS

Hydramnios is a condition occurring in some pregnancies in which the amount of amniotic fluid exceeds what is usually present. It occurs about once in every 200 pregnancies. In spite of a vast amount of research that has been undertaken to discover its cause its etiology remains a mystery. It is well known that certain maternal condition such as diabetes mellitus and Rh isoimmunization predispose to hydramnios. It is also known that certain fetal abnormalities are frequently associated with excessive accumulation of fluid. Fetal abnormalities are present in 25–30% of pregnancies complicated by hydramnios.

Because of this the ability to detect fetal abnormalities associated with hydramnios would be extremely useful, especially when diabetes mellitus, Rh isoimmunization, and multiple pregnancy are ruled out. Means of accomplishing this purpose rely on visualizing the fetus, and roentgenograms have been shown to be useful for the prenatal detection of a number of congenital malformations. Among them the technique of fetography described here is an extremely valuable aid.

Before fetography can become an acceptable procedure, the several possible complication from amniocentesis, X ray, ultrasound, and contrast media must be resolved.

Amniocentesis has potential hazards to the maternal-fetal unit. Penetration of the placenta, fetal puncture, fetal or maternal hemorrhage, and premature labor are

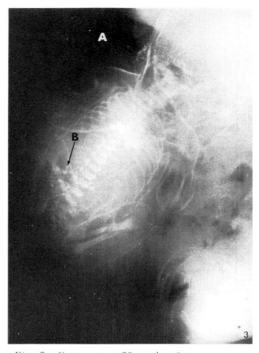

Fig. 3   Fetogram at 39 weeks of gestation. Note low-set malformed ears (indicated by arrow A). Arrow B indicates opacified gastrointestinal tract.

commonly considered to be possible consequences. To avoid them placental localization by ultrasonography prior to amniocentesis is very important in ensuring a safe percutaneous approach. After we identified the placental site the needle was inserted into the amniotic cavity so as to avoid the placenta. Usually we used the triangle adjacent to the nape of the fetus. The fetal head was displaced laterally and held in position. The needle was introduced close to the fingers. Possible damage to umbilical cord, fetal blood vessels on the surface of placenta, or fetal puncture were reduced by this method. Our experience suggests that transabdominal amniocentesis performed in this way carries a very low risk of either fetal or maternal complication.

Much investigation has been performed to assess the genetic effects of diagnostic X ray and ultrasound. It is calculated that the amount of radiation for a single X ray of the abdomen is only 150–300 mR. This small dose of X ray may theoretically in-

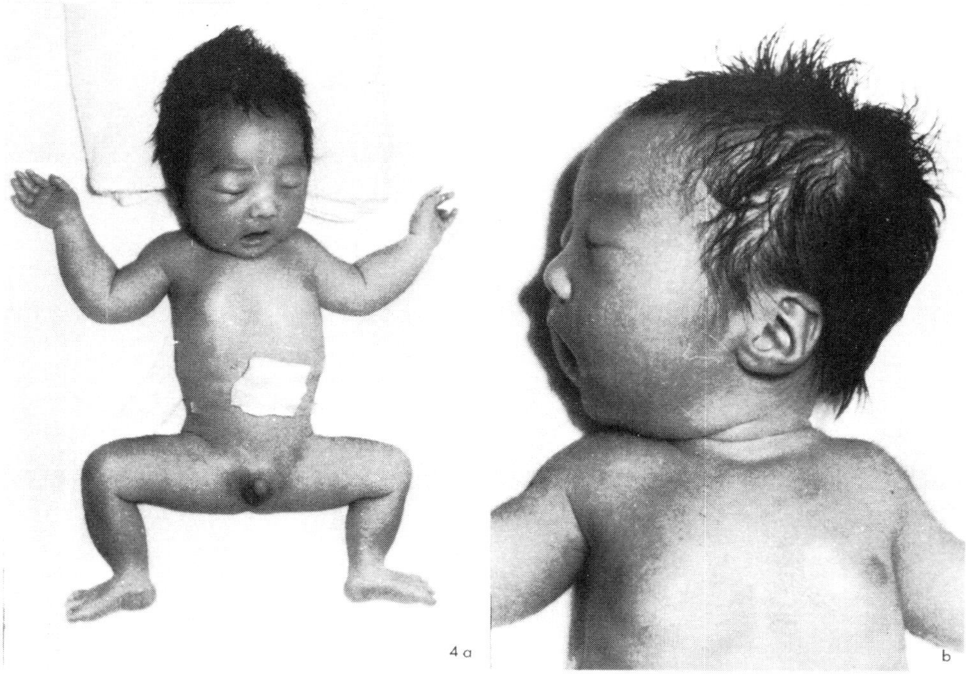

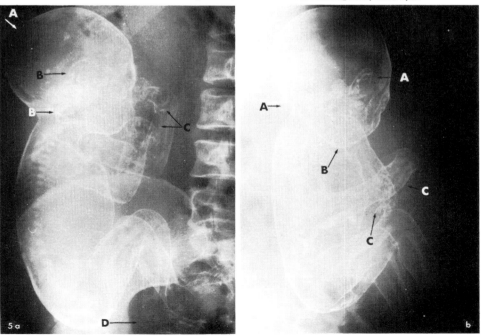

Fig. 4 Photographs of the infant with the Smith-Lemli-Opitz syndrome. a, frontal view; note hypotonicity, small phallus, and cryptorchidism. b, lateral view of the face; note ptosis, short nose with anteverted nares, micrognathia, and low-set ears slanting away from eyes.

Fig. 5 Fetograms of fetus with trisomy 18 taken at 32 weeks. a, lateral view; arrow A shows a prominent occiput; B, low-set malformed ears; C, abnormal bending of the wrist joints; and arrow D, rocker bottom feet. b, oblique view; arrow A indicates low-set malformed ears; B, micrognathia; C, abnormal bending of the wrist joints and flexion deformities of fingers.

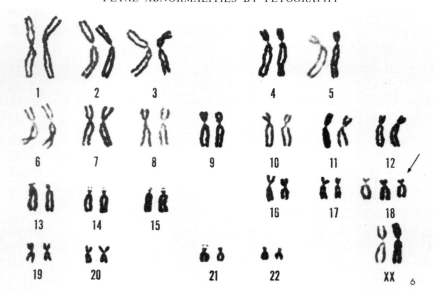

Fig. 6 Karyotype from the cultured amniotic fluid cells showing 47,XX, + 18.

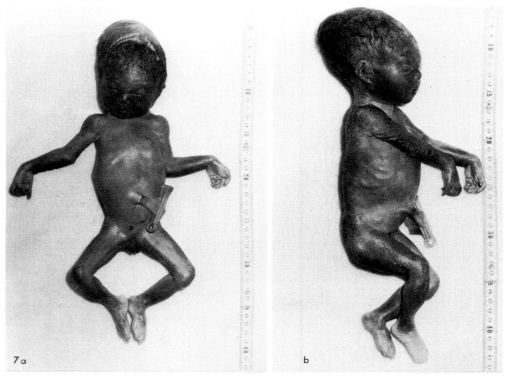

Fig. 7 Photographs of the stillborn infant weighing 980 g; a, frontal view, b, lateral view. Note the prominent occiput, low-set malformed ears, micrognathia, small mouth, clubhand, flexion deformities of fingers, rocker-bottom feet, short sternum, widespread nipples, small pelvis, and hypoplasia of external genitalia.

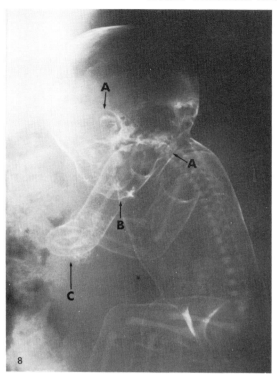 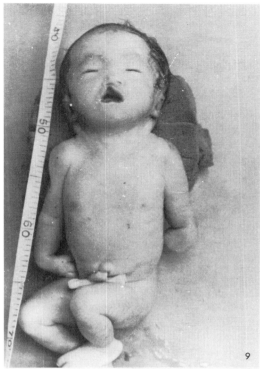

Fig. 8 Fetogram of trisomy 18 with esophageal atresia taken at 36 weeks. Low-set malformed ears (arrow A), micrognathia (B), and abnormal bending of the wrist joints (C) were noted. Note lack of intestinal opacification.

Fig. 9 Photograph of newborn infant with trisomy 18. Small oral opening, cleft lip, micrognathia, wide chest and widespread nipples, and rocker-bottom feet were indicated.

duce hereditary defects in mother and child. However, we feel that the advantage of the fetography seems to be greater than the risks of radiation in such special circumstances. On the other hand there has been no report of the deleterious genetic and somatic effects with the use of pulsed ultrasound at diagnostic levels.

Two different liposoluble and hydrosoluble contrast media were injected. Contrast media may have irritative effects to the patient. Sensitivity to the dye should be tested prior to the procedure. Fetal gasping of the oily contrast medium may result in lipid pneumonia, but no such occurrence has been recorded. No fetal mortality or morbidity directly attributable to this procedure has been encountered. In the light of these facts it can be assumed that the immediate risk to mother or fetus is extremely low.

Liposoluble contrast medium injected into the amniotic cavity adheres to the surface of the fetus, permitting visualization of its outline, and of intrauterine detection of fetal external abnormalities. The swallowed hydrosoluble contrast medium outlines the fetal gastrointestinal tract, facilitating diagnosis of esophageal atresia and diaphragmatic hernia. When correctable congenital malformations such as gastrointestinal atresia and diaphragmatic hernia are found they may be corrected by prompt surgery after birth; if noncorrectable abnormalities are found interruption of the pregnancy may be indicated.

There exists a considerable literature on antenatal detection of fetal abnormality by roentgenogram (Russell, '69; Queenan and Gadow, '70), but little work has been done to detect chromosomal abnormality radiologically. So far as we know,

Birnbaum ('71) was the first to diagnose a fetus with Down syndrome by finding extreme hyperextention of the head with dorsoflexion of the cervicodorsal vertebrae in roentgenogram. Later Ogita et al. ('74) succeeded in prenatally diagnosing trisomy 18 by fetography; they described that the findings of bent contracture of wrist joints and characteristic condition of fingers led to the successful prenatal diagnosis. In our experiments we experienced 2 cases of trisomy 18. Our findings are essentially in accord with those of Ogita et al. These results indicate it is possible that other chromosomal abnormalities will be diagnosed by detecting associated morphological abnormalities of the face and extremities through fetography.

Prenatal diagnosis of the Smith-Lemli-Opitz syndrome is difficult, and was unsuccessful for lack of characteristic findings on the fetogram as diagnostic bases. A further study of the prenatal detection of the Smith-Lemli-Opitz syndrome seems justified.

ACKNOWLEDGMENTS

The authors are grateful to Drs. K. Koike, S. Nakane, O. Waki, and S. Ishida for their assistance and collaboration. We also appreciate the technical assistance provided by midwives and nurses in our maternity unit.

LITERATURE CITED

Birnbaum, S. T. 1071 Prenatal diagnosis of mongolism by X-ray. Obst. Gyn., 37: 394–395.

Ogita, S., H. Hasegawa, M. Matsumoto, T. Takei, T. Shimamoto, M. Ohnishi and T. Sugawa 1974 Prenatal diagnosis of E trisomy syndrome by fetography. Obst. Gyn., 43: 887–892.

Queenan, J. T., and E. C. Gadow 1970 Amniography for detection of congenital malformations. Obst. Gyn., 35: 648–657.

Russell, J. G. B. 1971 Radiology in the diagnosis of fetal abnormalities. J. Obst. Gyn. Br. Comm., 76: 345–350.

Ruvalcava, R. H. A., A. Reichert and D. W. Smith 1968 Smith-Lemli-Opitz syndrome. Arch. Dis. Child., 43: 620–623.

Smith, D. W., L. Lemli and J. M. Opitz 1964 A newly recognized syndrome of multiple congenital anomalies. J. Pediat., 64: 210–217.

Wiesenhaan, P. F. 1972 Fetography. Am. J. Obst. Gyn., 113: 819–822.

PAPERS 52 AND 53

52. Emery A. E. H. (1974). Genetic counselling—or what can we tell parents? *Practitioner*, **213**, 641–646
53. Hagberg, B. (1975). Pre-, peri- and postnatal prevention of major neuropediatric handicaps. *Neuropädiatrie*, **6**, 331–338

COMMENTARY

Congenital genetic diseases are often associated with an increased incidence of infant mortality, developmental defects, and in many cases severe mental retardation. Because there is no effective way to treat the majority of these conditions, prevention remains the most rational approach in their management. Papers 52 and 53 are concerned with this difficult problem.

Identifying parents who run a high risk of conceiving a child with severe physical and mental handicaps, and also determining the risk of recurrence in cases where the parents already have an affected child, are the primary objectives of genetic counselling. Having established the correct diagnosis, the risk involved is estimated, and on this basis the parents are guided to make an informed decision. The practice of genetic counselling and some of the problems involved are discussed by Emery (Paper 52).

If an affected fetus is diagnosed or suspected as a result of amniocentesis or any other technique, the pregnancy is almost invariably terminated. Few attempts have been made to treat the diseased fetus *in utero*, and the practice of surgery offers little prospect for the correction of all major structural defects (Wilkinson, 1975). Intrauterine transfusion in fetal erythroblastosis is now a well-established procedure to prevent haemolytic disease of the newborn. More recently, Ampola and her colleagues (1975) have reported a case of methylmalonic acidaemia treated prenatally with large doses of vitamin B_{12}. Undoubtedly, attempts will be made to treat before birth other metabolic diseases in the fetus.

For children born with major congenital malformations and severe mental deficiency. institutional care represents the only real source of comfort. Surgical treatment is feasible only in specific cases, e.g. duodenal atresia and certain congenital heart diseases. Major neural tube defects invariably lead to early death, others to a disabling condition.

REFERENCES

Ampola, M. G. *et al.* (1975). Prenatal therapy of a patient with vitamin-B_{12}-responsive methylmalonic acidemia. *N. Engl. J. Med.*, **293**, 314–317

Wilkinson, A. W. (1975). Fetal surgery. *Dev. Med. Child. Neurol.*, **17**, 795–796

From A. E. H. Emery (1974). *Practitioner*, **213**, 641–646. *Copyright* (1974),
by kind permission of the author and The Practitioner

Symposium on: Practical Genetics

GENETIC COUNSELLING – OR WHAT CAN WE TELL PARENTS?

ALAN E. H. EMERY, M.D., PH.D., D.SC., F.R.S.ED., F.R.C.P.ED.

Professor of Human Genetics, University of Edinburgh,
Western General Hospital, Edinburgh

'How it comes—let doctors tell'—*Duncan Gray:* Robert Burns

A QUESTION I am often asked by medical friends is 'But if it is genetic, what can you do about it?'. Certainly in the past there was not a great deal one could do, but the situation is changing. In this short article I should like to discuss one aspect of this problem, namely genetic counselling and its importance in the prevention of genetic disease.

NATURE OF GENETIC DISEASE

It is useful to consider disease as being a spectrum. At one end we have those diseases such as nutritional deficiencies and infectious diseases which are caused by factors in the environment. At the other end we have those diseases which are largely genetic in origin. This latter group comprises the so-called *unifactorial* and *chromosomal* disorders. The former are due to single gene (Mendelian) defects. They are individually rare but the risks of recurrence in a family are often high. They include such conditions as muscular dystrophy, haemophilia and Huntington's chorea. Those disorders in which there is a chromosomal abnormality include Down's syndrome and certain disorders associated with male infertility (Klinefelter's syndrome) or primary amenorrhoea (Turner's syndrome). Towards the middle of the spectrum are those conditions which are partly genetic and partly environmental in causation. These are referred to as *multifactorial* disorders. They are comparatively common but the risks to relatives are usually low and include many congenital malformations and many so-called 'diseases of modern society' such as hypertension, diabetes mellitus, and peptic ulcer. Multifactorial disorders account for a great deal of ill-health both in children and in adults (table I).

EXTENT OF THE PROBLEM

The extent of the problem can be judged from the data in table I. Roughly 1 in 20 children admitted to hospital have a disorder which is entirely genetic in origin, and such disorders account for about 1 in 10 of childhood deaths in hospital. Only about 1 in 100 adult inpatients have a unifactorial or chromosome disorder, but then many of these disorders lead to early death or if they are compatible with survival to adulthood they usually do not warrant hospital admission. In any event there seems little doubt that nowadays genetic disorders contribute significantly to morbidity and mortality in childhood. Unfortunately only a relatively small proportion

Region	Year	Patients surveyed	Total No. of patients	Percentage of cases		
				UF	CHR	MF
Montreal[1]	1970	Paediatric inpatients	1145	6·7	0·4	3·9
Los Angeles[2]	1971–72	Paediatric inpatients	1500	3·0	0·5	15·0
Boston[3]	1970	Paediatric inpatients	200	5·0	0·0	16·5
		Paediatric outpatients	200	2·5	0·0	14·5
		Adult inpatients	200	1·5	0·0	—
		Adult outpatients	200	1·0	0·5	—
London[4]	1954	Childhood deaths in hospital	200	12·0	25·5	
Newcastle[5]	1960–66	Childhood deaths in hospital	1041	8·5	2·5	31·0
Edinburgh[6]	1971	Adult inpatients*	7126	0·3	0·2	11

[1]Clow et al., 1973; [2]Shinno et al., 1973; [3]Day and Holmes, 1973; [4]Carter, 1956; [5]Roberts et al., 1970; [6]unpublished data. *excludes obstetrics, gynaecology and psychiatry.

TABLE I.—Incidence of genetic disorders among various groups of patients (UF = unifactorial; CHR = chromosomal; MF = multifactorial).

of individuals at risk of having a child with a serious genetic disorder are referred for counselling (Emery, 1972). There is therefore an important need for the medical practitioner to be aware of this problem and to recognize when a particular disorder may recur in future children.

WHAT DOES GENETIC COUNSELLING INVOLVE?

Genetic counselling involves determining the risks of recurrence of a particular disorder in various relatives and explaining possibilities open to a couple in view of these risks, the prognosis and availability of treatment. A recurrence risk may be presented as the chance of (e.g. 1 in 10 or 10 per cent.), or as odds for (e.g. 1 to 9), or as odds against (e.g. 9 to 1) a disorder being transmitted to a child. Personally, I prefer to express risks as the chance of an event occurring and illustrate this with coloured beads when necessary. It is also important to present such risks in perspective. For example, after the birth of a child with anencephaly or spina bifida the chance of recurrence of either of these conditions in any subsequent children is roughly 1 in 20. This is roughly 10 times the risk for a couple who have not had an affected child, and must be compared with a risk of 1 in 50 that any newborn child may have a congenital malformation. In practice, risk figures need only be approximate. A discussion of the implications for the individual couple is more important.

PROBLEMS ENCOUNTERED IN GENETIC COUNSELLING

The problems often encountered when genetic advice is requested include congenital malformations, mental disorders, diabetes mellitus, profound childhood deafness, rare unifactorial disorders, abnormalities of sexual development and cousin marriages. The risks of recurrence for various congenital malformations are discussed elsewhere in this symposium (Carter, 1974).

Down's syndrome is a special case. Very few of these patients have an *inherited* translocation but all patients should have their chromosomes studied in order to exclude this possibility. Most patients with Down's syndrome have trisomy-21. The risks of recurrence in future children after the birth of such a child may be as high as 1 in 50, which is roughly the risk of having a child with Down's syndrome in a mother who has previously not had an affected child but is over 40 years of age.

With regard to mental disorders the most common problems in genetic counselling are mental handicap, schizophrenia, manic-depressive psychosis and epilepsy (table II). Provided there is no apparent cause for the con-

Disorder	Normal parents having a second affected child	Affected parent having an affected child
Epilepsy ('idiopathic')	1 in 20	1 in 20
Mental handicap	1 in 20	—
Manic-depressive psychosis	—	1 in 7
Schizophrenia	—	1 in 7
Profound childhood deafness	1 in 10	1 in 16
Diabetes mellitus:		
Early onset	1 in 12	1 in 12
Late onset	—	1 in 10

TABLE II.—Approximate risks of recurrence for some common disorders.

dition (e.g. birth injury, a metabolic or chromosomal defect or a genetic syndrome) the chance of recurrence of severe mental handicap in subsequent children is roughly 1 in 20 which is also the risk of 'idiopathic' epilepsy recurring in future children provided in both instances the parents are healthy. The picture is quite different in the case of manic-depressive psychosis and schizophrenia, in which the risk to the children of an affected parent is as high as 1 in 7 (Emery, 1974).

With regard to diabetes mellitus it is useful to consider the disorder in regard to early (childhood) or late (adult) onset, when the risks to the children of an affected parent are respectively 1 in 12 and 1 in 10.

Another common problem is that of profound childhood deafness (deaf-mutism). In the absence of a family history, and if the deafness is not associated with a recognized genetic syndrome and cannot be accounted for by any environmental factor, the chance of recurrence in subsequent children is approximately 1 in 10, whereas the chance of an affected parent having an affected child is approximately 1 in 16.

Genetic counselling in rare unifactorial disorders is usually easy because the risks of recurrence can be calculated on the basis of Mendelian principles (table III). There is, however, considerable heterogeneity in this group of disorders, and without a precise diagnosis it is often not possible to give reliable genetic counselling. Individuals in this group may therefore have to be advised by a specialist.

A proportion of patients with abnormalities of sexual development have a chromosomal abnormality such as the XO sex chromosome consti-

AUTOSOMAL DOMINANT TRAITS
Risk to offspring of affected individuals is 1 in 2
Achondroplasia (classical)
Huntington's chorea
Marfan's syndrome
Neurofibromatosis
Osteogenesis imperfecta
Polyposis coli
Tuberous sclerosis (epiloia)
AUTOSOMAL RECESSIVE TRAITS
Risk to further children of healthy parents is 1 in 4
Risk to offspring of affected individuals is usually negligible
Fibrocystic disease
Friedreich's ataxia
Galactosaemia
Glycogen storage diseases
Homocystinuria
Hurler's syndrome
Phenylketonuria
Sickle-cell anaemia
Tay-Sachs disease
Thalassaemia
Werdnig-Hoffmann's disease
Wilson's disease
SEX-LINKED RECESSIVE TRAITS
Risk to male offspring of healthy carrier females is 1 in 2
(there is a 1 in 2 chance that a daughter will also be a carrier)
Duchenne muscular dystrophy
Glucose-6-phosphate dehydrogenase deficiency
Haemophilia

TABLE III.—Examples of unifactorial disorders.

tution in Turner's syndrome and the XXY sex chromosome constitution in Klinefelter's syndrome. Such cases are rarely familial and parents can be reassured.

The subject of cousin marriages is dealt with in another article in this symposium (Roberts, 1974).

WHAT ADVICE TO GIVE

Apart from explaining the risk of recurrence the physician should take the opportunity to discuss the prognosis and availability of treatment, since parents are often influenced as much by the 'burden' of a disease as they are by the chances of recurrence (Emery *et al.*, 1973). The amount and nature of the information imparted should clearly be related to the educational background of the parents. Genetic mechanisms are often best explained only in the simplest terms. Principles should be emphasized rather than mathematical probabilities. If the parents decide that the risks are unacceptable then the possibilities of artificial insemination by donor (A.I.D.), sterilization and antenatal diagnosis (Ferguson-Smith, 1974) should be discussed with them. The physician should guide the parents in their decision-making, and it is in this regard that the science of genetic counselling becomes more an art. The more the physician understands the background of his patients the more he will be able to help them with difficult problems.

Immediately after the birth of an affected child, or when the diagnosis of a genetic disorder is first made, the parents are often confused and may be resentful. This is therefore not the time to give genetic counselling. It is best to wait a few weeks, by which time the parents are usually better able to cope with discussing the genetic implications.

A problem which often arises is whether parents should be told that they are at risk of having an affected child if this information has not been requested by them. For example, following the diagnosis of Huntington's chorea in the father or mother of a would-be parent. I feel that parents have a right to know these risks if it might prevent the birth of an affected child. The family doctor is a good guardian of the individual's interest in this regard. I have found that in situations like this it is best to discuss the genetic risks and their implications with the family doctor in the first instance.

A rather disturbing finding in our own studies has been the number of cases of failed contraception and of serious marital disharmony resulting from the fear of having an affected child (Emery *et al.*, 1973). These results clearly indicate that expert contraceptive as well as genetic advice is needed in such cases.

RESPONSE TO GENETIC COUNSELLING

There have been several recent studies in which the response of parents to genetic counselling has been investigated (Carter *et al.*, 1971; Leonard *et al.*, 1972; Emery *et al.*, 1973). The results of two of these studies (Carter *et al.*, 1971; Emery *et al.*, 1973) indicate that in general parents do react 'responsibly' to genetic counselling: when told that they are at high risk of having a child with a serious genetic disorder they are often deterred from having further children. There is no place for complacency in this regard, however, for genetic counsellors know of many instances in which, despite being told of the high risks, parents have gone ahead and had a child which has been affected. Though this may be the prerogative of parents in a free society it is no less disturbing. Perhaps as society becomes more aware of these problems, as a consequence of improvements in education, particularly in regard to human biology, the acceptance of genetic advice will increase.

THE ROLE OF THE FAMILY DOCTOR

There is no doubt that the help and advice of family doctors is often of great assistance in genetic counselling. In straightforward situations they are well suited to give such advice. After all they often know a great deal about the parents' background, and for this reason are often better equipped than the specialist to give guidance in these situations. Even with more complex problems, in which a geneticist may be asked to determine the risks—perhaps having to base such calculations on the results of special tests on the parents—the role of the family doctor is important. He can reinforce the advice given by the geneticist and probably make it more meaningful to the parents.

MANAGEMENT OF A FAMILY WITH A GENETIC DISORDER

The first priority is to establish a precise diagnosis which may mean hospital admission and investigation, or access to death certificates and pathology reports. Secondly the chances of recurrence must be established. In this regard there are a number of publications which can be helpful (Motulsky and Hecht, 1964; Emery, 1969; Stevenson and Davison, 1970; McKusick, 1971). If expert advice is required this may be obtained from one of the Genetic Advisory Centres. A list of these is contained in a publication entitled 'Human Genetics', issued by the Department of Health and Social Security, the Scottish Home and Health Department, and the Welsh Office, and obtainable from H.M. Stationery Office.

There is no doubt that there are situations in which specialist advice is essential, but in the case of congenital malformations in which the diagnosis is clear (e.g. spina bifida, anencephaly, congenital pyloric stenosis, cleft palate), in 'idiopathic' epilepsy, mental handicap, schizophrenia, manic-depressive psychosis, and clearly defined unifactorial disorders (such as Huntington's chorea, Marfan's syndrome, polyposis coli, fibrocystic disease and Werdnig-Hoffmann's disease) genetic counselling can be given by the family doctor. It has to be remembered, however, that the effects of genetic counselling on a family may be profound and therefore such advice should never be given lightly and must always be given with due regard to the possible problems involved.

References

Carter, C. O. (1956): *Gt Ormond Str. J.*, **11**, 65.
—— (1974): *The Practitioner*, **213**, 667.
——, Roberts, J. A. F., Evans, K. A., and Buck, A. R. (1971): *Lancet*, **i**, 281.
Clow, C. L., *et al.* (1973): *Progr. med. Genet.*, **9**, 159.
Day, N., and Holmes, L. B. (1973): *Amer. J. hum. Genet.*, **25**, 237.
Emery, A. E. H. (1969): *Scot. med. J.*, **14**, 335.
—— (1972): *Int. J. Environ. Studies*, **3**, 37.
—— (1974): 'Elements of Medical Genetics', third edition, Churchill Livingstone, Edinburgh and London.
——, Watt, M. S., and Clack, E. R. (1973): *Brit. med. J.*, **i**, 724.
Ferguson-Smith, M. A. (1974): *The Practitioner*, **213**, 655.
Leonard, C. O., Chase, G. A., and Childs, B. (1972): *New Engl. J. Med.*, **287**, 433.
McKusick, V. A. (1971): 'Mendelian Inheritance in Man', third edition, Johns Hopkins Press, Baltimore and London.
Motulsky, A. G., and Hecht, F. (1964): *Amer. J. Obstet. Gynec.*, **90**, 1227.
Roberts, D. F. (1974): *The Practitioner*, **213**, 675.
——, Chavez, J., and Court, S. D. M. (1970): *Arch. Dis. Childh.*, **45**, 33.
Shinno, N. W., *et al.* (1973): *Amer. J. hum. Genet.*, **25**, 70A.
Stevenson, A. C., and Davison, B. C. Clare (1970): 'Genetic Counselling', William Heinemann Medical Books Ltd, London.

354

From B. Hagberg (1975). Neuropadiätrie, **6**, 331–338. *Copyright* (1975),
by kind permission of the author and Hippokrates Verlag, Stuttgart, Germany

PRE-, PERI- AND POSTNATAL PREVENTION OF MAJOR NEUROPEDIATRIC HANDICAPS

B. Hagberg

Department of Pediatrics University Göteborg/Sweden

Hagberg, B.: Pre-, peri- and postnatal prevention of major neuropediatric handicaps. Neuropädiatrie 6: 331—338 (1975). Actual preventive aspects on major neuropediatric handicaps —
particularly cerebral palsy and severe mental retardation — are surveyed. Based on Swedish
epidemiologic studies on the changing pattern through 1954—70 it has been possible to conclude
that postnatal preventive measures are largely completed, and that perinatal brain damage syndromes have significantly decreased, while prenatal mechanisms now dominate and still constitute
mainly unsolved problems. The study has convincingly revealed that modern neonatal intensive
care does pay and has given favorable gains not only in surviving but in undamaged babies.

Prevention of handicaps   neonatal intensive care   cerebral palsy   mental retardation

It is important that habilitation programs be provided for all disabled children. But in the long run our chief goal must be to obtain effective tools to prevent mental and motor handicaps at their source. Table I demonstrates the magnitude of our main neuropediatric handicaps in Sweden today. It is seen that quantitatively mental retardation is the largest problem of our society. The heterogeneous group of severely mentally retarded is, at the same time, the one which is the most difficult to defeat through preventive measures.

Prevention against disabling conditions is a modern branch of medicine and has mainly developed during the last 40 to 50 years. It started with postnatal prevention, and switched over to mostly perinatal in the early fifties, while today there is increasing awareness of the vast prenatal aspects.

The *postnatal* preventive measures have been mainly social and in the northern parts of Europe are largely completed. Decreasing poverty, family planning and improved infant nutrition have all been of essential importance, with further support from child health services, organized vaccination programs and the development of potent antibiotics.

Table I   Main neuropediatric handicaps

(per 1000 live born Swedes)	
Mental retardation	9
severe: IQ < 50	3
Epilepsy	4
Cerebral palsy	1.5
Hydrocephalus	1.3
MMC	0.8
MBD (no epidemiologic study available!)	< 10 ??

Address: B. H., Department of Pediatrics, Östra Sjukhuset University of Göteborg, Smörslottsgatan 1, S-416 85 Göte-
borg/Sweden

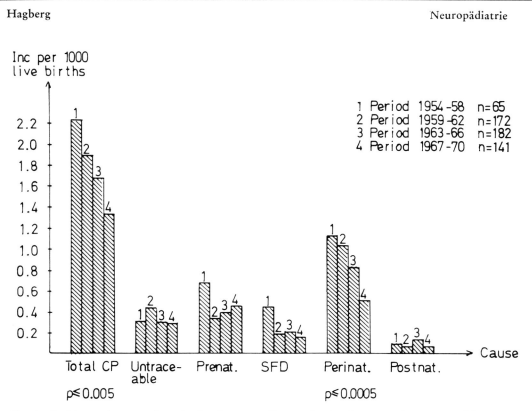

Fig. 1　Incidence changes of cerebral palsy according to dominating causative group of factors. From *Hagberg* et al. Acta Paediat. Scand. 1975, I

Today, postnatal factors are only responsible for a very modest percentage of severe neuropediatric handicaps, comprising the causes in not more than 5 % each of cerebral palsied and severely mentally retarded children. Future antiviral drugs might press the figures to an even lower level, as virus encephalopathies compose one of the more important remaining groups.

The pattern of the *perinatally* acquired chronic brain syndromes has shown very dynamic changes over the last 25 years. This is particularly reflected in the changing incidence and distribution of the different cerebral palsy syndromes. In the early fifties about 75 % of the cerebral palsy cases had a perinatal origin. Today the corresponding figure in Sweden is 40 % (*Hagberg* et al. 1975, I). Still it is a high figure when compared with mental retardation, where, perinatal factors play a modest role, not constituting more than about 10 % of obvious causes (*Hagberg* 1975, *Kaveggia* et al. 1970).

Recently our group in Gothenburg presented an unselected series of 560 cases of cerebral palsy, born in 1954 to 1970 (*Hagberg* et al. 1975, I and II). In this series, the total incidence had decreased gradually and significantly

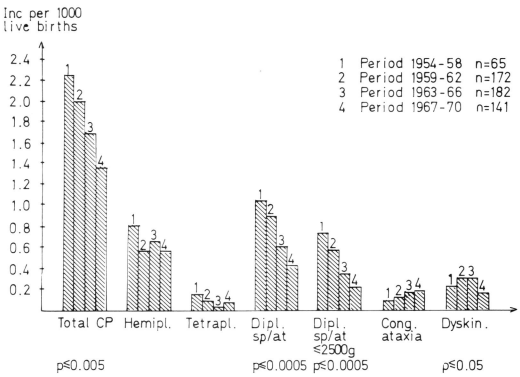

Fig. 2 Incidence changes of cerebral palsy according to syndromes. Sp/at = spastic/ataxic. From *Hagberg* et al. Acta Paediat. Scand. 1975, I

from 2.2 ⁰/oo in the first period to 1.3 ⁰/oo in the last. This decrease was exclusively related to perinatal causes (Fig. 1).

Further analyses revealed (Fig. 2) that the decrease was mainly related to diplegic syndromes among low birth weight babies, and to a minor extent during the last period also to dyskinetic syndromes, mainly due to hypoxia alone or combined with slight to moderate icterus.

Very gratifyingly, we found in addition that a gradual decrease had taken place both among the children with a normal and borderline intelligence quotient and among the mentally retarded ones (Fig. 3). We concluded that the

very active efforts during recent years to prevent brain damage caused by neonatal jaundice, asphyxia, acidosis and perhaps also severe birth trauma had given more profit in the form of undamaged babies than loss in the form of surviving severely disabled children who would have died with the less active approach of earlier years.

The perinatal preventive measures are summarized in Table II. With the support of animal experiments it can be postulated that the prevention of hypoxia and acidosis — particularly the combination of the two — has probably been of special importance (*Hrbek* et al. 1974, *Kjellmer* et al. 1974). Recently

Davies and *Tizard* (1975) in their follow-up studies of very low birth weight babies — confirming the Gothenburg decrease of diplegias — also provided evidence of the significance of disturbed body temperature, a factor which we have not closely analyzed. The additive effect of many interacting negative factors seem to be of major importance.

Growing evidence in recent years has increasingly discriminated *prenatal* mechanisms as the quantitively most im-

Table II   Perinatal preventive measures

Improved obstetric techniques
   Less hypoxia
   Less trauma
Improved neonatal regimens
   Less hypoxia
   Less acidosis
   Less hypoglycemia
   Less hyperbilirubinemia
   Less hypocaloremia
   Less hypothermia
   Less hypernatremia

Table III   Prenatal pathogenetic factors in:

Cerebral palsy	30 %	+ (25 % ?)
Mental retard. (IQ < 50)	45 %	+ (40 % ?)
Hydrocephalus (Sweden)	40 %	+ (?? %)

Table IV   Mental retardation

Conjectured distribution of causes 1975	
Prenatal forms	85—90 %
chromosomal syndromes	35 % ?
known malformations	10 % ?
unexplained malformations	20 % ?
foetal infections	10 % ??
biochemical disorders	3—5 % ?
other degenerative	
disorders	< 3 % ?
Perinatal/postnatal forms	10—15 %

portant pathogenetic factors today in both cerebral palsy and severe mental retardation. In Table III it is seen that perhaps up to 85 to 90 % of all cases of severe mental retardation *(Hagberg 1975, Kaveggia* et al. 1970) and up to about 55 % of the cerebral palsy *(Hagberg* et al. 1975, II) cases have a probably prenatal origin. Half of the cases in both groups have clearly prenatal histories and have clinical signs obviously acquired prenatally. In half of them, on the other hand, the pathogenesis and etiology are quite impossible to trace, in spite of the detailed obstetric and neonatologic information obtained today. Thus, no peri- or postnatal causative factors can be distinguished and it must be highly suspected that prenatal mechanisms must have been at work.

Cases of retardation with an IQ beneath 50 comprise a very heterogeneous and multifacetted group, with perhaps 400—500 different conditions involved. Table IV represents a tentative guess at the present etiologic/pathogenetic distribution, based on a review of the literature and on our experiences from an unselected Swedish series. In this context, it is only possible here to consider a few large groups which are attracting increasing interest from prevention aspects. Chromosomal aberrations, 3rd trimester foetopathies and defined biochemical disorders will be discussed in particular.

With the findings at new banding techniques *(Lubs* and *Lubs* 1973) added to conventional karyotype examination of unselected series *(Wallin* 1974), it has been revealed during recent years that at

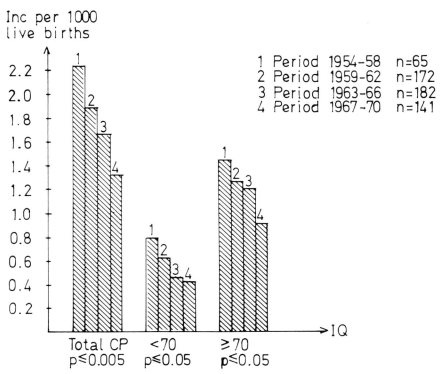

Fig. 3 Incidence changes of cerebral palsy according to intellectual capacity. From *Hagberg* et al. Acta Paediat. Scand. 1975, I

least one third of all cases of severe mental retardation are associated with different *chromosomal* syndromes. Some of these cases are preventable by systematic prenatal screening of all pregnant mothers over 35, and all mothers who have already had an affected child or are known to have had repeated stillbirths.

Late *fetal infections:* Toxoplasmosis, Rubella, CMV and Herpes are probably responsible for more brain damaged babies than was ever believed a few years ago. This particularly applies to CMV! If the figures of the London researchers *Elek* and *Stern* (1974) were applicable to Swedish conditions, up to 10—20% of the yearly contribution to severely mentally retarded children could be caused by silent CMV infections late in pregnancy. In other words, this number of mentally retarded infants could be as large as our total number of additional cerebral palsy infants in the whole of Sweden per year. If so, the challenging demand: "Vaccination against mental retardation" appearing in the Lancet in January 1974 would really be a correct approach.

Defined *neurochemical disorders* constitute a very limited but more and more preventable group of causes of severe mental retardation. For the neurolipidoses, the possibility of prevention after the first diagnosed key case is now excellent. All well-defined familial disorders within this group can be diagnosed by enzymatic tests on amniotic fluid or cultured cells taken by amniocentesis in the 16th week of pregnancy (*Svennerholm* 1975). Heterozygot screening of families or even population groups at risk, as well as more extensive genetic counselling, might further improve the prevention of these disorders.

The significance of prenatal factors associated with *fetal and placental dysfunction* has recently been analyzed in two studies from our department. *Sabel* and collaborators (1975) found in a nonselected population of 6500 children born in 1969 to 1970 at one Swedish hospital that babies who had shown various signs of intrauterine growth retardation were the major remaining group at risk for brain damage syndromes causing mental retardation and/or cerebral palsy. Two-thirds of these handicaps were recruited from the 16 per cent of newborns with birth weights below 1 SD in relation to gestational age.

On the basis of our own series of 560 unselected cerebral palsy cases it was shown (*Hagberg* et al., III) that during the last two gestational months cerebral palsied children — all along the line — had a significantly retarded intrauterine growth rate compared with a normal series. From gestational week 35 onwards the weights were significantly decreased throughout, indicating depressed fetal growth.

In the same Swedish cerebral palsy series a highly significant overrepresentation of data compatible with toxicosis and repeated bleeding during pregnancy was also noted, as well as a significantly larger number of twin births when compared with the Swedish birth data register.

Furthermore, it was quite obvious that a combination of fetal growth retardation/placental dysfunction and perinatal factors such as signs of intracranial hemorrhages and asphyxia played a more than statistically expected role in the development of cerebral palsy syndromes. This finding supports the importance not only of fetal and placental dysfunction per se but also, in particular, of polyfactorial pathogenetic mechanisms, especially for multihandicap syndromes. Perinatal processes that are usually uneventful after normal pregnancies may prove to result in or add to brain damage in a certain number of prenatally disfavored fetuses.

Thus it has become more and more obvious that preventive measures directed towards the often forgotten 3rd trimester are of utmost importance in our efforts to further minimize the number of cerebral palsied children. Accumulating information concerning the causes of severe forms of mental retardation points in the same direction. Our knowledge concerning the underlying mechanisms is as yet insufficient, however, and our tools not sharp enough for effective prevention.

It is evident that the battle against prenatal injurious factors and mechanisms is essential and must be reinforced to provide further significant success in pediatric handicap prevention. In Table V the prenatal preventive measures are presented at their different levels.

In Table VI the present-day situation in Sweden concerning the preventive battle against major neuropediatric handicapping conditions is summarized.

Preventive programs directed towards brain damaging factors occurring after the neonatal period are more or less completed, leaving only limited additional possibilities of decreasing major handicaps in a significant way.

Further gains, however moderate, should be attainable perinatally through yet more refined delivery techniques and neonatal care. Among other things, preventive cesaerean section in all breech presentations should be seriously considered. The factor, or more likely the combination of factors, causing the complex disturbance of brain homeostasis in low gestational age infants must be further analyzed and might also be

Table V   Prenatal preventive measures

I. Pre-pregnancy prevention
   genetic counselling
   heterozygote "hunting"
   vaccination of girls against rubella (CMV?)
   anti-D prophylaxis
II. Prenatal diagnostics
   chromosomal
   biochemical/enzymatic
   α-foetoprotein examination
III. Obstetric care
   vascular disorders
   diabetes
   twin birth
   polyhydramnios
   Rh supervision
   fetal growth control

Table VI   Summary of prevention 1950—75 in Sweden

A. Completed programs:
   vaccination of infants
   exchange transfusions
   anti-D prophylaxis
B. Uncompleted programs:
   improving delivery techniques
   improving neonatal regimens
   LBW (LGA, AGA)
   fetal growth control
C. Programs just developing:
   1. Pre-pregnancy care
      genetic counselling
      heterozygote "hunting"
      vaccination of mothers (CMV?)
   2. 16th week supervision
      chromosomal aberrations
      neurochemical disorders
      neural tube defects
   3. 3rd trimester care
      maternal disorders
      placental dysfunction
      fetal undernutrition

a key to the understanding of handicaps affecting small for gestational age babies.

The largest number of unsolved problems, and today the most challenging, refer to fetal brain damage during the prenatal period. Our present interest is particularly concentrated on brain damaging factors and mechanisms during the 3rd trimester, i.e. fetal growth retarding factors, placental dysfunction mechanisms and fetal infections retarding the CNS development. Additional important sectors refer to pre-pregnancy care — genetic counselling, heterozygote "hunting", vaccination programs directed towards selected agents proven to be dangerous for the fetus, and amnion fluid diagnostics in the 16th week; the latter include chromosomal aberrations, neurochemical disorders and neural tube defects.

Thus many promising new aspects and approaches have opened the doors for further research on preventive measures which in the long run should decrease even congenital disabling conditions.

References

1. Davies, P. A. and Tizard, J. P. M.: Very low birth weight and subsequent neurological defect (with special reference to spastic diplegia). Developm. Med. and Child Neurol. 17: 3 (1975).
2. Elek, S. D. and Stern, H.: Development of a vaccine against mental retardation caused by cytomegalovirus infection in utero. Lancet i: 1 (1974).
3. Hagberg, B.: Unpublished observations.
4. Hagberg, B., Olow, I. and Hagberg, G.: Decreasing incidence of low birth weight diplegia — an achievement of modern neonatal care? Acta Paediat. Scand. 62: 199 (1973).
5. Hagberg, B., Hagberg, G. and Olow, I.: The changing panorama of cerebral palsy in Sweden 1954—1970. I. Analysis of the general changes. Acta Paediat. Scand. 64: 187 (1975).
6. Hagberg, B., Hagberg, G. and Olow, I.: The changing panorama of cerebral palsy in Sweden 1954—1970. II. Analysis of the various syndromes. Acta Paediat. Scand. 64: 193 (1975).
7. Hagberg, G., Hagberg, B. and Olow, I.: The changing panorama of cerebral palsy in Sweden 1954—1970. III. The importance of fetal deprivation of supply. Acta Paediat. Scand. (to be published).
8. Hrbek, A., Karlsson, K., Kjellmer, I. and Riha, M.: Cerebral reactions during intrauterine asphyxia in the sheep. II. Evoked responses. Pediat. Res. 8: 58 (1974).
9. Kaveggia, E., Opitz, J. M. and Pallister, P. D.: Diagnostic/genetic studies in severe mental retardation. Proceed. 2nd Int. Ass. Scientif. Study Ment. Retard. p. 305 (1970).
10. Kjellmer, I., Karlsson, K., Olsson, T. and Rosén, K. G.: Cerebral reactions during intrauterine asphyxia in the sheep. I. Circulation and oxygen consumption in the fetal brain. Pediat. Res. 8: 50 (1974).
11. Lubs, H. A. and Lubs, M.-L.: New cytogenetic technics applied to a series of children with mental retardation. Chromosome Identification. Nobel Symposium 23, p. 241 (1973).
12. Sabel, K. G., Olegård, R. and Victorin, L.: Remaining sequelae with modern perinatal care. Pediatrics (accepted for print).
13. Svennerholm, L.: personal communication.
14. Wallin, L.: Severe mental retardation in a Swedish industrial town. An epidemiological and clinical investigation. Scandinavian University Books, Stockholm, Esselte Studium (1974).

PART VIII

SOCIAL, ETHICAL, AND MEDICO-LEGAL PROBLEMS

54. Fletcher, J. (1975). Moral and ethical problems of pre-natal diagnosis. *Clin. Genet.*, **8**, 251–257

55. Fletcher, J. (1974). Attitudes toward defective newborns. *Hastings Cent. Stud.*, **2**, 21–32

56. Zachary, R. B. (1968). Ethical and social aspects of treatment of spina bifida. *Lancet*, **ii**, 274–276

57. Duff, R. S. and Campbell, A. G. M. (1973). Moral and ethical dilemmas in the special-care nursery. *N. Engl. J. Med.*, **289**, 890–894

COMMENTARY

These related articles examine important moral, ethical, and medico-legal issues arising from the pre-natal diagnosis of defective fetuses and from the birth of children with severe physical and mental handicaps.

What are the rights of the unborn child? What decisions should be taken when a defective fetus is detected antenatally? Who should make these decisions and what criteria should be used? What is society's attitude at present to children born with severe handicapping conditions? Should such infants be permitted to live or encouraged to die? Is human life devalued when medical and surgical treatment are withheld from infants with severe congenital defects and 'a poor or hopeless prognosis for meaningful life'? Does the newborn have the right to sue for 'injuries' received before birth? Who should be held responsible in these circumstances? These vexing questions pose problems with considerable social and legal implications and, despite the urgency of the situation, will be difficult to resolve immediately. The four articles in this section (Papers 54, 55, 56 and 57) provide a good starting point for further discussions relating to the issues involved.

From J. Fletcher (1975). Clin. Genet., **8**, 251–257. *Copyright* (1975), *by kind permission of the author and Munksgaard, Copenhagen, Denmark*

Moral and ethical problems of pre-natal diagnosis

JOHN FLETCHER

Interfaith Metropolitan Theological Education, Inc.
Washington, D.C. 20009, U.S.A.

The moral and ethical problems resulting from application of pre-natal diagnosis are identified: abortion, questions about euthanasia for defective newborns, and the concept of genetic health. A holistic approach to ethical problems is presented that includes attention to both principles and consequences.

Received 19 March, accepted for publication 2 May 1975

On the spectrum of the possible interventions in applied human genetics, pre-natal diagnosis is currently the most prominent. If a fetus is at risk for genetic disease, an increasing number of diseases are diagnosable early in the pregnancy. Amniocentesis, fetoscopy, amnioscopy and ultrasound techniques constitute an impressive and growing set of means for pre-natal diagnosis. The medical literature has increasingly reported the utility and versatility of pre-natal diagnosis for the detection of a variety of inborn errors of metabolism, chromosomal abnormalities, and diseases which have complex causation, such as spina bifida and anencephaly (Milunsky 1974). In each instance, the information gained about the fetus affords the parents and attending physicians data which they may use to decide whether or not to abort the fetus.

There are a number of moral and ethical considerations involved in allowing a widespread use of pre-natal diagnosis for detection of genetic disease. These considerations arise for the following reasons:

a) Parents are now expected to help physicians make life and death decisions about their child-to-be. Parents' decisions about abortion create moral conflict with an earlier moral structure of parental caring for the unborn, inasmuch as the earlier norms of parental caring for the unborn permitted abortion only when life of the mother was threatened.

b) Decisions to prevent the birth of a fetus diagnosed for a crippling or fatal disease raise questions about the value of the lives of existing persons who have the disease (should they be kept alive?) and also about the value of newborn infants with the disease whose births are not prevented (should they live?).

c) Decisions to prevent new life which is crippled by genetic disease may presuppose a vision of health and particularly "genetic health", which is as yet an undefined and problematic concept.

If we look at problems in morality only from the standpoint of the particular persons involved (parents and physicians), we cannot do justice to the consideration of consequences which flow from their decisions. Individual decisions have social consequences. Social consequences influence individual decisions. In this discussion, I shall move back and forth between consideration of the concrete problems in morality of particular parents and physicians and the larger ethical issues raised for society by the possible consequences of applied human genetics.

In the heat of making decisions in genetic counseling what we most often debate is "morality". Should I and my wife decide for the abortion of our fetus, our child-to-be, when we know that it will have Down's syndrome or some other form of mental retardation? Should the physician or genetic counselor take a position on abortion of a fetus which will be a crippled infant? Morality it always concrete. Concern for morality appeals for guidance to inform *what* we should do or avoid in specific situations.

When we get at some distance from decisions and pressures, we can envision the possible effects or consequences of our decision-making on the ethical structure of society and raise questions about the meaning of these decisions. Do we want to have a society in which genetic health considerations have a high priority, since each of us carries a certain number of deleterious genes? Does an increasing number of parental decisions about abortion and withdrawal of medical care of defective newborn life seriously impair the beginning of a trustful bond between parents and children? Will increasing application of technology advance or undermine the formation of moral development in society? Seeking and giving guidance in the light of what we believe about the meaning of life and death, good and evil, is ethics. *Ethical* consideration involves developing the whys and wherefores which uphold or deny certain courses of action by individuals and groups in society.

Moral Problems of Genetic Counseling

It is important to understand parental decision-making about abortion following pre-natal diagnosis as one event in the process of genetic counseling. Counseling with a physician or specialist prior to pregnancy or shortly after pregnancy in which risks are recognized should precede decision-making about abortion. It is safe to assume that parents enter genetic counseling predisposed to abortion in case a serious disease is diagnosed. It is not safe to assume that predisposition to abortion is the same thing as a decision for abortion. Occasionally, parents change their minds, although this reversal appears to be rare. Most parents seek amniocentesis in the first place because one of their children or family members has a genetic disease, or because they are known to be carriers of a deleterious gene, or have been exposed to some environmental hazard.

On the basis of interviews with parents in genetic counseling, I concluded that abortion was the most serious moral problem associated with the process, though it was not the only problem (Fletcher 1972). It is easy to see why parents experience moral suffering in considering abortion of their own fetus. They are caught between two right avenues of action: caring for the life of the unborn child and caring for the lives of their existing children, their own lives and, in a wider sense, caring for the quality of human life in their society. Moral suffering occurs when highly motivated parents who desire children intensely, even desperately (since one other ill child is usually involved), are caught between the rightness of protecting their families from the great strains which genetic disease may place upon them, and the rightness of caring for the life of their conceived child.

Prior to the development of amniocentesis for genetic diagnosis of the fetus, the role of parental caring for the fetus did not

MORAL AND ETHICAL PROBLEMS OF PRE-NATAL DIAGNOSIS

include acting upon knowledge which could be made available in the first trimester or early in the second trimester of pregnancy. The norms of parenthood, informed by religious and humanistic sources, conditioned new parents to care without reserve for the nascent life they conceived. Christian and Jewish religious sources see parents as deputies of the Creator-God, representing the unconditional love of God to the growing child before and after birth. To personalize this fact, I can say that I was taught as a younger man that my role as a father of an expected child was to care for my spouse and the child unconditionally, to obtain the best care available, and if there were birth injuries or health problems of the child after birth, decision-making following birth would begin with the best interests of the child. The only imaginable situation in which I would be expected to decide against the life of my unborn child would be if, through the accidents of birth, the presence of the child was a threat to the life of my spouse.

Now the situation has changed. A prenatal diagnosis can inform us, if we have good reason to inquire, of the presence of a genetic condition which leads to certain consequences. Some conditions (Tay Sachs disease, anencephaly, etc.) lead to certain death, and there is no therapy available. Other conditions lead to "twilight" circumstances of medical care, in which the child may be supported, but no real cure is now feasible (e.g. spina bifida). A range of certain mental retardation states can be diagnosed, especially for Down's syndrome. And there are other conditions (hemophilia) which can be diagnosed and for which there are palliatives or drugs to support the child's life, but at a very high financial cost to the family.

Obviously, there are ranges and grades of seriousness of disease and seriousness of economic and social threat to families. At this point, one's basic orientation about good and evil, right and wrong, comes strongly into play. From one viewpoint, in which rules and principles upholding the parental and social care of newly conceived life are virtually exceptionless (Ramsey 1970), a parent should not consider abortion for his or her case unless there is also a willingness to extend the same action to an infant born with the same problem. Would it be right to do the same thing in every case which had the same moral and social features? In this view, if we cannot morally uphold the universalization of an action, then we should not be doing it. To employ an immoral means to an end demoralizes society as much as seeking an immoral end. Thus, working from the first principle that the right to life of a fetus cannot be ethically compromised by the needs of parents and society, this view disapproves of any abortion except to save the physical life of the mother and further disapproves of any intervention in the fetal-maternal unit except to save the life of the fetus. No nontherapeutic fetal research on a living fetus can be allowed.

From another viewpoint in ethics (Fletcher 1974), we should approach the decision with the features of the particular situation in mind and not be strongly concerned to find grounds upon which the actions (pro or con) could be universalized. Each situation is unique and the human needs within that situation should be addressed with compassion and reasonableness. In this view, our decisions about right and wrong must be made in the context of each new situation, and we should be guided by the consequences of our action. To engage in the ethical reasoning of universalization is to withdraw energy and love necessary to respond to the human needs in the particular case. Needs and consequences should be the moral guides. Using this approach, Joseph Fletcher finds support for the policy that unwanted pregnancy is a disease and that there should be no compulsory pregnancies. If we could not justify any compulsory pregnancies, then we can certainly justify abortion when the woman desires it, as a purely personal and private matter (Fletcher 1974, p. 142).

From another ethical approach, which I favor, there is a more holistic shape to our moral decisions when they reflect both careful attention to consequences (costs of all kinds), and the relevance of moral principles. These two elements are usually opposed in ethical debate, but in a wider sense, each is dependent on the other. Exclusive attention to consequences alone begs the question of what kind of principles one uses to help evaluate the good and bad consequences. Attention to principles alone begs the question of what kind of illumination they provide for concrete, moral struggles. The essence of the holistic approach to ethics is the inclusion of as many contending values, principles and forces as possible in the appraisal of policy and decisions. Holism resists the absolutizing of any particular value (e.g. the life of the fetus, or the desires of the mother) to the exclusion of other values in tension or conflict with the particular value in question. In this view, society (like nature) is seen as an irreducible whole, in which decisions that affect one realm inevitably affect all realms. Responsible decision-making seeks to balance the welfare of the individuals involved with the well-being of society. When these values come into conflict, as they obviously do in the debate about abortion, compensatory means must be found to reduce and resolve the conflicts.

To be specific about the individual and social conflicts involved in applying the practice of pre-natal diagnosis and selective abortion:

1) Abortion can be ethically justified when, with accurate medical advice, parents know that the diagnosed disease state in the fetus would be so serious as to deprive its human future and the family's future through the sheer struggle for survival. Yet, there can be serious disagreement about what would constitute deprivation of a "human future" and about how much the economic dimension of the family's welfare should be an element in the decision. In my view, there is more ethical justification for abortion based on the seriousness of the disease and less justification when economic factors are the principal concern. Tay-Sachs disease and hemophilia make interesting comparative case studies when one reviews the ethical warrants for abortion. In societies like the United States, where little or no financial aid is given to families to care for children with birth defects, the economic dimension of an expected defective child can be overwhelming. There needs to be a system of compensation for families so at-risk, especially in the face of unequal medical facilities, so that the medical and economic values in abortion decisions can be kept in reasonable balance. Risks of abortion for less than serious or for trivial reasons will be minimized when there are not heavy economic penalties associated with birth defects. The operative policy of no financial assistance makes a social mockery of many families' attempts to care for their handicapped children in a dignified way.

2) Decisions for abortion can be justified when there is no therapy for the diagnosed disease state, or when the therapy available is severely limited for the most serious cases (Lorber 1971). One would be hard pressed to justify a decision to bring a fetus to term that was at risk for Lesch-Nyhan syndrome. Selective abortion is the preferred policy. Yet, this policy is in tension with the need to develop therapies for inborn errors of metabolism and chromosomal defects. Abortion prevents the birth,

but it does not cure. The values of medicine itself are more enhanced when society supports the basic and applied research for the development of therapy rather than withholds support for such research because of concern about fetal experimentation and abortion.

3) Parents who conscientiously object to a policy of selective abortion should be respected and helped to cope with the personal and social rejection which come as a result of their objection. An ethics of *persuasion* and never coercion should dominate the climate of negotiations between parents, physicians, and the health-care institutions. Insurance carriers and governmental agencies may need to be restrained in the future from employing coercive strategies in order to reduce the genetically at-risk population. For example, insurance companies could decide to encourage selective abortion through a policy of refusing to pay hospital costs and follow-up care for any infant born to a couple already having a child with a serious genetic disease that was diagnosable in any subsequent pregnancy. Especially when the religious and moral convictions of parents are the basis for their opposition to abortion, society must be flexible and resourceful enough to protect their right to object, even though harm may ensue for the infant and for society. At the same time, parents should be able to recover damages from genetic counselors or physicians who do not provide adequate information about pre-natal diagnosis because their religious views prohibit abortion.

I hope that the three examples provided reveal the complex tensions between individual and social priorities. No one ethical system alone is adequate to resolve the conflicts between individual and society, especially in a pluralistic society that is open to the development of new values. Every ethical system will have a contribution to make to the careful balancing of interests required to guide applied pre-natal diagnosis towards the maximum of social and individual fulfillment.

Living with the Consequences of
Pre-natal Diagnosis

Among the various consequences of any new application of technology are its possible abuses. Pre-natal diagnosis will reveal the sex of a fetus early in pregnancy. Would it be right to seek the knowledge of sex because one was planning to have a male rather than a female baby? Other than in cases of sex-linked genetic diseases (e.g. hemophilia), sex can hardly be considered a disease. It is hard to imagine how trustful existing children would feel towards parents who they knew to elect abortion because of sex. In my view, physicians should not admit persons to amniocentesis when sex choice is the basis for decision. The more arguments are based on choices bordering on convenience or taste, the more trivialized applied human genetics may become.

How ought we now understand our obligation to care for the newborn defective infant when the moral case for genetically indicated abortion following amniocentesis has been successfully made? Do the arguments which support abortion of genetic disease also support infanticide of the same infants who slip through that screen and are born? A "consistent" person might well ask this question. The debate in ethics is at present polarized between a view which tends to equate genetically indicated abortion with infanticide, and a view which tends towards approving the morality of abortion and selective euthanasia of the defective newborn (Fletcher 1975).

Infanticide has been widely practiced in ancient and pre-modern times in every quarter of the world. Economic, population, superstitious and eugenic reasons have been used to justify infanticide. No "modern" nation can sanction the approval of infanticide, because the values of modernization (individualism, freedom, rationality) would be grossly contradicted by deliberate and conscious infanticide.

The "modern" attitude towards defective children is that they should be saved, where reasonable and possible, and that they should be raised by their parents or persons in caring institutions. Health care professionals actively work with parents of newborn defective children to accept them, where reasonably possible, as acceptable substitutes for the lost, healthy child.

New developments in applied human genetics and physicians' involvement of parents in life and death decisions about their newborn infants have a high likelihood of affecting the "modern" attitude towards defective infants. If an infant is born with a severe genetic defect which might have been diagnosed pre-natally, will it not occur to the physicians and parents that this infant might have been tested and aborted? Such thoughts will, presumably, intensify the rejection of the infant. The parents might reason "why not leave this baby in the hospital with orders not to feed, since we can have genetic counseling and amniocentesis with the next child?"

The ethical problems of care of the newborn defective are not cut from exactly the same cloth as care of the dying elderly or abortion. Ethicists who want to establish the similarities, rather than the differences, of these situations may be vulnerable to the problem of seeking to justify a particular solution (euthanasia) or block a solution (abortion) rather than undertake a painstaking evaluation of the needs of each situation. The newborn situation is different from the prenatal situation because the infant is a viable human being, separate from the mother and supportable. The newborn

can be reached for treatment, whereas the fetus cannot, with the single exception of Rh disease. When the infant is born, or when it becomes supportable apart from its mother, the full force of social and medical supports should become available.

If we enter the post-natal event with a too-easy conscience about what we allow in abortion, the ambience of caring which is so necessary for the healthy beginning of life might be seriously harmed. We should not be too simply disposed to the line of argument that because we allow for abortion in pre-natal situations it follows that we should or we will allow for selective infanticide. The "slippery slope" argument is not inevitable, and in my view, drawing a sharp moral line between the two situations is extremely important. Others have stated that the law is a method to reinforce the difference between the fetus and the infant (Shaw 1974). Drawing a line enables physicians and parents who are faced with difficult life and death situations, with fetal life at stake, to do so with freedom to approach the newborn situation from a different standpoint than the approach to the fetus before viability.

Genetic Disease and Genetic Health
Because of the vast unknowns underlying the nature of genetic disease and the infinite varieties of interactions between environmental and genetic factors in disease, the concept of genetic disease is only now beginning to be formulated. Even more indistinct is a concept of genetic health, since every individual carries a certain number of deleterious genes. We must, above all, be cautious about temptations towards perfectionism in a concept of genetic health and careful about movements to "eradicate" genetic diseases. There is no way to achieve the eradication of a genetic disease without political intervention in the very real life chances of existing persons and groups. I

am not suggesting that systematic efforts should not be made to reduce the incidence of genetic disease as well as the gene frequency of certain catastrophic gene states, but these efforts must be made with the utmost sensitivity to the rights of the individuals and groups involved. Because the movement towards cultural pluralism is much stronger than in the recent past, and "integration" is not the preferred ideal, leaders of the various ethnic and racial communities are more motivated to concentrate on reducing every obstacle to progress of their particular community, especially in the area of health. Yet, the cultural situation will not allow for monochromatic definitions of genetic health, anymore than it will allow for monopolies of any cultural resource. Insofar as many genetic diseases are culturally specific, and because early social experience with the status of carriers makes these persons liable to stigmatization, a great deal of patience and tolerance is required to allow groups and persons the education and freedom to work towards procedures for carrier detection and pre-natal diagnosis that are fitting for the groups or individuals concerned. At the present time, when there is so much more to be learned about human genetics, an attitude of ethical realism, if not skepticism, should obtain about plans for vast projects to improve the quality of human life through genetics. The promise of human genetics must not be derailed by premature and too hasty social experimentation.

Underlying my last remark is an assumption that human genetics will someday be more completely understood and that knowledge will lead to possibilities for genetic therapy and permanent prevention of genetic disease. Between today and that future, geneticists, their patients, and their non-scientific colleagues must negotiate their way through the cultural and ethical complexities of the application of technical insights to human genetic problems without sacrificing the humanity which justifies the scientific quest itself.

References

Fletcher, J. C. (1972). The brink: The parent-child bond in the genetic revolution. *Theological Stud.* **33**, 457–485.

Fletcher, J. C. (1975). Abortion, euthanasia, and care of defective newborns. *New Engl. J. Med.* **292**, 75–78.

Fletcher, J. F. (1974). *The Ethics of Genetic Control.* Garden City, N. Y., Doubleday.

Lorber, J. (1971). Results of treatment of myelomeningocele. *Develop. Med. Child Neurol.* **13**, 279–303.

Milunsky, A. (1974). *The Prenatal Diagnosis of Hereditary Disorders.* Springfield, Ill., Charles C Thomas.

Ramsey, P. (1970). Reference points in deciding about abortion. *The Morality of Abortion,* ed. Noonan, J. T. Cambridge, Harvard University Press.

Shaw, M. W. (1974). Genetic counseling (editorial). *Science* **184**, No. 4138.

Address:
Interfaith Metropolitan Theological Education, Inc. 1419 V Street NW Washington, D.C. 20009 U.S.A.

From J. Fletcher (1974). Hastings Cent. Stud., **2**, 21–32. *Copyright* (1974),
by kind permission of the author and the Institute of Society, Ethics and the Life Sciences

THE END OF THE 'MODERN' OUTLOOK?

Attitudes toward defective newborns
JOHN FLETCHER

THE PURPOSE of this paper is to further an understanding of the shape and meaning of developing attitudes toward the congenitally abnormal newborn infant. The social context of my own research in this area is the United States, and my comments are limited to reports on attitudes in Great Britain and the United States. However, a full discussion of the subject should include a much wider spectrum of countries and social arrangements.

The basic thesis presented here is that a prevailing "modern" attitude toward releasing human compassion and medical care for the defective newborn, where reasonably possible, has developed into a more complex and differentiated attitude. More precisely, through the impact of genetic counseling, pre-natal diagnosis of some inherited chromosomal and metabolic disorders, and the selective abortion of at-risk fetuses, a "feedback" is occurring upon attitudes toward the defective newborn. The shape of the newly emerging attitudes and their possible meanings will be discussed. As an introduction to the main discussion, a historical sketch of the understandings and attitudes toward congenital malformations will follow.

Historical Introduction

Attitudes towards the defective newborn in history derive from the prevailing understanding of congenital malformations.[1] The profound ambivalence which we experience towards defective children is not a modern phenomenon. Josef Warkany, a medical historian of congenital malformations, noted that ancient societies were both repelled and fascinated by monstrous births, and these societies often both exterminated and adored the newborn abnormal.[2] The earliest societies to record attitudes on abnormalities, Babylonian, Assyrian, and Egyptian, show that defects were taken to be portents, events

---

[1] The best collections of historical research into teratology and its etiology are: G. M. Gould and W. L. Pyle, *Anomalies and Curiosities in Medicine* (Philadelphia: W. B. Saunders, 1897); Josef Warkany, *Congenital Malformations* (Chicago: Year Book Medical Publishers, 1971); and Josef Warkany, "Congenital Malformation in the Past," *Journal of Chronic Diseases* 10 (1959), 84 ff.

[2] Warkany, *Congenital Malformations*, p. 6.

which were useful for divination, predictions of good or evil events. For example, one Chaldean tablet was uncovered with the message that "when a woman gives birth to an infant that has the heart open, and that has no skin, the country will suffer from calamities."[3] From North Africa, belief in the supernatural origin and meaning of defects spread to Greece, Rome and Europe. Cicero was a staunch believer in divination, and he wrote an entire tract upon the subject which contains discussion of abnormalities as signs of fate and providence.[1] Augury played a special role in Roman history. It was from the Latin that words "portent," "monster," and "prodigy" came into English. The relation of defects to divination continued through the Middle Ages and even into the Protestant Reformation. In 1523, the noted reformers Luther and Melanchthon published a tract named *Der Papstesel*. The discovery of a strange ass-like monster floating in the Tiber prompted them to interpret a sign from God meaning the downfall of the papacy.

Another widely found theory of birth defects was based on the belief in maternal impressions or frights. European, Middle Eastern, Eskimo, and African societies have been found to believe that pre-natal mental impressions of the mother can influence the formation of the child, or a sudden shock produce a defect. Being frightened by a rabbit has long been considered the cause of harelip. Positive impressions could produce healthy children. In Greece, expectant mothers in Sparta were ordered to gaze at statues of Castor and Pollux to make the babies more perfect, and it is still a custom in France for expectant mothers to visit the Louvre. This psychogenic explanation of defects was believed by no less a person than Montaigne, one of the most prominent intellectuals of the 16th century. In his essay on the "Power of Imagination," Montaigne accounted for the rough and hairy appearance of a girl presented to the King of Bohemia by explaining that her mother had said that an image of St. John the Baptist hung within the curtains of her bed.

Birth defects were also associated with theories of demons and witches. Many unfortunate mothers and fathers of defective newborns were persecuted and killed for this reason. Also, a hybridity theory developed, which accounted for defects due to coupling between humans and animals. In the New Haven colony in 1642, an innocent one-eyed servant named George Spencer was executed due to his being found guilty of the birth of a cyclopic pig with proboscis.[5]

Infanticide has been widely practiced in ancient and pre-modern times in every quarter of the world.[6] Destruction of defective newborns, especially those whose defects made them resemble animals or who were hermaphroditic, has been widespread. Some protection was offered by the Jews to androgynes, as recorded by the Hebrew book, *Tosefta*, "whoever slays him intentionally is slain and whoever does so unwittingly is exiled." Historically infanticide was pursued for a number of reasons: economic, demographic, superstitious and eugenic. Although recommended by Plato in his *Republic*, it remained for the Spartans to make eugenic infanticide constitutional. Plutarch described Lycurgus as believing that children "were not so much the property of their parents as of the whole commonwealth."[7]

[3]J. W. Ballantyne, "The Teratological Records of Chaldea," *Teratologia* 1 (1894), 12.

[4]Cicero, *De Senectute, de Amicita, de Divinatione*, trans. W. A. Falconer (Cambridge: Harvard University Press, 1908).

[5]W. Landover, "Hybridization Between Animals and Man as a Cause of Congenital Malformations," *Archives of Anatomy* 44 (1962), 155.

[6]"Infanticide," *Encyclopedia Britannica*, Vol. 12 (Chicago: Encyclopedia Britannica, Inc., 1964).

[7]Plutarch, *Lives of Noble Grecians and Romans*, trans. J. Dryden (New York: Modern Library, 1934).

THE DEFECTIVE NEWBORN

The biologic theories of the past and the superstitions relating to them were largely overcome in the nineteenth century, through a wide interest in comparative anatomy and the environmental causes of malformations. Mendel's laws of heredity, when applied to human genetics, provided the second great thrust of understanding. Even with the addition of new scientific knowledge of the origins of congenital defects, it is still fair to say that ancient superstitions still plague modern parents. It is as if the lore of the past goes underground and surfaces to haunt modern parents of defective children.

The "modern" attitude towards congenital defects stems from a scientific understanding of the genetic, environmental, or combined causes of defects. There was a great interest in the last century, continuing into our century, in rescuing children (especially deformed children) from cruel views and barbarism of the past. Leo Kanner recorded the history of the first pioneers in caring for the congenitally malformed, and the story of special institutions for the mentally retarded.[8] With the growth of state and philanthropic interests in treating and preventing congenital malformations, legislation and public attitudes combined to build a reservoir of care and resources to extend to defective children. Better medical care, surgery, and disease control enabled many more to live, but there had to be a receptivity to acceptance of defective children in society before a "modern" attitude became possible. Awe and superstition have been officially replaced by scientific theories of abnormalities, and a major interest in extending care to the defective lies in the hope of curing and ultimately preventing these conditions. Warkany observed at the end of his treatment of modern attitudes towards de-

fects that laws in developed countries are set up to protect human life, perfect or imperfect, and that there may be more of a threat to civilization from the strong than from the weak.[9] Although knowledge about congenital malformations is much more extensive, much more is unknown than known. The extent of the problem is signified in Nishimura's estimation that "an anomalous baby is born somewhere in the world every thirty seconds."[10]

Attitudes of Parents and Health Professionals

The literature on experience with parents and defective newborns shows that there is evidence of a cumulative process of attempting, where possible, to care for and treat the child. There has been a growing movement among health professionals towards home care of defective children and away from large institutional care. This process, taken as a whole, is what I have called a "modern" consciousness about the newborn defective. An initially negative attitude about the defective newborn is gradually overcome and built into a more complex attitude of acceptance wherever possible. The attitude of leading health professionals who are directly involved with the birth of defective children is to attempt to implement an acceptance of the child, wherever possible, on the part of the family, and to attempt to overcome the guilt and denial of the child on the part of their colleagues. There are three identifiable points in the process or structuring of the attitude change:

1. An initial experience of rejection by parents and possibly, health professionals.

2. A "working through" of denial, defenses, and anger against child and self, often with the aid of health professionals.

---

[8]Leo Kanner, *History of the Case and Study of Mental Retardation* (Springfield, Ill.: Charles C. Thomas, 1964).

[9]Warkany, *Congenital Malformations,* p. 22.
[10]A. L. Villumsen, *Environmental Factors in Congenital Abnormality," Obstetrical & Gynecological Survey* 26 (1971), 635-37.

3. An attempt to present the defective child, where reasonably possible, as an acceptable substitute for the lost child and to restore parental readiness to accept and raise the child caringly, often with reinforcement from health professionals. Given the choice, it is desirable that parents keep the defective child.

Each of the points will be discussed below.

Initial Rejection

Despite a readiness in modern consciousness to accept a scientific explanation of congenital defects, both literature about and experience with parents of defective newborns in the United States and Great Britain shows almost a universally negative initial reaction to the child and a personal assumption of guilt on the part of parents.

The experience of learning that your child is defective immediately after birth can still be categorized among the most painful and stigmatizing experiences of modern people. It is as if the parents' *raison d'etre* were called into question before an imagined parental bar of justice and an ontological blow dealt to their hopes of continuing their identities. Only

---

The experience of learning that your child is defective immediately after birth can still be categorized among the most painful and stigmatizing experiences of modern people.

---

a few of the many studies of this excruciating experience will be cited here, in order to attempt to gain a sense of the reasons for self-rejection and the consequences for the newborn.

Pauline Cohen, in discussing the reactions of parents to births of abnormal children, states that "grief and anger" at the blow that life has dealt them are almost universal reactions.[11] The grief reaction, followed by a long period of mourning for the loss of a normal child and the particular loss of the healthy limb, gene, or enzyme, has been noted by many other specialists in this field.[12] A detailed analysis of modern parental response to the defective newborn, which is not possible here, would include five major lines: (1) to the child, (2) the self, (3) the marriage partner, (4) society, (5) the fate or God which allows the event.

The parental response to the newborn defective usually represents an initial rejection based upon disappointed hope, and the rejection may be conditioned by two factors: (1) the nature of the defect, and (2) the social status of the parents. The process of pregnancy involves stages in which both parents undergo profound changes to prepare them for accepting their roles. Energy and commitment must be released from other objects and persons in order to ready themselves to care

---

[11]P. Cohen, "The Impact of the Handicapped on the Family," *Social Casework* 43 (1962), 137.

[12]Among the most valuable recent reports about parental reactions to defective newborns are: A. Bentovim, "Emotional Disturbances of Handicapped Pre-School Children and Their Families—Attitudes to the Child," *British Medical Journal* 2 (1972), 579-81; J. H. Kennell and M. H. Klaus, "Care of the Mother of the High-Risk Infant," *Clinical Obstetrics and Gynecology* 14 (1971), 928-40; J. H. Walker, M. Thomas and J. T. Russell, "Spina Bifida—and the Parents," *Developmental Medicine and Child Neurology* 13 (1971), 462-76; N. Johns, "Family Reactions to the Birth of a Child with Congenital Abnormality," *Obstetrical & Gynecological Survey* 26 (1971), 635-37.

for the child. Especially the mother identifies with the growing child as a separate individual. Pregnancy is one among many life crises in a marriage in which the positive side of parenthood must be projected upon the awaited child. Bentovim describes the initial response to the newborn defective:

> The initial responses are those of an intense crisis, instead of the feeling of relief that the baby is apparently normal. Numbness, grief, disgust, waves of helplessness, rage, disbelief are felt; the expected perfect child is lost, and the feared damaged, deformed child is born. Parents may wish at first to "get rid" of the child, followed by feelings of guilt, self-blame, and intense anxiety.[13]

Certain conclusions can be drawn from studies of the variations in the parental response to the child. The visibility and the social acceptability of the defect will be decisive. Nan Johns noted that:

> Any abnormality involving the head or neck, however slight, was regarded as of more serious significance for the child's future development than one involving other parts of the body.[14]

James Sorenson, a sociologist studying modern human genetics, assembled data on the social acceptability of genetic diseases. He concluded:

> ... genetic disorders which impair physical functioning in a non-cosmetic way are the most acceptable, such as diabetes, followed by genetic disorders which effect cosmetic physical disorders, and finally, the least acceptable are (those) which impair mental functioning, such as mental retardation.[15]

Research on the potential for stigmatization of disease, genetic and non-genetic, has shown that the most serious cultural responses are related to (1) visibility, (2) "physicalness," as opposed to mental handicap, (3) social disruption, and (4) fear, or the degree to which there may be harm to the non-disabled as a function of the disabling problem.[16]

The social class position of the parents may also be an intensely conditioning factor. Giannini and Goodman reported on their study of parents' attitude toward newborn mongoloid infants:

> All families react to a retarded child in terms of their own life experiences and the values and attitudes of their own immediate environment. The mongoloid child, the most stigmatized of the retarded, physically and socially, represents an assault to middle class strivings and aspirations and culturally determined goals. He is seen as a serious impediment to social mobility. The child is retarded for all the world to see—the family cannot find solace in euphemisms like brain damage or post-encephalitis—and as a result the family's self concept becomes seriously threatened. At the same time this is antithetical to the family's sense of justice and responsibility, which adds to the dilemma. Families with less status concern seem to be far less traumatized.[17]

A plausible hypothesis is that there is an initial parental rejection of the defective newborn upon seeing or hearing that it is not "all right," and that the degree of rejection is conditioned by multiple factors: socio-economic status, education, religion, and sex. Zuk's studies of attitudes of Protestant and Catholic mothers of retarded children showed the latter to be

---

[13]Bentovim, "Emotional Disturbances," p. 580.

[14]Johns, "Family Reactions," p. 636.

[15]James R. Sorenson, "Some Social and Psychological Risks in Genetic Screening" (unpublished paper for the Genetics Research Group, Institute of Society, Ethics and the Life Sciences, Hastings-on-Hudson, N.Y., 1973), p. 6.

[16]S. Horasymiw, "Prejudice Toward Minority Groups and Familiarity With Disabilities: Their Relationship to Attitudes Toward the Disabled" (unpublished manuscript, New England Special Education Instructional Material Center, Boston University, 1971).

[17]M. J. Giannini and L. Goodman, "Counselling Families During the Crisis Reaction to Mongolism," *American Journal of Mental Deficiency* 67 (1963), 743-44.

far more accepting of their children than the former. He concluded that Catholics were more accepting "due to the explicit absolution from personal guilt offered by their religious belief," and that a mother could accept the child in a framework of "a test of her religious faith . . . a special gift of God."[18]

Women have been found consistently to be more accepting of defective children than men. Lazar and Orpet recently presented the fascinating results of a study of attitudes of young gifted boys and girls toward handicapped individuals. Using an instrument designed to identify negative reactions and the sex of the respondent, it was found that in a group of fifteen gifted girls (mean I.Q. 136.7) and fifteen gifted boys (mean I.Q. 140.1), the girls scored higher in acceptance. The young boys closely approximated their normative male counterparts in thirteen other trials of the test. In each trial the women proved more accepting.[19]

The readiness to reject the defective is dramatically portrayed in a case of self-fulling prophecy reported by David Freedman.[20] During her second and third pregnancies a mother with no family history of mental retardation, married to a man also in good health, developed the conviction that each of these children would be defective. She isolated them almost immediately, keeping them in a bare room, feeding them a minimum, until the first isolated child, a girl, was almost six years old. After being discovered by authorities, the devastating effects of maternal isolation were there for all to see. She had treated the first and fourth children quite warmly, fed them well, and they were robust. The six-year-old weighed thirty pounds and measured 42.5 inches. Neither child could talk beyond a few incoherent words, and neither could feed itself. After sixteen months in a foster home, each had made dramatic physical progress, but each was still seriously retarded. Freedman concluded that we should not always assume biochemical abnormalities are inborn errors of metabolism, since in this case maternal deprivation results in a syndrome which "includes failure of either production or utilization of growth hormone."[21]

There are also indications in the literature of initial rejection on the part of health professionals, although no careful study of the attitudes of health professionals towards the newborn defective has been done. Giannini and Goodman indicate that the behavior of the physician involved may vary according to the social class of the parents. Since middle-class families use private physicians, pediatricians and obstetricians, these doctors become identified with the family.

> The physician may feel a sense of having failed the family with whom he has a relationship—and his own emotions and feelings come into play—seemingly to a greater extent than with lower class families. His recommendations may be influenced unconsciously by his discomfort with the situation and his strong desire to "save" the family.[22]

Since most physicians in the United States and Great Britain are male, one would expect them to reflect the finding about masculine proclivity to reject defective persons, and the feeling of physicians reported above to stem initially

[18]G. H. Zuk, "Religious Factor and Role of Guilt in Parental Acceptance of the Retarded Child," *American Journal of Mental Deficiency* 64 (1959), 145.

[19]A. L. Lazar and R. E. Orpet, "Attitudes of Young Gifted Boys and Girls Toward Handicapped Individuals," *Exceptional Children* 38 (1972), 489-90.

[20]D. Freedman, "The Role of Early Mother/Child Relations in the Etiology of Some Cases of Mental Retardation," in *Congenital Mental Retardation,* A Symposium, ed. by Gordon Farrell (Austin, Tex.: University of Texas Press, 1969).

[21]*Ibid.,* p. 256.

[22]Giannini and Goodman, "Counselling Families," p. 744.

from an experience of rejection of defective newborns. The doctor would not feel himself a failure unless he had previously been affected by characteristics in the child he did not initially accept.

In their study of British parents' and health professionals' handling of newborns with spina bifida, Walker and his colleagues stated:

> We gained the impression that immediately after the birth, staff devoted more energy to making arrangements for the transfer of the child for surgical care than they did to dealing with the shocked bewilderment of the parents.[23]

The busy avoidance of communication with the parents can also be related hypothetically to an initial disappointment and rejection experience.

The initial experience of rejection appears to evolve into an attitude of profound ambivalence towards the child, with increased feelings of guilt and self-rejection on the part of the parents. Schild described her understanding of the reason for ambivalence:

> A factor accounting for sustained ambivalence toward a retarded child is that the parents are deprived of the opportunity to project any blame for the problem onto the child himself. It is too difficult in any rational way to blame the child for his own defect.[24]

Pinkerton described the non-rational side of ambivalence.

> Sometimes the unfortunate child himself becomes the target of "censure" and is thus consciously or unconsciously rejected . . . his handicap may represent a slight on the father's germplasm or serve to confirm the hostility felt about his covert illegitimate status. The term ambivalence might best be used to convey the sense of such neg-

atively charged parental attitudes which militate against acceptance.[25]

P arents, especially in the middle class, expect more intimacy and perfection in their children. The appearance of a defective newborn is more self-devastating than in an earlier time, when a famliy needed many children, and when children were not so regarded as expressions of the selves of the parents.

An adequate explanation of the tendency to initial rejection of a newborn defective would include both psychological and cultural factors. The history of the family in the industrial countries shows an increasing reduction of broad activities to those involved with the personal fulfillment of the adults. Parents, especially in the middle class, expect more intimacy and perfection in their children.[26] Thus, the appearance of a defective newborn is more self-devastating than in an earlier time, when a family needed many children, and when children were not so regarded as expressions of the selves of the parents. The psychological meaning of initial rejection was summed up by a mother carrying Lesch-Nyhan

---

[23]Walker, et al., "Spina Bifida—and the Parents," p. 465-66.

[24]S. Schild, "Counseling with Parents of Retarded Children Living at Home," *Social Work,* January 1964, p. 87.

[25]P. Pinkerton, "Parental Acceptance of the Handicapped Child," *Developmental Medicine and Child Neurology* 12 (1970), 209.

[26]Philippe Ariès, *Centuries of Childhood* (New York: Vintage Books, 1962), p. 413.

syndrome in an interview with the author:

> You spend all your life looking at pictures of pretty babies and their mothers and growing up thinking that will be you. It is pretty gruesome when you are the one who is different.[27]

Working Through

Many of the studies cited here counsel a process of "working through" feelings of denial, anger, and helplessness on the part of the parents of a defective child. A report of a special working-party set up by the British National Association for Mental Health goes into detail on the dynamics of informing the parents of the birth of an abnormal child and working with them to make an adjustment to the child.[28] The assumption behind the report is clearly that although a severe blow has been struck at the self-esteem of the parents, the informant will be committed to working through feelings rather than ignoring them. The goal is clearly to restore the defective child to the care of the parents. Goodman reports on a whole series of counseling measures for parents of newborn retarded children.[29]

Re-Presentation of the Defective Child

In effect, the transactions at this stage between parents and health professionals amount to a "re-presentation" of the newborn defective. A certain amount of time has elapsed, and the basic choice about keeping the child has to be faced. The literature is almost unanimous in encouraging that the defective child be raised with parents wherever possible, and within the proviso that the capacity to nurture the child can be seen in the parents. The British report cited above stated:

> Somewhat different skills (than those required by the informant) are required to foster an attachment between the parents and the handicapped child. Psychologically it is important that the abnormal child be presented as an acceptable but different substitute for the lost normal baby. If the child is regarded as a 'piece of damaged goods,' it is unlikely that he will be accepted, but if shown as a human dependent individual with a capacity to grow and develop in his own way there will usually be a parental response to his needs.[30]

The basic norms for what I have called the "modern" attitude towards the defective newborn are contained within the last passage. The hospital, the parents, and the health professionals form an alliance on behalf of care of the child. The evidence is clear that abnormal children cared for at home do better physically and emotionally than institutionalized children, and that the isolation of mothers from their newborns is a very damaging problem.[31] Furthermore, there is some evidence that the potential for child abuse is greatest among parents who were both emotionally deprived through lack of early mothering.[32] Thus, a cruel vicious circle may be set up when parents do not keep their newborn children, or feel forced to institutionalize them. Such children may be found in the next generation's child abusers. Kempe studied over 400 battering parents and found them in

[27]John C. Fletcher, "Parents in Genetic Counseling: The Moral Shape of Decision-Making," in *Ethical Issues in Human Genetics,* ed. by Bruce Hilton, Daniel Callahan, et al. (New York: Plenum Press, 1973), p. 319.

[28]National Association for Mental Health, "The Birth of an Abnormal Child: Telling the Parents," *Lancet,* November 13, 1971, 1075-77.

[29]L. Goodman, "Continuing Treatment of Parents with Congenitally Defective Infants," *Social Work,* January 1964, 93-94.

[30]National Association for Mental Health, "Birth of an Abnormal Child," p. 1076.

[31]C. Barnett, et al., "Neo-natal Separation: The Maternal Side of Interactional Deprivation," *Pediatrics* 45 (1970), 197.

[32]C. H. Kempe, "Pediatric Implications of the Battered Baby Syndrome," *Archives of Disease in Childhood* 46 (1971), 33.

all classes, races and creeds. The basic attitude towards infants which he discerned was the "conviction, largely unconscious, that children exist to satisfy parental needs."[33] I suggest that this attitude in the infantile battering parent is very close to the initial negative response to the newborn. Hopefully, in more mature and loving parents, the disappointment in a child who does not meet one's needs can be transformed into service to the child rather than punishment.

On the basis of the evidence presented here, one must conclude that a very impressive and compassionate attitude has gradually come into being in the modern period on behalf of the defective newborn who is not too ill to be saved.

New Developments in Genetics

I am advancing the thesis that new developments in genetics, namely, prenatal diagnosis of genetic diseases and the option of selective abortion are already showing signs of affecting the attitude described earlier and will cause even more differentiation in that attitude in the near future.

The list of inherited disorders which are subject to pre-natal diagnosis is growing steadily.[34] This procedure is producing more demand for it in the public, as parents become aware of the benefits. The benefits are especially impressive where a family already has one or more defective children. The test is technically safe, and my own research into the moral experience of a sample of parents of tested children showed that despite the fact that abortion was the most severe moral problem for the parents (since they desperately wanted children), they were willing to take the risk in order to have a healthy child.[35] I also found that when given the chance to assume personal responsibility for having contemplated the abortion of a tested and healthy child, the parents did not feel that this action would erode the trust required for a strong parent-child bond to thrive.[36]

Among the effects of amniocentesis and selective abortion on society we must now evaluate its effects on (1) attitudes towards the defective newborn and (2) attitudes towards the present generation of growing defective children and adults in the society.

When a newborn appears with a defect for which it was possible to obtain a pre-natal diagnosis and thus, on evidence, abort earlier, we must expect the newborn to be seen in a new light. The thought will occur to the physician, the parents, and other health professionals: "this child might have been prevented from birth if it had been tested." The more successful amniocentesis becomes, the more we can expect its feedback effect on the attitude described earlier in this paper. The "modern" attitude towards the defective newborn developed before amniocentesis, and it represents the best that an earlier society could do in terms of organizing care for vulnerable newborns. The basic question is, will the initial proclivity to reject the child, which we studied earlier, be reinforced by the obvious conclusion that the child might have (or "should have") been prevented? Will a desire to overcome the technical lag in "delivering" amniocentesis absorb much of the reservoir of care which can be called on in the health services for the defective newborn? Will parents of defective newborns be more inclined to abandon them because they feel more guilty than ever because of omitting an opportunity to diagnose? Will these par-

[33]*Ibid.*, p. 30.

[34]A good recent summary shows thirty-three. J. W. Littlefield, et al., "Pre-natal Genetic Diagnosis: Status and Problems," in Hilton and Callahan (eds.), *Ethical Issues in Human Genetics*, p. 46.

[35]John C. Fletcher, "The Parent-Child Bond in the Genetic Revolution," *Theological Studies* 33 (1972), 457-85.

[36]*Ibid.*, p. 479.

ents feel censure or punishment? I raise these questions not because I see massive evidence with which to answer them, but I do see signs of an alteration in attitudes towards the newborn defective because of amniocentesis.

Joseph Fletcher, certainly a bellwether of the most advanced liberal attitudes in medical ethics, observed recently in an article on euthanasia, that

> it is ridiculous to give ethical approval to the positive ending of subhuman life *in utero,* as we do in therapeutic abortions for reasons of mercy and compassion, but refuse to approve of positively ending a sub-human life *in extremis.*

and further

> if we are morally obliged to put an end to a pregnancy when an amniocentesis reveals a terribly defective fetus, we are equally obliged to put an end to a patient's hopeless misery when a brain scan reveals that a patient with cancer has advanced brain metastases.

He criticizes those who use amniocentesis to end a defective fetus and then avoid euthanasia, and states: "This contradiction has equal force whether the euthanasia comes at the fetal point on life's spectrum or at some terminal point post-natally."[37] Thus, for this ethicist, the feedback from amniocentesis not only affects the status of the newborn defective, but makes more plausible its euthanasia. Another smaller sign of this feedback effect occurs in an article by Heese, a pediatrician who is organizing the alternatives facing a physician with the defective newborn:

> (1) Kill the foetus or newborn—an unacceptable course of action at present as far as the newborn is concerned, but permissible in the eyes of many in the case of the foetus in which . . . biochemical defects can be diagnosed antenatally.[38]

Obviously, the thought has occurred to him, since he qualifies the first declaration with "at present."

There are signs of this changing attitude in remarks of James Crow in discussing the claims of society upon the prevention of birth defects:

> But does society have a larger responsibility? How far should we defend the right of a parent to produce a child that is painfully diseased, condemned to an early death, or mentally retarded? In our society, a parent does not have the right to withhold an education from his children. Does he then have an inalienable right to produce a child that is uneducable?[39]

The values in this passage do not agree with the values about the newborn defective which we examined in the previous section, especially those related to the mentally retarded. It is reasonable to expect attitudes towards newborn defective children to be affected more negatively than positively by amniocentesis. This means that the initial reaction towards the child will be more complex than it already is. Not only will the perception of the child be colored by the cultural and psychological factors discussed earlier, but also by the wish for an earlier diagnosis. Whether this wish will lead to more abandonments of defective children, or to more "neo-naticide,"[40] only time and careful study will tell. It does seem apparent that the missed opportunity for diagnosis would tend to erode parental willingness to care for the child. Perhaps selective abortion will feed back even more upon the delicate emotional problems of selecting a defective baby for the lost baby. The parents might reason as

[37]Joseph Fletcher, "Ethics and Euthanasia," *American Journal of Nursing* 73 (1973), 673.

[38]H. Heese, "Thoughts on the Ethics of Treating or Operating on New Borns With Congenital Abnormalities," *Medical Journal of South Africa* 45 (1971), 631.

[39]J. F. Crow, "Conclusion, Advances in Human Genetics and Their Impact on Society," *Birth Defects* 8 (1972), 116.

[40]"Neo-naticide" is a term coined by Philip Resnick to identify a murder of a child in the first 24 hours of life. Cf. "Child-Murder by Parents: A Psychiatric Review of Filicide," *American Journal of Psychiatry* 126 (1969), 325-334.

follows: "Why not leave this baby at the hospital, since we can have genetic counseling and amniocentesis with the next child?" Through such feedback on the modern attitude towards defective children, the reservoir of care which, along with better medical care of defective children, was the best an earlier society could offer, may be slowly emptied. One might predict a rise in the number of parents who attempt to instruct physicians not to elect to keep a seriously defective child alive. A quite telling indication, in my opinion, is the following statement by Motulsky and colleagues:

> Most parents in our society if given the choice would prefer abortion of an affected fetus to a sick child who requires any but the most trivial treatment. This preference is likely to become more definite with rapidly changing attitudes to abortion at a time when the low risks of amniocentesis will become fully established and when simple abortion technics become available.[41]

If this statement is accurate, then one should also expect a change in attitude toward the newborn defective "who requires any but the most trivial treatment." The moral problem of abortion has been successfully argued, in my opinion, with reference to serious genetic defects. Would it seem so difficult for modern persons to withdraw care from the defective newborn, when they know that they might have done it only a few months earlier?

The second area of concern lies in possible threats to the adequate care and safety of existing defective persons because of the knowledge that they "might have been" detected and prevented if the technique had only been available. I saw some evidence in my research with couples in amniocentesis that there was a perceived threat to existing family members with the disease. Two mothers electing hysterotomy had living children or family members suffering from genetic disease. They were acutely aware that aborting a fetus affected by the same problem amounted to a type of "rejection" of the relative. One mother talked of her child:

> He knows what's going on. I wonder what he thinks about the baby. He could think . . . they want to put me out of the way, too. And he could think, no one should have to suffer the way I do. I suppose it would be more the second.[42]

If the effect of pre-natal diagnosis on the defective newborn might be to decrease the success of health professionals in helping parents care for their own children, the results would be an increase on the already strained and money-starved institutions for the care of genetically handicapped individuals. It is conceivable that struggles over funds for extending pre-natal diagnosis will further deprive existing sick persons of adequate care. It will take extraordinary measures of compassion to care adequately for existing persons, accept newborns where possible, and extend amniocentesis, too. Yet the morality which has controlled the relations between medicine and society in the modern era would not condone a depletion of the fund of justice which has been won for the handicapped in order to extend new control over in-born handicaps through early diagnosis. New pressure groups are emerging around both sides of this tension: those who represent the individual interests of the newborn as over against those who represent the interests of society. The tensions within this conflict must be maintained and not shredded apart. We must beware of ex-

[41]Arno G. Motulsky, et al., "Public Health and Long-Term Genetic Implications of Intra-Uterine Diagnosis and Selective Abortion," *Birth Defects* 7 (1971), 31.

[42]John C. Fletcher, "The Parent-Child Bond," p. 470.

tending our technical capabilities at the expense of our humanity and hard-won achievements. Students of the ethics of medicine should continue to take close readings of the real effects of advances in genetics on our attitudes towards the newborn defective and their predecessors to guard against arbitrary and unreasonable erosion of the trust which must exist between newborn and parents if the basic moral health of a society is to be maintained.

*From R. B. Zachary (1968). Lancet, **ii**, 274–276. Copyright (1968), by kind permission of the author and The Lancet Ltd*

ETHICAL AND SOCIAL ASPECTS OF TREATMENT OF SPINA BIFIDA *

R. B. ZACHARY
M.B. Leeds, F.R.C.S.
CONSULTANT PÆDIATRIC SURGEON,
CHILDREN'S HOSPITAL, SHEFFIELD S10 3BR

IN our society the actions of one individual towards another are not without their effect on the rest of the community. Our plans of action in the treatment of myelomeningocele and their attainment are directed in the first place to the patient, but there are also important and significant effects on the family and on the community. Although we acknowledge and accept these wider effects of our treatment, we have always thought that our primary duty is to the patient, and that the most important decision is to do what is right and best for him.

I shall therefore consider first the question of the treatment of the patient and afterwards the important social implications of this treatment.

THE CHILD

The first and the most serious ethical problem arising in the case of a child with myelomeningocele is whether he should receive medical treatment or not. The relative merits of early operation, secondary operation, or no operation at all, can only be decided when this basic principle has been established.

When a baby is born with a serious spina bifida (i.e., a myelomeningocele with a plaque of neural tissue exposed on the surface and with all the associated complications) there are three possible lines of thought: (1) he should be killed; (2) he should be encouraged to die, either by giving no treatment at all (e.g., no feeding) or by not treating complications (e.g., no treatment of infection by antibiotics); or (3) he should be encouraged to live.

* Extended from an address given to the Société Française de Chirurgie Infantile, in Lausanne, on June 8.

The ethical principle that the direct and deliberate killing of a human being is wrong is widely accepted on a religious and philosophical basis, and has been the basis of medical practice since the time of Hippocrates, and even earlier. (I am talking of medical matters here, not of crime and war.) The second alternative has no better justification. To leave a child without food is to kill it as deliberately and directly as if one was cutting its throat. Even the prescribing of antibiotics for infection, such as pneumonia, must now be considered as ordinary care of patients.

Once the principle has been established that the child should be encouraged to live, we are then in a position to consider which method of management gives the child the best chance to live, and secondly, which method of treatment will reduce the handicap to a minimum.

There is a widely held but mistaken view that the purpose of early operation in myelomeningocele is to save the child's life—that if operation is undertaken the child will live, and if operation is not undertaken the child will die. Pædiatric surgeons will at once recognise that this is untrue, and that it contrasts with the treatment of many other congenital abnormalities. For example, in œsophageal atresia we know for certain that the child will die unless a neonatal operation is undertaken, but quite a number of patients with myelomeningocele survive without any operation at all on the back, and some die as a direct result of operation when otherwise they might have survived.

In other words, there is no necessary connection between early operation and survival. It is true that in a large series of cases treated with and without operation, the results favour surgery as far as mortality is concerned. Yet this is probably not a valid reflection of the effect of operation on survival-rates. Surgical patients are receiving active treatment from all points of view: infections are treated vigorously whether they are local infections, systemic infections, or ventriculitis, and the child will probably be getting better attention to the renal tract than those who are receiving no treatment at all. I do not think it has been proved, from a concurrent study of two large series of cases, that the mortality is less in those receiving early operation than in those who do not have early operation but, in every other respect, receive the same care and attention as the surgical series.

The question at issue is whether there are advantages of early operation which outweigh any possible extra risks that such operation might have for the life of the child.

The surgeon who operates on such a child in the neonatal period has a continuing concern for the fullest development of the child; and I think it is right to emphasise the maximum development of the child, rather than the reduction of handicaps to the minimum, for this will influence the whole attitude to the child and his future.

The doctor who accepts the responsibility for the early treatment of the child, whether he be pædiatrician, or pædiatric surgeon, or neurosurgeon, has a duty to see that the long-term total development of the child is always kept in mind. The treatment of the hydrocephalus is only a part of the total care of these children, and we have no hesitation in calling upon other specialists to help in those aspects of the total care of the child in which we ourselves are not competent. The amount of outside help required will vary from one centre to another, but we must be quite certain that the child's orthopædic difficulties, those of the lower limbs and the spine, his renal-tract problems, and his ophthalmic problems, are dealt with competently.

What will be the effect of this treatment on the child himself? Most of the survivors who have had a severe myelomeningocele will still remain severely handicapped —they will have considerable weakness of the lower limbs and will probably be wearing callipers. About 10% will be permanently in a wheelchair, but others may use a wheelchair for most of the time, but will be able to walk a little. Few will have normal renal tracts, either because of poor control of the bladder or because of renal-tract infection and renal damage, and there will be many with urinary diversions. In most cases the hydrocephalus will be well controlled, but even as the children approach school age it may still be necessary for revision operations on the ventriculocaval shunt.

As the child grows up, therefore, his disabilities are mainly those of the lower part of the body—his arms are normal, and his head circumference will usually be within the normal range or only slightly above, and 90% of the children will be educable. In fact it is likely that between two-thirds and three-quarters of them will have an intelligence quotient within the normal range, and from this point of view be capable of receiving normal education.

THE FAMILY

But the child is not going to develop in vacuo, he is going to be brought up in a family as part of a community, and his prospects will depend very much on his integration into the life of the family and the possibility of the community supplying any special needs.

We should consider first the effect on the family of the birth of a seriously handicapped child such as one with serious myelomeningocele. Such an event is not merely a disappointment after nine months of pregnancy, it is a shattering blow to the confidence of the parents in themselves, and one which we must understand if we are to be able to help. It is strange that in these days of equality of the sexes, there is a very common and frequent feeling among the mothers that they have failed their husbands by producing a baby who is not perfect, and there is an immediate searching back in the memory for any event in the early part of pregnancy which could have contributed to this catastrophe. Later comes the recognition on the part of each parent that this may be not entirely due to them, that perhaps the other partner is partly or mainly to blame, and I think it is very important to foresee these doubts, particularly when the parents ask whether there is an hereditary factor concerned with the deformity. If parents ask me whether it is likely that another child in the family will also have spina bifida my immediate answer is that it is most unlikely to happen. If they would like some further information on this point, I give them the figures that we have used for a long time as the basis of our advice, namely, that there is, perhaps, a $5-10\%$ chance of another child having this congenital anomaly. This is, of course, about 20-30 times the incidence in the rest of the community, and such a risk would deter some parents from having further children. However, I think it should be pointed out to them that this means that there is perhaps a $90-95\%$ chance of a subsequent child being normal in this respect: strangely, this alternative way of expressing the same facts seems much more promising to them (indeed, compared with the odds that they get on the football pools, the prospects seem very good indeed).

Parents are entitled to have this information, but it can produce a serious rift in domestic harmony unless some further explanation is given. Very soon you will find that the wife's knowledge about her husband's ancestors is only equalled by that of the husband's knowledge of the wife's ancestors, and

I think it is vital to make clear two aspects of family incidence: firstly, that there is a genetic factor which is almost certainly derived from both sides of the family and, secondly, that the genetic factor is not the only one, there must be some environmental factor which may be of great importance. The clearest way of explaining this to the parents is to tell them that it is possible for one of a pair of identical twins to have spina bifida and the other to be perfectly normal; indeed, there is some evidence to show that the incidence among twins is less than the incidence among non-twin siblings.

A most important step in integrating the handicapped child into the life of the family is the acceptance of the child back home by the parents at the earliest possible moment. In many cases the child will only have been shown to the mother for a brief moment and the father may not have seen him at all before he is sent to a special centre for treatment. This may involve a child travelling a long distance from home, and separation from the mother at this stage will do harm unless special efforts are made to prevent it. Firstly, the mere fact of the child going to a special centre for treatment should in itself give the parents some hope that the child can be helped to overcome his disability. If there is no attempt to send the child for special treatment, if the parents are told that the case is hopeless, that the baby will not survive, that he will be mentally defective, or that he will never be able to walk or go to school or earn his living, the parents are left without any hope at all and their morale drops to zero.

If, on the other hand, they are told that their child is seriously handicapped but active treatment is to be undertaken to help the child to develop himself more fully, and to reduce the handicaps to the minimum, they look forward to having the child back home to do what they can to help him. The child should not be kept in hospital any longer than is absolutely necessary, and if there are to be delays of even two or three weeks between operations it is most important that he should be allowed home. Moreover, if at all possible, the mother should be encouraged to visit the child in hospital, and to learn how to feed him and take care of him under the supervision of the sister. With this attitude of optimistic realism, with the encouragement of visiting by the mother and the early discharge of the patient, it is very seldom indeed that the child is rejected by the parents, no matter how serious his disabilities. The rejection-rate is far greater in those areas where there is no policy of active treatment, and, even if the child is not left for months in the hospital or in an institution, the family has a heavy burden of unhappiness because they have been given no hope.

Besides the anxieties which the parents have about the survival of their child, his disabilities, and their feelings of guilt, there are also other heavy burdens which they must bear.

During infancy the task of the mother may not be very much greater than with a normal child, but as he grows older there is considerable extra work which the parents accept so very willingly. They find themselves tied to the household very much more than the parents of normal children, for they feel a grave responsibility which will not permit them to leave the child in the care of a baby-sitter, so that free evenings and even holidays become very difficult indeed, unless the parents get help from outside.

There is also a considerable financial burden which is sometimes overlooked. Although apparatus and special shoes may be supplied by the Health Service, the wear and tear on clothing is very much greater than with other children, as a result of the apparatus and appliances which they wear. In addition, the frequent admissions to hospital for the various operations which are going to be required mean that the parents have to spend quite a lot of money on travelling to the hospital, for which they may have to give up some of the ordinary dangerous habits such as smoking.

As the children grow the anxiety of the parents does not diminish, and they are extremely worried about the prospects of education for their children, and about their chances of being accepted by the community.

THE COMMUNITY

What are the responsibilities of the community in the care of the children with myelomeningocele? I think the health authorities in Britain are only now becoming aware of the size of this problem and of its gravity. It has taken a considerable time to obtain a clear idea of the incidence of serious spina bifida in our country, and of the survival-rates to be expected. We know that there is a considerable variation in incidence from one country to another, and even in different parts of the same country—for example, in South Wales and in the area around Liverpool the incidence is about twice as great as in some other parts of England. For the country as a whole it seems likely that a figure approaching 2 per 1000 live births is not very far off the mark. Survival-rates are even more difficult to assess, but when all cases are accepted for treatment it seems likely that at least 70% will be surviving at the end of one year, and probably between 50% and 60% will be alive at five years of age.

In the first place the health authorities should make themselves aware of the extent of the problem. It will be necessary to provide treatment centres, and we have found in this special type of neonatal surgery that there are very great advantages in operations being undertaken in special units designed for neonatal surgery, where the whole hospital is geared to the special needs of seriously ill neonates and infants. There are also many advantages in concentrating this work so that not merely 5 or 6 cases are done in the course of a year, but perhaps a minimum of 20 or 30. I think the maximum that we have had has been 170 in a year, and I think this is too many, and we have now persuaded other centres to undertake this work and we do about 120 a year at present.

An adult who sustains a spinal injury causing paraplegia has already received his education, and in many countries there are opportunities for retraining of the adult paraplegic. The child paraplegic, the child with a serious myelomeningocele, has many handicaps in his struggle to obtain even a basic education.

How can these children be fitted into the educational system of the country? In the first place, if the intelligence quotient of a child is normal, he should go to an ordinary school if at all possible. His two major problems are difficulty in walking and incontinence. Many modern schools are built on one floor and have no steps, and so children can attend them even though they spend most of their time in a wheelchair or use callipers; but if there are many steps in a school, it is quite impossible for the child to attend.

A more serious barrier to attendance at a normal school is incontinence, and it is largely for this reason that special day-schools are needed, where frequent attention can be given to the children and, most important, where the child does not feel embarrassed and become emotionally disturbed by being the only incontinent child in the class.

A small number of residential schools for the seriously handicapped are important when parents live too far away from a day-school for handicapped children, or when the child's condition needs very frequent supervision, and I think there are advantages in having such a residential school closely related to a centre for treatment.

We must also look forward to the time when they are about to leave school and consider in what way they are going to make their living. Education is even more important than for those children who have no handicap at all, and vocational training should be specially directed towards the needs of the seriously handicapped.

They will have to rely on their brains and their arms and hands to earn a living, and I think it is most important that the vocational training should not be narrow, simply learning how to undertake mechanical procedures with the hands; it should also have a wide scope, with the possibilities of developing the talents and abilities of these young people in many directions. Simple clerical and manual mechanical work is well within the capacity of most of these young people, but there must be many who are potentially great authors, artists, linguists, musicians, scientists, and philosophers, and yet they may have no opportunity to advance themselves in this way because of the lack of educational opportunities and the lack of vocational training.

It is here, I think, that the parents' associations have proved most valuable. These associations are now scattered widely throughout Great Britain, and although their aim at first was to provide moral support for the parents in the management and care of their children, it has now become clear that a major concern of the parents is education.

In helping these children the community is helping itself. If it provides adequate treatment these children will be less handicapped than they would otherwise be: if it provides adequate educational and vocational training, they will be able to earn their living. In simple economic terms the potential for a child with myelomeningocele must be very much greater than that of the old person with carcinoma of the lung or stomach. Let us be fair to children born with myelomeningocele. Let us plan their treatment so that their handicap is minimal. Let us develop their minds and bodies so as to compensate for their serious disability, and give them education and vocational training to fit them for a career.

A shortened version of this paper is to be published in the *Annales de Chirugie Infantile*.

From R. S. Duff and A. G. M. Campbell (1973). N. Engl. J. Med., **289**, 890–894.
Copyright (1973), *by kind permission of the authors and the Massachusetts Medical Society*

MORAL AND ETHICAL DILEMMAS IN THE SPECIAL-CARE NURSERY

Raymond S. Duff, M.D., and A.G.M. Campbell, M.B., F.R.C.P. (Edin.)

Abstract Of 299 consecutive deaths occurring in a special-care nursery, 43 (14 per cent) were related to withholding treatment. In this group were 15 with multiple anomalies, eight with trisomy, eight with cardiopulmonary disease, seven with meningomyelocele, three with other central-nervous-system disorders, and two with short-bowel syndrome. After careful consideration of each of these 43 infants, parents and physicians in a group decision concluded that prognosis for meaningful life was extremely poor or hopeless, and therefore rejected further treatment. The awesome finality of these decisions, combined with a potential for error in prognosis, made the choice agonizing for families and health professionals. Nevertheless, the issue has to be faced, for not to decide is an arbitrary and potentially devastating decision of default. (N Engl J Med 289:890-894, 1973)

Between 1940 and 1970 there was a 58 per cent decrease in the infant death rate in the United States.[1] This reduction was related in part to the application of new knowledge to the care of infants. Neonatal mortality rates in hospitals having infant intensive-care units have been about ½ those reported in hospitals without such units.[2] There is now evidence that in many conditions of early infancy the long-term morbidity may also be reduced.[3] Survivors of these units may be healthy, and their parents grateful, but some infants continue to suffer from such conditions as chronic cardiopulmonary disease, short-bowel-syndrome or various manifestations of brain damage; others are severely handicapped by a myriad of congenital malformations that in previous times would have resulted in early death. Recently, both lay and professional persons have expressed increasing concern about the quality of life for these severely impaired survivors and their families.[4,5] Many pediatricians and others are distressed with the long-term results of pressing on and on to save life at all costs and in all circumstances. Eliot Slater[6] stated, "If this is one of the consequences of the sanctity-of-life ethic, perhaps our formulation of the principle should be revised."

The experiences described in this communication document some of the grave moral and ethical dilemmas now faced by physicians and families. They indicate some of the problems in a large special-care nursery where medical technology has prolonged life and where "informed" parents influence the management decisions concerning their infants.

Background and Methods

The special-care nursery of the Yale–New Haven Hospital not only serves an obstetric service for over 4000 live births annually but also acts as the principal referral center in Connecticut for infants with major problems of the newborn period. From January 1, 1970, through June 30, 1972, 1615 infants born at the Hospital were admitted, and 556 others were transferred for specialized care from community hospitals. During this interval, the average daily census was 26, with a range of 14 to 37.

For some years the unit has had a liberal policy for parental visiting, with the staff placing particular emphasis on helping parents adjust to and participate in the care of their infants with special problems. By encouraging visiting, attempting to create a relaxed at-

From the Department of Pediatrics, Yale University School of Medicine. 333 Cedar St., New Haven. Conn. 06510. where reprint requests should be addressed to Dr. Duff.

mosphere within the unit, exploring carefully the special needs of the infants, and familiarizing parents with various aspects of care, it was hoped to remove much of the apprehension — indeed, fear — with which parents at first view an intensive-care nursery.[7] At any time, parents may see and handle their babies. They commonly observe or participate in most routine aspects of care and are often present when some infant is critically ill or moribund. They may attend, as they choose, the death of their own infant. Since an average of two to three deaths occur each week and many infants are critically ill for long periods, it is obvious that the concentrated, intimate social interactions between personnel, infants and parents in an emotionally charged atmosphere often make the work of the staff very difficult and demanding. However, such participation and recognition of parents' rights to information about their infant appear to be the chief foundations of "informed consent" for treatment.

Each staff member must know how to cope with many questions and problems brought up by parents, and if he or she cannot help, they must have access to those who can. These requirements can be met only when staff members work closely with each other in all the varied circumstances from simple to complex, from triumph to tragedy. Formal and informal meetings take place regularly to discuss the technical and family aspects of care. As a given problem may require, some or all of several persons (including families, nurses, social workers, physicians, chaplains and others) may convene to exchange information and reach decisions. Thus, staff and parents function more or less as a small community in which a concerted attempt is made to ensure that each member may participate in and know about the major decisions that concern him or her. However, the physician takes appropriate initiative in final decision making, so that the family will not have to bear that heavy burden alone.

For several years, the responsibilities of attending pediatrician have been assumed chiefly by ourselves, who, as a result, have become acquainted intimately with the problems of the infants, the staff, and the parents. Our almost constant availability to staff, private pediatricians and parents has resulted in the raising of more and more ethical questions about various aspects of intensive care for critically ill and congenitally deformed infants. The penetrating questions and challenges, particularly of knowledgeable parents (such as physicians, nurses, or lawyers), brought increasing doubts about the wisdom of many of the decisions that seemed to parents to be predicated chiefly on technical considerations. Some thought their child had a right to die since he could not live well or effectively. Others thought that society should pay the costs of care that may be so destructive to the family economy. Often, too, the parents' or siblings' rights to relief from the seemingly pointless, crushing burdens were important considerations. It seemed right to yield to parent wishes in several cases as physicians have done for generations. As a result, some treatments were withheld or stopped with the knowledge that earlier death and relief from suffering would result. Such options were explored with the less knowledgeable parents to ensure that their consent for treatment of their defective children was truly informed. As Eisenberg[8] pointed out regarding the application of technology, "At long last, we are beginning to ask, not *can* it be done, but *should* it be done?" In lengthy, frank discussions, the anguish of the parents was shared, and attempts were made to support fully the reasoned choices, whether for active treatment and rehabilitation or for an early death.

To determine the extent to which death resulted from withdrawing or with-holding treatment, we examined the hospital records of all children who died from January 1, 1970, through June 30, 1972.

RESULTS

In total, there were 299 deaths; each was classified in one of two categories; deaths in Category 1 resulted from pathologic conditions in spite of the treatment given; 256 (86 per cent) were in this category. Of these, 66 per cent were the result of respiratory problems or complications associated with extreme prematurity (birth weight under 1000 g). Congenital heart disease and other anomalies accounted for an additional 22 per cent (Table 1).

Deaths in Category 2 were associated with severe impairment, usually from congenital disorders (Table 2): 43 (14 per cent) were in this group. These deaths or their timing was associated with discontinuance or withdrawal of treatment. The mean duration of life in Category 2 (Table 3) was greater than that in Category 1. This was the result of a mean life of 55 days for eight infants who became chronic cardiopulmonary cripples

Table 1. Problems Causing Death in Category 1.

PROBLEM	NO. OF DEATHS	PERCENTAGE
Respiratory	108	42.2
Extreme prematurity	60	23.4
Heart disease	42	16.4
Multiple anomalies	14	5.5
Other	32	12.5
Totals	256	100.0

but for whom prolonged and intensive efforts were made in the hope of eventual recovery. They were infants who were dependent on oxygen, digoxin and diuretics, and most of them had been treated for the idiopathic respiratory-distress syndrome with high oxygen concentrations and positive-pressure ventilation.

Some examples of management choices in Category 2 illustrate the problems. An infant with Down's syn-

Table 2. Problems Associated with Death in Category 2.

PROBLEM	NO. OF DEATHS	PERCENTAGE
Multiple anomalies	15	34.9
Trisomy	8	18.6
Cardiopulmonary	8	18.6
Meningomyelocele	7	16.3
Other central-nervous-system defects	3	7.0
Short-bowel syndrome	2	4.6
Totals	43	100.0

after positive-pressure ventilation with high oxygen concentrations for treatment of severe idiopathic respidrome and intestinal atresia, like the much-publicized one at Johns Hopkins Hospital,[9] was not treated because his parents thought that surgery was wrong for their baby and themselves. He died seven days after birth. Another child had chronic pulmonary disease

ratory-distress syndrome. By five months of age, he still required 40 per cent oxygen to survive, and even then, he was chronically dyspneic and cyanotic. He also suffered from cor pulmonale, which was difficult to control with digoxin and diuretics. The nurses, parents and physicians considered it cruel to continue, and yet difficult to stop. All were attached to this child, whose life they had tried so hard to make worthwhile. The family had endured high expenses (the hospital bill exceeding $15,000), and the strains of the illness were believed to be threatening the marriage bonds and to be causing sibling behavioral disturbances. Oxygen sup-

Table 3. Selected Comparisons of 256 Cases in Category 1 and 43 in Category 2.

ATTRIBUTE	CATEGORY 1	CATEGORY 2
Mean length of life	4.8 days	7.5 days
Standard deviation	8.8	34.3
Range	1-69	1-150
Portion living for < 2 days	50.0%	12.0%

plementation was stopped, and the child died in about three hours. The family settled down and 18 months later had another baby, who was healthy.

A third child had meningomyelocele, hydrocephalus and major anomalies of every organ in the pelvis. When the parents understood the limits of medical care and rehabilitation, they believed no treatment should be given. She died at five days of age.

We have maintained contact with most families of children in Category 2. Thus far, these families appear to have experienced a normal mourning for their losses. Although some have exhibited doubts that the choices were correct, all appear to be as effective in their lives as they were before this experience. Some claim that their profoundly moving experience has provided a deeper meaning in life, and from this they believe they have become more effective people.

Members of all religious faiths and atheists were participants as parents and as staff in these experiences. There appeared to be no relation between participation and a person's religion. Repeated participation in these troubling events did not appear to reduce the worry of the staff about the awesome nature of the decisions.

DISCUSSION

That decisions are made not to treat severely defective infants may be no surprise to those familiar with special-care facilities. All laymen and professionals familiar with our nursery appeared to set some limits upon their application of treatment to extend life or to investigate a pathologic process. For example, an experienced nurse said about one child, "We lost him several weeks ago. Isn't it time to quit?" In another case, a house officer said to a physician investigating an aspect of a child's disease, "For this child, don't you think it's time to turn off your curiosity so you can turn on your kindness?" Like many others, these children eventually acquired the "right to die."

Arguments among staff members and families for and against such decisions were based on varied notions of the rights and interests of defective infants, their families, professionals and society. They were also related to varying ideas about prognosis. Regarding the infants, some contended that individuals should have a right to die in some circumstances such as anencephaly, hydranencephaly, and some severely deforming and incapacitating conditions. Such very defective individuals were considered to have little or no hope of achieving meaningful "humanhood."[10] For example, they have little or no capacity to love or be loved. They are often cared for in facilities that have been characterized as "hardly more than dying bins,"[11] an assessment with which, in our experience, knowledgeable parents (those who visited chronic-care facilities for placement of their children) agreed. With institutionalized well children, social participation may be essentially nonexistent, and maternal deprivation severe; this is known to have an adverse, usually disastrous, effect upon the child.[12] The situation for the defective child is probably worse, for he is restricted socially both by his need for care and by his defects. To escape "wrongful life,"[13] a fate rated as worse than death, seemed right. In this regard, Lasagna[14] notes, "We may, as a society, scorn the civilizations that slaughtered their infants, but our present treatment of the retarded is in some ways more cruel."

Others considered allowing a child to die wrong for several reasons. The person most involved, the infant, had no voice in the decision. Prognosis was not always exact, and a few children with extensive care might live for months, and occasionally years. Some might survive and function satisfactorily. To a few persons, withholding treatment and accepting death was condemned as criminal.

Families had strong but mixed feelings about management decisions. Living with the handicapped is clearly a family affair, and families of deformed infants thought there were limits to what they could bear or should be expected to bear. Most of them wanted maximal efforts to sustain life and to rehabilitate the handicapped; in such cases, they were supported fully. However, some families, especially those having children with severe defects, feared that they and their other children would become socially enslaved, economically deprived, and permanently stigmatized, all perhaps for a lost cause. Such a state of "chronic sorrow" until death has been described by Olshansky.[15] In some cases, families considered the death of the child right both for the child and for the family. They asked if that choice could be theirs or their doctors.

As Feifel has reported,[16] physicians on the whole are reluctant to deal with the issues. Some, particularly specialists based in the medical center, gave specific reasons for this disinclination. There was a feeling that to "give up" was disloyal to the cause of the profession. Since major research, teaching and patient-care efforts were being made, professionals expected to discover, transmit and apply knowledge and skills; patients and

families were supposed to co-operate fully even if they were not always grateful. Some physicians recognized that the wishes of families went against their own, but they were resolute. They commonly agreed that if they were the parents of very defective children, with-holding treatment would be most desirable for them. However, they argued that aggressive management was indicated for others. Some believed that allowing death as a management option was euthanasia and must be stopped for fear of setting a "poor ethical example" or for fear of personal prosecution or damage to their clinical departments or to the medical center as a whole. Alexander's report on Nazi Germany[17] was cited in some cases as providing justification for pressing the effort to combat disease. Some persons were concerned about the loss through death of "teaching material." They feared the training of professionals for the care of defective children in the future and the advancing of the state of the art would be compromised. Some parents who became aware of this concern thought their children should not become experimental subjects.

Practicing pediatricians, general practitioners and obstetricians were often familiar with these families and were usually sympathetic with their views. However, since they were more distant from the special-care nursery than the specialists of the medical center, their influence was often minimal. As a result, families received little support from them, and tension in community-medical relations was a recurring problem.

Infants with severe types of meningomyelocele precipitated the most controversial decisions. Several decades ago, those who survived this condition beyond a few weeks usually became hydrocephalic and retarded, in addition to being crippled and deformed. Without modern treatment, they died earlier.[18] Some may have been killed or at least not resuscitated at birth.[19] From the early 1960's, the tendency has been to treat vigorously all infants with meningomyelocele. As advocated by Zachary[20] and Shurtleff,[21] aggressive management of these children became the rule in our unit as in many others. Infants were usually referred quickly. Parents routinely signed permits for operation though rarely had they seen their children's defects or had the nature of various management plans and their respective prognoses clearly explained to them. Some physicians believed that parents were too upset to understand the nature of the problems and the options for care. Since they believed informed consent had no meaning in these circumstances, they either ignored the parents or simply told them that the child needed an operation on the back as the first step in correcting several defects. As a result, parents often felt completely left out while the activities of care proceeded at a brisk pace.

Some physicians experienced in the care of these children and familiar with the impact of such conditions upon families had early reservations about this plan of care.[22] More recently, they were influenced by the pessimistic appraisal of vigorous management schemes in some cases.[5] Meningomyelocele, when treated vigorously, is associated with higher survival rates,[21] but the achievement of satisfactory rehabilitation is at best difficult and usually impossible for almost all who are severely affected. Knowing this, some physicians and some families[23] decide against treatment of the most severely affected. If treatment is not carried out, the child's condition will usually deteriorate from further brain damage, urinary-tract infections and orthopedic difficulties, and death can be expected much earlier. Two thirds may be dead by three months, and over 90 per cent by one year of age. However, the quality of life during that time is poor, and the strains on families are great, but not necessarily greater than with treatment.[24] Thus, both treatment and nontreatment constitute unsatisfactory dilemmas for everyone, especially for the child and his family. When maximum treatment was viewed as unacceptable by families and physicians in our unit, there was a growing tendency to seek early death as a management option, to avoid that cruel choice of gradual, often slow, but progressive deterioration of the child who was required under these circumstances in effect to kill himself. Parents and the staff then asked if his dying needed to be prolonged. If not, what were the most appropriate medical responses?

Is it possible that some physicians and some families may join in a conspiracy to deny the right of a defective child to live or to die? Either could occur. Prolongation of the dying process by resident physicians having a vested interest in their careers has been described by Sudnow.[25] On the other hand, from the fatigue of working long and hard some physicians may give up too soon, assuming that their cause is lost. Families, similarly, may have mixed motives. They may demand death to obtain relief from the high costs and the tensions inherent in suffering, but their sense of guilt in this thought may produce the opposite demand, perhaps in violation of the sick person's rights. Thus, the challenge of deciding what course to take can be most tormenting for the family and the physician. Unquestionably, not facing the issue would appear to be the easier course, at least temporarily; no doubt many patients, families, and physicians decline to join in an effort to solve the problems. They can readily assume that what is being done is right and sufficient and ask no questions. But pretending there is no decision to be made is an arbitrary and potentially devastating decision of default. Since families and patients must live with the problems one way or another in any case, the physician's failure to face the issues may constitute a victimizing abandonment of patients and their families in times of greatest need. As Lasagna[14] pointed out, "There is no place for the physician to hide."

Can families in the shock resulting from the birth of a defective child understand what faces them? Can they give truly "informed consent" for treatment or with-holding treatment? Some of our colleagues answer no to both questions. In our opinion, if families regardless of background are heard sympathetically and

at length and are given information and answers to their questions in words they understand, the problems of their children as well as the expected benefits and limits of any proposed care can be understood clearly in practically all instances. Parents *are* able to understand the implications of such things as chronic dyspnea, oxygen dependency, incontinence, paralysis, contractures, sexual handicaps and mental retardation.

Another problem concerns who decides for a child. It may be acceptable for a person to reject treatment and bring about his own death. But it is quite a different situation when others are doing this for him. We do not know how often families and their physicians will make just decisions for severely handicapped children. Clearly, this issue is central in evaluation of the process of decision making that we have described. But we also ask, if these parties cannot make such decisions justly, who can?

We recognize great variability and often much uncertainty in prognoses and in family capacities to deal with defective newborn infants. We also acknowledge that there are limits of support that society can or will give to assist handicapped persons and their families. Severely deforming conditions that are associated with little or no hope of a functional existence pose painful dilemmas for the laymen and professionals who must decide how to cope with severe handicaps. We believe the burdens of decision making must be borne by families and their professional advisers because they are most familiar with the respective situations. Since families primarily must live with and are most affected by the decisions, it therefore appears that society and the health professions should provide only general guidelines for decision making. Moreover, since variations between situations are so great, and the situations themselves so complex, it follows that much latitude in decision making should be expected and tolerated. Otherwise, the rules of society or the policies most convenient for medical technologists may become cruel masters of human beings instead of their servants. Regarding any "allocation of death"[26] policy we readily acknowledge that the extreme excesses of Hegelian "rational utility" under dictatorships must be avoided.[17] Perhaps it is less recognized that the uncontrolled application of medical technology may be detrimental to individuals and families. In this regard, our views are similar to those of Waitzkin and Stoekle.[27] Physicians may hold excessive power over decision making by limiting or controlling the information made available to patients or families. It seems appropriate that the profession be held accountable for presenting fully all management options and their expected consequences. Also, the public should be aware that professionals often face conflicts of interest that may result in decisions against individual preferences.

What are the legal implications of actions like those described in this paper? Some persons may argue that the law has been broken, and others would contend otherwise. Perhaps more than anything else, the public and professional silence on a major social taboo and some common practices has been broken further. That seems appropriate, for out of the ensuing dialogue perhaps better choices for patients and families can be made. If working out these dilemmas in ways such as those we suggest is in violation of the law, we believe the law should be changed.

REFERENCES

1. Wegman ME: Annual summary of vital statistics — 1970. Pediatrics 48:979-983, 1971
2. Swyer PR: The regional organization of special care for the neonate. Pediatr Clin North Am 17:761-776, 1970
3. Rawlings G, Reynold EOR, Stewart A, et al: Changing prognosis for infants of very low birth weight. Lancet 1:516-519, 1971
4. Freeman E: The god committee. New York Times Magazine, May 21, 1972, pp 84-90
5. Lorber J: Results of treatment of myelomeningocele. Dev Med Child Neurol 13:279-303, 1971
6. Slater E: Health service or sickness service. Br Med J 4:734-736, 1971
7. Klaus MH, Kennell JH: Mothers separated from their newborn infants. Pediatr Clin North Am 17:1015-1037, 1970
8. Eisenberg L: The human nature of human nature. Science 176:123-128, 1972
9. Report of the Joseph P. Kennedy Foundation International Symposium on Human Rights, Retardation and Research. Washington, DC, The John F. Kennedy Center for the Performing Arts, October 16, 1971
10. Fletcher J: Indicators of humanhood: a tentative profile of man, The Hastings Center Report Vol 2, No 5. Hastings-on-Hudson, New York, Institute of Society, Ethics and the Life Sciences, November, 1972, pp 1-4
11. Freeman HE, Brim OG Jr, Williams G: New dimensions of dying, The Dying Patient. Edited by OG Brim Jr. New York, Russell Sage Foundation, 1970, pp xiii-xxvi
12. Spitz RA: Hospitalism: an inquiry into the genesis of psychiatric conditions in early childhood. Psychoanal Study Child 1:53-74, 1945
13. Engelhardt HT Jr: Euthanasia and children: the injury of continued existence. J Pediatr 83:170-171, 1973
14. Lasagna L: Life, Death and the Doctor. New York, Alfred A Knopf, 1968
15. Olshansky S: Chronic sorrow: a response to having a mentally defective child. Soc Casework 43:190-193, 1962
16. Feifel H: Perception of death. Ann NY Acad Sci 164:669-677, 1969
17. Alexander L: Medical science under dictatorship. N Engl J Med 241:39-47, 1949
18. Laurence KM and Tew BJ: Natural history of spina bifida cystica and cranium bifidum cysticum: major central nervous system malformations in South Wales. Part IV. Arch Dis Child 46:127-138, 1971
19. Forrest DM: Modern trends in the treatment of spina bifida: early closure in spina bifida: results and problems. Proc R Soc Med 60:763-767, 1967
20. Zachary RB: Ethical and social aspects of treatment of spina bifida. Lancet 2:274-276, 1968
21. Shurtleff DB: Care of the myelodysplastic patient, Ambulatory Pediatrics. Edited by M Green, R Haggerty. Philadelphia, WB Saunders Company, 1968, pp 726-741
22. Matson DD: Surgical treatment of myelomeningocele. Pediatrics 42:225-227, 1968
23. Mac Keith RC: A new look at spina bifida aperta. Dev Med Child Neurol 13:277-278, 1971
24. Hide DW, Williams HP, Ellis HL: The outlook for the child with a myelomeningocele for whom early surgery was considered inadvisable. Dev Med Child Neurol 14:304-307, 1972
25. Sudnow D: Passing On. Englewood Cliffs, New Jersey, Prentice Hall, 1967
26. Manning B: Legal and policy issues in the allocation of death, The Dying Patient. Edited by OG Brim Jr. New York, Russell Sage Foundation, 1970, pp 253-274
27. Waitzkin H, Stoeckle JD: The communication of information about illness. Adv Psychosom Med 8:180-215, 1972

FURTHER REFERENCES

I. BELIEFS, MYTHOLOGY, MAGIC AND SUPERSTITION

Ballantyne, J. W. (1904). *Manual of Antenatal Pathology and Hygiene. The Embryo.* (Edinburgh: William Green & Sons)

Brodsky, I. (1943). Congenital abnormalities, teratology and embryology: some evidence of primitive man's knowledge as expressed in art and lore in Oceania. *Med. J. Aust.,* **1,** 417–420

Gruber, G. B. (1964). Studien zur Historik der Teratologie. *Zbl. Allg. Pathol.,* **105,** 219–237, 293–316 (Teil I); **106,** 512–562 (Teil II)

Hickey, M. F. (1953). Genes and mermaids: changing theories of the causation of congenital abnormalities. *Med. J. Aust.,* **1,** 649–667

Needham, J. (1934). *A History of Embryology.* (Cambridge, England: Cambridge University Press)

Persaud, T. V. N. (1970). Congenital malformations: from Hippocrates to thalidomide. *West Ind. Med. J.,* **19,** 240–246

Warkany, J. (1971). *Congenital Malformations,* pp. 6–20. (Chicago: Year Book Medical Publishers, Inc.)

Warkany, J. and Kalter, H. (1962). Maternal impressions and congenital malformations. *Plast. Reconstruct. Surg.,* **30,** 628–637

II. EPIDEMIOLOGY OF BIRTH DEFECTS

Buckfield, P. (1973). Major congenital faults in newborn infants: a pilot study in New Zealand. *N.Z. Med. J.,* **78,** 195–204

Carter, C. O. (1974). Recurrence risk of common congenital malformations. *Practitioner,* **213,** 667–683

Chung, C. S. and Myrianthopoulos, N. C. (1968). Racial and prenatal factors in major congenital malformations. *Am. J. Hum. Genet.,* **20,** 44–60

Coffey, V. P. (1974). Twenty-one years' study of anencephaly in Dublin. *J. Irish Med. Assoc.,* **67,** 553–558

Fitzgerald, R. J. and Healy, B. (1974). The spina bifida problem. *J. Irish Med. Assoc.,* **67,** 565–567

Gerfeldt, E. (1964). Frequenz, Ätiologie und Prophylaxe von angeborenen Entwicklungsstörungen. *Med. Klin.,* **59,** 1287–1292

Harris, L. E., Stayura, L. A., Ramirez-Talavera, P. F. and Annegers, J. F. (1975). Congenital and acquired abnormalities observed in live-born and stillborn neonates. *Mayo Clin. Proc.,* **50,** 85–90

Hay, S. and Ionascia, S. (1968). *A Classification of Congenital Malformations.* (San Francisco: US Dept. of Health, Education and Welfare Public Health Service, Dental Health Center)

Hook, E. B., Marden, P. M., Reiss, N. P. and Smith, D. W. (1976). Some aspects of the epidemiology of human minor birth defects and morphological variants in a completely ascertained new born population (Madison study). *Teratology,* **13,** 47–56

Knox, E. G. (1974). Twins and neural tube defects. *Br. J. Prev. Soc. Med.,* **28,** 73–80

Knutzen, V. K., Baillie, P. and Malan, A. F. (1975). Clinical classification of perinatal deaths. *S. Afr. Med. J.,* **49,** 1434–1436

Leck, I. (1974). Causation of neural tube defects: clues from epidemiology. *Br. Med. Bull.,* **30,** 158–163

Leck, I. (1976). Descriptive epidemiology of common malformations (excluding central nervous system defects). *Br. Med. Bull.,* **32,** 45–52

Liban, E. and Salzberger, M. (1976). A prospective clinicopathological study of 1,108 cases of antenatal fetal death. *Isr. J. Med. Sci.,* **12,** 34–44

Marden, P. M., Smith, D. W. and McDonald, M. J. (1964). Congenital anomalies in the newborn infant, including minor variations. *J. Pediatr.,* **64,** 357–371

Molz, G. (1973). Perinatal and newborn deaths. In E. Grundmann and W. H. Kirsten (eds.). *Current Topics in Pathology*, Vol. 58, pp. 149–164. (Berlin: Springer Verlag)

Polani, P. E. (1973). The incidence of developmental and other genetic abnormalities. *Guy's Hosp. Rep.*, **122**, 53–63

Potter, E. (1964). Classification and pathology of congenital anomalies. *Am. J. Obstet. Gynecol.*, **90**, 985–993

Renwick, D. H. G. (1968). The combined use of a central registry and vital records for incidence studies of congenital defects. *Br. J. Prev. Soc. Med.*, **22**, 61–67

Richards, I. D. G. (1973). Fetal and infant mortality associated with congenital malformations. *Br. J. Prev. Soc. Med.*, **27**, 85–90

Roberts, C. J., Laurence, K. M. and Lloyd, S. (1975). An investigation of space and space-time clustering in a large sample of infants with neural tube defects born in Cardiff. *Br. J. Prev. Soc. Med.*, **29**, 202–204

Scriver, C. R., Neal, J. L., Saginur, R. and Clow, A. (1973). The frequency of genetic disease and congenital malformation among patients in a pediatric hospital. *Can. Med. Assoc. J.*, **108**, 1111–1115

Smith, D. W. (1975). Classification, nomenclature, and naming of morphologic defects. *J. Pediatr.*, **87**, 162–164

Smithells, R. W. (1974). Epidemiology of malformations: inspiration and perspiration. *Teratology*, **10**, 217–220

Weatherall, J. A. C. and Haskey, J. C. (1976). Surveillance of malformations. *Br. Med. Bull.*, **32**, 39–44

III. TERATOLOGICAL MECHANISMS

Burnet, F. M. (1974). *Intrinsic Mutagenesis: A Genetic Approach to Ageing.* (Lancaster: MTP Press Limited)

Carter, C. O. (1976). Genetics of common single malformations. *Br. Med. Bull.*, **32**, 21–26

Edwards, R. G. (1974). Advances in reproductive biology and their implication for studies of human congenital defects. In A. G. Motulsky and W. Lenz (eds.). *Birth Defects*, pp. 92–104. (Amsterdam: Excerpta Medica)

Goldman, A. S. (1973). Developmental defects: a final common pathway of teratogenicity. *Clin. Pediatr.*, **12**, 637–648

Hughes, A. F. W. (1976). Developmental biology and the study of malformations. *Biol. Rev.*, **51**, 143–179

Janerich, D. T. (1972). Anencephaly and maternal age. *Am. J. Epidemiol.*, **95**, 319–326

Johnston, M. C. and Pratt, R. M. (1975). A developmental approach to teratology. In C. L. Berry and D. E. Poswillo (eds.). *Teratology. Trends and Applications*, pp. 2–16. (New York: Springer Verlag)

Kennedy, L. A. and Persaud, T. V. N. (1976). Pathogenesis of developmental defects induced in the rat by amniotic sac puncture. *Acta Anat.* (in press)

Kretchmer, N. (1972). Teratology and development. In E. V. Perrin and M. J. Finegold (eds.). *Pathobiology of Development — or Ontogeny Revisited*, pp. 65–75. (Baltimore: The Williams & Wilkins Co)

Kushnick, T. (1975). Immunologic rejection of chromosomally abnormal fetuses. *Perspect. Biol. Med.*, **18**, 292–293

McCredie, J. (1976). Mechanism of the teratogenic effect of thalidomide. *Med. Hypoth.*, **2**, 63–69

Melnick, M. and Shields, E. D. (1976). Allelic restriction: a biologic alternative to multifactorial threshold inheritance. *Lancet*, **i**, 176–179

Poswillo, D. (1976). Mechanisms and pathogenesis of malformation. *Br. Med. Bull.*, **32**, 59–64

Runner, M. N. (1965). General mechanisms of teratogenesis. In J. G. Wilson and J. Warkany (eds.). *Teratology: Principles and Techniques*, pp. 95–103. (Chicago: University of Chicago Press)

Saxen, L. (1972). Tissue interactions and teratogenesis. In E. V. Perrin and M. J. Finegold (eds.). *Pathobiology of Development — or Ontogeny Revisited*, pp. 31–51. (Baltimore: The Williams & Wilkins Co.)

Snow, H. C. (1976). Maternal effects on development. *Nature (London)*, **260**, 94

Wilson, J. G. (1973). *Environment and Birth Defects*, pp. 83–96. (New York: Academic Press)

IV. CYTOGENETIC AND CHROMOSOMAL STUDIES

Bergsma, D. (1975). New chromosomal and malformation syndromes. *Birth Defects: Original Article Series*, Vol. XI, No. 5. (New York: National Foundation—March of Dimes)

Bishun, N. P., Williams, D. C., Mills, J., Lloyd, N., Raven, R. W. and Parke, D. V. (1973). Chromosome damage induced by chemicals. *Chem. Biol. Interactions*, **6**, 375–392

Cohen, M. M., Dahan, S. and Shaham, M. (1975). Cytogenetic evaluation of 500 Jerusalem newborn infants. *Isr. J. Med. Sci.*, **11**, 969–977

Erbe, R. W. (1976). Principles of medical genetics. *N. Engl. J. Med.*, **294**, 381–383, 480–482

Erdtmann, B., Salzano, F. M. and Mattevi, M. S. (1975). Chromosome studies in patients with congenital malformations and mental retardation. *Humangenetik*, **26**, 297–306

Fraser, F. C. and Nora, J. J. (1975). *Genetics of Man.* (Philadelphia: Lea & Febiger)

Freire-Maia, N. (1975). Some epidemiological and genetic aspects of congenital heart diseases. *Acta Genet. Med. Gemellol.*, **24**, 151–158

Gerald, P. S. (1976). Sex chromosome disorders. *N. Engl. J. Med.*, **294**, 706–708

Grosset, L., Barrelet, V. and Odartchenko, N. (1974). Antenatal fetal sex determination from maternal blood during early pregnancy. *Am. J. Obstet. Gynecol.*, **120**, 60–63

Gustavson, K.-H. and Jorulf, H. (1976). Recurrence risks in a consecutive series of congenitally malformed children dying in the perinatal period. *Clin. Genet.*, **9**, 307–314

Hamerton, J. L., Canning, N., Ray, M. and Smith, S. (1975). A cytogenetic survey of 14,069 newborn infants. I. Incidence of chromosome abnormalities. *Clin. Genet.*, **8**, 223–243

Karjalainen, O. and Aula, P. (1975). Intrauterine diagnosis of chromosome anomalies. *Ann. Chir. Gynaecol. Fenn.*, **64**, 146–151

Manuel, M., Park, I. J. and Jones Jr., H. W. (1974). Prenatal sex determination by fluorescent staining of cells for the presence of Y chromatin. *Am. J. Obstet. Gynecol.*, **119**, 853–854

Milunsky, A. (1975). *The Prevention of Genetic Disease and Mental Retardation.* (Philadelphia: W. B. Saunders Co.)

Montagu, M. F. A. (1961). *Genetic Mechanisms in Human Disease. Chromosomal Aberrations.* (Springfield, Ill.: Charles C. Thomas

Moore, K. L. (1974). Sex determination. Normal and abnormal sexual development. *J. Obstet. Gynecol. Nursing*, **3**, 61–69

Scriver, C. R., Neal, J. L., Saginur, R. and Clow, A. (1973). The frequency of genetic disease and congenital malformation among patients in a pediatric hospital. *Can. Med. Assoc. J.*, **108**, 1111–1116

Siebers, J. W., Knauf, I. and Hillemanns, H. G. (1975). Antenatal sex determination in blood from pregnant women. *Humangenetik*, **28**, 273–280

Smith, D. W. and Aase, J. M. (1970). Polygenic inheritance of certain common malformations. *J. Pediatr.*, **76**, 653–659

Woolf, C. M. (1975). A genetic study of spina bifida cystica in Utah. *Soc. Biol.*, **22**, 216–220

V. ENVIRONMENTAL INFLUENCES AND CONGENITAL ABNORMALITIES

Barlow, S. M. and Sullivan, F. M. (1975). Behavioral teratology. In C. L. Berry and D. E. Poswillo (eds.). *Teratology. Trends and Applications*, pp. 103–120. (New York: Springer Verlag)

Blattner, R. J. (1974). The role of viruses in congenital defects. *Am. J. Dis. Child.*, **128**, 781–786

Connors, T. A. (1975). Cytotoxic agents in teratologic research. In C. L. Berry and D. E. Poswillo (eds.). *Teratology. Trends and Applications*, pp. 49–79. (New York: Springer Verlag)

Coyle, I., Wayner, M. J. and Singer, G. (1976). Behavioral teratogenesis: a critical evaluation. *Pharmacol. Biochem. Behav.*, **4**, 191–200

Dudgeon, J. A. (1976). Infective causes of human malformations. *Br. Med. Bull.*, **32**, 77–83

Fuccillo, D. A. and Sever, J. L. (1973). Viral teratology. *Bacteriol. Rev.*, **37**, 19–31

Hale, F. (1935). The relation of vitamin A to anophthalmos in pigs. *Am. J. Ophthalmol.*, **18**, 1087–1093

Jaffe, S. J. (1975). A clinical look at the problem of drugs in pregnancy and their effect on the fetus. *Can. Med. Assoc. J.*, **112**, 728–731

Klassen, R. W. and Persaud, T. V. N. (1976). Experimental studies on the influence of male alcoholism on pregnancy and progeny. *Exp. Pathol.*, **12**, 38–45

Langman, J., Webster, W. and Rodier, P. (1975). Morphological and behavioral abnormalities caused by insults to the CNS in the perinatal period. In C. L. Berry and D. E. Poswillo (eds.). *Teratology. Trends and Applications*, pp. 182–200. (New York: Springer Verlag)

Lanier, A. P., Noller, K. L., Decker, D. G., Elveback, L. R. and Kurland, L. T. (1973). Cancer and stilbestrol. A follow-up of 1,719 persons exposed to estrogens *in utero* and born 1943–1959. *Mayo Clin. Proc.*, **48**, 793–799

Levine, M. M., Edsall, G. and Bruce-Chwatt, L. J. (1974). Live-virus vaccines in pregnancy. Risks and recommendations. *Lancet*, **i**, 34–37

Magee, P. N. (1975). Transplacental carcinogenesis. *Proc. R. Soc. Med.*, **68**, 655–657

McBride, J. (1973). Thalidomide and congenital Charcot's joints. *Lancet*, **ii**, 1058–1061

Miller, H. C., Hassanein, K. and Hensleigh, P. A. (1976). Fetal growth retardation in relation to maternal smoking and weight gain in pregnancy. *Am. J. Obstet. Gynecol.*, **125**, 55–60

Mofenson, H. C., Greensher, J. and Horowitz, R. (1974). Hazards of maternally administered drugs. *Clin. Toxicol.*, **7**, 59–68

Persaud, T. V. N. and Moore, K. L. (1974). Causes and prenatal diagnosis of congenital abnormalities. *J. Obstet. Gynecol. Nursing*, **3**, 50–55

Plotkin, S. A. (1975). Routes of fetal infection and mechanisms of fetal damage. *Am. J. Dis. Child.*, **129**, 444–450

Sallomi, S. J. (1966). Rubella in pregnancy. A review of prospective studies from the literature. *Obstet. Gynecol.*, **27**, 252–256

Shepard, T. H. (1976). *Catalog of Teratogenic Agents.* (Baltimore: The Johns Hopkins University Press)

Stevenson, R. E. (1973). *The Fetus and Newly Born Infant: Influences of the Prenatal Environment.* (St. Louis: The C. V. Mosby Co.)

Tuchmann-Duplessis, H. (1976). *Drug Effects on the Fetus.* Monographs on Drugs, Vol. 12. (Netherlands: ADIS Press)

Ilumsen, A. L. (1970). *Environmental Factors in Congenital Malformations. A Prospective Study of 9,006 Human Pregnancies.* (Copenhagen: F.A.D.L.s Forlag)

Weiss, B. and Spyker, J. M. (1974). Behavioral implications of prenatal and early postnatal exposure to chemical pollutants. *Pediatrics.*, **53**, 851–856

Wilson, J. G. (1973). *Environment and Birth Defects.* (New York: Academic Press)

VI. DETECTION OF ENVIRONMENTAL TERATOGENS

Beck, F. (1976). Model systems in teratology. *Br. Med. Bull.*, **32**, 53–58

Berry, C. L. and Barlow, S. (1976). Reproductive toxicity testing of drugs. *Br. Med. Bull.*, **32**, 34–38

Hook, E. B., Janerich, D. T. and Porter, I. H. (1971). *Monitoring, Birth Defects and Environment.* (New York: Academic Press)

Kochhar, D. M. (1975). The use of *in vitro* procedures in teratology. *Teratology*, **11**, 273–287

Leck, I. (1974). Causation of neural tube defects: clues from epidemiology. *Br. Med. Bull.*, **30**, 158–163

Palmer, A. K. (1974). Problems associated with the screening of drugs for possible teratogenic activity. In D. H. M. Woollam and G. M. Morris (eds.). *Experimental Embryology and Teratology*, Vol. 1, 16–33

Persaud, T. V. N. and Boehm, P. (1976). A technique for the teratological testing of drugs in the rabbit following intra-amniotic administration. In T. Antikatzides, S. Erichsen and A. Spiegel (eds.). *The Laboratory Animal in the Study of Reproduction*, pp. 83–88. (Stuttgart: Gustav Fischer Verlag)

Poswillo, D. E. and Phillips, I. R. (1975). Teratological investigations in laboratory primates: why, when and how to use them. In C. L. Berry and D. E. Poswillo (eds.). *Teratology. Trends and Applications*, pp. 121–135. (New York: Springer Verlag)

Rajan, K. T. (1974). Human organ culture: applications in the screening of teratogenic drugs. In D. H. M. Woollam and G. M. Morris (eds.).

Experimental Embryology and Teratology, Vol. 1, 65–89. (London: Paul Elek (Scientific Books) Ltd)

Smithells, R. W. (1974). Epidemiology of malformations: inspiration and perspiration. *Teratology*, **10**, 217–220

Weatherall, J. A. C. and Haskey, J. C. (1976). Surveillance of malformations. *Br. Med. Bull.*, **32**, 39–44

VII. PRENATAL DIAGNOSIS AND MANAGEMENT OF CONGENITAL ABNORMALITIES

Alberman, E. (1975). The prevention of Down's syndrome. *Dev. Med. Child. Neurol.*, **17**, 793–801

Benzie, R. J. and Doran, T. A. (1975). The 'fetoscope' —a new clinical tool for prenatal genetic diagnosis. *Am. J. Obstet. Gynecol.*, **121**, 460–464

Burton, B. K., Gerbie, A. B. and Nadler, H. L. (1974). Present status of intrauterine diagnosis of genetic defects. *Am. J. Obstet. Gynecol.*, **118**, 718–746

Chaube, S. and Swinyard, C. A. (1975). The present status of prenatal detection of neural tube defects. *Am. J. Obstet. Gynecol.*, **121**, 429–438

Chez, R. A. and Fleischman, A. R. (1973). Fetal therapeutics—challenges and responsibilities. *Clin. Pharmacol. Ther.*, **14**, 754–761

Cowchock, F. S. and Jackson, L. G. (1976). Diagnostic use of maternal serum alpha-fetoprotein levels. *Obstet. Gynecol.*, **47**, 63–68

Emery, A. E. H. (1973). *Antenatal Diagnosis of Genetic Disease*. (Edinburgh and London: Churchill Livingstone)

Fuhrmann, W. and Vogel, F. (1976). *Genetic Counseling*, 2nd Ed. (New York: Springer Verlag)

Goldstein, A., Dumars, K. W. and Kent, D. R. (1976). Prenatal diagnosis of chromosomal and enzymatic defects. *Obstet. Gynecol.*, **47**, 503–506

Hobbins, J. C., Mahoney, M. J. and Goldstein, L. A. (1974). New method of intrauterine evaluation by the combined use of fetoscopy and ultrasound. *Am. J. Obstet. Gynecol.*, **118**, 1069–1072

Karjalainen, O. (1975). Antenatal assessment of fetal maturity. *Ann. Chir. Gynaecol. Fenn.*, **64**, 138–145

Nadler, H. L. (1975). Present status of the prevention of neural tube defects. *Pediatrics.*, **55**, 751–753

Pueschel, S. and Murphy, A. (1975). Counseling parents of infants with Down's syndrome. *Postgrad. Med.*, **58**, 90–95

Ramzin, M. S., Meudt, R. O. and Hinselmann, M. J. (1973). Prognostic significance of abnormal ultrasonographic findings during the second trimester of gestation. *J. Perinat. Med.*, **1**, 60–64

Reynolds, B. D., Puck, M. H. and Robinson, A. (1974). Genetic counseling: an appraisal. *Clin. Genet.*, **5**, 177–187

Robinson, J., Tennes, K. and Robinson, A. (1975). Amniocentesis: its impact on mothers and infants. A 1-year follow-up study. *Clin. Genet.*, **8**, 97–106

Rossman, D. L. and Schull, W. J. (1973). Genetic counseling: past, present and future. *Am. J. Publ. Health*, **63**, 925–926

Stocker, J., Desjardins, P. and Deleon, A. (1975). Ultrasonography: its usefulness and reliability in early pregnancy. *Am. J. Obstet. Gynecol.*, **121**, 1084–1088

Turnbull, A. C. and Woodford, F. P. (1976). *Prevention of Handicap Through Antenatal Care.* (Amsterdam: Excerpta Medica)

Weiss, R. R. *et al.* (1976). Amniotic fluid α-fetoprotein as a marker in prenatal diagnosis of neural tube defects. *Obstet. Gynecol.*, **47**, 148–151

Wiesenhaan, P. F. (1972). Fetography. *Am. J. Obstet. Gynecol.*, **113**, 819–822

VIII. SOCIAL, ETHICAL, AND MEDICO-LEGAL PROBLEMS

Anonymous (1973). Having a congenitally deformed baby. *Lancet*, **i**, 1499–1501

Arnold, A. and Moseley, R. (1976). Ethical issues arising from human genetics. *J. Med. Ethics*, **2**, 12–17

Blumberg, B. D., Golbus, M. S. and Hanson, K. H. (1975). The psychological sequelae of abortion performed for a genetic indication. *Am. J. Obstet. Gynecol.*, **122**, 799–808

Brent, R. L. (1967). Medicolegal aspects of teratology. *J. Pediatr.*, **71**, 288–298

Carter, G. (1976). Legal responses and the right to compensation. *Br. Med. Bull.*, **32**, 89–94

Chez, R. A. and Fleischman, A. R. (1973). Fetal therapeutics—challenges and responsibilities. *Clin. Pharmacol. Ther.*, **14**, 754–761

Cullinan, T. R. (1973). Clinical and social aspects of congenital abnormality with reference to at risk registers. *Proc. R. Soc. Med.*, **66**, 1113–1118

Dorner, S. (1975). The relationship of physical handicap to stress in families with an adolescent with spina bifida. *Dev. Med. Child Neurol.*, **17**, 765–776

Editorial (1976). Compensation for congenital defects. *Br. Med. J.*, **1**, 482–483

Etzioni, A. (1976). Issues of public policy in the USA raised by amniocentesis. *J. Med. Ethics*, **2**, 8–11

Heese, H. De V. (1971). Thoughts on the ethics of treating or operating on newborns and infants with congenital abnormalities. *S. Afr. Med. J.*, **45**, 631–632

Laurence, K. M. (1974). Effect of early surgery for spina bifida cystica on survival and quality of life. *Lancet*, **i**, 301–304

Law Commission. (1974). *Report on Injuries to Unborn Children.* (London: HMSO)

Martin, P. (1975). Marital breakdown in families of patients with spina bifida cystica. *Dev. Med. Child Neurol.*, **17**, 757–764

Record, R. G. and Armstrong, E. (1975). The influence of the birth of a malformed child on the mother's further reproduction. *Br. J. Prev. Soc. Med.*, **29**, 267–273

Tiefel, H. O. (1976). The cost of fetal research: ethical considerations. *N. Engl. J. Med.*, **294**, 85–90

Waldman, A. M. (1976). Medical ethics and the hopelessly ill child. *J. Pediatr.*, **88**, 890–892